*Edited by*
*Jarkko Rautio*

**Prodrugs and Targeted Delivery**

## *Methods and Principles in Medicinal Chemistry*



## *Previous Volumes of this Series:*

Smit, Martine J. / Lira, Sergio A. / Leurs, Rob (Eds.)

**Chemokine Receptors as Drug Targets**

2011

ISBN: 978-3-527-32118-6

Vol. 46

Ghosh, Arun K. (Ed.)

**Aspartic Acid Proteases as Therapeutic Targets**

2010

ISBN: 978-3-527-31811-7

Vol. 45

Ecker, Gerhard F. / Chiba, Peter (Eds.)

**Transporters as Drug Carriers**

**Structure, Function, Substrates**

2009

ISBN: 978-3-527-31661-8

Vol. 44

Faller, Bernhard / Urban, Laszlo (Eds.)

**Hit and Lead Profiling**

**Identification and Optimization of Drug-like Molecules**

2009

ISBN: 978-3-527-32331-9

Vol. 43

Sippl, Wolfgang / Jung, Manfred (Eds.)

**Epigenetic Targets in Drug Discovery**

2009

ISBN: 978-3-527-32355-5

Vol. 42

Todeschini, Roberto / Consonni, Viviana

**Molecular Descriptors for Chemoinformatics**

**Volume I: Alphabetical Listing / Volume II: Appendices, References**

2009

ISBN: 978-3-527-31852-0

Vol. 41

van de Waterbeemd, Han / Testa, Bernard (Eds.)

**Drug Bioavailability**

**Estimation of Solubility, Permeability, Absorption and Bioavailability**

Second, Completely Revised Edition

2008

ISBN: 978-3-527-32051-6

Vol. 40

Ottow, Eckhard / Weinmann, Hilmar (Eds.)

**Nuclear Receptors as Drug Targets**

2008

ISBN: 978-3-527-31872-8

Vol. 39

Vaz, Roy J. / Klabunde, Thomas (Eds.)

**Antitargets**

**Prediction and Prevention of Drug Side Effects**

2008

ISBN: 978-3-527-31821-6

Vol. 38

Mannhold, Raimund (Ed.)

**Molecular Drug Properties**

**Measurement and Prediction**

2007

ISBN: 978-3-527-31755-4

Vol. 37

*Edited by*
*Jarkko Rautio*

# Prodrugs and Targeted Delivery

Towards Better ADME Properties

WILEY-VCH

WILEY-VCH Verlag GmbH & Co. KGaA

**Series Editors**

***Prof. Dr. Raimund Mannhold***
Molecular Drug Research Group
Heinrich-Heine-Universität
Universitätsstrasse 1
40225 Düsseldorf
Germany
mannhold@uni-duesseldorf.de

***Prof. Dr. Hugo Kubinyi***
Donnersbergstrasse 9
67256 Weisenheim am Sand
Germany
kubinyi@t-online.de

***Prof. Dr. Gerd Folkers***
Collegium Helveticum
STW/ETH Zurich
8092 Zurich
Switzerland
folkers@collegium.ethz.ch

**Volume Editor**

***Prof. Dr. Jarkko Rautio***
University of Eastern Finland
School of Pharmacy
Yliopistonranta 1
70211 Kuopio
Finland


**Cover Description**

Prodrugs are bioreversible derivatives of drug molecules that can address ADME issues ("backbone") and must undergo an enzymatic and/or chemical transformation *in vivo* to release the pharmacologically active parent drug. A representative prodrug is oseltamivir (Tamiflu®).
(Laskowski anatomy taken with courtesy of the U.S. National Library of Medicine)




**Library of Congress Card No.:** applied for

**British Library Cataloguing-in-Publication Data**
A catalogue record for this book is available from the British Library.

**Bibliographic information published by the Deutsche Nationalbibliothek**
The Deutsche Nationalbibliothek lists this publication in the Deutsche Nationalbibliografie; detailed bibliographic data are available on the Internet at http://dnb.d-nb.de.





**Typesetting** Thomson Digital, Noida, India
**Printing and Binding** CPI Group (UK) Ltd, Croydon, CR0 4YY
**Cover Design** Grafik-Design Schulz, Fußgönheim

Printed on acid-free paper

**ISBN:** 978-3-527-32603-7

C9783527326037_201125

The manufacturer's authorized representative according to the EU General Product Safety Regulation is Wiley-VCH GmbH, Boschstr. 12, 69469 Weinheim, Germany, e-mail: Product_Safety@wiley.com.

# Contents



*Prodrugs and Targeted Delivery: Towards Better ADME Properties.* Edited by Jarkko Rautio

ISBN: 978-3-527-32603-7

# List of Contributors

*Jane P.F. Bai*
US Food and Drug Administration
Center for Drug Evaluation and Research
Office of Translational Science
Office of Clinical Pharmacology
10903 New Hampshire, Ave.
Silver Spring
MD 20993
USA

*Eyal H. Barash*
Barash Law LLC
3000 Kent Avenue
West Lafayette
IN 47906
USA

*Ujjwal Chakraborty*
University of Kentucky
Department of Chemistry
Lexington
KY 40536-0082
USA

*Peter A. Crooks*
University of Kentucky
College of Pharmacy
Department of Pharmaceutical Sciences
Lexington
KY 40536-0082
USA

*Harpreet K. Dhooper*
University of Kentucky
Department of Chemistry
Lexington
KY 40536-0082
USA

*Paul W. Erhardt*
The University of Toledo College of Pharmacy
Center for Drug Design and Development
Toledo
OH
USA

*Ripal Gaudana*
University of Missouri-Kansas City
School of Pharmacy
Division of Pharmaceutical Sciences
Kansas City
MO
USA

*Prodrugs and Targeted Delivery: Towards Better ADME Properties.* Edited by Jarkko Rautio

ISBN: 978-3-527-32603-7

***Victor R. Guarino***
Bristol-Myers Squibb
Pharmaceutical Candidate
Optimization
Princeton
NJ 08543
USA

***Douglas Hedley***
Institute of Cancer Research
CRC Centre for Cancer Therapeutics
15 Cotswold Road
Sutton
Surrey SM2 5NG
UK

***Kristiina Huttunen***
University of Eastern Finland
School of Pharmacy
Yliopistonranta 1
FI-70211 Kuopio
Finland

***Jwala Jwala***
University of Missouri-Kansas City
School of Pharmacy
Division of Pharmaceutical Sciences
Kansas City
MO
USA

***Deep Kwatra***
University of Missouri-Kansas City
School of Pharmacy
Division of Pharmaceutical Sciences
Kansas City
MO
USA

***Krista Laine***
University of Eastern Finland
School of Pharmacy
Yliopistonranta 1
FI-70211 Kuopio
Finland

***Lawrence L. Lesko***
US Food and Drug Administration
Center for Drug Evaluation and
Research
Office of Translational Science
Office of Clinical Pharmacology
10903 New Hampshire, Ave.
Silver Spring
MD 20993
USA

***Paul R. Lockman***
Texas Tech University Health Sciences
Center
Department of Pharmaceutical Sciences
1406 Coulter
Amarillo
TX 79106
USA

***Susruta Majumdar***
Memorial Sloan
Kettering Cancer Center
Laboratory of Chemistry, Pharmacology,
and Neuroscience
1275 York Avenue
New York
NY 10021
USA

***Ashim K. Mitra***
University of Missouri-Kansas City
School of Pharmacy
Division of Pharmaceutical Sciences
Kansas City
MO
USA

***Majid Y. Moridani***
Texas Tech University
Health Sciences Center
Amarillo
TX 79106
USA

***Gabriel Negoita-Giras***
Institute of Cancer Research
CRC Centre for Cancer Therapeutics
15 Cotswold Road
Sutton
Surrey SM2 5NG
UK

***Dan Niculescu-Duvaz***
Institute of Cancer Research
CRC Centre for Cancer Therapeutics
15 Cotswold Road
Sutton
Surrey SM2 5NG
UK

***John P. O'Donnell***
Pfizer Global Research and
Development
Department of Antibacterials Research
Eastern Point Road
Groton
CT 06340
USA

***Mike Pacanowski***
US Food and Drug Administration
Center for Drug Evaluation and
Research
Office of Translational Science
Office of Clinical Pharmacology
10903 New Hampshire, Ave.
Silver Spring
MD 20993
USA

***Atiqur Rahman***
US Food and Drug Administration
Center for Drug Evaluation and
Research
Office of Translational Science
Office of Clinical Pharmacology
10903 New Hampshire, Ave.
Silver Spring
MD 20993
USA

***Jarkko Rautio***
University of Eastern Finland
School of Pharmacy
Yliopistonranta 1
FI-70211 Kuopio
Finland

***Michael D. Reese***
The University of Toledo College of
Pharmacy
Center for Drug Design and
Development
Toledo
OH
USA

***Kenneth Sloan***
University of Florida
Department of Medicinal Chemistry
1600 SW Archer Road P6-20
Gainesville
FL 32610
USA

***Quentin R. Smith***
Texas Tech University
Health Sciences Center
Department of Pharmaceutical Sciences
1406 Coulter
Amarillo
TX 79106
USA

***Caroline J. Springer***
Institute of Cancer Research
CRC Centre for Cancer Therapeutics
15 Cotswold Road
Sutton
Surrey SM2 5NG
UK

***Ravi Vaishya***
University of Missouri-Kansas City
School of Pharmacy
Division of Pharmaceutical Sciences
Kansas City
MO
USA

***Scott C. Wasdo***
University of Florida
Department of Anesthesiology
1600 SW Archer Road M5-16
Gainesville
FL 32610
USA

***Mark S. Warren***
XenoPort, Inc.
3410 Central Expressway
Santa Clara
CA 95051
USA

# Preface

Historically, biological screening of new compounds was performed in animals. Application by the enteral route automatically provided a first overview on bioavailability and biological half-life. Nowadays, lead structure search and optimization are dominated by *in vitro* screening systems. Correspondingly, problems in compound liberation, oral absorption, organ distribution, metabolism, and excretion (LADME) are often observed at a relatively late stage. The problems may already result either from inappropriate lead structure selection or from unidirectional affinity optimization, without sufficient consideration for solubility, permeation properties, and metabolic stability. However, there are many options to rescue a preclinical candidate with such problems. Liberation can be enhanced by increasing the solubility via the formation of polar derivatives, for example, phosphates, reduction of carbonyl to hydroxyl groups, or introduction of polar, most often basic residues, where they do not negatively interfere with binding. Absorption can be enhanced by making the compound more lipophilic in first line by the conversion of acids into esters. Distribution can be influenced by using transporters, for example, for the blood–brain barrier penetration of L-DOPA, or by designing compounds that are preferentially metabolized in a certain organ or tumor, for example, omeprazole or capecitabine. Metabolism can be easily controlled by avoiding or introducing metabolically labile groups.

Prodrugs are inactive or less active drug analogues or derivatives that have better physicochemical or pharmacokinetic properties than their parent drugs. They are more or less specifically metabolized to the active form of the drug. There are manifold reasons for the development of a prodrug. In most cases, prodrugs are designed for a drug that is not sufficiently bioavailable. Other reasons are that the drug does not permeate the blood–brain barrier, the drug has poor solubility or taste, the drug has no sufficient chemical stability, or the drug has no sufficient organ or cell specificity. Soft drugs (sometimes also called antedrugs) are drugs with very short half-life or without systemic activity. Some esters of corticosteroid carboxylic acids are topically active; after dermal absorption, they are metabolically degraded to inactive analogues, in this manner avoiding systemic side effects. Targeted drugs are drugs or prodrugs that exert their biological action only in certain organs or cells.

*Prodrugs and Targeted Delivery: Towards Better ADME Properties.* Edited by Jarkko Rautio

ISBN: 978-3-527-32603-7

We are very grateful to Jarkko Rautio, who assembled a team of leading experts to discuss all these concepts. In a comprehensive manner, strategies are presented to rescue a drug candidate with insufficient ADME properties. For this purpose, the book is well suited both for all practitioners in medicinal chemistry and for graduate students who want to learn about rational concepts of lead structure optimization. We are also grateful to Frank Weinreich and Nicola Oberbeckmann-Winter for their ongoing support and enthusiasm for our book series, *Methods and Principles in Medicinal Chemistry*, of which this book is another highlight.

October 2010

*Raimund Mannhold*, Düsseldorf
*Hugo Kubinyi*, Weisenheim am Sand
*Gerd Folkers*, Zurich

## A Personal Foreword

The prodrug concept, as first introduced by Adrian Albert in the 1950s, defines a prodrug as a pharmacologically inactive agent that undergoes an enzymatic and/or chemical transformation *in vivo* to a therapeutically active drug. Prodrug strategies have traditionally been used to address ADMET (absorption, distribution, metabolism, excretion, and toxicity) properties and risks of marketed drugs or as a tool in late-stage problem solving for drug development candidates. However, prodrugs are now increasingly being integrated into early drug discovery. Indeed, the successful application of prodrug strategies over the past two decades has significantly increased the percentage of drugs approved as prodrugs to an eye-catching 10%. In addition, the percentage of prodrugs among the world's top-selling drugs is particularly high, including blockbusters such as all the proton pump inhibitor "prazoles," the antiplatelet agent clopidogrel, and the hypercholesterolemia drugs simvastatin and fenofibrate, to name a few.

The success of prodrugs can also be seen in the literature. Books, book chapters, and numerous research and review articles have been published in recent years, with the compilation of the prodrug two-volume book in 2007 by AAPS Press/Springer and edited by Professor Valentino Stella *et al.* certainly providing the most comprehensive overview of early and current prodrug strategies. So why do we need a new book on prodrugs so soon? The idea of this new prodrug book was mulled over by several prodrug enthusiasts, and it soon became obvious that there are topics that are not really addressed in the existing works. Moreover, I think the more perspectives we can explore on strategies suitable for a prodrug approach, or when they should not be pursued, the better off we will be scientifically. Thus, with some trepidation regarding content, especially trying to avoid extensive redundancy, the task was indeed found worth rewarding and invigorating.

This volume of *Methods and Principles in Medicinal Chemistry* contains various strategies for prodrug design and highlights many examples of prodrugs that either have been launched or are undergoing experimental assessment. Part One begins with a historical overview and is followed by approaches of prodrug design and the concepts of prodrug patentability. Part Two focuses on the ADMET issues that can be addressed by prodrugs, ranging from permeability and solubility to targeting. In Part

*Prodrugs and Targeted Delivery: Towards Better ADME Properties.* Edited by Jarkko Rautio

ISBN: 978-3-527-32603-7

Three, the emphasis is on codrugs, which consist of two active drugs incorporated into a single chemical entity, and soft drugs, which in contrast to prodrugs are designed to undergo inactivation after their biotransformation. Both prodrugs and soft drugs rely upon biotransformation to dictate their course of activation and are worth discussing in the same context. Part Four is devoted to preclinical and clinical considerations for prodrugs providing a discovery screening strategy for evaluation of prodrugs and pharmacogenetic focus for prodrugs.

I want to express my sincere gratitude to all authors for their excellent efforts and cooperation. It has been a pleasure for me to be involved with all of these high-profile prodrug enthusiasts. I also want to acknowledge the people at Wiley-VCH, namely, Dr Nicola Oberbeckmann-Winter for her tireless support in the production of this book and Dr Hugo Kubinyi for his valuable advice on its content. I truly hope that this book will stimulate multidisciplinary teams of medicinal chemists, biologists, and other scientists in drug design and development process to consider a prodrug approach as a rational tool in drug discovery that will ultimately lead to better drugs.

October 2010 *Jarkko Rautio*, Kuopio

# Part One
# Prodrug Design and Intellectual Property

*Prodrugs and Targeted Delivery: Towards Better ADME Properties.* Edited by Jarkko Rautio

ISBN: 978-3-527-32603-7

# 1 Prodrug Strategies in Drug Design

*Jarkko Rautio*

## 1.1 Prodrug Concept

Prodrugs are bioreversible derivatives of pharmacologically active agents that must undergo an enzymatic and/or chemical transformation *in vivo* to release the active parent drug, which can then elicit its desired pharmacological effect [1–4]. According to this strict definition, active agents whose metabolites contribute to a pharmacological response and salts of active drugs, which have sometimes mistakenly been referred to as prodrugs, are not considered to be prodrugs. In most cases, prodrugs are simple chemical derivatives that are one or two chemical or enzymatic steps away from the active parent drug. Some prodrugs lack an obvious carrier or promoiety, but result from a molecular modification of the active drug itself *in vivo*. Such a modification can be, for example, a metabolic oxidation or reduction that generates a new and active compound. These prodrugs are usually referred to as "bioprecursor prodrugs." In some cases, a prodrug may consist of two pharmacologically active drugs that are coupled together in a single molecule, so that each drug acts as a promoiety for the other. Such derivatives are called "codrugs" [5]. Finally, "soft drugs," which are often confused with prodrugs, also find applications in tissue targeting. In contrast to prodrugs, soft drugs are active drugs as such but are designed to transform into an inactive form *in vivo* after achieving their therapeutic effect [6]. The prodrug concept is illustrated in Figure 1.1.

Prodrugs have been classified according to several criteria; these being, for example, based on therapeutic categories, or based on categories of chemical linkages between the parent drug and the promoiety, or based on mechanism of action of a prodrug. A recently proposed more systematic approach categorizes prodrugs on the basis of their two cellular sites of conversion: intracellular (e.g., antiviral nucleoside analogues and statins) and extracellular be it in digestive fluids or the systemic circulation (e.g., valganciclovir, fosamprenavir, and antibody-, gene-, or virus-directed enzyme prodrugs) [7, 8]. Both types can be further categorized into subtypes depending on whether or not the intracellular converting location is also the site of therapeutic action, or the conversion occurs in the gastrointestinal fluids or

*Prodrugs and Targeted Delivery: Towards Better ADME Properties.* Edited by Jarkko Rautio

ISBN: 978-3-527-32603-7

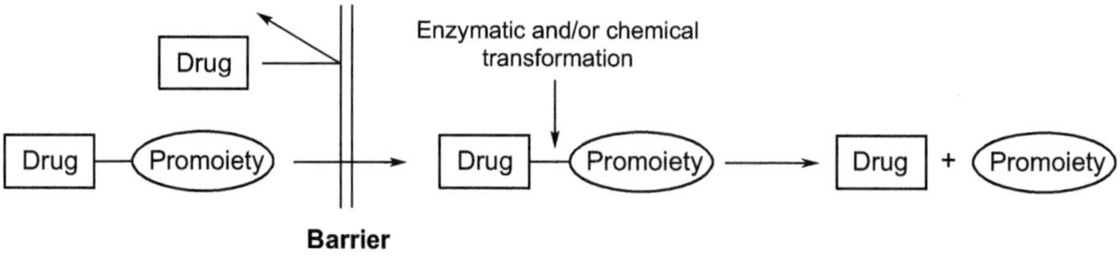


**Figure 1.1** Simplified representation of the prodrug concept. The drug–promoiety molecule is the prodrug that is typically inactive pharmacologically. In broad terms, the barrier can be thought of as any biological liability for a parent drug that prevents optimal (bio)pharmaceutical or pharmacokinetic performance. This barrier must be overcome in order to achieve a marketable drug.

systemic circulation. From a regulatory perspective, this new classification system will certainly help in the understanding of a prodrug's pharmacokinetics and safety.

## 1.2
## Basics of Prodrug Design

The design of an appropriate prodrug structure should be considered in the early stages of preclinical development, bearing in mind that prodrugs may alter the tissue distribution, efficacy, and even the toxicity of the parent drug. Although designing a prodrug so as to include all important factors in one molecule is admittedly very challenging, it can still be more feasible than searching for an entirely new therapeutic agent that has the desired properties. Moreover, the prodrug approach can enable the selection of a suitable drug candidate faster. The main factors that should be carefully considered when designing a prodrug structure are as follows:

- Which functional groups on the parent drug are amenable to chemical derivatization?
- Chemical modifications made to the parent drug must be reversible and allow the prodrug to be converted back into the parent drug by an *in vivo* chemical and/or enzymatic reaction.
- The promoiety should be safe and rapidly excreted from the body. The choice of promoiety and relative safety should be considered with respect to the disease state, the dose, and the duration of therapy.
- The absorption, distribution, metabolism, and excretion (ADME) properties of parent drug and prodrug require a comprehensive understanding.
- Possible degradation by-products can affect both chemical and physical stability that lead to the formation of new degradation products.

Arguably, the most common approaches for prodrug design are aimed at prodrugs undergoing metabolic bioconversion to the active parent molecule by functionally prominent and diversity-tolerant hydrolase enzymes such as peptidases, phosphatases, and, especially, carboxylesterases [9]. Because they are distributed throughout the body, the potential for carboxylesterases to become saturated or the potential for their substrates to become involved in drug–drug interactions is generally insignificant [10], but not unprecedented [11]. Although esterases in general provide a good starting point for prodrug design strategy, premature bioconversion by first-pass metabolism may hinder the success of prodrugs that rely on esterase activation. Moreover, *in vitro* assessments of the hydrolysis rates are not always good predictors of the relative rates of the *in vivo* conversion of a prodrug because of confounding physiological processes that cannot be completely controlled in such studies. Cytochrome P450 (CYP450) enzymes, which are prominent in the liver and are also present in the intestine and lung, have been both intentional [12–14] and unintentional [15] targets for some prodrug strategies; however, these enzymes are not as reliable as esterases in prodrug design due to individual variations in liver functions. Finally, there is a growing interest to design prodrugs that are devoid of a detachable promoiety; in other words, bioprecursor prodrugs that are activated by oxidative or reductive metabolism [16, 17]. Figure 1.2 illustrates prodrug structures for the most common parent drug functionalities. Further discussion of functional group approaches in prodrug design, with representative examples, is given in Chapter 3.

## 1.3 Rationale for Prodrug Design

Drug discovery is an exceedingly complex and demanding enterprise. During the drug discovery process, new molecular entities (NMEs) are identified by using various techniques that include rational and receptor-based drug design, combinatorial chemistry, and high-throughput screens, or isolating and characterizing active components from living organisms, such as plants, fungi, or bacteria. These technologies can produce novel lead structures with high pharmacological potency. However, until the mid-1990s these technologies frequently ignored important physicochemical and biopharmaceutical aspects of the discovered molecules. These classical drug discovery paradigms often led to drug candidates with poor "drug-like" properties and faced significant problems in later drug development [18, 19]. The term "drug-like" is defined as those compounds that have sufficiently acceptable absorption, distribution, metabolism, excretion, and toxicity (ADMET) properties [19, 20]. Poor outcome resulted in a high attrition rate of potential drug candidates in initial clinical studies when ADMET parameters were not thoroughly studied during preclinical phases. This poor outcome eventually prompted an emphasis to prioritize ADMET-related parameters into the HTS format at earlier decision points, which has enabled the optimization of lead compounds for ADMET properties during the early stages of drug discovery.

The process of developing a prodrug is now more focused also on optimizing the ADMET properties of potential pharmacological compounds, which consequently increases the eventual utility of potential drug candidates [1, 21–26]. Some of the main barriers, which are not limited to a drug's ADMET properties yet may be

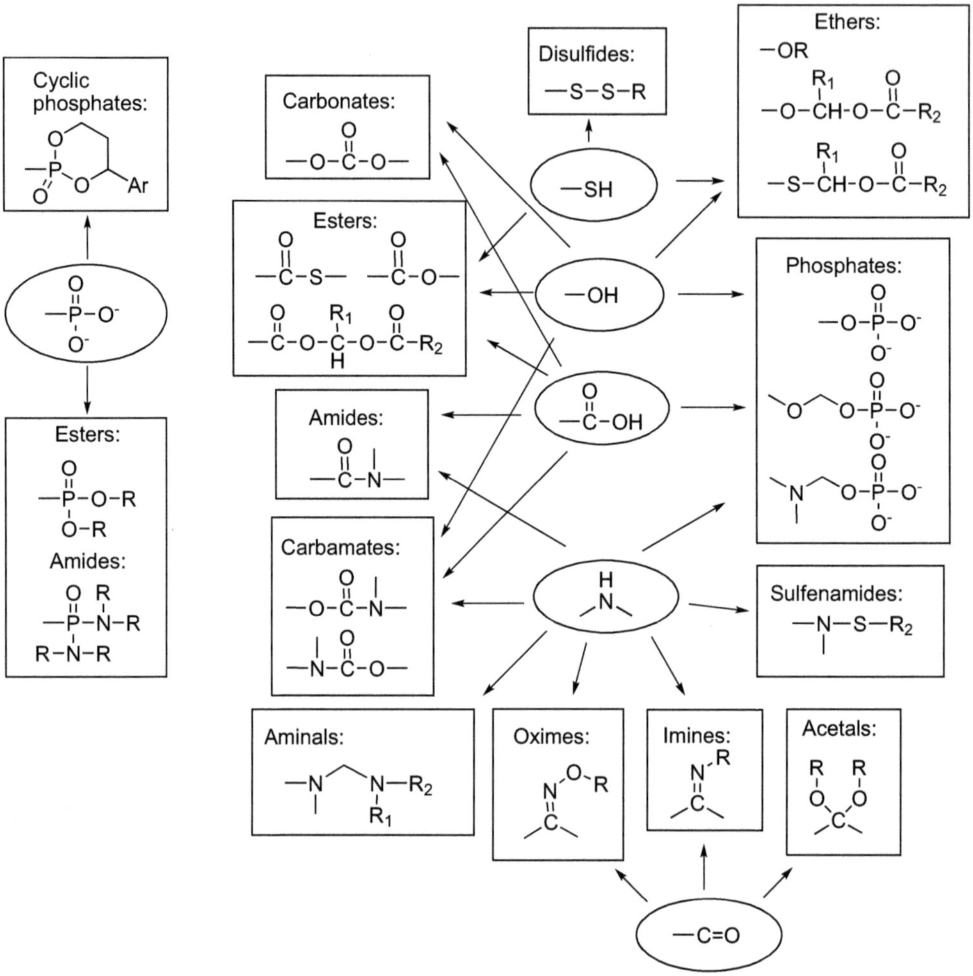


**Figure 1.2** Common functional groups amenable to prodrug design. Most prodrugs require "synthetic handles," which are typically heteroatomic combinations.

overcome by a prodrug modification, are listed in Table 1.1 [4, 24]. It should be understood that these obstacles are often intertwined. Several of these issues are also briefly discussed in the following sections.

### 1.3.1
### Overcoming Formulation and Administration Problems

Sufficient aqueous solubility of a drug is a prerequisite for the preparation of aqueous-based solutions for parenteral or injectable drug dosing. When conventional formulation techniques are not always successful or even possible, such as salt

**Table 1.1** Prodrugs can be used to address the following barriers to a drug's usefulness.

Formulation and administration
- Inadequate aqueous solubility for liquid dosage forms
- Inadequate shelf life for solid or liquid dosage forms
- Pain or irritation after local administration*
- Unpleasant taste or odor

Absorption
- Inadequate dissolution rate due to low aqueous solubility
- Poor membrane permeation and low oral or topical (e.g., dermal and ocular) bioavailability due to poor lipophilicity
- Inadequate stability in acidic gastric juices or during first-pass metabolism
- Inadequate availability due to efflux mechanisms

Distribution
- Lack of site specificity (e.g., poor brain or tumor targeting)*
- Need to decrease plasma protein binding or deposition in lipophilic compartments

Metabolism and excretion
- Lack or need of site-specific bioactivation*
- Short duration of action

Toxicity
- See entries above marked with asterisk* (typically associated with lack of site specificity)
- Need to temporarily mask a reactive, inherently active, functional group

Life cycle management
- Development of a prodrug from an existing drug, to achieve improved properties that may represent a life cycle management opportunity.

formation, a prodrug strategy becomes an extremely valuable option. From a technical and a commercial point of view, there are several successful prodrugs with improved aqueous solubility properties that serve as solved examples of formulation and administration problems with parenteral administration [27, 28]. The most common approach has been to increase water solubility by introducing an ionizable/polar promoiety to the parent drug. A number of phosphoric acid esters have been developed as potential water-soluble prodrugs, especially for parenteral administration, as the increase in solubility imparted by the dianionic phosphate group is often several orders of magnitude [27].

An excellent example of this is fosphenytoin (**1**), a phosphate ester prodrug of the poorly water-soluble anticonvulsant phenytoin (**3**), which can be used in both intravenous and intramuscular administration [29, 30]. Although the simple sodium salt of this weakly acidic ($pK_a = 8.3$) drug also exhibits good water solubility at high pH values, it can cause local irritation at the injection site, which is due to drug precipitation as the pH adjusts to the physiological range. With fosphenytoin, a phosphate ester is attached to an acidic amine functionality of phenytoin via an oxymethylene spacer. Therefore, this prodrug example demonstrates the use of "spacer" or "linker" group in prodrug design, which can be a viable option to form prodrug if there are no functional groups on the parent drug amenable to direct chemical derivatization. With fosphenytoin this modification leads to a remarkable increase in aqueous solubility (from 20–25 μg/ml for phenytoin to 140 mg/ml for fosphenytoin) [31]. While being stable at neutral pH values, fosphenytoin is completely converted back to phenytoin *in vivo* by alkaline phosphatases through a chemically unstable aminol intermediate (**2**), with half-lives ranging from 7 to 15 min in humans [30, 31].

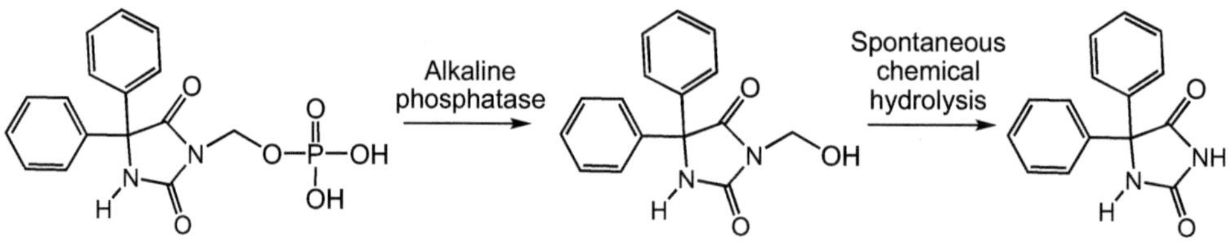


**1** **2** **3**

## 1.3.2
## Overcoming Absorption Barriers

The most successful area of prodrug research has so far been the improvement of passive drug permeation across various epithelial cell membranes, and a majority of these prodrugs have been developed to improve absorption from the GI tract. Similarly, the prodrug approach has been used to improve topical absorption through transdermal and ocular administration. These two approaches are discussed in Chapters 7 and 8.

The oral bioavailability of a drug may be limited by its aqueous solubility, low permeability, propensity to be an efflux substrate, and both rapid and extensive hepatic metabolism followed by biliary excretion. Since unfacilitated and largely nonspecific passive transport mechanisms are the most common absorption routes in oral drug delivery, better diffusion across the biologic phospholipid bilayers, and thus better oral bioavailability, can be achieved by increasing the lipophilicity of an active agent by masking polar ionized or nonionized functional groups.

Several lipophilic alkyl and aryl ester prodrugs are in clinical use [22], of which oseltamivir (Tamiflu®) represents a very recent and successful example. Oseltamivir (**4**) is an orally active prodrug of oseltamivir carboxylate (**5**, GS4071, Ro 64-0802), which is a selective inhibitor of viral neuraminidase glycoprotein in both influenza A and B [32–34] and has some antiviral activity against the H1N1 influenza virus ("swine" flu). As an ethyl ester, oseltamivir is both rapidly and well absorbed, and this modification also increases the oral bioavailability of oseltamivir carboxylate from 5 to 79% [34, 35]. Oseltamivir undergoes fast bioconversion to oseltamivir carboxylate, mostly by human carboxylesterase 1, and maximum plasma levels of oseltamivir carboxylate are reached within 3–4 h after oral dosing [32, 35]. It is interesting to mention another neuraminidase inhibitor in this context: zanamivir (Relenza®), which was the first of the two to be marketed, but was available only in an inhaled form due to its hydrophilicity, and was soon outsold by oseltamivir as an oral tablet formulation.

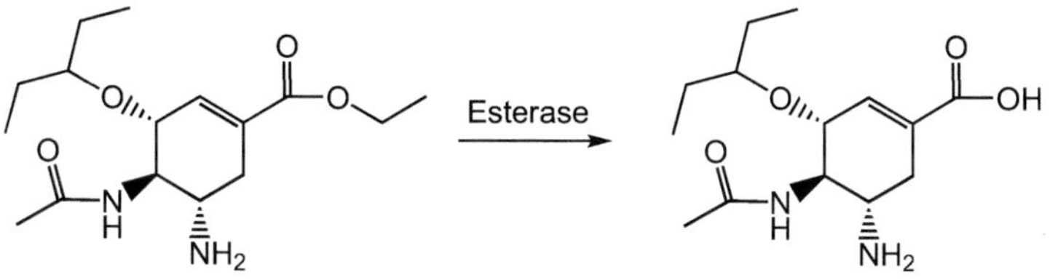


4 5

An alternative means of increasing oral absorption of a drug is carrier-mediated transport, which is particularly important where a drug is either polar or charged and where passive transcellular absorption is negligible. While surprisingly many drugs already take advantage of gastrointestinal tract transporters [36], a number of prodrugs have been designed to have structural features that would allow them to be recognized and taken up by one of these transporters. A good example that exploits carrier-mediated transport is midodrine (**6**), which is an oral prodrug of desglymidodrine (**7**, DMAE), a selective α1-receptor agonist for the treatment of orthostatic hypotension [37, 38]. Midodrine contains a glycine promoiety that is attached to the amine functionality of DMAE, and it is converted into its parent active drug primarily in the liver and in the systemic circulation by unknown peptidases [37]. Midodrine is a substrate for the di- and tripeptide transporter (hPEPT1), and this carrier-mediated transport raises the bioavailability of midodrine to 93% from 50% for that of DMAE [38].

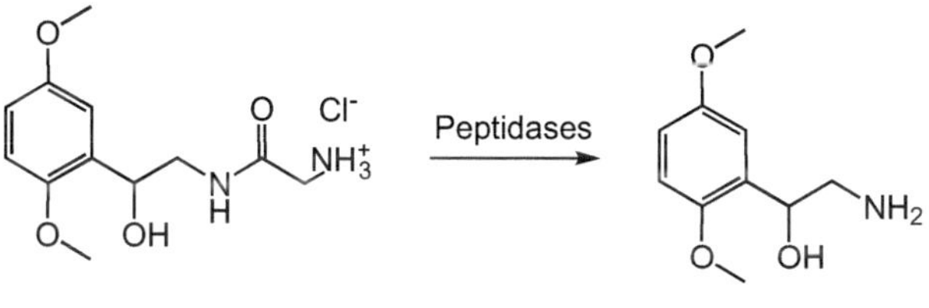


6 7

### 1.3.3
### Overcoming Distribution Problems

There are several prodrugs that have been able to successfully alter the distribution of an active parent drug by achieving site selective delivery. While most of these examples also address side effects and toxicity issues associated with a parent drug, and are discussed in more detail in Section 1.3.5, a classic yet still interesting example of directing distribution by a prodrug is given by levodopa (**8**, L-dopa). The neurotransmitter dopamine (**9**) is not able to cross the blood–brain barrier and is poorly distributed in the brain because of its hydrophilic nature. However, the conversion of dopamine into its α-amino acid, levodopa, enables the uptake of dopamine into the brain via the large neutral amino acid transporter (LAT1) [39, 40]. After entering the brain tissue, levodopa is rapidly converted back to dopamine by dopa decarboxylase, and being a very hydrophilic molecule, it is trapped close to the active site, thus enabling its pharmacodynamic effects. Because decarboxylation also takes place prematurely in the peripheral tissues, a polar dopa decarboxylase inhibitor, carbidopa, is consequently coadministered with levodopa.

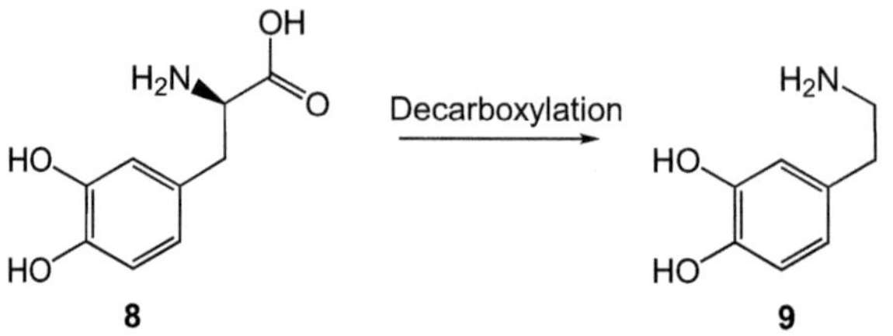


### 1.3.4
### Overcoming Metabolism and Excretion Problems

The use of prodrugs to attenuate the rapid elimination of a drug caused by metabolism and/or excretion is not as frequently used strategy as various controlled release formulations or making drug analogues, but a few examples exist that use prodrugs. The rationale for making a prodrug derivative is often to mask that metabolically labile but pharmacologically essential functional group(s) in order to avoid rapid metabolism. In the case of the bronchodilator and $\beta_2$-agonist terbutaline (**11**), a sustained drug action is achieved with its bis-dimethylcarbamate derivative, bambuterol (**10**). Protection of the phenolic moieties, which are susceptible to rapid and extensive presystemic metabolism, results in some avoidance of first-pass intestinal and hepatic metabolism. After oral administration, bambuterol is slowly bioconverted to terbutaline, predominantly by nonspecific butyrylcholinesterase, and also by lung tissue that is capable of the same metabolism [41–43]. As a result of slower release and prolonged action, a once-daily bambuterol treatment provides relief from asthma with a lower incidence of side effects than terbutaline taken three times a day [44].

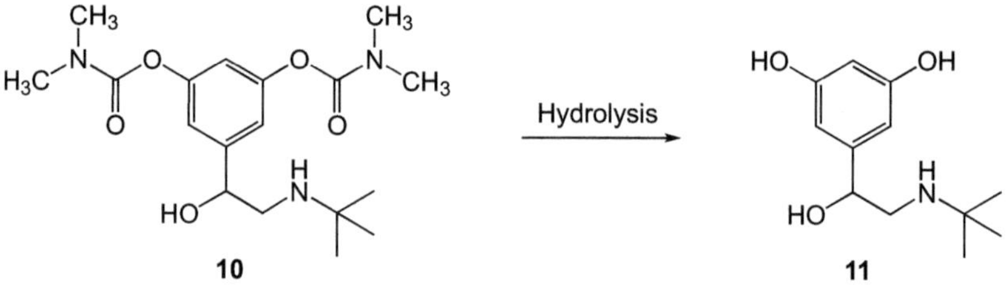


### 1.3.5
### Overcoming Toxicity Problems

Overcoming a parent drug's toxicity can sometimes be accomplished through prodrug strategies that alter one or more of the ADME barriers discussed earlier (see also Table 1.1). Of particular interest is the exclusive, and often elusive, site-selective drug delivery to a particular target, also known as the "magic bullet," to minimize toxicity associated with "freely" distributed drug. In a prodrug approach, such site selectivity can generally be achieved either by site-specific drug bioactivation or site-directed drug delivery. While site-directed drug delivery consists of the selective or primary transport of the intact prodrug to the site of drug action, as in the case of ocular and dermal administration, in site-specific bioactivation the prodrug releases the active drug predominantly at the desired site by a selective metabolic activation reaction.

There are several excellent prodrugs that undergo site-specific activation by exploiting endogenous enzymes of the target tissue. A recent and clinically significant example is capecitabine, an orally active prodrug of the anticancer drug 5-fluorouracil, which requires a cascade of three enzymes for its bioconversion. Capecitabine and several other interesting site-selective prodrugs are discussed in more detail in Chapter 11.

The ubiquitous distribution of most endogenous enzymes that are responsible for bioactivating a prodrug diminishes the opportunities for selective activation and, consequently, targeting. Therefore, prodrugs that rely on bioactivation by exogenous enzymes selectively delivered via monoclonal antibodies (i.e., antibody-directed enzyme prodrug therapy, ADEPT) or generated from genes encoding an exogenous enzyme (i.e., gene-directed enzyme prodrug therapy, GDEPT) have received considerable attention over the past decade, especially in cancer therapy. These approaches are described in more detail in Chapter 12. The rest of this chapter will focus on other examples of site-activated prodrugs.

Nucleoside analogues and nucleoside phosphonates are widely used for the treatment of antiviral infections, and some also have antineoplastic properties. A representative example of selectivity for viral infected cells is acyclovir (**13**) [45, 46]. This prodrug requires intracellular phosphorylation by kinases to produce the active triphosphate nucleotide form (**15**), which cannot be administered as such due to its high polarity and consequently its poor absorption. Desirable site activation is obtained by viral thymidine kinase, which is far more effective (3000 times) in the monophosphorylation of acyclovir than thymidine kinase in uninfected cells. Subsequently, the monophosphate form (**14**) must be further phosphorylated to the triphosphate by cellular kinases in order to become active. This triphosphorylated form has demonstrated a very potent inhibition of viral DNA polymerase and shown approximately 100 times greater affinity for viral than cellular polymerases. However, due to the low oral bioavailability of acyclovir itself (only 10–30%), a valine derivative of acyclovir (**12**) with 3–5 times higher oral bioavailability was also eventually developed for clinical use [47, 48]. Typically, it has been more common to think of these derivatives of nucleoside analogues, such as valacyclovir, which get metabolized into their respective nucleosides to become nucleosidic prodrugs. However, to be more precise, these are prodrugs of prodrugs (or, pro-prodrugs).

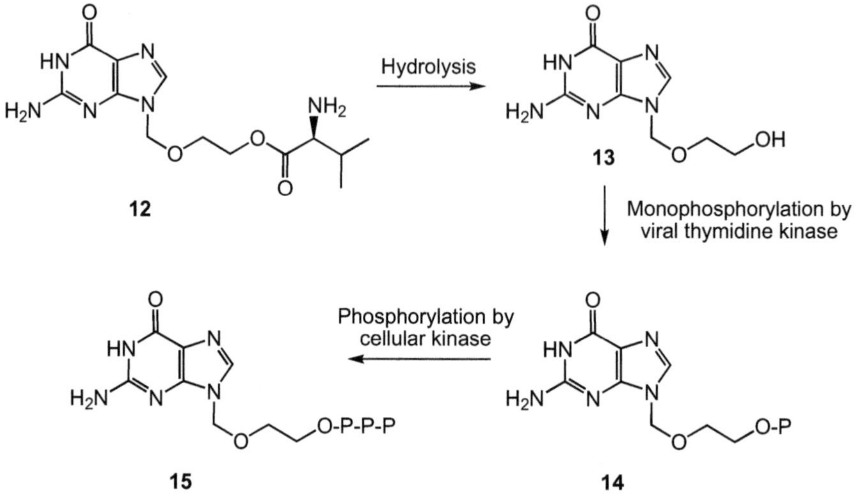


Although the proton pump inhibitor omeprazole (**16**) was initially not designed to behave as a prodrug, it offers another excellent example of a site-activated prodrug. Omeprazole has a basic p$K_a$ of 3.97, which causes it to accumulate in the acidic secretory parietal cells due to pyridine protonation [49]. In the acidic conditions of parietal cells, omeprazole is converted to its active sulfenamide (**17**), followed by irreversible binding with a cysteine group in $H^+/K^+$ ATPase (**18**), thereby inhibiting the ability of the parietal cells to produce gastric acid [50]. The excellent safety profile of omeprazole can be attributed to the fact that nongastric $H^+/K^+$ ATPases lack the highly acidic compartment seen in the parietal cells and are thus unable to convert omeprazole to its active form. Therefore, omeprazole is converted to its active form by molecular rearrangement under acidic conditions that are only close to the acid-producing enzyme it inhibits. Other proton pump inhibitors such as lansoprazole, pantoprazole, rabeprazole, esomeprazole, and tenatoprazole share the same activation mechanism as omeprazole.

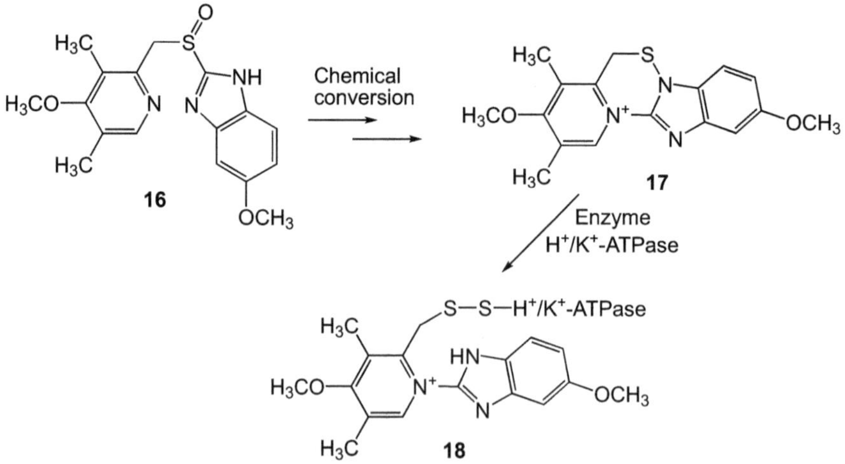

More examples of prodrugs with decreasing systemic toxicities include the antiplatelet drugs clopidogrel (**19**) and prasugrel (**20**), which are converted to their active species at or close to their site of action. Clopidogrel must be metabolized by CYP450 enzymes to produce the active metabolite (**22**), which selectively inhibits platelet aggregation by forming an irreversible disulfide bond with the platelet adenosine diphosphate (ADP) receptor, and thus prevents ADP binding [51]. This *in situ* biological effect takes place primarily at the bioconversion site, in the liver, and thus accounts for the absence of an antiaggregating action in the plasma. Interestingly, only a small proportion of administered clopidogrel is metabolized by CYP450 enzymes to the active species, whereas about 85% of the clopidogrel dose is hydrolyzed by esterases to an inactive carboxylic acid derivative (**21**) [17, 52]. This drawback has led to the design of prasugrel that is primarily bioconverted to the active thiol in a cascade of events that involve enzymatic hydrolysis by carboxylesterases 1 and 2, and oxidation reactions by CYP450 enzymes [16, 53]. It is also worth noting that genetic polymorphism in CYP450 enzymes is known to significantly affect the disposition and response of many drugs. For example, variability in the response to clopidogrel is well documented (see Chapter 16).

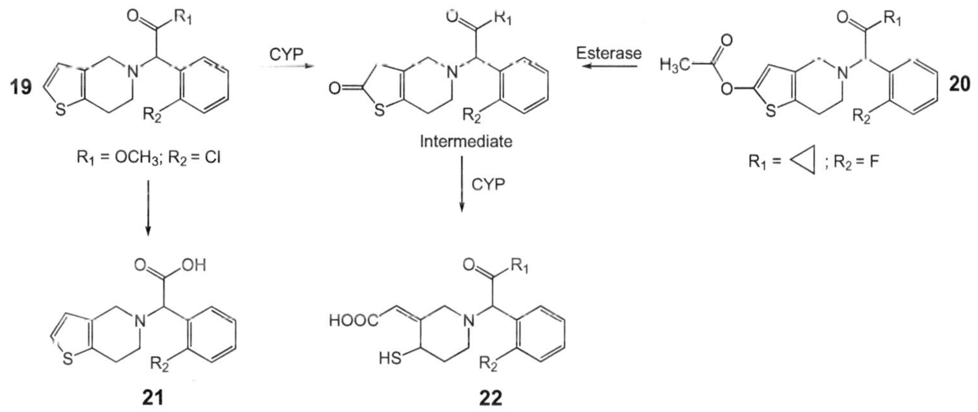


## 1.3.6 Life Cycle Management

As new chemical entities (NCEs), prodrugs are likely to have the added benefit of being considered as intellectual property (IP). Therefore, the development of a prodrug from an existing drug, with improved properties, represents an opportunity for life cycle management. For example, fosphenytoin is a prodrug of the older off-patent phenytoin and has recaptured a market position that was essentially lost when injectable sodium phenytoin became generic [54]. Similarly, as the protection for the fosamprenavir patent will continue up to at least 2017, the protection by the composition of matter patent for its parent drug, amprenavir, will expire in 2013 (*FDA Orange Book*). Therefore, the additional costs to develop fosamprenavir will probably be leveraged by revenues created by its extended patent life.

## 1.4
## History of Prodrug Design

After giving a modern rationale for prodrug design, a glimpse into the history of and very early examples of prodrugs is worthwhile, and it may be surprising to learn that many are still in clinical use. The term "prodrug" itself was first introduced by Albert in 1958 to describe compounds that undergo biotransformation prior to exhibiting their pharmacological effects [55]. For such compounds, the term "drug latentiation" was also introduced at nearly the same time by Harper [56, 57], which further promoted the concept. Prodrugs have also been called reversible or bioreversible derivatives and biolabile drug–carrier conjugates [58], but at present the term prodrug is both standard and simple.

Several examples of prodrugs precede the formal introduction of the concept. While most of these examples were intentionally designed to function as prodrugs, the actual mechanisms of many were discovered later. Methenamine (**23**), one of the first prodrugs, was introduced in 1899 and intentionally relied on the formation of antibacterial formaldehyde in urine. Because of the relatively selective conversion of methenamine at urinary acidic pH and not in plasma or other tissues, it also serves as an early example of site-activated prodrugs.

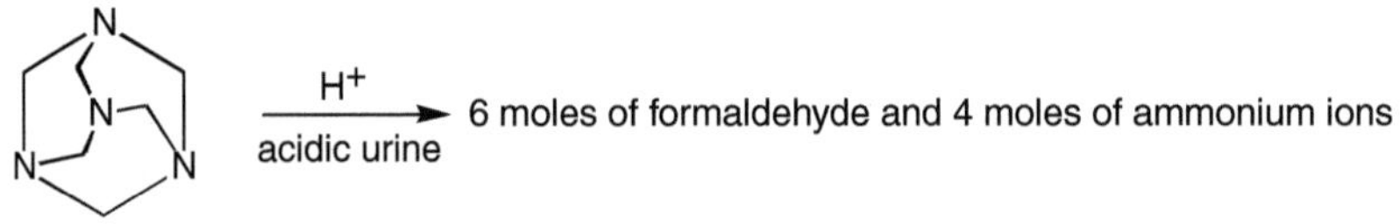


**23**

In the very same year, another prodrug was introduced that certainly falls into the category of the best-known and the most widely used prodrug ever, namely, aspirin (or acetylsalicylic acid, **24**), which was intentionally designed to be a less-irritating replacement for the common salicylate medicines of that time. Aspirin has a relatively short half-life in circulation and it hydrolyzes to both salicylic acid (**25**) and an acetate. Much of aspirin's mechanism of action is due to its ability to suppress the production of prostaglandins and thromboxanes by an irreversible inactivation of cyclooxygenase (COX). While released salicylic acid is a weak COX inhibitor, the released acetyl group is mainly responsible for aspirin's pharmacological effects by covalently and irreversibly attaching to a serine residue on an active site of the COX enzyme [59].

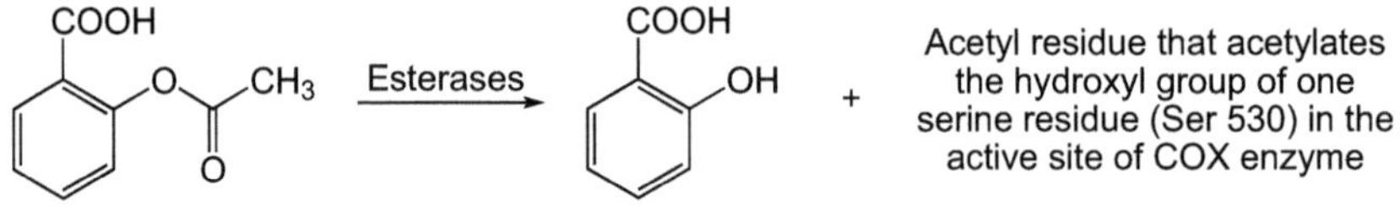


**24** **25**

Another very popular analgesic and antipyretic drug with a weak anti-inflammatory action, paracetamol (**27** or acetaminophen in the United States), may also function via the metabolite *para*-aminophenol (**29**), which makes it a prodrug (the exact mechanism by which paracetamol reduces fever and pain is still debated). *para*-Aminophenol reacts further with arachidonic acid to form *N*-arachidonoylphenolamine, which is responsible for most of the paracetamol's analgesic action [60]. The predecessors of paracetamol, acetanilide (**26**) (introduced in 1886) and phenacetin (**28**) (introduced in 1887), were the first aniline derivatives found to provide both analgesic and antipyretic properties, but were later discovered to provide their therapeutic efficacy via their common major metabolite, paracetamol. In this way, both acetanilide and phenacetin may be considered to be unintentional prodrugs of paracetamol.

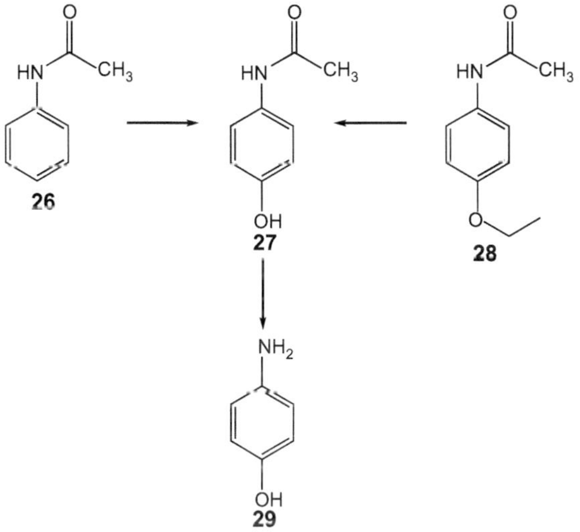


In a similar way, the prodrug activity of the antituberculosis drug isoniazid (**30**) was recently discovered in hindsight. For decades, after its introduction in the early 1950s, the mechanisms of action of isoniazid remained unclear. Developments in late 1990s have shown that isoniazid is activated by the mycobacterial catalase–peroxidase enzyme called KatG. This activation generates the reactive species (**31**) that form adducts with $NAD^+$ and $NADP^+$ (**32**), which are potent inhibitors of lipid and nucleic acid biosynthetic enzymes [61].

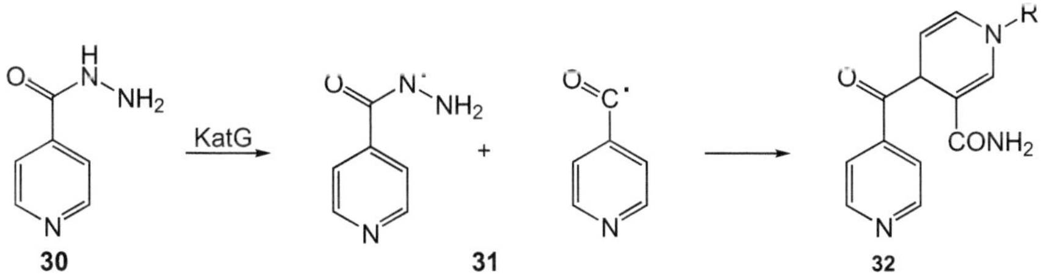

More examples of such hindsight recognition are given by the antibacterial prontosil (**33**) and prodrugs of morphine (**35**), namely, heroin (**34**) and codeine (**36**). The discovery in 1935 of sulfanilamide as the active metabolite of prontosil ushered in the era of sulfonamide antibiotics [62].

Diacetylmorphine was synthesized in 1874 and subsequently marketed as an over-the-counter drug in 1895 under the name heroin and used as a morphine substitute for treating coughs and as a cure for both cocaine and morphine addictions. Interestingly, it is still available by prescription in the United Kingdom and other European countries. However, the discovery of rapid metabolism of heroin into morphine became eventually a historic blunder for Bayer.

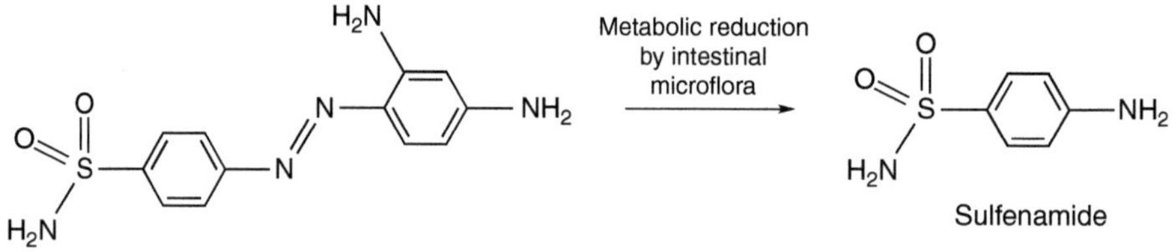


**33**

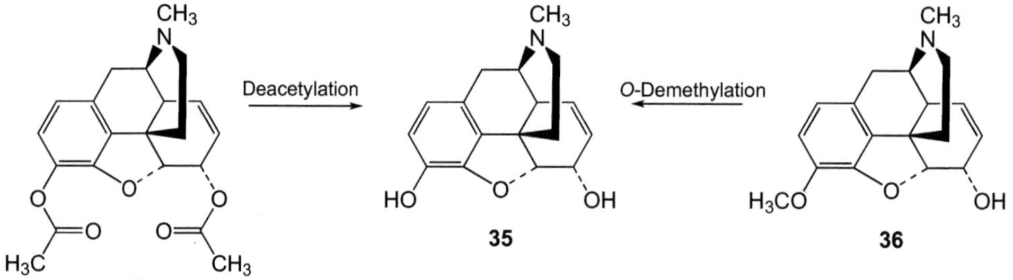


**34**

The pioneering research on chloramphenicol derivatives in the 1950s by Glazko and coworkers at Parke-Davis is also worth recognizing. Both a sparingly water-soluble palmitate ester (**39**), to mask the bitter taste of chloramphenicol (**38**) in pediatric use [63], and a more water-soluble chloramphenicol sodium hemisuccinate (**37**) [64], for aqueous-based formulations, are early examples of rationally developed prodrugs by a pharmaceutical company.

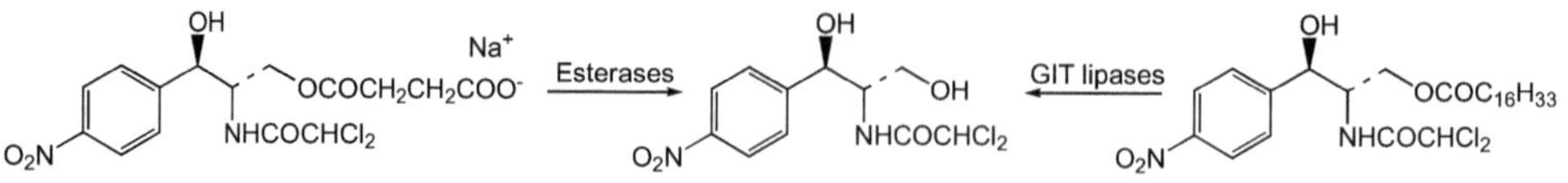


**37** **38** **39**

## 1.5 Recently Marketed Prodrugs

### 1.5.1 Prodrug Prevalence

A review of pharmacologically active, new chemical entities approved by the US FDA between 2004 and 2008 shows 6 prodrugs (Table 1.2) out of the total 84 NCEs entering the market. Therefore, 7% of the recently approved drugs can be classified as prodrugs, which is very similar to a value of 5–7% estimated by Stella in 2007 for all drugs approved worldwide [54]. However, these numbers do not include the previously discussed nucleoside analogues, which require intracellular phosphorylation by kinases to produce the active nucleotide analogues capable of inhibiting RNA or DNA polymerases. When drugs such as azacitidine (introduced in 2004), clofarabine (2005), entecavir (2005), decitabine (2006), nelarabine (2006), telbivudine (2006), and clevudine (2007) are included, as well as those nucleoside analogues brought to market earlier, a prodrug prevalence of about 15% is seen between 2004 and 2008, which raises the prodrug market share closer to 10%.

The prevalence of prodrugs among world's 100 top selling pharmaceuticals is also substantial (data from 2008; http://www.drugs.com/top200.html). Out of the 100 blockbuster drugs, 9 are biologics and 91 small molecules. Of the small molecules, 14 can be classified as prodrugs (Table 1.3), which gives a prodrug prevalence of 15.4% among the 100 best selling small molecular weight drugs. These 14 prodrugs include only one nucleosidal analogue (emtricitabine), therefore further demonstrating the extent of the successful implementation of the prodrug approach.

### 1.5.2 Recent Prodrug Approvals

Several prodrugs were launched worldwide during 2004–2008, and these are summarized in Table 1.2 (FDA approved) and Table 1.4 (approved elsewhere, excluding prodrugs in Table 1.2). These products demonstrate the versatility of the prodrug approach. They include four different routes of administration (oral, inhalation, ocular, and intravenous), many types of activity (anticoagulant, anti-inflammatory, stimulant, antimuscarinic, sedative, and reduction of ocular hypertension), and other indications (thrombin inhibition, asthma, ocular pain, attention deficit hyperactivity disorder (ADHD), overactive bladder, sedation, and glaucoma). The common feature for all these recently approved prodrugs is their bioconversion mechanisms, as they all rely on hydrolase activation. This is not a total surprise; by estimation half of all marketed prodrugs are hydrolytically bioconverted to their parent drugs [23].

The two most recently approved prodrugs are dexlansoprazole and prasugrel, which were both launched in 2009. Dexlansoprazole is the slower metabolized *R*-enantiomer of the proton pump inhibitor lansoprazole. The main advantage of this prodrug is not based on chemistry but rather on a dual-release formulation tech-

**Table 1.2** Prodrugs approved by the US FDA during 2004–2008.

| Prodrug, approval year, therapeutic area | Functional group | Prodrug structure (dashed lines indicate site of bioconversion) | Prodrug strategy |
|---|---|---|---|
| Ciclesonide, 2005, anti-inflammatory corticosteroid | Isobutyryl ester of des-isobutyryl ciclesonide | 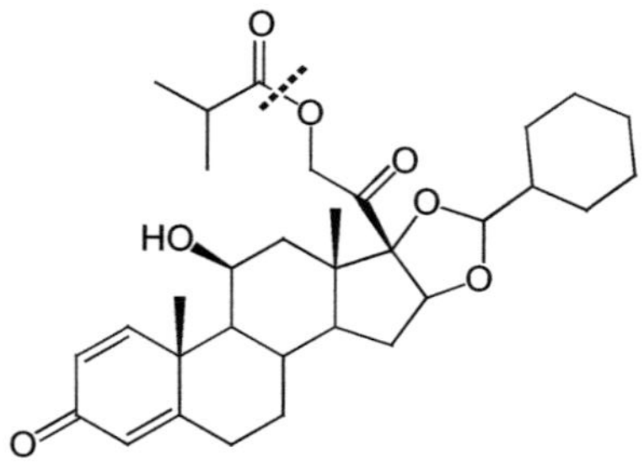 | Bioconversion by lung esterases [65]<br><br>Reduced systemic exposure and consequently reduced risk of adverse effects [66] |
| Nepafenac, 2005, anti-inflammatory | Amide of amfenac | 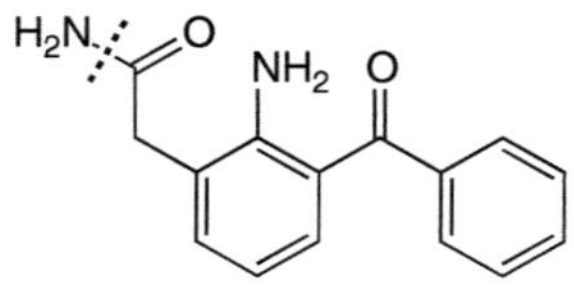 | Bioconversion by intraocular hydrolases [67]<br><br>Improved ocular absorption and prolonged duration of activity [68] |

| | | | |
|---|---|---|---|
| Lisdexamfetamine, 2007, psychostimulant (ADHD) | L-Lysyl amide of D-amphetamine | 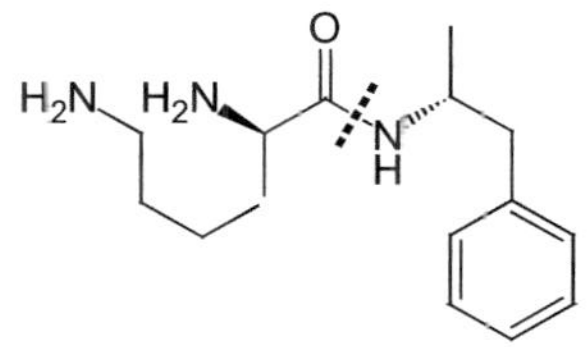 | Bioconversion by intestinal or hepatic hydrolases [69]<br><br>Reduced potential for abuse due to prolonged release of active drug [70] |
| Fesoterodine, 2008, antimuscarinic (overactive bladder) | Isobutyryl ester of 5-hydroxymethyl tolterodine | 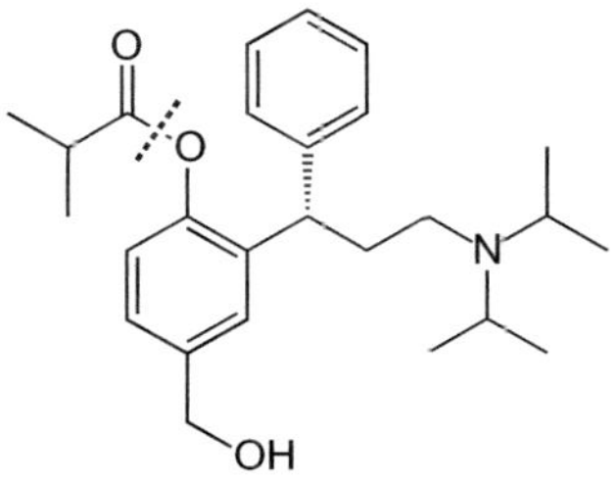 | Bioconversion by esterases<br><br>Reduced interpatient pharmacokinetic variability [71, 72] |
| Fospropofol, 2008, anesthetic | Phosphonooxymethyl ether of propofol | 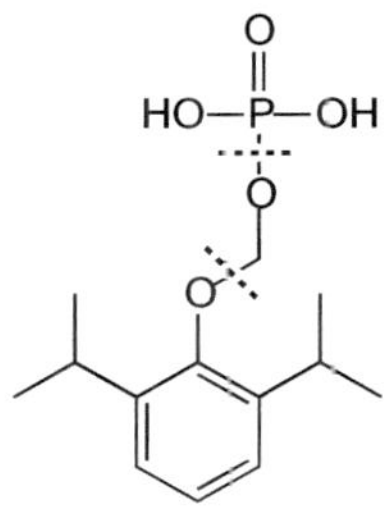 | Is rapidly converted to propofol after intravenous administration by alkaline phosphatases [73, 74]<br><br>Significantly increases the aqueous solubility of propofol from 150 μg/ml to ~500 mg/ml |

(*Continued*)

**Table 1.2** (*Continued*)

| Prodrug, approval year, therapeutic area | Functional group | Prodrug structure (dashed lines indicate site of bioconversion) | Prodrug strategy |
|---|---|---|---|
| Fosaprepitant, 2008, antiemetic | *N*-Phosphono aprepitant | 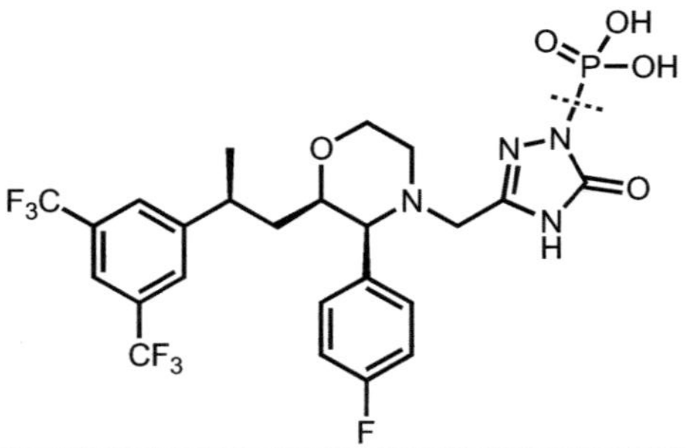 | Reduced injection site pain [75]<br>Is rapidly converted to aprepitant after intravenous administration by alkaline phosphate<br>The prodrug enabled the development of a liquid formulation |

**Table 1.3** The occurrence of prodrugs among the world's 100 top selling pharmaceuticals in 2008.

| Prodrug name (therapeutic area) | Functional group | Prodrug strategy |
|---|---|---|
| Esomeprazole, lansoprazole, pantoprazole, rabeprazole (proton pump inhibitors) | Formation of active sulfenamide form | Bioprecursor prodrugs that are converted into their respective active sulfenamide forms site selectively under acidic conditions of stomach [50] |
| Clopidogrel (antiplatelet) | Formation of the active thiol | Bioprecursor prodrug that selectively inhibits platelet aggregation [51] |
| Simvastatin (hypercholesterolemia) | Inactive lactones | Bioprecursor prodrug that is converted into the active hydroxyl acids in the liver [76] |
| Fenofibrate (hypercholesterolemia) | Isopropyl ester of fenofibric acid | Lipophilic ester of fenofibric acid [77] |
| Olmesartan medoxomil (hypertension) | Cyclic carbonate ester of olmesartan | Improved bioavailability compared to olmesartan, allowing oral administration [78] |
| Mycophenolate mofetil (immunosuppressant) | Morpholinyl ethyl ester of mycophenolic acid | Improved oral bioavailability with less variability [79] |
| Valacyclovir (antiviral) | L-Valyl ester of acyclovir | Bioconversion by valacyclovir hydrolase (valacyclovirase). Transported predominantly by hPEPT1. Oral bioavailability improved from 12–20% (acyclovir) to 54% (valacyclovir) [80–83] |
| Latanoprost (glaucoma) | Isopropyl ester of latanoprost acid | Bioconversion by esterases. Improved lipophilicity to achieve better ocular absorption and safety [84, 85] |
| Tenofovir disoproxil (antiviral) | Bis(isopropyloxycarbonyloxymethyl) ester of tenofovir | Bioconversion by esterases and phosphodiesterases. The oral bioavailability of tenofovir from tenofovir disoproxil is 39% after food [86–88] |

nology that produces two peaks in plasma drug concentration, which subsequently prolongs exposure to the proton pumps [93]. Prasugrel is a novel platelet inhibitor that was described earlier in this chapter.

Both ciclesonide and fesoterodine are isobutyryl ester prodrugs of their parent active drugs, des-isobutyryl ciclesonide and 5-hydroxymethyl tolterodine, respectively. While ciclesonide is an inhaled corticosteroid used in the preventative treatment of asthma, fesoterodine is a new orally administered antimuscarinic agent for the treatment of overactive bladder. The bioconversion of ciclesonide to its active species takes place in the target organ, that is, the lung, by endogenous esterases located both on airway epithelial cells and on lung fibroblasts [65]. The minimal oral bioavailability

**Table 1.4** Prodrugs approved outside the United States during 2004–2008 (excluding the FDA approvals).

| Prodrug, approval year, therapeutic area | Functional group | Prodrug structure (dashed lines indicate site of bioconversion) | Prodrug strategy |
|---|---|---|---|
| Ximelagatran, 2004, anticoagulant | Hydroxyamidine and the ethyl ester of melagatran | 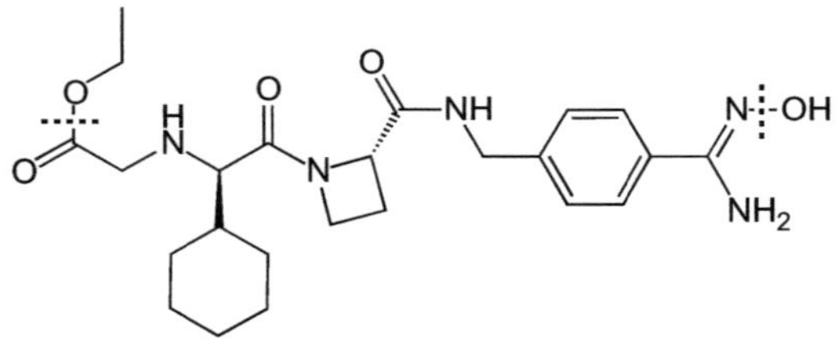 | Bioconversion by esterases and reductive enzymes<br><br>Increased oral bioavailability of 3–7% for melagatran to 20% for ximelagatran [89, 90] |
| Dabigatran etexilate, 2008, anticoagulant | Hexyloxycarbonylamidine and ethyl ester of dabigatran | 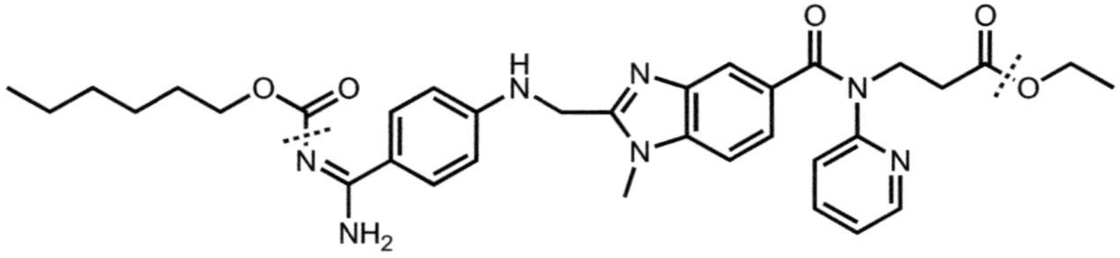 | Bioconversion by esterases<br><br>Oral bioavailability of 7%, measured for dabigatran [91] |

| | | | |
|---|---|---|---|
| Tafluprost, 2008, glaucoma | Isopropyl ester of tafluprost acid | 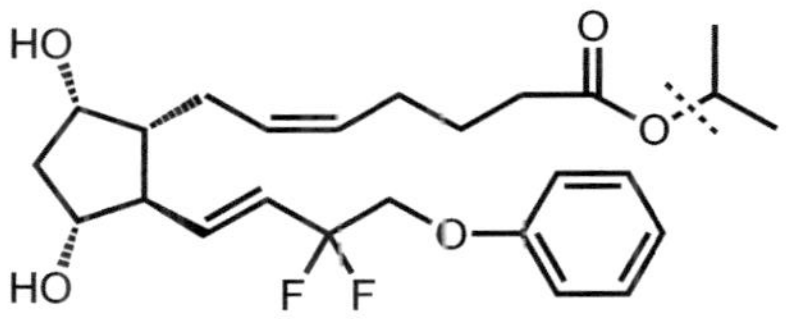 | Bioconversion by esterases<br><br>Improved lipophilicity achieves better ocular absorption and safety [92] |

of ciclesonide and des-isobutyryl ciclesonide, which is normally less than 1% for both drugs, combined with a pulmonary bioavailability of about 50%, supports the favorable risk–benefit profile observed in clinical trials for ciclesonide [66]. Fesoterodine is also rapidly and extensively hydrolyzed by nonspecific esterases after oral administration, and no intact prodrug can be detected in plasma. As the oral bioavailability of fesoterodine is 52% [94], a value commonly seen with esterified drugs [22], at least part of the bioconversion probably occurs prematurely during absorption.

Stimulants such as amphetamine have remained the most effective treatment of ADHD for decades. The recently approved lisdexamfetamine dimesylate (**40**) is a prodrug of dextroamphetamine (**41**) covalently attached to the essential amino acid L-lysine, via an amide bond [95]. It was designed to have less abuse potential than other amphetamines, as it is not rapidly converted to the active form if inhaled or injected, compared to amphetamine, and thus reduces the potential for euphoric effects. The bioconversion of lisdexamfetamine occurs through first-pass intestinal and/or hepatic metabolism after oral administration to provide a time-released effect dose [96]. Of course, lisdexamfetamine can still be used illicitly when taken orally, yet the rewarding effects are substantially attenuated when compared to amphetamine. As a consequence, another amino acid prodrug has been introduced: homoarginine dextroamphetamine (**42**), which has maintained similar blood levels of amphetamine in preclinical species compared to lisdexamfetamine, but with a delayed onset and a longer duration of action, which contribute to a lower abuse potential [97].

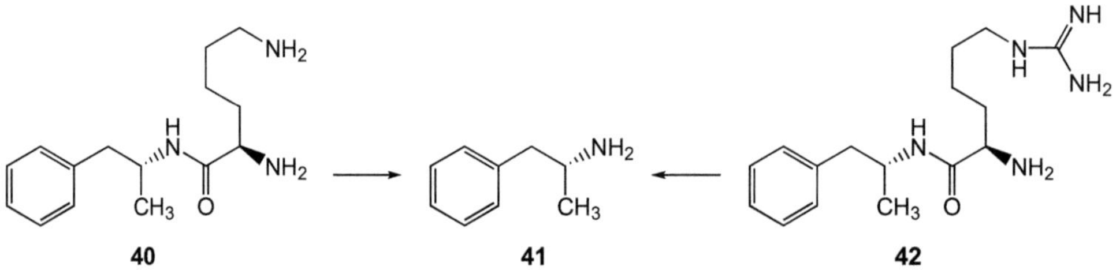

**40** **41** **42**

Nepafenac is an amide prodrug of the NSAID amfenac, which is indicated for the treatment of ocular pain and inflammation [67, 68]. It efficiently permeates the external ocular barriers, cornea, and scleral tissues and has a penetration coefficient that is 4–28 times greater than that achieved with conventional NSAIDs such as diclofenac and ketorolac. This efficient ocular penetration is followed by rapid hydrolysis to amfenac by ocular tissue hydrolases, specifically in the iris, ciliary body, retina, and choroid.

There are several successful phosphate prodrugs in clinical use with improved aqueous solubility properties for parenteral administration. The most recent entrants are phosphonooxymethyl prodrug fospropofol and the *N*-phosphono prodrug fosaprepitant, which were both approved in 2008. The widely used, and unfortunately abused, anesthetic propofol is formulated as an oil-in-water emulsion because of its high lipophilicity and referred to as "milk of amnesia" in some circles due to its physical appearance and recreational effects. However, pain on injection, inherent emulsion instability, and hyperlipidemia after prolonged administration are major drawbacks, which eventually encouraged the development of fospropofol. Being significantly more water soluble, fospropofol is formulated as a purely aqueous solution, thus avoiding some of the problems associated with propofol. Fospropofol releases propofol rapidly after intravenous administration by alkaline phosphatases [73, 74]. This highly water-soluble phosphate prodrug strategy was also applied to the antiemetic aprepitant. Plasma concentrations of fosaprepitant are below the limits of quantification (10 ng/ml) within 30 min after infusion, which indicates rapid bioconversion by alkaline phosphatases. This is also demonstrated by the similarity in aprepitant plasma concentrations at 24 h postdose for 125 mg of oral aprepitant and 115 mg of intravenous fosaprepitant.

Ximelagatran is an ethoxyl prodrug of melagatran and represents the first example of an orally administered direct thrombin inhibitor [89]. It was approved for the European market in 2004 but was withdrawn in early 2006 after an extended clinical trial confirmed initial concerns of severe liver toxicity. Another anticoagulant, dabigatran etexilate, was approved in some European countries and Canada in 2008. Both ximelagatran and dabigatran etexilate are double prodrugs with an ethyl ester on the carboxylic acid and *N*-hydroxyamidine or *N*-hexyloxycarbonylamidine groups, respectively, on the amidine function. The subsequent formation of the respective parent drugs, melagatran and dabigatran, requires two metabolic reactions, where the *N* hydroxy group in ximelagatran is reduced to an amidine, mainly in the liver by CYP450 enzymes [89, 98], and *N*-hexyloxycarbonyl is primarily metabolized by esterases [99]. The ethyl ester in both prodrugs is hydrolyzed to provide the free carboxylic acid in the liver. The masking of two ionizable groups in the parent drugs results in more lipophilic prodrugs that have oral bioavailability of 20% for melagatran from ximelagatran [90] and 7% for dabigatran from dabigatran etexilate [99].

## 1.6 Concluding Remarks

The prodrug strategy is a versatile and powerful method that can be applied to a wide variety of pharmaceuticals whose pharmacologic limitations compromise their clinical use. The development of prodrugs is now well established as a strategy to improve ADMET properties of pharmacologically potent compounds already in the early phases of drug discovery. Also, the economic importance of extending patent protection for an existing pharmaceutical can be significant. These reasons have already led to an increasing number of approved prodrugs that are on the market. About 10% of all approved drugs worldwide can be classified as prodrugs. In addition, the percentage of prodrugs among the most successful drugs is particularly high.

The majority of clinical prodrugs are based on enhanced drug permeation and delivery to the active site via increased drug lipophilicity and, more recently, improved water solubility. However, there are also unmet needs that have not yet been adequately addressed by prodrugs. It is surprising how few prodrugs exist for cancer therapy, even though the side effects of antineoplastic agents are considerable and potentially lethal. Perhaps, this means that the easier problems have been resolved while more complex issues remain unaddressed. More creative prodrug strategies will be required to address drug delivery issues that are related to site-selective drug delivery with reduced side effects, prevention of presystemic drug metabolism, and circumvention of efflux-limited drug absorption.

I hope that this chapter has provided useful examples of potential applications for using prodrugs and will encourage creative prodrug research to solve some of the unmet drug delivery needs. Prodrugs will certainly be an exciting area of research in the future.

## References


1 Stella, V., Hageman, M., Oliyai, R., Tilley, J., and Maag, H. (eds) (2007) *Prodrugs: Challenges and Rewards*, AAPS Press/Springer, New York.

2 Rautio, J. *et al.* (2008) Prodrugs: design and clinical applications. *Nature Reviews. Drug Discovery*, **7**, 255–270.

3 Stella, V.J., Charman, W.N., and Naringrekar, V.H. (1985) Prodrugs. Do they have advantages in clinical practice? *Drugs*, **29**, 455–473.

4 Erhardt, P.W., Khupse, R., Sarver, J.G., and Trendel, J.A.,in *Burger's Medicinal Chemistry, Drug Discovery and Development* (ed. D. Abraham), John Wiley & Sons, Inc., New York, pp. 1–71, in press.

5 Leppanen, J. *et al.* (2002) Design and synthesis of a novel L-dopa-entacapone codrug. *Journal of Medicinal Chemistry*, **45**, 1379–1382.

6 Bodor, N. and Buchwald, P. (2000) Soft drug design: general principles and recent applications. *Medicinal Research Reviews*, **20**, 58–101.

7 Wu, K.-M. (2009) A new classification of prodrugs: regulatory perspective. *Pharmaceuticals*, **2**, 77–81.

8 Wu, K.M. and Farrelly, J.G. (2007) Regulatory perspectives of type II prodrug development and time-dependent toxicity management: nonclinical Pharm/Tox analysis and the role of comparative toxicology. *Toxicology*, **236**, 1–6.

9 Testa, B. and Mayer, J.M. (2003) *Hydrolysis in Drug and Prodrug Metabolism*, Wiley-VCH Verlag GmbH, Weinheim.

10 Liederer, B.M. and Borchardt, R.T. (2006) Enzymes involved in the bioconversion of ester-based prodrugs. *Journal of Pharmaceutical Sciences*, **95**, 1177–1195.

11 Bellott, R. *et al.* (2008) Functional study of the 830C>G polymorphism of the human carboxylesterase 2 gene. *Cancer Chemotherapy and Pharmacology*, **61**, 481–488.

12 Reddy, K.R. *et al.* (2008) Pradefovir: a prodrug that targets adefovir to the liver for the treatment of hepatitis B. *Journal of Medicinal Chemistry*, **51**, 666–676.

13 Kumpulainen, H. *et al.* (2006) Evaluation of hydroxyimine as cytochrome P450-selective prodrug structure. *Journal of Medicinal Chemistry*, **49**, 1207–1211.

14 Saunders, M.P., Patterson, A.V., Chinje, E.C., Harris, A.L., and Stratford, I.J. (2000) NADPH:cytochrome *c* (P450) reductase activates tirapazamine (SR4233) to restore hypoxic and oxic cytotoxicity in an aerobic resistant derivative of the A549 lung cancer cell line. *British Journal of Cancer*, **82**, 651–656.

15 Boddy, A.V. and Yule, S.M. (2000) Metabolism and pharmacokinetics of

oxazaphosphorines. *Clinical Pharmacokinetics*, **38**, 291–304.
16 Dobesh, P.P. (2009) Pharmacokinetics and pharmacodynamics of prasugrel, a thienopyridine P2Y12 inhibitor. *Pharmacotherapy*, **29**, 1089–1102.
17 Pereillo, J.M. *et al.* (2002) Structure and stereochemistry of the active metabolite of clopidogrel. *Drug Metabolism and Disposition: The Biological Fate of Chemicals*, **30**, 1288–1295.
18 Erhardt, P.W. (2002) Medicinal chemistry in the new millennium: a glance into the future. *Pure and Applied Chemistry*, **74**, 703–785.
19 Venkatesh, S. and Lipper, R.A. (2000) Role of the development scientist in compound lead selection and optimization. *Journal of Pharmaceutical Sciences*, **89**, 145–154.
20 Kerns, E.H. and Di, L. (2008) *Drug-Like Properties: Concepts, Structure Design and Methods*, Academic Press, New York.
21 Stella, V. (2006) in *Optimizing the "Drug-Like" Properties of Leads in Drug Discovery* (eds R. Borchardt, M. Hageman, J. Stevens, E. Kerns, and D. Thakker), Springer, New York, pp. 221–242.
22 Beaumont, K., Webster, R., Gardner, I., and Dack, K. (2003) Design of ester prodrugs to enhance oral absorption of poorly permeable compounds: challenges to the discovery scientist. *Current Drug Metabolism*, **4**, 461–485.
23 Ettmayer, P., Amidon, G.L., Clement, B., and Testa, B. (2004) Lessons learned from marketed and investigational prodrugs. *Journal of Medicinal Chemistry*, **47**, 2393–2404.
24 Järvinen, T., Rautio, J., Masson, M., and Loftsson, T. (2005) in *Drug Discovery Handbook* (ed. S. Gad), John Wiley & Sons, Inc., Hoboken, NJ, pp. 733–796.
25 Stella, V.J. (2004) Prodrugs as therapeutics. *Expert Opinion on Therapeutic Patents*, **14**, 277–280.
26 Testa, B. (2004) Prodrug research: futile or fertile? *Biochemical Pharmacology*, **68**, 2097–2106.
27 Stella, V.J. and Nti-Addae, K.W. (2007) Prodrug strategies to overcome poor water solubility. *Advanced Drug Delivery Reviews*, **59**, 677–694.
28 Muller, C.E. (2009) Prodrug approaches for enhancing the bioavailability of drugs with low solubility. *Chemistry & Biodiversity*, **6**, 2071–2083.
29 Boucher, B.A. (1996) Fosphenytoin: a novel phenytoin prodrug. *Pharmacotherapy*, **16**, 777–791.
30 Browne, T.R., Kugler, A.R., and Eldon, M.A. (1996) Pharmacology and pharmacokinetics of fosphenytoin. *Neurology*, **46**, S3–S7.
31 Varia, S.A., Schuller, S., Sloan, K.B., and Stella, V.J. (1984) Phenytoin prodrugs III: water-soluble prodrugs for oral and/or parenteral use. *Journal of Pharmaceutical Sciences*, **73**, 1068–1073.
32 Bardsley-Elliot, A. and Noble, S. (1999) Oseltamivir. *Drugs*, **58**, 851–860; discussion 861–862.
33 Doucette, K.E. and Aoki, F.Y. (2001) Oseltamivir: a clinical and pharmacological perspective. *Expert Opinion on Pharmacotherapy*, **2**, 1671–1683.
34 McClellan, K. and Perry, C.M. (2001) Oseltamivir: a review of its use in influenza. *Drugs*, **61**, 263–283.
35 Shi, D. *et al.* (2006) Anti-influenza prodrug oseltamivir is activated by carboxylesterase human carboxylesterase 1, and the activation is inhibited by antiplatelet agent clopidogrel. *The Journal of Pharmacology and Experimental Therapeutics*, **319**, 1477–1481.
36 Dobson, P.D. and Kell, D.B. (2008) Carrier-mediated cellular uptake of pharmaceutical drugs: an exception or the rule? *Nature Reviews. Drug Discovery*, **7**, 205–220.
37 Cruz, D.N. (2000) Midodrine: a selective alpha-adrenergic agonist for orthostatic hypotension and dialysis hypotension. *Expert Opinion on Pharmacotherapy*, **1**, 835–840.
38 Tsuda, M. *et al.* (2006) Transport characteristics of a novel peptide transporter 1 substrate, antihypotensive drug midodrine, and its amino acid derivatives. *The Journal of Pharmacology and Experimental Therapeutics*, **318**, 455–460.
39 Nutt, J.G. and Woodward, W.R. (1986) Levodopa pharmacokinetics and

pharmacodynamics in fluctuating parkinsonian patients. *Neurology*, **36**, 739–744.

40 Nutt, J.G., Woodward, W.R., Hammerstad, J.P., Carter, J.H., and Anderson, J.L. (1984) The "on–off" phenomenon in Parkinson's disease: relation to levodopa absorption and transport. *The New England Journal of Medicine*, **310**, 483–488.

41 Svensson, L. and Tunek, A. (1988) The design and bioactivation of presystemically stable prodrugs. *Drug Metabolism Reviews*, **19**, 165–194.

42 Tunek, A., Levin, E., and Svensson, L. (1988) Hydrolysis of 3H-bambuterol, a carbamate prodrug of terbutaline, in blood from humans and laboratory animals *in vitro*. *Biochemical Pharmacology*, **37**, 3867–3876.

43 Sitar, D.S. (1996) Clinical pharmacokinetics of bambuterol. *Clinical Pharmacokinetics*, **31**, 246–256.

44 Persson, G., Pahlm, O., and Gnosspelius, Y. (1995) Oral bambuterol versus terbutaline in patients with asthma. *Current Therapeutic Research*, **56**, 457–465.

45 Richards, D.M. *et al.* (1983) Acyclovir: a review of its pharmacodynamic properties and therapeutic efficacy. *Drugs*, **26**, 378–438.

46 O'Brien, J.J. and Campoli-Richards, D.M. (1989) Acyclovir: an updated review of its antiviral activity, pharmacokinetic properties and therapeutic efficacy. *Drugs*, **37**, 233–309.

47 Weller, S. *et al.* (1993) Pharmacokinetics of the acyclovir pro-drug valaciclovir after escalating single- and multiple-dose administration to normal volunteers. *Clinical Pharmacology and Therapeutics*, **54**, 595–605.

48 Beutner, K.R., Friedman, D.J., Forszpaniak, C., Andersen, P.L., and Wood, M.J. (1995) Valaciclovir compared with acyclovir for improved therapy for herpes zoster in immunocompetent adults. *Antimicrobial Agents and Chemotherapy*, **39**, 1546–1553.

49 Sachs, G., Shin, J.M., Briving, C., Wallmark, B., and Hersey, S. (1995) The pharmacology of the gastric acid pump: the $H^+,K^+$ ATPase. *Annual Review of Pharmacology and Toxicology*, **35**, 277–305.

50 Shin, J.M., Cho, Y.M., and Sachs, G. (2004) Chemistry of covalent inhibition of the gastric ($H^+,K^+$)-ATPase by proton pump inhibitors. *Journal of the American Chemical Society*, **126**, 7800–7811.

51 Savi, P. *et al.* (2001) P2y(12), a new platelet ADP receptor, target of clopidogrel. *Biochemical and Biophysical Research Communications*, **283**, 379–383.

52 Dansette, P.M., Libraire, J., Bertho, G., and Mansuy, D. (2009) Metabolic oxidative cleavage of thioesters: evidence for the formation of sulfenic acid intermediates in the bioactivation of the antithrombotic prodrugs ticlopidine and clopidogrel. *Chemical Research in Toxicology*, **22**, 369–373.

53 Williams, E.T. *et al.* (2008) The biotransformation of prasugrel, a new thienopyridine prodrug, by the human carboxylesterases 1 and 2. *Drug Metabolism and Disposition: The Biological Fate of Chemicals*, **36**, 1227–1232.

54 Stella, V.J. (2007) in *Prodrugs: Challenges and Rewards. Part 1* (eds V.J. Stella *et al.*), AAPS Press/Springer, New York, pp. 3–33.

55 Albert, A. (1958) Chemical aspects of selective toxicity. *Nature*, **182**, 421–422.

56 Harper, N.J. (1959) Drug latentiation. *Journal of Medicinal and Pharmaceutical Chemistry*, **1**, 467–500.

57 Harper, N.J. (1962) Drug latentiation. *Progress in Drug Research*, **4**, 221–294.

58 Sinkula, A.A. and Yalkowsky, S.H. (1975) Rationale for design of biologically reversible drug derivatives: prodrugs. *Journal of Pharmaceutical Sciences*, **64**, 181–210.

59 Vane, J.R. and Botting, R.M. (2003) The mechanism of action of aspirin. *Thrombosis Research*, **110**, 255–258.

60 Aronoff, D.M., Oates, J.A., and Boutaud, O. (2006) New insights into the mechanism of action of acetaminophen: its clinical pharmacologic characteristics reflect its inhibition of the two prostaglandin H2 synthases. *Clinical Pharmacology and Therapeutics*, **79**, 9–19.

61 Timmins, G.S. and Deretic, V. (2006) Mechanisms of action of isoniazid. *Molecular Microbiology*, **62**, 1220–1227.

62 Bentley, R. (2009) Different roads to discovery: prontosil (hence sulfa drugs) and penicillin (hence beta-lactams). *Journal of Industrial Microbiology & Biotechnology*, **36**, 775–786.

63 Glazko, A.J., Edgerton, W.H., Dill, W.A., and Lenz, W.R. (1952) Chloromycetin palmitate: a synthetic ester of chloromycetin. *Antibiotics and Chemotherapy*, **2**, 234–242.

64 Glazko, A.J., Carnes, H.E., Kazenko, A., Wolf, L.M., and Reutner, T.F. (1957) Succinic acid esters of chloramphenicol. *Antibiotics Annual*, **5**, 792–802.

65 Boero, S. *et al.* (2007) Modulation of human lung fibroblast functions by ciclesonide: evidence for its conversion into the active metabolite desisobutyryl-ciclesonide. *Immunology Letters*, **112**, 39–46.

66 Derendorf, H. (2007) Pharmacokinetic and pharmacodynamic properties of inhaled ciclesonide. *Journal of Clinical Pharmacology*, **47**, 782–789.

67 Ke, T.L., Graff, G., Spellman, J.M., and Yanni, J.M. (2000) Nepafenac, a unique nonsteroidal prodrug with potential utility in the treatment of trauma-induced ocular inflammation: II. *In vitro* bioactivation and permeation of external ocular barriers. *Inflammation*, **24**, 371–384.

68 Gamache, D.A., Graff, G., Brady, M.T., Spellman, J.M., and Yanni, J.M. (2000) Nepafenac, a unique nonsteroidal prodrug with potential utility in the treatment of trauma-induced ocular inflammation: I. Assessment of anti-inflammatory efficacy. *Inflammation*, **24**, 357–370.

69 Suma, K., Pennick, M., and Stark, J. (2008) Metabolism, distribution and elimination of lisdexamfetamine dimesylate. *Clinical Drug Investigation*, **28**, 745–755.

70 Blick, S.K. and Keating, G.M. (2007) Lisdexamfetamine. *Paediatric Drugs*, **9**, 129–135; discussion 136–138.

71 Ney, P. *et al.* (2008) Pharmacological characterization of a novel investigational antimuscarinic drug, fesoterodine, *in vitro* and *in vivo*. *BJU International*, **101**, 1036–1042.

72 Michel, M.C. (2008) Fesoterodine: a novel muscarinic receptor antagonist for the treatment of overactive bladder syndrome. *Expert Opinion on Pharmacotherapy*, **9**, 1787–1796.

73 Schywalsky, M. *et al.* (2003) Pharmacokinetics and pharmacodynamics of the new propofol prodrug GPI 15715 in rats. *European Journal of Anaesthesiology*, **20**, 182–190.

74 Stella, V., Zygmunt, J., Georg, I., and MS, S. (2005) US Patent 19980131385.

75 Fechner, J., Schwilden, H., and Schuttler, J. (2008) Pharmacokinetics and pharmacodynamics of GPI 15715 or fospropofol (Aquavan injection): a water-soluble propofol prodrug. *Handbook of Experimental Pharmacology*, 253–266.

76 Mauro, V.F. (1993) Clinical pharmacokinetics and practical applications of simvastatin. *Clinical Pharmacokinetics*, **24**, 195–202.

77 Chapman, M.J. (1987) Pharmacology of fenofibrate. *The American Journal of Medicine*, **83**, 21–25.

78 Gardner, S.F. and Franks, A.M. (2003) Olmesartan medoxomil: the seventh angiotensin receptor antagonist. *Annals of Pharmacotherapy*, **37**, 99–105.

79 Lee, W.A. *et al.* (1990) Bioavailability improvement of mycophenolic acid through amino ester derivatization. *Pharmaceutical Research*, **7**, 161–166.

80 Balimane, P.V. *et al.* (1998) Direct evidence for peptide transporter (PepT1)-mediated uptake of a nonpeptide prodrug, valacyclovir. *Biochemical and Biophysical Research Communications*, **250**, 246–251.

81 de Vrueh, R.L., Smith, P.L., and Lee, C.P. (1998) Transport of L-valine-acyclovir via the oligopeptide transporter in the human intestinal cell line, Caco-2. *The Journal of Pharmacology and Experimental Therapeutics*, **286**, 1166–1170.

82 Guo, A., Hu, P., Balimane, P.V., Leibach, F.H., and Sinko, P.J. (1999) Interactions of a nonpeptidic drug, valacyclovir, with the human intestinal peptide transporter (hPEPT1) expressed in a mammalian cell line. *The Journal of Pharmacology and Experimental Therapeutics*, **289**, 448–454.

83 Perry, C.M. and Faulds, D. (1996) Valaciclovir: a review of its antiviral

activity, pharmacokinetic properties and therapeutic efficacy in herpes virus infections. *Drugs*, **52**, 754–772.

**84** Järvinen, T. and Niemi, R. (2007) in *Prodrugs: Challenges and Rewards. Part 1* (ed V.J. Stella *et al.*), AAPS Press/Springer, New York, pp. 125–155.

**85** Netland, P.A. *et al.* (2001) Travoprost compared with latanoprost and timolol in patients with open-angle glaucoma or ocular hypertension. *American Journal of Ophthalmology*, **132**, 472–484.

**86** Chapman, T., McGavin, J., and Noble, S. (2003) Tenofovir disoproxil fumarate. *Drugs*, **63**, 1597–1608.

**87** Gallant, J.E. and Deresinski, S. (2003) Tenofovir disoproxil fumarate. *Clinical Infectious Diseases*, **37**, 944–950.

**88** Shaw, J.P. *et al.* (1997) Metabolism and pharmacokinetics of novel oral prodrugs of 9-[(*R*)-2-(phosphonomethoxy)propyl] adenine (PMPA) in dogs. *Pharmaceutical Research*, **14**, 1824–1829.

**89** Eriksson, U.G. *et al.* (2003) Absorption, distribution, metabolism, and excretion of ximelagatran, an oral direct thrombin inhibitor, in rats, dogs, and humans. *Drug Metabolism and Disposition: The Biological Fate of Chemicals*, **31**, 294–305.

**90** Gustafsson, D. *et al.* (2001) The direct thrombin inhibitor melagatran and its oral prodrug H 376/95: intestinal absorption properties, biochemical and pharmacodynamic effects. *Thrombosis Research*, **101**, 171–181.

**91** Gustafsson, D. (2003) Oral direct thrombin inhibitors in clinical development. *Journal of Internal Medicine*, **254**, 322–334.

**92** Fukano, Y. and Kawazu, K. (2009) Disposition and metabolism of a novel prostanoid antiglaucoma medication, tafluprost, following ocular administration to rats. *Drug Metabolism and Disposition: The Biological Fate of Chemicals*, **37**, 1622–1634.

**93** DeVault, K.R. and Talley, N.J. (2009) Insights into the future of gastric acid suppression. *Nature Reviews. Gastroenterology & Hepatology*, **6**, 524–532.

**94** Pfizer Labs, Division of Pfizer Inc; http://media.pfizer.com/files/products/uspi_toviaz.pdf, 2008.

**95** Najib, J. (2009) The efficacy and safety profile of lisdexamfetamine dimesylate, a prodrug of D-amphetamine, for the treatment of attention-deficit/hyperactivity disorder in children and adults. *Clinical Therapeutics*, **31**, 142–176.

**96** Krishnan, S.M., Pennick, M., and Stark, J.G. (2008) Metabolism, distribution and elimination of lisdexamfetamine dimesylate: open-label, single-centre, phase I study in healthy adult volunteers. *Clinical Drug Investigation*, **28**, 745–755.

**97** Mickle, T.C. (2008) Polar hydrophilic prodrugs of amphetamine and other stimulants and processes for making and using the same. WO 2008/098151.

**98** Clement, B. and Lopian, K. (2003) Characterization of *in vitro* biotransformation of new, orally active, direct thrombin inhibitor ximelagatran, an amidoxime and ester prodrug. *Drug Metabolism and Disposition: The Biological Fate of Chemicals*, **31**, 645–651.

**99** Blech, S., Ebner, T., Ludwig-Schwellinger, E., Stangier, J., and Roth, W. (2008) The metabolism and disposition of the oral direct thrombin inhibitor, dabigatran, in humans. *Drug Metabolism and Disposition: The Biological Fate of Chemicals*, **36**, 386–399.

# 2
# The Molecular Design of Prodrugs by Functional Group

*Victor R. Guarino*

## 2.1
## Introduction

Drug design in pharmaceutical companies continues to evolve toward a more multidisciplinary effort aiming to balance multiple factors during optimization, with the end goal of selecting a drug candidate for clinical trials that displays promising signs of efficacy, safety, and market potential. Today's commonly practiced "target-based" approach for drug discovery aims for a molecule that is potent against a chosen biological target of assumed therapeutic relevance (receptor, enzyme, DNA, etc.) while being sufficiently inactive against targets of assumed and/or known liability; furthermore, as with any drug discovery approach, the chosen molecule needs both to possess sufficient biopharmaceutical and pharmacokinetic properties allowing a viable drug delivery strategy and to appear safe and efficacious in preclinical models. Even in cases where this can be achieved, the actual process of designing one molecule that possesses all of these desired properties can be a resource-intensive and time-consuming activity. According to an estimate, it requires roughly US$ 1.3 billion[1)] [1] and 12–15 years [2, 3] to produce one approved new molecular entity drug product; the extended time lines and high costs that might be required in order to design a drug candidate *intrinsically* possessing all of the desired properties can serve to inevitably diminish the original market potential that once existed for the therapeutic concept.

Prodrugs [4–7], when used appropriately, are one of the many drug delivery tools that can enable a *suitable* candidate molecule to be selected for development more quickly and with less overall resources. Since effective prodrugs enable the delivery of otherwise problematic molecules, they can serve to relax some of the biopharmaceutical and/or pharmacokinetic "criteria" that a molecule would otherwise need to intrinsically fulfill. Therefore, appropriate use of the prodrug concept can directly affect the operational efficiency of a pharmaceutical company by allowing faster and less costly candidate selection. This chapter will highlight various chemical technologies available for designing prodrugs. Given the recently published two-volume

1) Cost estimate is in "2005" US dollars.

*Prodrugs and Targeted Delivery: Towards Better ADME Properties.* Edited by Jarkko Rautio

ISBN: 978-3-527-32603-7

prodrug text [4], part of which contains an extensive review of functional group modifications, the goal of this chapter is to act more as a general tool by distilling the wide-ranging prodrug literature down to some basic and commonly used functional group approaches as well as to illustrate the promise and limitations of each approach through a *representative* selection of examples. It is hoped that the reader can use this chapter to more quickly gain a basic overview of the established approaches for functional group modification, and if more details are still desired, the reader can then search the more comprehensive reviews with better focus to gain a deeper appreciation of the desired approach. The remaining chapter is divided into two primary sections, listed as follows:

1) The prodrug concept and basics of design
2) Common functional group approaches to prodrug design.

## 2.2 The Prodrug Concept and Basics of Design

The prodrug concept is one approach that can enable the selection of a suitable candidate for development in the least amount of time. As illustrated in Figure 2.1, this concept involves the chemical modification of the parent drug into a totally new molecule with a different set of intrinsic properties (illustrated in the figure through different shapes) that improve the suboptimal nature of the parent drug that was limiting its delivery (e.g., improved solubility, improved permeability, etc.). As a direct result of the enhanced "delivery" properties, the prodrug does not experience the same delivery barrier as exists for the parent drug. However, typically the

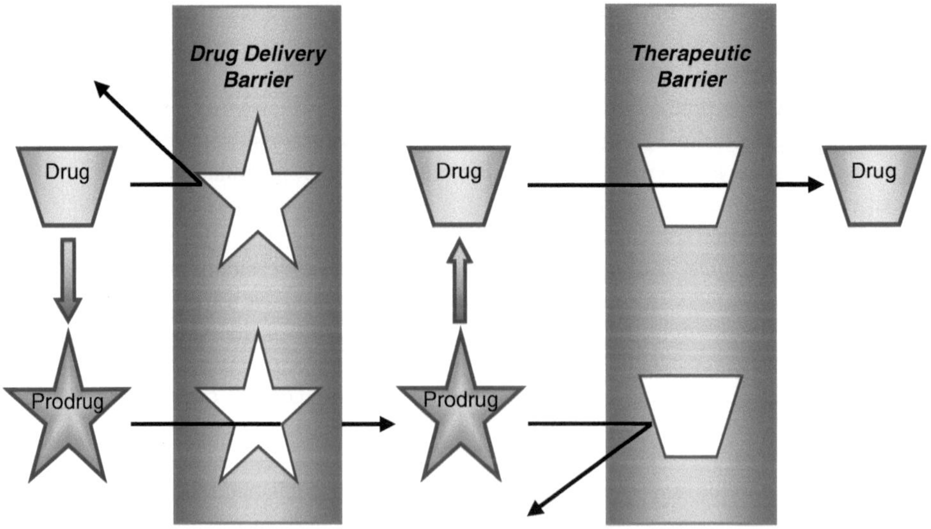


**Figure 2.1** The prodrug concept for improved drug delivery.

enhanced "delivery" properties of the prodrug also mask the parent drug's therapeutic nature, thereby presenting a "therapeutic barrier" to the prodrug. Because of this resulting therapeutic barrier, the modifications employed to design the prodrug must be reversible, allowing the prodrug to eventually convert back to the parent drug (by chemical and/or biochemical reaction) such that the parent drug can interact with the therapeutic target. Finally, if byproducts are produced during reconversion, they should have an acceptable level of safety within the context of the therapeutic concept and level of unmet medical need. Admittedly, designing all of this into a prodrug can certainly present its own challenges, but depending on the chemical nature of the parent drug and the therapeutic target, many times the prodrug design can represent a comparably smaller challenge than the alternative of searching for a new therapeutically active molecule that also inherently possesses the desired delivery properties.

Regarding the design of bioreversibility, the most common approaches to date are either to "target" *in vivo* hydrolases, of which there are a wide variety [5], and/or to design a reconversion process that is strictly "chemical" in nature (not enzymatic). Some hydrolases commonly targeted are carboxylesterases, peptidases, and phosphatases. These enzymes are located in various places throughout the body, and many times, the exact identity of the enzyme(s) responsible for the prodrug reconversion is not known. This ambiguity in enzyme conversion can present significant challenges to those attempting to *predict* prodrug *in vivo* performance from *in vitro* enzyme-containing surrogate systems since those systems might not contain the relevant enzyme(s), and therefore the designer could easily disregard what would have been a high-performing prodrug due to an inappropriate surrogate model; moreover, the definition of "relevant enzyme(s)" could change from prodrug to prodrug, further adding complexity to attempts at prediction and design based on *in vitro* surrogate models. This is not to trivialize the potential value that surrogate models can bring when used appropriately, but rather to emphasize that there is often more value in just dosing the *in vivo* model and letting that system indicate whether the prodrug performs or not. Of course, even the animal model in itself is a surrogate for humans, so appreciating the limitations of any surrogate system is very helpful in predicting performance translation to humans.

Both the advantages and the limitations of the prodrug concept stem from its chemical nature. One main limitation is that the prodrug approach will naturally be very compound specific in both the modifications possible and the strategy for ultimate bioconversion. On the other hand, an advantage of the prodrug approach is that a very wide range of property modulation is possible, allowing dramatic enhancements in drug delivery. As more viable strategies are continually established for bioreversibly derivatizing functional groups, the more generically applicable the prodrug concept will become, but there will always be some molecules that are not realistically amenable to the approach, as is the case with any drug delivery approach.

Finally, since there is a heavy emphasis in this chapter on molecular design, it is useful to briefly define the terminology related to the structure and design of a prodrug. The term prodrug refers to the chemical derivative of a drug that is often formed by covalently attaching some moiety (promoiety) to the drug (Figure 2.2).

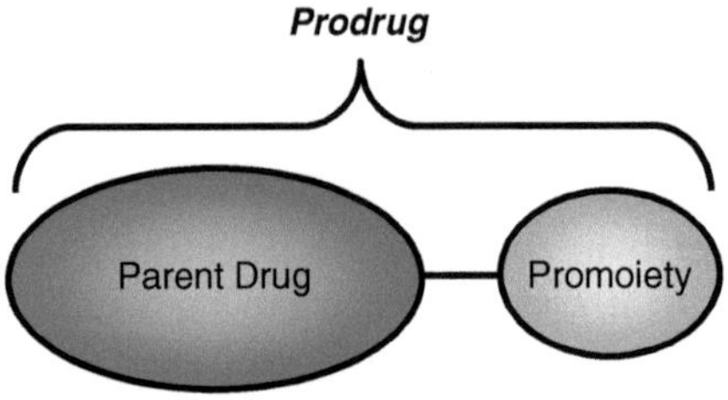


**Figure 2.2** A simplified representation of a prodrug.

While Figure 2.2 is a commonly used representation of a generic prodrug, it is also an oversimplification of the greater flexibility inherent in the prodrug concept, and it is useful to realize that prodrugs can also be designed by the addition of more than one promoiety, the addition of one promoiety across multiple attachment sites, or even through a rearrangement that does not involve promoiety attachment; furthermore, a prodrug can even be designed by the subtraction of atoms from the parent drug, such that a later "addition" of some type is required to re-form the parent drug. So in essence, any type of chemical transformation can result in a successful prodrug as long as that new molecule can convert back to the parent drug while not releasing any unacceptable byproducts. The following sections will illustrate some typical functional groups and common modifications for prodrug design.

## 2.3
## Common Functional Group Approaches in Prodrug Design

Historically, ester formation in some fashion has been a common theme in prodrug design. Sections 2.3.1 and 2.3.2 cover alcohols and carboxylic acids since these two functionalities are the *direct* building blocks of an ester functionality; furthermore, one common approach used to modify other functional groups is to first alter them into a new moiety that resembles a simple alcohol or carboxylic acid, and then employ the established modification strategies for alcohols and carboxylic acids. This alteration of one functional group into another is usually done through the addition of a "spacer" group, which generally provides a "space" between the drug and the section of the promoiety that triggers the reconversion process; in addition to the chemical transformation advantages, a spacer group can also be used to spatially extend the reactive section of the promoiety from the bulk molecule where it is less sterically hindered from reacting with either the enzyme or the chemical reactant responsible for reconversion.

### 2.3.1
### Aliphatic and Aromatic Alcohols

The hydroxyl group tends to be a favorite "handle" for the prodrug designer since it is usually synthetically accessible and able to be *directly* derivatized into a bioreversible ester-based linkage to join the promoiety and the drug. In addition to typically being straightforward to derivatize, the hydroxyl is also a good leaving group that allows aldehyde-based spacer moieties (e.g., formaldehyde and acetaldehyde) to be used to spatially extend bioreversible esters with confidence that the hemiacetal reconversion intermediate following ester hydrolysis will degrade quickly. Below are some common ester-based approaches for modifying the hydroxyl group.

#### 2.3.1.1 Phosphate Monoesters

Phosphorylating a hydroxyl group in a nonpolar drug creates a phosphate monoester prodrug that can be dramatically more soluble, or at least can possess a very different pH-solubility relationship, in aqueous media due to the ionization afforded by the phosphate promoiety. The phosphate monoester linkage to the parent drug is typically bioreversible through reaction with alkaline phosphatase, a nonspecific esterase found in many parts of the body, including the liver, kidneys, and apical membrane of enterocytes [5, 8]. The potential for dramatic solubility modulation can be useful for satisfying either the high solubility requirements of many parenteral solution formulations or the necessary solubility and dissolution properties to allow effective drug delivery from oral solid formulations (e.g., conventional tablets). Also, because of the location of alkaline phosphatase at the intestinal brush border, phosphate prodrugs have the potential to create supersaturated concentrations of the poorly soluble parent drug at what is typically considered the main oral absorption site, which can serve to drive flux across the enterocytes, as long as the parent drug demonstrates slow precipitation kinetics and sufficient permeability [8].

A dramatic example of the promise in the phosphate monoester technology for improved drug delivery is fosamprenavir (**1**, Lexiva®) [9–11], the phosphate monoester of the HIV protease inhibitor amprenavir (**2**, Agenerase®). In this case, amprenavir was marketed first, but due to a very high dose (1200 mg twice daily) combined with limited aqueous solubility, the drug was formulated in soft gelatin capsules as a solubilized liquid formulation[2)] containing just 150 mg of amprenavir per capsule, and therefore requiring a dosing regimen of eight capsules taken twice daily. On the other hand, the improved solubility and delivery attributes of fosamprenavir allow it to be formulated as the calcium salt in a solid tablet formulation that contains the molar equivalent of 600 mg of amprenavir, both allowing the same 1200 mg dose to be taken with just two tablets and avoiding the continual exposure to cosolvents such as propylene glycol.

2) Formulation vehicle contained propylene glycol, polyethylene glycol 400, and vitamin E TPGS.

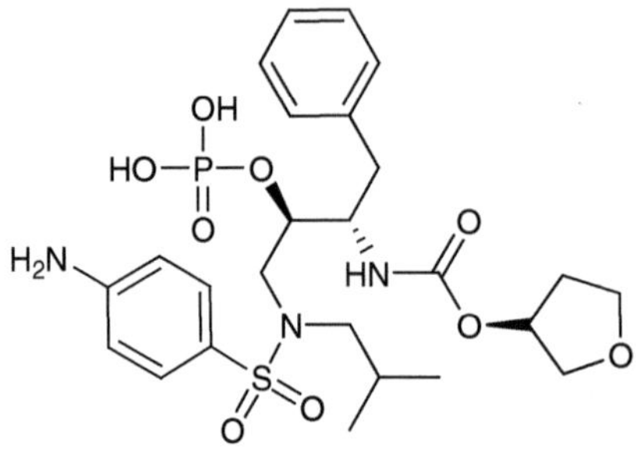


1

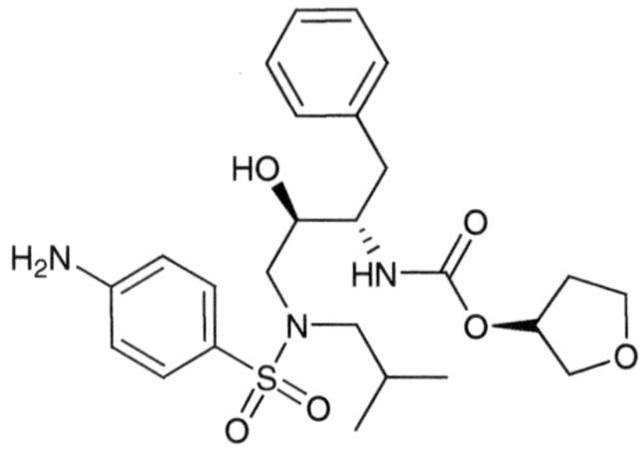


2

While fosamprenavir could effectively perform as a simple direct phosphate monoester, other drugs can contain hydroxyl groups that are more sterically hindered, and effective prodrug performance requires that the phosphate ester be further separated in space from the rest of the drug molecule to allow improved access to alkaline phosphatase. To relieve steric hindrance, a common spacer strategy is to incorporate simple aldehydes into the promoiety such as formaldehyde [12] or acetaldehyde. Once the phosphate monoester is enzymatically cleaved, the resulting hydroxyalkyl derivative collapses in a unimolecular fashion to form the corresponding aldehyde and the hydroxyl-containing parent drug. An example of this reconversion is illustrated in Scheme 2.1 using fospropofol (**3**, Lusedra®) [13, 14], a recently approved phosphoryloxymethyl prodrug of the sterically hindered phenol-containing anesthetic propofol (**4**, Diprivan®). Due to its enhanced aqueous solubility, fospropofol can be formulated in a convenient aqueous ready-to-use formulation, as opposed to the oil/water emulsion formulation that is used for the parent. Fospropofol has even been found to greatly reduce the local pain observed upon injection of propofol and is not as prone to either the bacterial contamination potential of the emulsion or the lipid load concerns that can exist if continual administration is needed. A comparison of

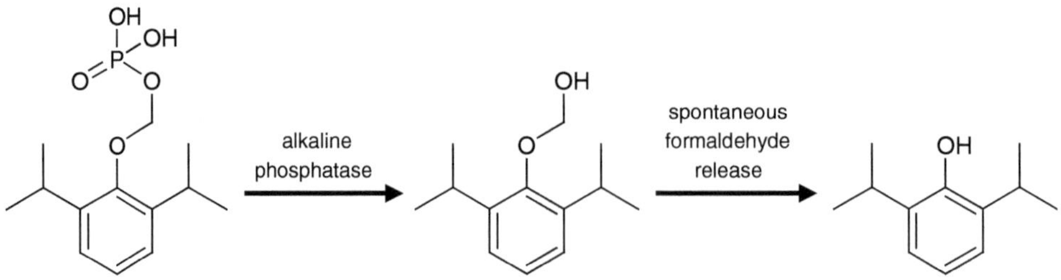


3 **Transient Intermediate** 4

**Scheme 2.1** The proposed reconversion of fospropofol to propofol.

phosphoryloxyalkyl prodrugs of propofol using acetaldehyde versus formaldehyde as the linker has recently been reported [15]. The use of acetaldehyde allows the designer to avoid potential safety questions regarding formaldehyde release [12], but at the cost of adding chirality to the prodrug. While the *in vivo* reconversion kinetics of the two phosphoryloxyalkyl propofol prodrugs in rats were reported to be comparable, it is useful to note that the acetaldehyde-based prodrug was found to possess less hydrolytic stability than the formaldehyde-based prodrug, which might add complexity to formulation design and manufacture if the acetaldehyde-based prodrug was selected for further development. This comparison study [15] illustrates some of the potential competing factors that can impact the choice of which prodrug to ultimately develop; more specifically in this case, while the use of acetaldehyde would avoid potential safety concerns regarding formaldehyde release [12], that potential benefit comes at a cost of greater structural complexity combined with a potentially more challenging prodrug to process and formulate.

#### 2.3.1.2 **Simple Acyl Esters**

Another modification technique for hydroxyl compounds is the use of simple acyl esters. Although the phosphate esters mentioned above work well for aqueous solubility modulations, they typically do not allow lipophilicity enhancement that might be used to increase membrane permeability. Simple aliphatic and aromatic esters can serve as prodrugs to increase the lipophilicity and sometimes even to simultaneously gain a solubility enhancement (aqueous and/or oil solubility) due to the potential for disruption of possible solid-state crystal lattice interactions; furthermore, because these ester prodrugs, at least in theory, have the chance to permeate through the enterocytes and reach the portal vein intact, this approach can conceivably be used to disguise parent drugs that are subject to first-pass metabolism and/or elimination by transporters. Various enzymes capable of hydrolyzing esters are present throughout the body [5], and many times the identity and/or location of the enzyme(s) involved in the *in vivo* reconversion process is not clear. Also, simple acyl esters can often be less hydrolytically stable than the analogous phosphate esters and therefore simple chemical hydrolysis can play at least a partial role in their *in vivo* reconversion.

One simple acyl ester approach for alcohols is to attach an acetyl moiety, which will release acetic acid upon reconversion *in vivo*. It is useful to note that one of the oldest examples displaying this approach is aspirin (**5**), or acetylsalicylic acid, which could be viewed as an acetate prodrug of salicylic acid (**6**) that is less irritating to the GI tract (for the mechanism of action of acetylsalicylic acid see p. 14). In a different application, an *O*-acetyl propanolol prodrug (**7**) was observed to enhance the drug delivery of propanolol (**8**) following oral dosing, presumably because the prodrug avoided the significant first-pass effect experienced by the parent drug [16]. To affect first-pass metabolism, or transporter activity, the prodrug would likely need to possess sufficient stability to bypass the location of these issues, which can be a significant challenge with an ester modification due to the common presence of esterases *in vivo*.

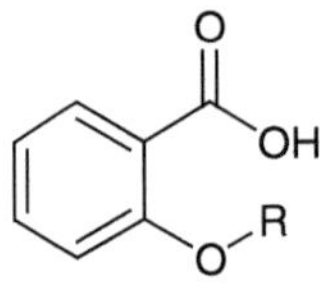


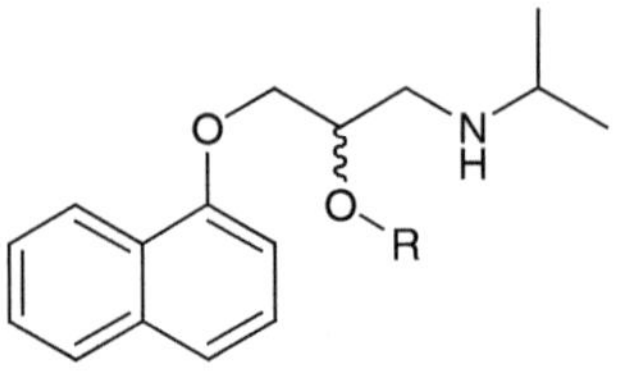


**5** R = Acetyl ($COCH_3$)
**6** R = H

**7** R = Acetyl ($COCH_3$)
**8** R = H

In contrast to the short-chain alkyl esters, long-chain fatty acids have been used to dramatically increase lipophilicity, not only potentially increasing oil solubility but also modulating the *in vivo* distribution properties of the prodrug (protein binding, tissue distribution, etc.) that can affect the elimination half-life of the compound. One example of this approach is the decanoate ester prodrug (**9**) of the antipsychotic drug haloperidol (**10**), which is available as a sustained release intramuscular product where the prodrug is dissolved in sesame oil and often requires only an injection once every 4 weeks, which is particularly helpful for noncompliant patients [17].

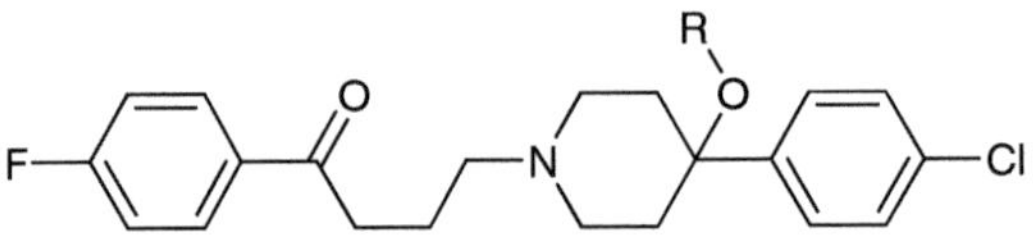


**9** R = Decanoyl ($COC_9H_{19}$)
**10** R = H

### 2.3.1.3 **Amino Acid Esters**

The amino acid ester approach builds on the simple acyl ester approach by introducing an ionizable amine into the promoiety to modulate solubility. One benefit of using endogenous amino acids is that they are expected to carry less safety concerns; however, there can be some other complications introduced by using amino acids. One complication can arise from the additional chiral center that is introduced, except of course when glycine is selected as the promoiety. Another complication is that amino acid esters can often exhibit less hydrolytic stability, especially when compared to the phosphate esters, and this chemical instability could result in significant formulation and/or handling challenges. However, as long as they have suitable stability in the GI tract, the amino acid prodrugs do have a potential advantage over phosphates in that they can potentially permeate into, and possibly even through, the enterocytes, both due to the passive permeation of the neutral fraction (assuming drug is neutral) and due to potentially being recognized by an active transporter in the intestine (e.g., the peptide transporter PEPT1). An example demonstrating this latter scenario is valganciclovir (**11**, Valcyte®), a valine-based prodrug of the antiviral drug ganciclovir (**12**, Cytovene®) [18]. And because amino acid esters can potentially permeate through the enterocytes, they could at least conceivably have the potential to mask the drug from first-pass metabolism or elimination transporters in the enterocytes and/or the liver. However, it should also be noted that many discovery efforts would view prodrug systemic exposure as a disadvantage since it would raise concerns around characterizing the pharmacokinetics of the prodrug to understand its safety profile. This type of concern would suggest that the designer use the phosphate ester approach as long as the parent molecule can permeate through the enterocytes and sufficiently survive first-pass elimination.

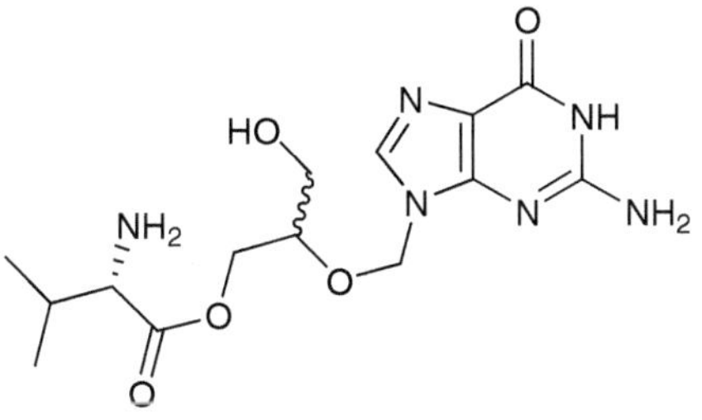


**11**

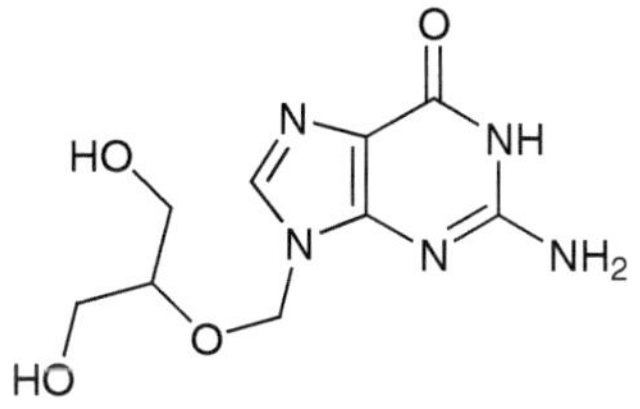


**12**

#### 2.3.1.4 **Other Ester-Based Approaches**

Before concluding this section on alcohol modification strategies, it is worth briefly pointing out some other approaches that can possess value in certain situations. The first is a solubilizing approach where a dicarboxylic acid is attached through an ester bond to make a prodrug with a terminal carboxylic acid, which is expected to add solubilization potential at a more neutral pH relative to amine-based promoieties. Hemisuccinate esters of alcohols have been employed as found in chloramphenicol succinate (**13**), a prodrug of chloramphenicol (**14**) designed for IV administration [19]. This approach, however, can sometimes suffer from both reconversion inefficiency and chemical stability issues that might be a concern for certain delivery strategies [19, 20].

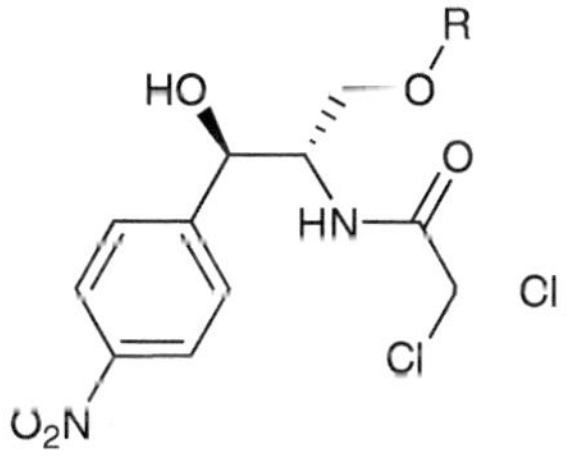


**13** R = $COCH_2CH_2COOH$
**14** R = H

Another approach worth mentioning is the formation of carbamates, instead of simple acyl esters. Because carbamates can tend to be more chemically stable, and not as reactive to reconversion enzymes, these prodrugs can have higher and longer systemic exposures and display slower reconversion kinetics; furthermore, this approach is likely to be more successful for the phenol functionality, given its better leaving group capability. While circulating levels of a prodrug are often considered a disadvantage in prodrug design efforts due to the complexity introduced into their characterization, there are times when a more stable prodrug is desired, such as when trying to disguise a drug from first-pass elimination by the liver/enterocytes following oral administration or when trying to target a prodrug to a certain location in the body. One notable carbamate-based prodrug example that reduces presystemic elimination and whose slow release kinetics produces a more sustained plasma concentration profile of parent drug is bambuterol (**15**, Bambec®) [21], a bis-dimethylcarbamate prodrug of the asthma drug terbutaline (**16**) that enables a once daily oral administration of terbutaline and can be particularly helpful in patients who are not able to easily use inhalers, such as children or the elderly. Another notable carbamate-based prodrug example is irinotecan (**17**, Camptosar®), a water-soluble carbamate prodrug of the antineoplastic agent SN-38 (**18**) designed for IV administration [22].

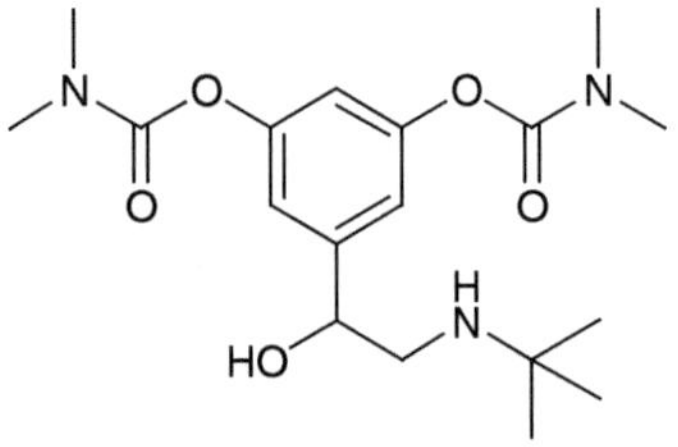

**15**

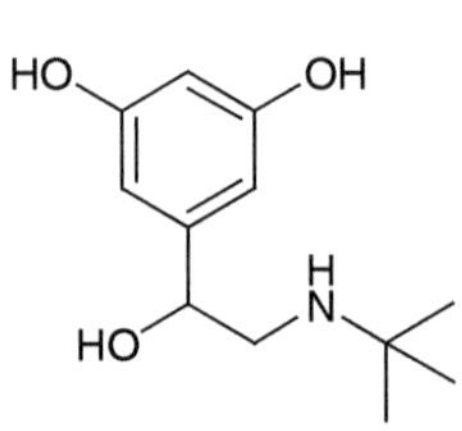

**16**

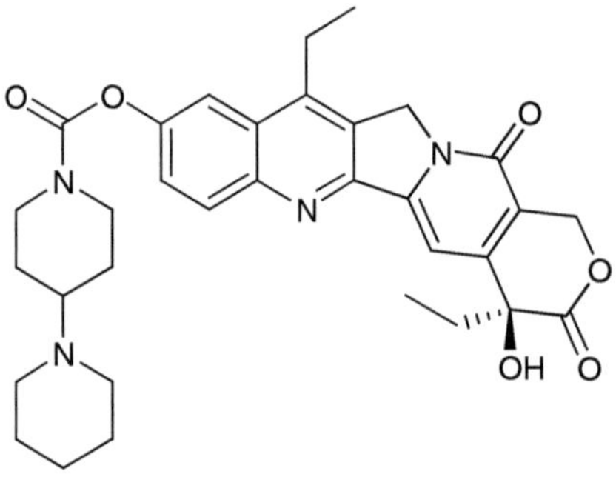

**17**

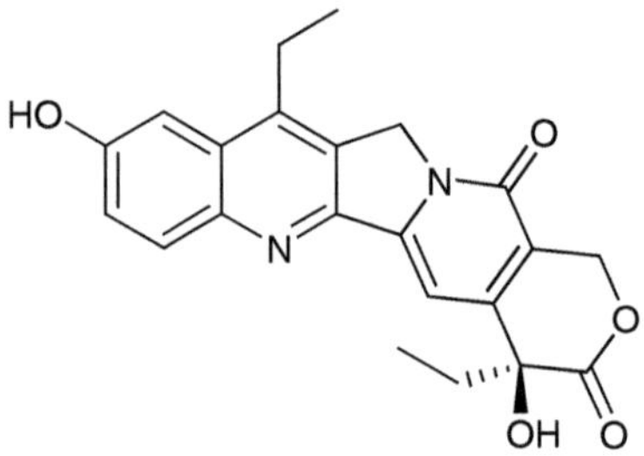

**18**

### 2.3.2 Carboxylic Acids

The other direct building block of an ester functionality is the carboxylic acid, which makes this moiety another favorite target in prodrug design due to the known bioreversibility of ester linked promoieties. However, the typical reason for needing a prodrug of a carboxylic acid can be quite different from that of alcohols. Because a carboxylic acid commonly has a $pK_a$ around 4–5, these functionalities are predominantly ionized when dissolved in the intestinal tract (from small intestine to colon). While this ionization can provide a significant boost to aqueous solubility, it can also become detrimental to the molecule's passive diffusion through the enterocytes. Therefore, unless the molecule happens to be a substrate for an intestinal influx transporter, the carboxylate can become a major limitation to the oral delivery strategy, and many times it cannot be easily removed from the drug molecule because it is needed for a selective and potent interaction with the biological target of interest. Therefore, oral prodrugs of carboxylic acids are often designed to mask the ionization of the carboxylate through formation of an ester, with the goal of increasing membrane permeability. Of course, if not careful in doing this, the prodrug designer can introduce too much lipophilicity, which might result in aqueous solubility becoming the new limiting issue for oral delivery (i.e., one problem solved and another one created). In the following sections, there are discussed some common prodrug approaches used to modify carboxylic acids that have found success in enabling oral drug delivery.

#### 2.3.2.1 Alkyl Esters

One way to remove the potential ionization of a carboxylate is to make a simple alkyl ester. A methyl ester, for instance, is a simple modification to make and has been successful as demonstrated with the prostaglandin prodrug efforts such as misoprostol (**19**, Cytotec®) [23]; however, the release of methanol during reconversion can be a safety concern [24, 25], particularly if the required prodrug dose is high. To avoid the methanol safety concern, the ethyl ester is typically the favorite choice for masking a carboxylate using a simple alkyl ester since the reconversion will instead release ethanol, which is considered safe at the levels being generated. A significant oral delivery enhancement using the ethyl ester approach can be seen in oseltamivir (**20**, Tamiflu®), where masking the carboxylate led to an oral bioavailability enhancement in man from less than 5% for the parent carboxylate to 80% for the prodrug, giving a competitive advantage by enabling an orally administered product [26, 27]. Finally, it is worthwhile to mention the transporter observations that came out of the ethyl ester prodrug work for the angiotensin-converting enzyme (ACE) inhibitors. This series of drug molecules typically possess two carboxylic acids, and one's first inclination might be to mask both groups thinking that these carboxylates are causing the oral bioavailability problem. However, studies suggest that one of the carboxylic acids is part of a structural motif that is recognized by an active intestinal influx transporter, PEPT1, and so it is actually advantageous to avoid masking that carboxylate and esterify just the other acid using an ethyl ester approach. A prodrug example that resulted from this extensive ACE inhibitor effort is enalapril (**21**, Vasotec®) [28, 29] and serves as a useful reminder for designers to be cautious when assuming that carboxylate masking will necessarily lead to a greater oral bioavailability since it might not only inadvertently tip the hydrophilic/lipophilic balance too far to the lipophilic side (potentially introducing solubility limitations) but it might also cover up a structural motif recognized by an active transporter.

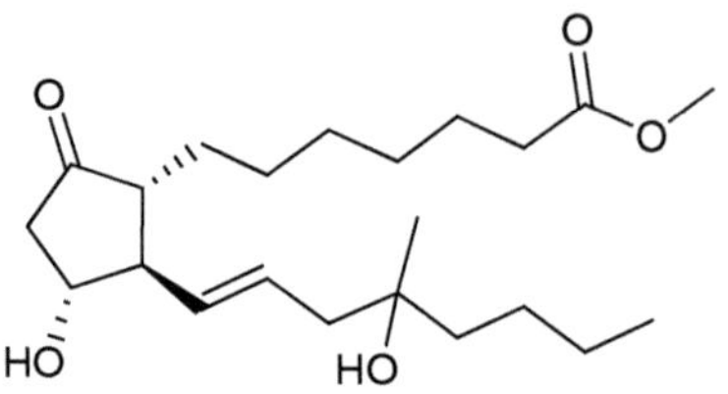

**19**

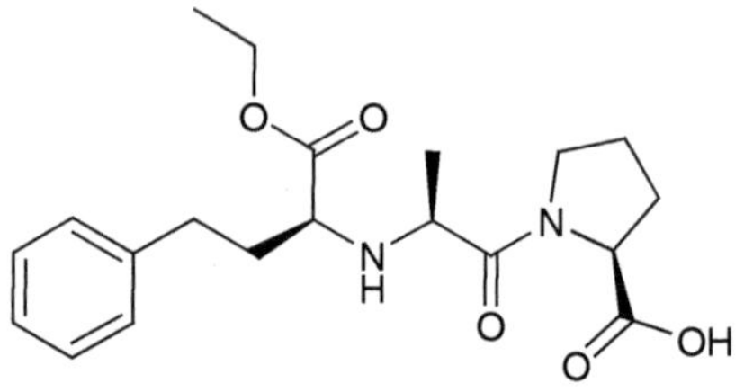

**21**

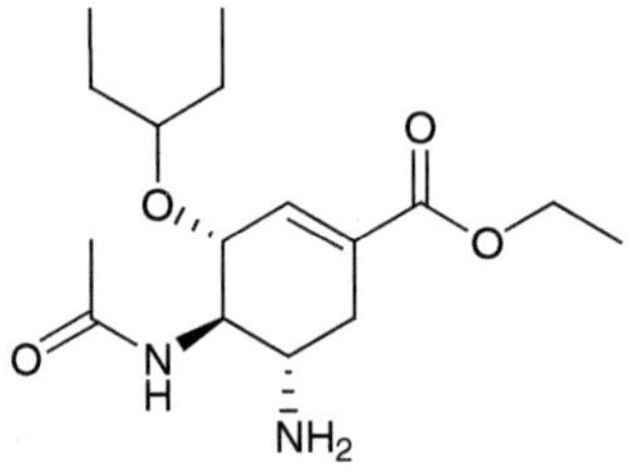

**20**

2.3.2.2 **Aminoalkyl Esters**

A potential risk when masking a carboxylate is adding too much lipophilicity such that aqueous solubility can become limiting to oral absorption. The aminoalkyl ester approach can potentially prevent that situation since it can allow the designer to mask the carboxylate through esterification while maintaining some amount of ionization potential in the promoiety to promote sufficient aqueous solubility. One successful example of this approach is mycophenolate mofetil (**22**, CellCept®), which uses a morpholinoethyl ester to mask the carboxylate of mycophenolic acid. The p$K_a$ of the morpholino moiety in this aminoalkyl ester prodrug is reported to be 5.6 [30], which should allow the prodrug to be predominantly neutral by the time it reaches the small intestine for absorption.

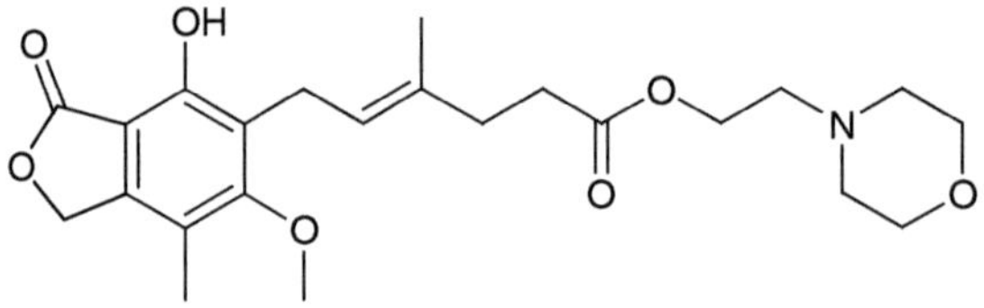

**22**

2.3.2.3 **Spacer Groups to Alleviate Steric Hindrance**

As discussed in Section 2.3.1, spacer groups can be used to spatially extend the "trigger" portion of the promoiety from the bulk molecule, so that an enzyme, or chemical reactant, can more easily access that trigger for prodrug reconversion. The same acyloxyalkyl approach mentioned in the alcohol/phenol section can be used for the carboxylic acids as well. One successful example using this type of spacer for a carboxylic acid drug is the antibiotic bacampicillin (**23**) [31], a prodrug of ampicillin (**24**), where a carbonate group serves as the initial trigger for reconversion that ultimately releases ethanol, carbon dioxide, and acetaldehyde as reconversion byproducts. As discussed in a previous section, while acetaldehyde can often replace formaldehyde, it is useful to note that acetaldehyde adds a chiral center to the promoiety, which can introduce synthetic and/or analytical issues depending on the characteristics present in the rest of the molecule, so it is probably worthwhile at least to question whether that added complexity is necessary in the prodrug design. Finally, another interesting spacer-based approach is the (oxodioxolyl)methyl ester that has also been used to modify carboxylates to promote oral absorption. A successful example of this approach can be seen with the antibiotic lenampicillin (**25**), another prodrug of ampicillin, where the reconversion byproducts in this case are carbon dioxide and dimethyl glyoxal [32].

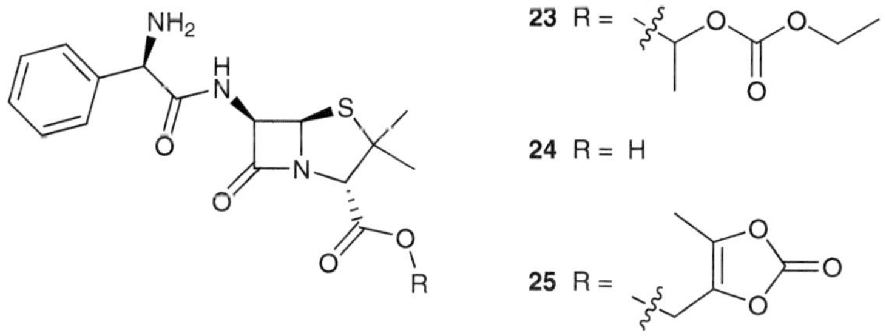


## 2.3.3
## Imides, Amides, and Other NH Acids

NH acids, particularly amide-like NH acids, are commonly found in drug molecules. The two previous sections covering the alcohols/phenols and carboxylic acids were purposely discussed first to introduce the general concept and utility of ester-based prodrug strategies. Sometimes, these ester-based strategies can be applied to other functional groups, such as certain NH acids, by first modifying them to more closely resemble either an alcohol or a carboxylic acid. However, depending on the NH acid, a "modified" ester-based approach cannot always be used to achieve a prodrug with desired performance, and fortunately there are nonester-based approaches also available that perform through chemical reconversion providing additional design options. Since the term NH acid encompasses a wide range of functional groups with very different characteristics in the context of prodrug design, a different organization is used in this section, where the information will be divided by NH acid type instead of by promoiety. The three main NH acid types will be the imide-type, the amide-type, and the sulfonamide NH acids, where one main distinction will be the p$K_a$ of the NH acid and another distinction will be whether the adjacent double bond to oxygen is based on carbon or another atom such as sulfur (e.g., a sulfonamide).

#### 2.3.3.1 Imide-Type NH Acids

The imide-type NH acids are defined as having a p$K_a$ in the range of a model imide, such as phthalimide (p$K_a$ 8.3). These imide-type NH acids are the most acidic and tend to have relatively good leaving group potential. Because of this, the acyloxyalkyl spacer-based approaches can be successfully used since the imide-type NH acid will rapidly release from the hydroxyalkyl intermediate that forms following initial ester hydrolysis. Therefore, all of the ester-based approaches presented in Sections 2.3.1 and 2.3.2 can be used for the imide-type NH acids, as long as a spacer-based approach is incorporated, which serves to modify the NH acid into an "alcohol" that can be esterified. A successful example of a spacer-based ester approach targeted toward hydrolase reconversion is fosphenytoin (**26**, Cerebyx®), the phosphoryloxymethyl prodrug of phenytoin, which has enhanced aqueous solubility allowing it to be formulated into a ready-to-use IV product using an inert aqueous vehicle that is safer than the vehicle[3] used for sodium phenytoin [33]. Similar to fospropofol (Section 2.3.1.1), the reconversion of fosphenytoin is triggered by the action of alkaline phosphatase on the terminal phosphate monoester forming the hydroxymethyl intermediate, which then rapidly forms phenytoin and one equivalent of formaldehyde [12].

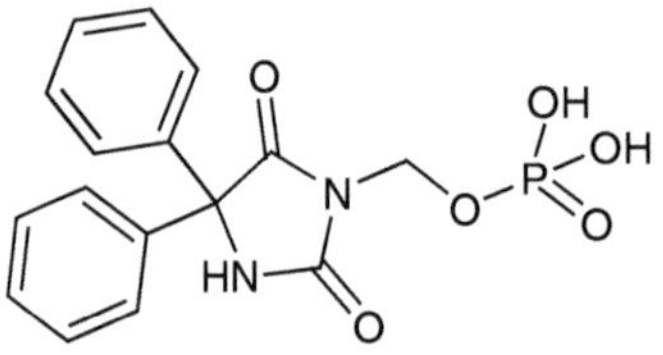


**26**

#### 2.3.3.2 Amide-Type NH Acids

Amide-type NH acids are defined in this chapter as functionalities where the NH acid is adjacent to just one carbonyl and the p$K_a$ is in the range of a simple model amide, such as benzamide. These more weakly acidic NH acids are poorer leaving groups compared to their imide-type counterparts, and they are not as amenable to the acyloxyalkyl approaches since the hydroxyalkyl intermediate does not rapidly degrade to release the amide-type NH acid.[4]

**N-Acyloxyalkoxycarbonyl Prodrugs** Despite the lower utility of *directly* using the acyloxyalkyl approach for amide-type NH acids, a similar ester-based reconversion approach can sometimes still be possible for amide-type NH acids by incorporating an initial carbon dioxide building block into the promoiety from which a subsequent acyloxyalkyl moiety can extend, forming an *N*-acyloxyalkoxycarbonyl promoiety. The carbon dioxide building block serves to locally convert the amide-type

3) Vehicle for sodium phenytoin contains 10% ethanol and 40% propylene glycol with a final pH of 12.

4) If a slow release of parent drug is desired, it is conceivable that the weaker leaving group potential of NH acids might not present a problem in using the acyloxyalkyl approach.

NH acid into a carbamic acid-type functionality, which is a better leaving group from the hydroxyalkyl intermediate that forms as a result of terminal ester bioreconversion; furthermore, the carbamic acid intermediate that is released from degradation of the hydroxyalkyl intermediate spontaneously releases the parent NH acid along with one molecule of carbon dioxide. This *N*-acyloxyalkoxycarbonyl approach was successfully applied to design a prodrug (**27**) of an oxazolidinone antiobiotic drug (**28**) that increased its oral bioavailability from 21 to 75% with an accompanying fivefold increase in maximum plasma concentration following a 10 mg/kg aqueous suspension dose to male beagle dogs [34]. Despite the success this approach sometimes offers, there is a risk of nonproductive degradation that can occur since the attachment of the acyloxyalkoxycarbonyl promoiety to the amide-type NH acid creates an imide, which could be hydrolyzed at the undesired carbonyl leading to a carboxylic acid compound that at the very least causes analytical and product potency concerns, and more seriously, might even result in safety issues (Figure 2.3).

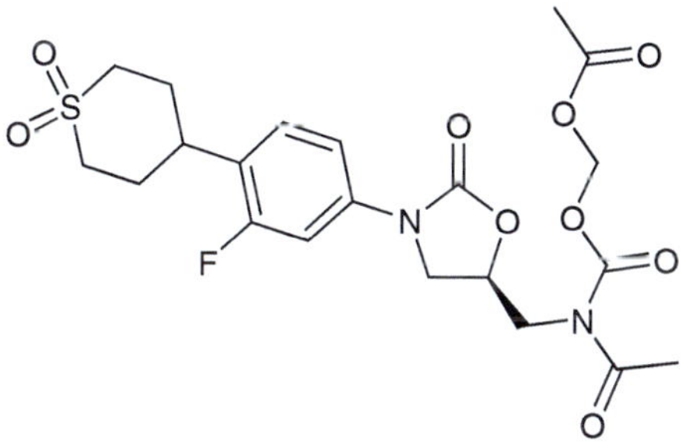

**27**

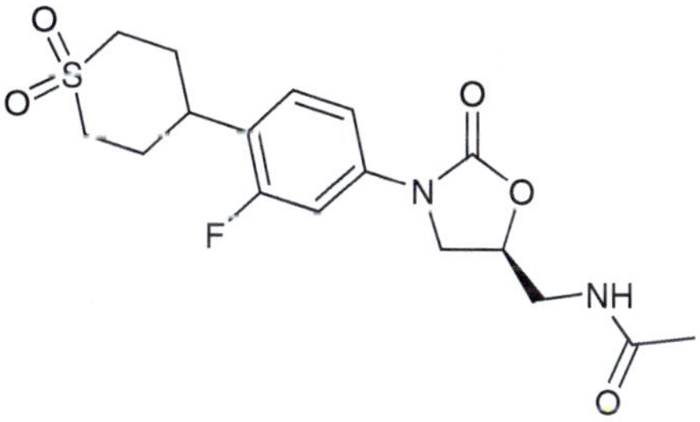

**28**

**N-Mannich Base Prodrugs** Fortunately, there are other approaches that can be successful for amide-type NH acids that rely on a chemical reconversion mechanism. One strategy is the *N*-Mannich base approach that was used to design the prodrug rolitetracycline (**29**), which can be administered parenterally given its enhanced aqueous solubility. As shown in Scheme 2.2 (using **29** as an example), the reconversion mechanism for an *N*-Mannich base is a unimolecular reaction where the most reactive species is typically the unprotonated form, and because of this, the

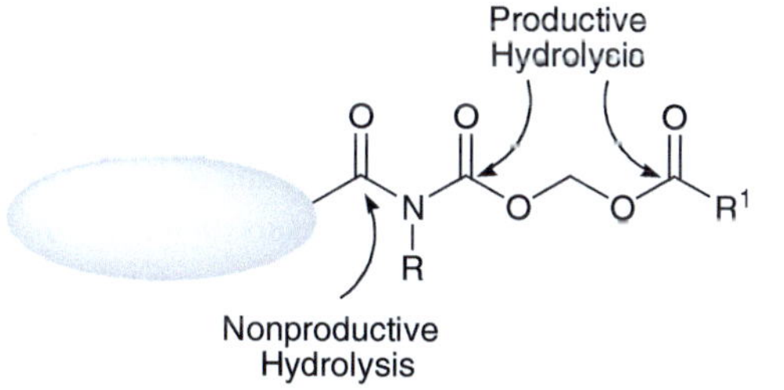


**Figure 2.3** The *N*-acyloxyalkoxycarbonyl prodrug approach for amide-type NH acids showing potential soft spots for productive and nonproductive prodrug degradation.

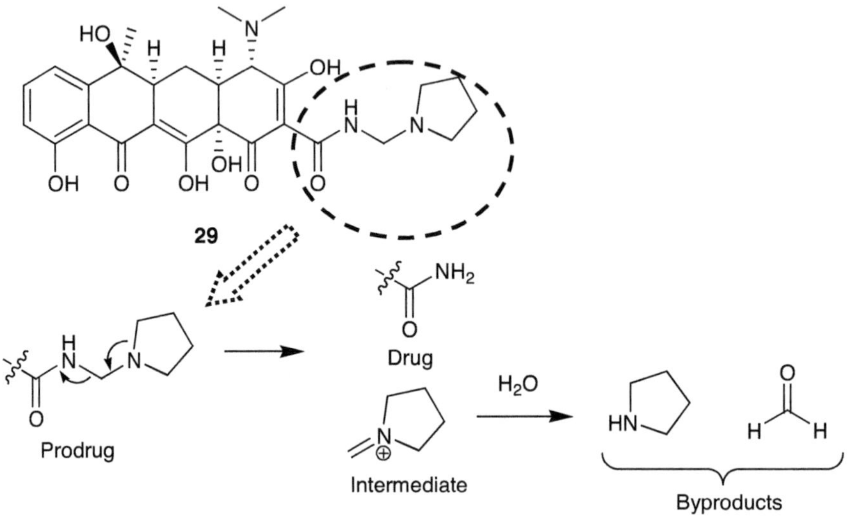


**Scheme 2.2** The general reconversion of an *N*-Mannich base prodrug using rolitetracycline as an example.

reconversion strongly depends on pH [35]. It should be noted that the protonated species does have its own intrinsic reactivity, and the pH rate profiles for hydrolysis of an *N*-Mannich base characteristically follow a sigmoidal shape that coincides with the $pK_a$ of the amine containing promoiety. Finally, because the reconversion releases both an amine and an NH acid, this prodrug approach can be used for amine functionalities as well. As with any chemical reconversion strategy, chemical stability can be a limiting factor that could result in formulation and/or general handling/ storage issues. To help address this, there is some flexibility for the designer to modulate the chemical stability of an *N*-Mannich base by choosing the $pK_a$ and steric nature of the amine in the promoiety.

**Sulfenamide Prodrugs** A second chemical-based prodrug approach for amide-type NH acids is the sulfenamide approach, which has been introduced only very recently [36–39] and therefore has no commercial examples to date. Sulfenamides are characterized by a single covalent bond between a bivalent sulfur and a nitrogen atom, and have historically been used both in the rubber and pesticide industries and in chemical syntheses as sulfenylating reagents (e.g., in the synthesis of asymmetrical disulfide bonds) [40–42]. However, only recently was it realized and reported that sulfenamides can successfully perform as *prodrugs* for NH acids [36–39], with particular promise realized for the weakly acidic amide-type NH acids. Given the general reactivity of sulfenamides with thiols to form disulfide bonds, the proposed reconversion of a sulfenamide prodrug *in vivo* is through nucleophilic attack from an endogenous thiol such as glutathione (Scheme 2.3). The advantage of sulfenamides as a prodrug approach is that the sulfenamide bond of a *weakly acidic* NH acid (e.g.,

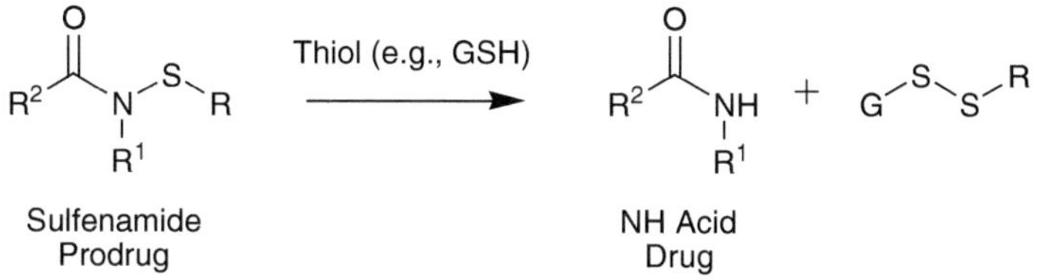


**Scheme 2.3** The proposed reconversion of a generic sulfenamide prodrug using glutathione as an example endogenous thiol-containing compound.

simple amides and ureas) can be quite hydrolytically stable while also possessing a selective and very high reactivity with thiols, allowing a rapid and quantitative reconversion in their presence [37, 38]. Furthermore, since it is the thiolate fraction that is most likely responsible for the rapid reconversion *in vivo*, the thiol-driven reconversion is expected to depend on pH and occur faster at neutral compared to acidic pH due to the higher thiolate fraction in the former. This point becomes particularly relevant when considering the likelihood of success for a sulfenamide prodrug in oral dosing, where there is a wide pH gradient ranging from acidic to neutral along the GI tract.

As alluded to in the beginning of this section, one void in the prodrug literature is related to the lack of viable approaches to design hydrolytically stable but rapidly bioreversible prodrugs of weakly acidic NH acids (simple amides, ureas, and carbamates), which has been unfortunate because these types of NH acids are commonly found in drug molecules but are rarely *generically* exploited through prodrugs. On the basis of the recent findings reported so far, sulfenamides appear to help fill that void for these amide-type NH acids. For example, a cysteine-based sulfenamide prodrug (**30**) of the weakly NH-acidic benzamide was quite hydrolytically stable not only displaying a projected 6.3-year half-life at pH 6.0 and 25 °C but also showing a quick and quantitative reconversion upon spiking cysteine into the same pH 6.0 buffer to release benzamide [37, 38]. As another example, a cysteine ethyl ester sulfenamide prodrug of carbamazepine (**31**) was synthesized and showed a 180-day half-life at pH 4.0 and 25 °C [37, 38]. Both of these examples clearly demonstrate that hydrolytically stable sulfenamides can be realized from derivatizing weakly acidic NH acids. Because both preclinical species and humans possess endogenous thiols, such as glutathione, the translation of sulfenamide performance across species might be more straightforward to predict; furthermore, because the reaction with thiols is so rapid, there would be a very low likelihood that a sulfenamide prodrug of an NH acid would be detected in systemic circulation, even if administered IV. This point was demonstrated in an experiment where aliquots of two sulfenamide-based linezolid prodrugs (**32–33**) were spiked directly into dog whole blood, which in both cases resulted in an *instantaneous* and *quantitative* conversion to release linezolid, and the presence of the sulfenamide prodrugs in the whole blood could not be detected. This whole blood study, along with the supporting buffer-based cysteine studies mentioned above, established the concept that sulfenamide prodrugs of weakly acidic NH acids will indeed instantaneously convert upon introduction into the blood [37, 38]. Providing further supporting evidence, a follow-up rat intravenously dosed PK study using a sulfenamide prodrug of carbamazepine demonstrated the expected *rapid* and *quantitative* reconversion to carbamazepine following introduction into the rat blood [43], which is consistent with the previous dog whole blood reconversion observations. Finally, from the designer's perspective, the sulfenamide approach offers a very wide range of potential chemical space since the promoiety can be made lipophilic or hydrophilic, as well as ionizable or nonionizable.

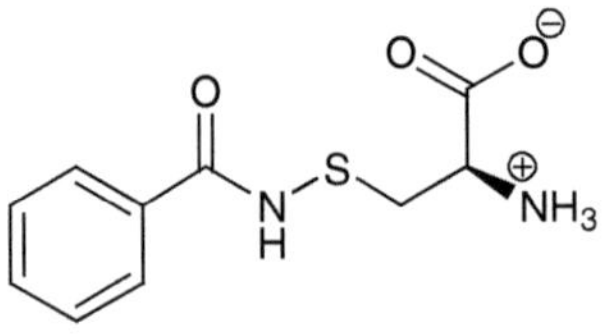

**30**

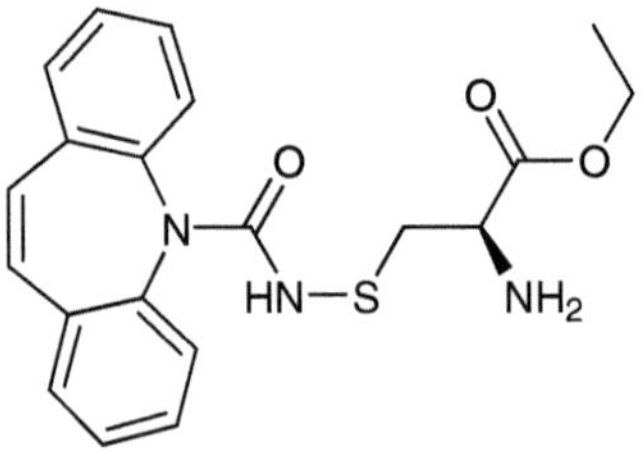

**31**

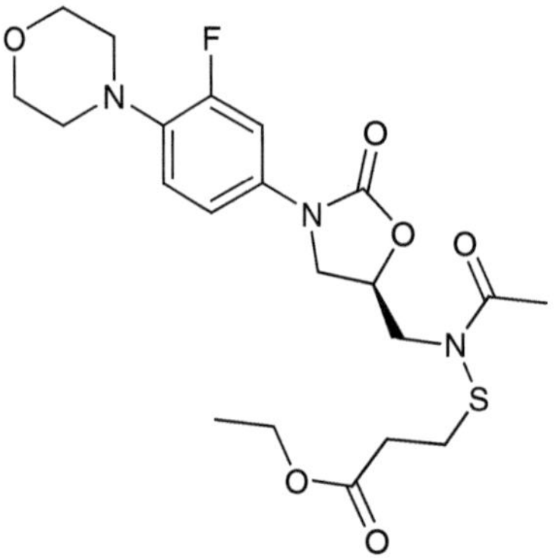

**32**

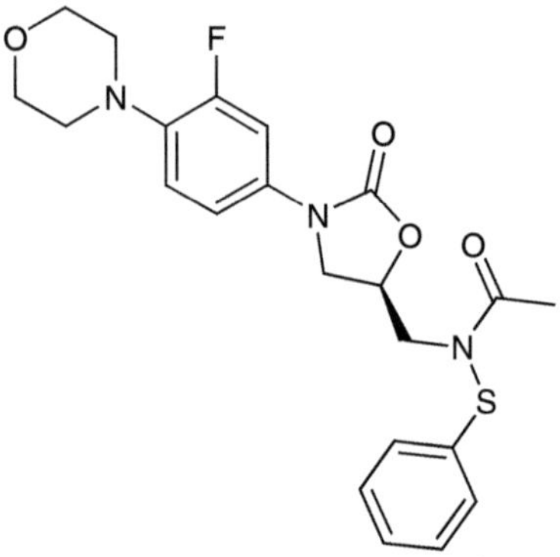

**33**

### 2.3.3.3 Sulfonamide NH Acids

Sulfonamide NH acids can be found with some frequency in drug molecules and offer a potential handle from which to design prodrugs. A successful example of a prodrug for a sulfonamide NH acid is parecoxib (**34**, Dynastat®), a highly water-soluble prodrug (22 mg/ml in phosphate-buffered saline at 25 °C) of the COX-2 selective inhibitor valdecoxib (**35**, Bextra®) [44]. The *N*-propanoylation dramatically drops the p$K_a$ of the sulfonamide NH such that a parenteral of the sodium salt is a viable option due to the great enhancement of solubility. It is interesting to recognize that the solubility enhancement in this case is not accomplished through a direct attachment of an ionizable group, but rather through an N-acylation with a neutral promoiety to make the sulfonamide NH itself more readily ionizable.

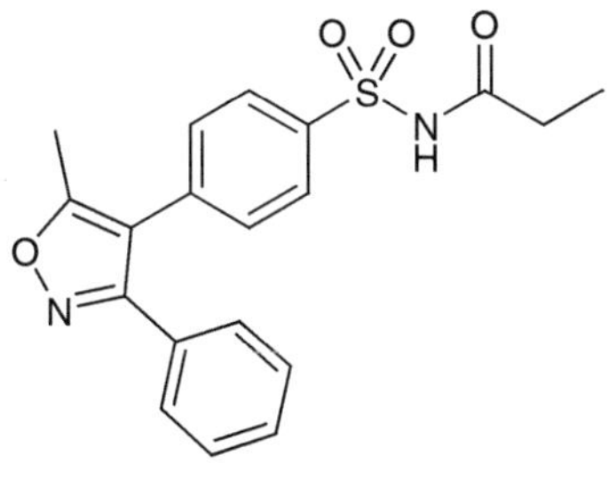

**34**

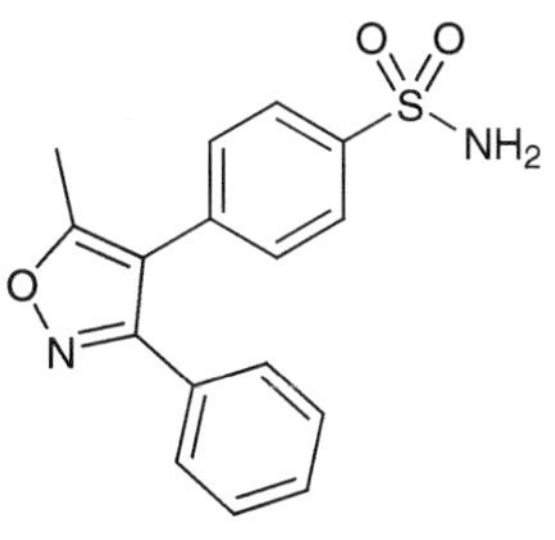

**35**

### 2.3.4 Phosphates, Phosphonates, and Phosphinates

A common characteristic of phosphates, phosphonates, and phosphinates is their ionization potential to predominantly form anionic species across the majority of the physiologically relevant pH range; furthermore, that ionization potential is more significant than the typical carboxylic acid, given the greater acidity of these phosphorus-based acids. This predominantly ionized state would typically not support passive membrane permeability, which can be detrimental to both oral absorption and intracellular access, the latter of which could prohibit efficacy at intracellular targets; therefore, masking this ionization potential through esterification (or other modification) is a common goal in designing prodrugs of these functional groups. Related to their poor passive membrane permeability, phosphates, phosphonates, and phosphinates can be good candidates for drug targeting to an intracellular space because if they can be released into the intracellular space, there is a reasonable chance that they would remain trapped in that cell because of a lower likelihood of diffusing back to the extracellular space; however, this aspect can also raise concerns if this same trapping phenomenon would result in an unintended toxicity for the cell. There are many approaches that have been taken to enhance the delivery of the highly charged phosphates, phosphonates, and phosphinates and there is not enough space available in this chapter to comprehensively cover them. Fortunately, there have been some very recent reviews that are quite comprehensive in their treatment of this wide-ranging area of prodrug research [45–47]. Finally, for simplification purposes, the term "phosph(on)ate" will be used subsequently to include phosphates, phosphonates, and phosphinates, unless otherwise specified (*note*: this nomenclature simplification might not be consistent with other texts).

#### 2.3.4.1 Simple Alkyl and Aryl Esters

Unlike phosphoric acid and various carboxylic acids, whose mono alkyl esters are good substrates for alkaline phosphatase and/or esterases, simple alkyl esters of the phosph(on)ate-based drugs are typically quite stable to these enzymes. Therefore, simple alkyl esterification is not typically promising for masking phosph(on)ate-based drugs in a *bioreversible* way. Given their better leaving group potential, aryl esters have displayed some level of relative promise for reversibly masking a phosph (on)ate, such as the diphenyl ester prodrug CGS-25 462 (**36**) of a phosphonate-based neutral endopeptidase inhibitor (**37**) [48]; however, given the relatively decent enzymatic stability of these esters, this is still not a commonly used approach. Furthermore, the potential toxicity of the aryl alcohol that is released should be considered in the context of dose level and length of treatment. Therefore, while the goal in making prodrugs of the phosph(on)ates and carboxylic acids can be the same (i.e., masking ionization), the approaches necessary for rapid bioconversion typically require a more complex promoiety than just a simple alkyl or aryl ester.

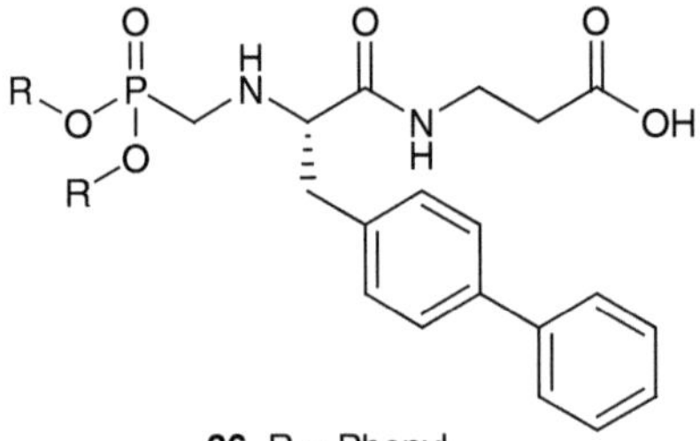

**36** R = Phenyl
**37** R = H

2.3.4.2 **Acyloxyalkyl and Alkoxycarbonyloxyalkyl Esters**

A very successful approach taken to increase membrane permeability for phosph(on) ate-based drugs is the acyloxyalkyl (or alkoxycarbonyloxyalkyl) approach that uses a terminal ester as the reconversion trigger for releasing the phosph(on)ate drug. To increase membrane permeability for enhanced oral absorption, a successful acyloxyalkyl prodrug of a phosph(on)ate drug requires the selection of a triggering ester moiety chemically and enzymatically stable enough to at least cross the apical membrane, and ideally the entire enterocyte, largely intact. A successful example of this prodrug approach can be seen in tenofovir disoproxil fumarate (**38**, Viread®), a prodrug of the antiviral tenofovir (**39**) [49, 50]. This is a dialkoxycarbonyloxyalkyl prodrug where the byproducts of reconversion are isopropyl alcohol, carbon dioxide, and formaldehyde. By derivatizing the phosphonate using the same moiety on both acidic groups, the potential chirality issues around the phosphorus atom can be avoided, which simplifies synthesis and isolation. Chiral issues are also avoided by using formaldehyde instead of another aldehyde. While the prodrug succeeds in masking both phosphonate ionization centers, the aqueous solubility of the prodrug fumarate still remains high at 13.4 mg/ml in water. The basic scheme for reconversion is similar to the other acyloxyalkyl-type moieties seen previously in the chapter (refer to Scheme 2.1). One aspect worth noting for diacyloxyalkyl approaches for phosphonates and phosphates is that while the first cleavage is thought to occur by esterase action on one of the terminal esters, the origin of the second promoiety cleavage is less certain and may partly involve both chemical reaction and potential action from phosphodiesterase. Either way, this prodrug of tenofovir successfully enhances the oral absorption of tenofovir, and dose proportional exposures were observed in the clinic using the prodrug fumarate salt across a dose range of

75–600 mg; furthermore, the bioavailability for the 300 mg dose in humans was estimated to be ~40% in the fed state [51]. Finally, it is worth noting that even the released tenofovir is a prodrug itself, in that it undergoes further intracellular phosphorylation to form the final active species [52].

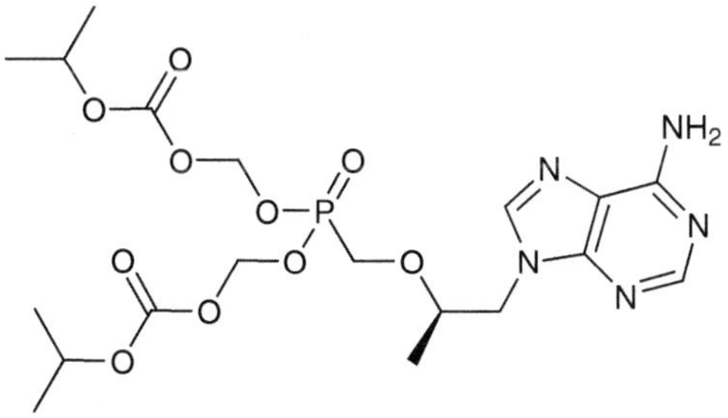

38

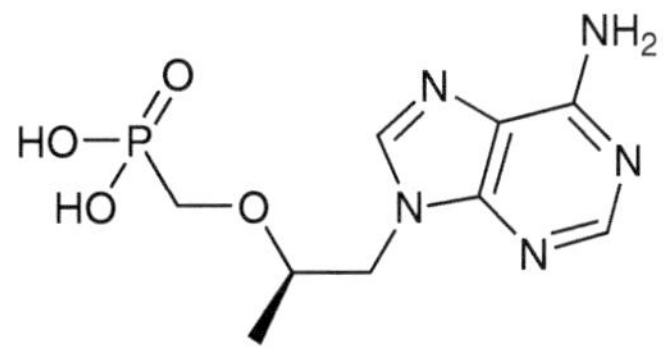

39

#### 2.3.4.3 **Aryl Phospho(n/r)amidates and Phospho(n/r)diamides**

Another design strategy for improving delivery across membranes that also carries some amount of targeting potential involves the replacement of one or both phosph(on)ate esters with either one or two phosphoramidate (for phosphate drug) or phosphonamidate (for phosphonate drug) bonds. The remainder of this section will focus on phosphate-based examples, but many of the concepts would apply to a phosphonate as well. One approach is to make aryl phosphoramidate prodrugs [53] that incorporate just one phosphoramidate bond that very commonly is a simple alkyl ester of an amino acid phosphoramide, where a common choice for the core amino acid is alanine. The other phosphoric acid group is esterified with a simple aryl ester, such as a phenyl ester. It is useful to notice that the incorporation of two different promoieties creates chirality at the phosphorus center; furthermore, the amino acid-based promoiety of the phosphoramide bond adds a second chiral center since alanine is a favorite choice for this technology (glycine would avoid this, but is not as commonly chosen). The reconversion of this type of prodrug is shown in Scheme 2.4, where the initial trigger is likely an esterase-based degradation and/or chemical hydrolysis of the simple alkyl terminal ester in the amino acid moiety forming a terminal carboxylic acid. This acid then attacks the phosphorus center forming a temporary five-membered cyclic mixed anhydride and releases the aryl ester to reform one of the phosphoric acid groups. The cyclic anhydride intermediate is unstable and degrades back to form an amino acid phosphoramide, and this phosphorus–nitrogen bond is then degraded chemically and/or enzymatically by an intracellular phosphoramidase to form the phosphate drug. A typical goal for using this technology is the intracellular delivery of a phosphate nucleotide where it can bypass the first kinase-based monophosphorylation of nucleotide drugs, which tends to be either slow or absent in cases of drug resistance; furthermore, the hope is that the continual phosphorylation of this delivered nucleotide monophosphate to the active species will occur more quickly than dephosphorylation by phosphatases since if the dephosphorylation occurs first, the kinase bypass advantage is lost. While there

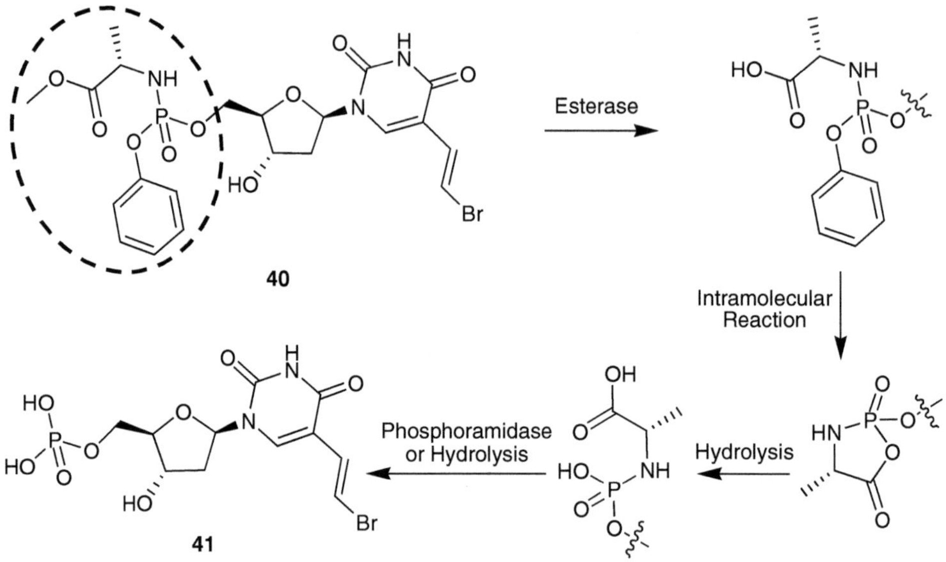


**Scheme 2.4** The proposed reconversion for an aryl phosphoramidate prodrug using thymectacin (**40**) as an example.

are no commercial examples of aryl phosphoramidates, one clinical example is thymectacin (**40**, Scheme 2.4), a prodrug of brivudine monophosphate (**41**), which entered clinical trials as a treatment for colon cancer [54].

Related in principle to the aryl phosphoramidate concept is the phosphordiamide approach that involves the replacement of the aryl alcohol promoiety with a second equivalent of the same esterified amino acid ester, as illustrated by the phosphordiamide prodrug (**42**) of the anti-HIV drug AZT (3′-azido-3′-deoxythymidine) monophosphate (**43**) [55]. Because the same promoiety is attached to both acidic groups, the creation of the phosphorus chiral center is avoided, as well as the release of an aryl alcohol (typically phenol), which is a typical toxicity concern with the aryl phosphoramidate approach. A common amino acid chosen for the diamide approach is also an esterified alanine and the initial trigger is still terminal ester cleavage. The proposed mechanism for the reconversion of these prodrugs is similar to that of aryl phosphoramidates (Scheme 2.4) and begins with hydrolysis at one of the terminal esters as the trigger to begin cyclization to the mixed anhydride and after a series of steps eventually ends with the release of the phosphate drug. Finally, with the same terminal ester cleavage serving as the initial reconversion trigger for both the aryl phosphoramidates and the phosphordiamides, dialing the appropriate level of stability into that terminal ester is an important factor for allowing effective drug delivery. Another thing worth re-emphasizing is that for phosphate drugs, if the prodrug reconversion occurs too early, the released phosphate "drug" will likely be short lived due to quick action by alkaline phosphatase and the kinase bypass potential will be lost. In comparison, an early release of a phosphonate drug should not be as damaging from a stability point of view, but its dianionic charge could still be detrimental to reaching an intracellular target unless it is recognized by a special uptake system.

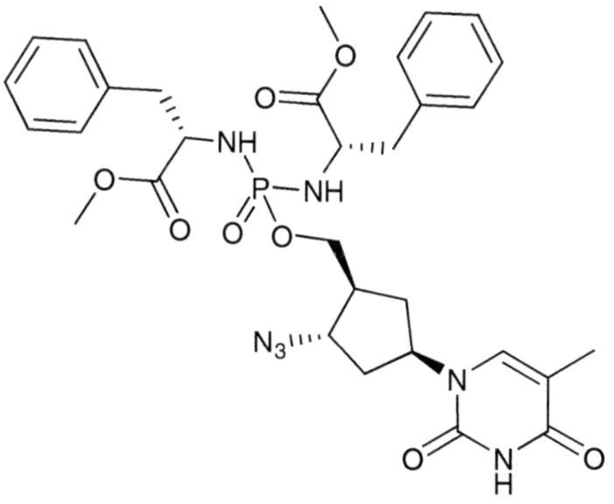

42

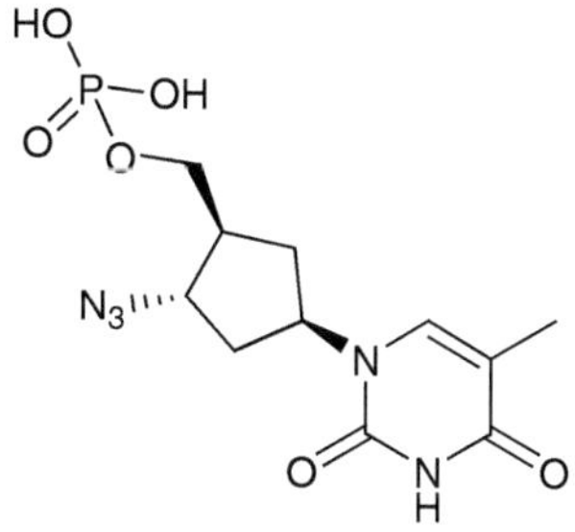

43

#### 2.3.4.4 HepDirect Technology

It is doubtful that any of the previous approaches can offer a *generic* and robust method for targeting phosph(on)ate drugs to the intracellular space because many of the reconversion steps could also occur outside the cell, or even worse, in the GI lumen and enterocytes. In contrast, the HepDirect approach [56] targets phosph(on) ate drugs to the liver by depending on a reconversion trigger that occurs to a great extent in hepatocytes. The HepDirect prodrug approach therefore holds promise for treating liver diseases in a targeted manner that could potentially increase the therapeutic index of the drug. Scheme 2.5 displays the proposed mechanism for the reconversion of a HepDirect prodrug. As shown, the trigger in this case is not hydrolysis, but oxidation, proposed to be driven primarily by CYP3A4, which leads to a hemiacetal intermediate that quickly collapses to release one of the acidic groups, and upon doing that, further undergoes a beta elimination to release the other acidic group forming an aryl vinyl ketone byproduct. This aryl vinyl ketone can certainly raise toxicity concerns given its electrophilic nature; however, it is assumed that the abundant levels of glutathione in hepatocytes will trap the reactive metabolite preventing it from alkylating a more problematic target. An example of a HepDirect prodrug that entered clinical trials is pradefovir (**44**) [57], the prodrug of adefovir (**45**) for the treatment of hepatitis B infection, intended to achieve an increased efficacy relative to adefovir dipivoxil (an acyloxyalkyl prodrug), which has to be dosed at a suboptimal level due to renal toxicity [58].

### 2.3.5 Amines and Benzamidines

This last section will describe some common approaches for amines and benzamidines. The term "amine" covers a very wide range of nitrogen bases ranging from the mildly basic aromatic amines, such as aniline, to the very basic amidines and

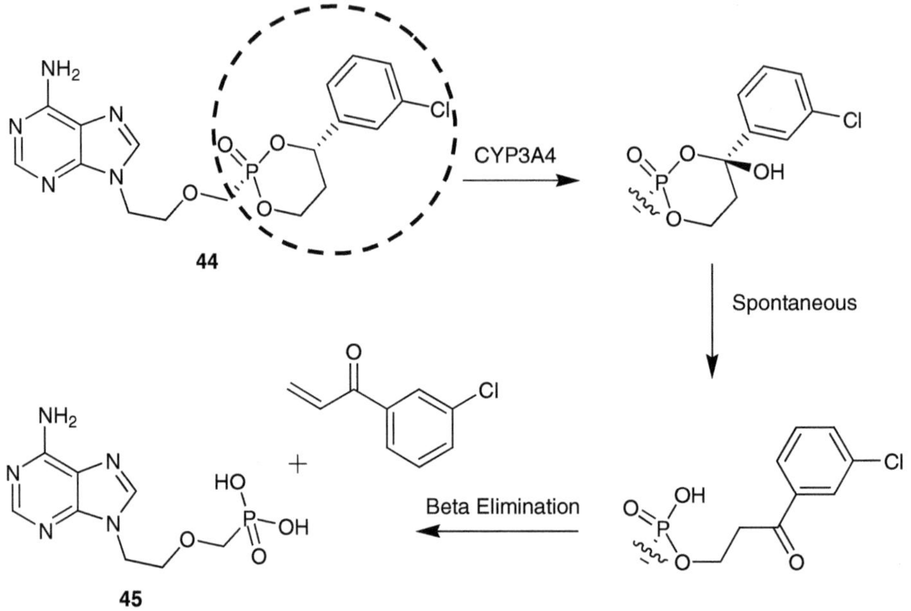


**Scheme 2.5** The proposed reconversion for a HepDirect prodrug using pradefovir (**44**) as an example.

guanidines. The p$K_a$ of an amine's conjugate acid can play a significant role in its ability to be orally delivered. A higher p$K_a$ results in a greater fraction of the drug being protonated in the intestine, and while the positive charge certainly allows an enhanced solubilization, it can also decrease the passive membrane permeability, which could be detrimental to oral absorption. In contrast to alcohols, the direct acylation of an amine creates an amide that is typically a more stable species than an ester. So while amines are typically easy to derivatize, it can be more challenging with amines to design a prodrug with the desired chemical stability and bioreconversion, and often a spacer group is required in the design.

### 2.3.5.1 ***N*-Acyloxyalkoxycarbonyl Prodrugs**

Because rapid *in vivo* conversion is a common goal in prodrug design, a promising approach is to chemically modify the amine into a terminal alcohol through a spacer group such that the alcohol can then be esterified to serve as a reconversion trigger from the action of esterases. It can be an advantage for chemical stability to attach an acyloxyalkyl moiety to the amine through a carbamic acid linker to make an acyloxyalkoxycarbonyl promoiety [59, 60]. Therefore, when the acyloxyalkyl promoiety is released *in vivo*, an unstable carbamic acid is created that immediately collapses to release the amine and carbon dioxide. It is important to note that if a terminal phosphate monoester is used for solubilization, a potential concern is whether the anionic phosphate will participate intramolecularly in the chemical hydrolysis of the prodrug, which could lead to a far lower chemical stability than initially anticipated [61].

### 2.3.5.2 *N*-Mannich Bases

As mentioned in Section 2.3.3.2, the *N*-Mannich base approach is equally valid for amines and NH acids. However, it is worth noting that while *N*-Mannich bases are commonly used to increase aqueous solubility for NH acid drugs, this approach is typically applied to amine drugs for $pK_a$ reduction (typically by 2–4 units) that can translate to better membrane permeability and oral absorption from the intestine. When designing an *N*-Mannich base prodrug for an amine, the acidity of the NH acid used in the promoiety will affect the overall stability and reconversion time *in vivo* [35].

### 2.3.5.3 *N*-Acyloxyalkyl and *N*-Phosphoryloxyalkyl Prodrugs of Tertiary Amines

Unlike the primary or secondary amines, it can be promising to directly attach an acyloxylalkyl [62–64] or phosphoryloxyalkyl [65–67] promoiety to a tertiary amine, which forms a quaternary ammonium prodrug that can have a reasonable chemical stability. This approach can lead to a dramatic solubilization due to the quaternary ammonium center as well as the ionization of the phosphate group if the phosphoryloxyalkyl approach is taken, although it is useful to recognize that the latter approach will result in a zwitterionic species at some pH values (not necessarily a problem, but useful to at least recognize). The phosphoryloxymethyl approach was applied to design water-soluble quaternary ammonium prodrugs of tertiary amines, which rapidly and quantitatively reconverted to the parent tertiary amines following IV administration to rats and dogs [65–67], an example of which was the phosphoryloxymethyl prodrug (**46**) of the antipsychotic drug loxapine (**47**). The solubilization potential afforded by this general approach can allow a more straightforward parenteral formulation and a dramatic modulation of the parent drug's pH-solubility profile. If this general quaternary amine approach were used to deliver drugs orally, the prodrug reconversion would likely need to occur no later than reaching the apical surface of the enterocytes, and the tertiary parent amine would need to possess sufficient intrinsic permeability to transport across the enterocytes. The phosphoryloxyalkyl approach could be particularly valuable for this latter purpose since the presence of alkaline phosphatase at the brush border membrane of the intestine should provide some assurance that prodrug reconversion process would be available in the intestine.

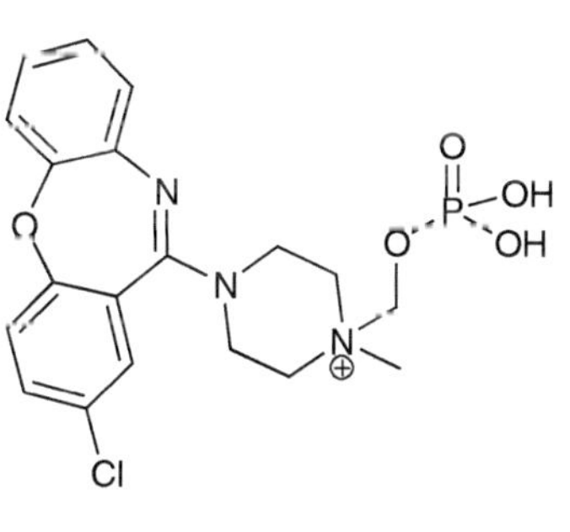


**46**

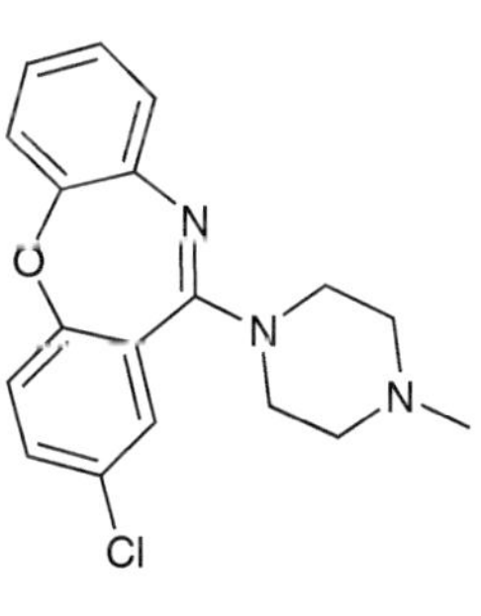


**47**

#### 2.3.5.4 **N-Hydroxy and Other Modifications for Benzamidines**

Benzamidines are one of the most basic groups ($pK_a$ can be 11–12 for conjugate acid) that have been incorporated into drugs. The positive ionization that is dominant across the entire physiological pH range can greatly inhibit passive membrane permeability resulting in poor oral absorption, and therefore significant effort has gone into bioreversible modifications that can dramatically lower the benzamidine basicity. Probably the most well-known approach is the *N*-hydroxybenzamidine strategy, an example being ximelagatran (**48**), which has a dramatically lower $pK_a$ allowing an improvement in the oral bioavailability of melagatran (**49**) in humans (from 6 to 20%) [68–70]. The bioreconversion of an *N*-hydroxybenzamidine prodrug is thought to involve the action of reductive enzymes [71] that can be commonly found in hepatocytes, among other places. As also mentioned in the sections on phosph(on) ates, it is useful to note that permeable prodrugs of very impermeable parent drugs (such as benzamidines) carry the risk (or benefit) of the parent drug becoming trapped (or targeted) intracellularly. Finally, in addition to the hydroxybenzamidine approach, there are other approaches for lowering the basicity of benzamidines that have found success, and these have been recently reviewed [72] for the reader with further interest in this area.

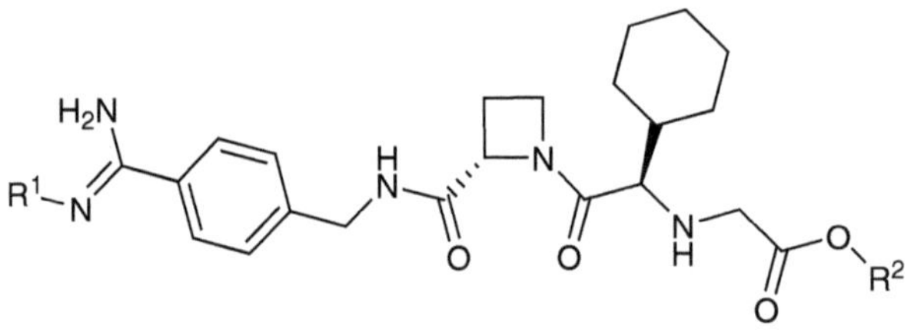

**48** $R^1$ = OH; $R^2$ = Ethyl
**49** $R^1$, $R^2$ = H

## 2.4 Conclusions

In summary, prodrugs can be a valuable drug delivery tool to temporarily enhance the problematic characteristics of a drug molecule, thereby allowing a viable drug delivery strategy by the desired route of administration. Because of the "chemical" nature of the prodrug approach, the design strategy will strongly depend on the available structural features in the drug molecule. Therefore, the more viable approaches that can be established, the more flexible and generic the prodrug approach can become, and it is useful for the designer to be aware of the already established approaches that exist from the many research efforts. It is hoped that this chapter can serve as a tool to both guide the designer toward strategies more likely to succeed and direct the designer to additional sources if more specific detail is desired.

## References


1 DiMasi, J.A. and Grabowski, H.G. (2007) The cost of biopharmaceutical R&D: is biotech different? *Managerial and Decision Economics*, **28**, 469.

2 From molecule to medicine, 2008, http://www.jnjpharmarnd.com/jnjpharmarnd/molMedVideo.html.

3 PhRMA (2008) What goes into the cost of prescription drugs, http://www.phrma.org/files/Cost_of_Prescription_Drugs.pdf.

4 Stella, V.J., Borchardt, R.T., Hageman, M.J., Oliyai, R., Maag, H., and Tilley, J.W. (eds) (2007) *Prodrugs: Challenges and Rewards*, AAPS Press/Springer, New York.

5 Testa, B. and Mayer, J.M. (2003) *Hydrolysis in Drug and Prodrug Metabolism*, Wiley-VCH Verlag GmbH, Weinheim.

6 Bundgaard, H. (ed.) (1985) *Design of Prodrugs*, Elsevier, Amsterdam.

7 Rautio, J., Kumpulainen, H., Heimbach, T., Oliyai, R., Oh, D., Jarvinen, T., and Savolainen, J. (2008) Prodrugs: design and clinical applications. *Nature Reviews. Drug Discovery*, **7**, 255.

8 Fleisher, D., Stewart, B.H., and Amidon, G.L. (1985) Design of prodrugs for improved gastrointestinal absorption by intestinal enzyme targeting. *Methods in Enzymology*, **112**, 360.

9 GlaxoSmithKline and Vertex (2009) Lexiva (fosamprenavir calcium): prescribing information, http://us.gsk.com/products/assets/us_lexiva.pdf, p. 45.

10 Furfine, E.S., Baker, C.T., Hale, M.R., Reynolds, D.J., Salisbury, J.A., Searle, A.D., Studenberg, S.D., Todd, D., Tung, R.D., and Spaltenstein, A. (2004) Preclinical pharmacology and pharmacokinetics of GW433908, a water-soluble prodrug of the human immunodeficiency virus protease inhibitor amprenavir. *Antimicrobial Agents and Chemotherapy*, **48**, 791.

11 Wire, M.B., Shelton, M.J., and Studenberg, S. (2006) Fosamprenavir: clinical pharmacokinetics and drug interactions of the amprenavir prodrug. *Clinical Pharmacokinetics*, **45**, 137.

12 Dhareshwar, S.S. and Stella, V.J. (2008) Your prodrug releases formaldehyde: should you be concerned? no! *Journal of Pharmaceutical Sciences*, **97**, 4184.

13 Stella, V.J., Zygmunt, J.J., Georg, I.G., and Safadi, M.S. (2005) Water-Soluble Prodrugs of Hindered Alcohols or Phenols, US Patent No. 19980131385.

14 Fechner, J., Schwilden, H., and Schuettler, J. (2008) Pharmacokinetics and pharmacodynamics of GPI 15715 or fospropofol (aquavan injection): a water-soluble propofol prodrug. *Handbook of Experimental Pharmacology*, **182**, 253.

15 Kumpulainen, H., Jarvinen, T., Mannila, A., Leppanen, J., Nevalainen, T., Mantyla, A., Vepsalainen, J., and Rautio, J. (2008) Synthesis, *in vitro* and *in vivo* characterization of novel ethyl dioxy phosphate prodrug of propofol. *European Journal of Pharmaceutical Sciences*, **34**, 110.

16 Anderson, B.D., Chu, W.W., and Galinsky, R.E. (1988) Reduction of first-pass metabolism of propanolol after oral administration of ester prodrugs. *International Journal of Pharmaceutics*, **43**, 261.

17 Beresford, R. and Ward, A. (1987) Haloperidol decanoate: a preliminary review of its pharmacodynamic and pharmacokinetic properties and therapeutic use in psychosis. *Drugs*, **33**, 31.

18 Sugawara, M., Huang, W., Fei, Y., Leibach, F., Ganapathy, V., and Ganapathy, M. (2000) Transport of valganciclovir, a ganciclovir prodrug, via peptide transporters PEPT1 and PEPT2. *Journal of Pharmaceutical Sciences*, **89**, 781.

19 Glazko, A.J., Carnes, H.E., Kazenk, A., Wolf, L.M., and Reutner, T.F. (1957–1958) Succinic acid esters of chloramphenicol. *Antibiotics Annual*, **5**, 792.

20 Anderson, B.D., Conradi, R.A., and Knuth, K.E. (1985) Strategies in the design of solution stable, water-soluble prodrugs. I: a physical-organic approach to pro-moiety selection for 21-esters of corticosteroids. *Journal of Pharmaceutical Sciences*, **74**, 365.

21 Persson, G., Pahlm, O., and Gnosspelius, Y. (1995) Oral bambuterol versus

terbutaline in patients with asthma. *Current Therapeutic Research*, **56**, 457.
22 Slatter, J.G., Schaaf, L.J., Sams, J.P., Feenstra, K.L., Johnson, M.G., Bombardt, P.A., Cathcart, K.S., Verburg, M.T., Pearson, L.K., Compton, L.D., Miller, L.L., Baker, D.S., Pesheck, C.V., and Lord, R.S. (2000) Pharmacokinetics, metabolism, and excretion of irinotecan (CPT-11) following I.V. Infusion of [$^{14}$C] CPT-11 in cancer patients. *Drug Metabolism and Disposition*, **28** 423.
23 Monk, J.P. and Clissold, S.P. (1987) Misoprostol: a preliminary review of its pharmacodynamic and pharmacokinetic properties, and therapeutic efficacy. *Drugs*, **33**, 1.
24 Kostic, M.A. and Dart, R.C. (2003) Rethinking the toxic methanol level. *Journal of Toxicology. Clinical Toxicology*, **41**, 793.
25 Tephly, T.R. (1991) The toxicity of methanol. *Life Sciences*, **48**, 1031.
26 He, G., Massarella, J., and Ward, P. (1999) Clinical pharmacokinetics of the prodrug oseltamivir and its active metabolite RO 64-0802. *Clinical Pharmacokinetics*, **37**, 471.
27 McClellan, K. and Perry, C.M. (2001) Oseltamivir: a review of its use in influenza. *Drugs*, **61**, 261.
28 Swaan, P.W., Stehouwer, M.C., and Tukker, J.J. (1995) Molecular mechanism for the relative binding affinity to the intestinal peptide carrier. Comparison of three ACE-inhibitors: enalapril, enalaprilat and lisinopril. *Biochimica et Biophysica Acta, Biomembranes*, **1236**, 31.
29 Todd, P.A. and Heel, R.C. (1986) Enalapril: a review of its pharmacodynamic and pharmacokinetic properties, and therapeutic use in hypertension and congestive heart failure. *Drugs*, **31**, 198.
30 Cellcept® Prescribing information, 2009, http://www.rocheusa.com/products/cellcept/pi.pdf.
31 Ehrnebo, M., Nilsson, S., and Boreus, L.O. (1979) Pharmacokinetics of ampicillin and its prodrugs bacampicillin and pivampicillin in man. *Journal of Pharmacokinetics and Biopharmaceutics*, **7**, 429.
32 Saito, A. and Nakashima, M. (1986) Pharmacokinetic study of lenampicillin (KBT-1585) in healthy volunteers. *Antimicrobial Agents and Chemotherapy*, **29**, 948.
33 Stella, V.J. (1996) A case for prodrugs, fosphenytoin. *Advanced Drug Delivery Reviews*, **19**, 311.
34 Josyula, V.P.V.N., Gadwood, R.C., Thomasco, L.M., Kim, J., Choy, A.L., and Boyer, F.E., Jr. (2005) Preparation of acyloxymethyl carbamate prodrugs of oxazolidinone bactericides with excellent oral bioavailability. PCT Int. Appl. WO 2005/028473 A1.
35 Bundgaard, H. and Johansen, M. (1980) Pro-drugs as drug delivery systems. X. *N*-Mannich bases as novel pro-drug candidates for amides, imides, urea derivatives, amines and other NH-acidic compounds. Kinetics and mechanisms of decomposition and structure–reactivity relationships. *Archiv for Pharmaciog Chemi, Scientific Edition*, **8**, 29.
36 Guarino, V.R., Karunaratne, V., and Stella, V.J. (2003) Novel Sulfenamide Prodrugs of N–H Bond-Containing Compounds. WO2002/US32957.
37 Guarino, V.R. (2004) Sulfenamide Prodrugs: A Novel Prodrug Approach for Amides, Imides and other NH-Acidic Compounds. Doctoral Dissertation, University of Kansas, 241 p.
38 Guarino, V.R., Karunaratne, V., and Stella, V.J. (2007) Sulfenamides as prodrugs of NH-acidic compounds: a new prodrug option for the amide bond. *Bioorganic and Medicinal Chemistry Letters*, **17**, 4910.
39 Guarino, V.R. and Stella, V.J. (2007) in Prodrugs of amides, imides and other NH-acidic compounds, in *Prodrugs: Challenges and Rewards*, Part 2, AAPS Press/Springer, New York, pp. 133–187.
40 Davis, E.A. (1973) Chemistry of the sulfur–nitrogen bond in sulfenamides. *International Journal of Sulfur Chemistry*, **8**, 71.
41 Craine, L. and Raban, M. (1989) The chemistry of sulfenamides. *Chemical Reviews*, **89**, 689.
42 Koval, I.V. (1996) Chemistry of sulfenamides. *Russian Journal of Organic Chemistry*, **32**, 1239.

43 Hemenway, J.N., Nti-Addae, K., Guarino, V.R., and Stella, V.J. (2007) Preparation, characterization and *in vivo* conversion of new water-soluble sulfenamide prodrugs of carbamazepine. *Bioorganic and Medicinal Chemistry Letters*, **17**, 6629.

44 Talley, J.J., Bertenshaw, S.R., Brown, D.L., Carter, J.S., Graneto, M.J., Kellogg, M.S., Koboldt, C.M., Yuan, J.H., Zhang, Y.Y., and Seibert, K. (2000) *N*-(5-Methyl-3-phenylisoxazol-4-yl)-phenyl sulfonyl propanamide, sodium salt, parecoxib sodium: a potent and selective inhibitor of COX-2 for parenteral administration. *Journal of Medicinal Chemistry*, **43**, 1661.

45 Hecker, S.J. and Erion, M.D. (2008) Prodrugs of phosphates and phosphonates. *Journal of Medicinal Chemistry*, **51**, 2328.

46 Hostetler, K.Y. (2009) Alkoxyalkyl prodrugs of acyclic nucleoside phosphonates enhance oral antiviral activity and reduce toxicity: current state of the art. *Antiviral Research*, **82**, A84.

47 He, G., Krise, J.P., and Oliyai, R. (2007) Prodrugs of phosphonates, phosphinates and phosphates, in *Prodrugs: Challenges and Rewards*, Part 2, AAPS Press/Springer, New York, pp. 223–264.

48 de Lombaert, S., Erion, M.D., Tan, J., Blanchard, L., el-Chehabi, L., Ghai, R.D., Sakane, Y., Berry, C., and Trapani, A.J. (1994) N-Phosphonomethyl dipeptides and their phosphonate prodrugs, a new generation of neutral endopeptidase (NEP, EC 3.4.24.11) inhibitors. *Journal of Medicinal Chemistry*, **37**, 498.

49 Shaw, J.-P., Sueoka, C.M., Oliyai, R., Lee, W.A., Arimilli, M.N., Kim, C.U., and Cundy, K.C. (1997) Metabolism and pharmacokinetics of novel oral prodrugs of 9-[(*R*)-2-(phosphonomethoxy)propyl] adenine (PMPA) in dogs. *Pharmaceutical Research*, **14**, 1824.

50 Yuan, L.-C., Dahl, T.C., and Oliyai, R. (2001) Degradation kinetics of oxycarbonyloxymethyl prodrugs of phosphonates in solution. *Pharmaceutical Research*, **18**, 234.

51 Barditch-Crovo, P., Deeks, S.G., Collier, A., Safrin, S., Coakley, D.F., Miller, M., Kearney, B.P., Coleman, R.L., Lamy, P.D., Kahn, J.O., McGowna, I., and Lietman, P.S. (2001) Phase I/II trial of the pharmacokinetics, safety, and antiretroviral activity of tenofovir disoproxil fumarate in HIV-1 infected adults. *Antimicrobial Agents and Chemotherapy*, **45**, 2733.

52 Naesens, L., Snoeck, R., Andrei, G., Balzarini, J., Neyts, J., and De Clercq, E. (1997) HPMPC (cidofovir), PMEA (adefovir) and related acyclic nucleoside phosphonate analogues: a review of their pharmacology and clinical potential in the treatment of viral infections. *Antiviral Chemistry and Chemotherapy*, **8**, 1.

53 Cahard, D., McGuigan, C., and Balzarini, J. (2004) Aryloxy phosphoramidate triesters as protides. *Mini-Reviews in Medicinal Chemistry*, **4**, 371.

54 Pegram, M., Ku, N., Shepard, M., Speid, L., and Lenz, H.-J. (2002) Enzyme-catalyzed therapeutic activation (ECTA) NB1011 (thymectacin) selectively targets thymidylate synthase (TS)-overexpressing tumor cells: preclinical and phase I clinical results. *European Journal of Cancer*, **38** (Suppl. 7), 99.

55 Jones, B.C.N.M., McGuigan, C., O'Connor, T.J., Jeffries, D.J., and Kinchington, D. (1991) Synthesis and anti-HIV activity of some novel phosphorodiamidate derivatives of 3′-azido-3′-deoxythymidine (AZT). *Antiviral Chemistry & Chemotherapy*, **2**, 35.

56 Erion, M.D., Reddy, K.R., Boyer, S.H., Matelich, M.C., Gomez-Galeno, J., Lemus, R.H., Ugarkar, B.G., Colby, T.J., Schanzer, J., and van Poelje, P.D. (2004) Design, synthesis, and characterization of a series of cytochrome P(450) 3A-activated prodrugs (HepDirect prodrugs) useful for targeting phosph(on)ate-based drugs to the liver. *Journal of the American Chemical Society*, **126**, 5154.

57 Sorbera, L.A., Serradell, N., and Bolos, J. (2007) Pradefovir mesilate treatment of hepatitis B. *Drugs of the Future*, **32**, 137.

58 Marcellin, P., Chang, T.T., Lim, S.G., Tong, M.J., Sievert, W., Shiffman, M.L., Jeffers, L., Goodman, Z., Wulfsohn, M.S., Xiong, S., Fry, J., and Brosgart, C.L. (2003) Adefovir dipivoxil for the treatment of hepatitis B e antigen-positive chronic

hepatitis B. *New England Journal of Medicine*, **348**, 808.

**59** Gogate, U.S., Repta, A.J., and Alexander, J. (1987) N-(Acyloxyalkoxycarbonyl) derivatives as potential prodrugs of amines. I. kinetics and mechanism of degradation in aqueous solutions. *International Journal of Pharmaceutics*, **40**, 235.

**60** Gogate, U.S. and Repta, A.J. (1987) N-(Acyloxyalkoxycarbonyl) derivatives as potential prodrugs of amines. II. Esterase-catalyzed release of parent amines from model prodrugs. *International Journal of Pharmaceutics*, **40**, 249.

**61** Safadi, M., Oliyai, R., and Stella, V.J. (1993) Phosphoaryloxymethyl carbamates and carbonates: novel water-soluble prodrugs for amines and hindered alcohols. *Pharmaceutical Research*, **10**, 1350.

**62** Vinogradova, N.D., Kuznetsov, S.G., and Chigareva, S.M. (1980) Quaternary ammonium salts with labile $(N^+)-C$ bonds as drug precursors. *Khimiko-Farmatsevticheskii Zhurnal*, **14**, 41.

**63** Davidsen, S.K., Summers, J.B., Albert, D.H., Holms, J.H., Heyman, H.R., Magoc, T.J., Conway, R.G., Rhein, D.A., and Carter, G.W. (1994) *N*-(Acyloxyalkyl) pyridinium salts as soluble prodrugs of a potent platelet activating factor antagonist. *Journal of Medicinal Chemistry*, **37**, 4423.

**64** Albert, D.H., Conway, R.G., Magoc, T.J., Tapang, P., Rhein, D.A., Luo, G., Holms, J.H., Davidsen, S.K., Summers, J.B., and Carter, G.W. (1996) Properties of ABT-299: a prodrug of A-85783, a highly potent platelet activating factor receptor antagonist. *Journal of Pharmacology and Experimental Therapeutics*, **277**, 1595.

**65** Krise, J.P., Zygmunt, J., Georg, G.I., and Stella, V.J. (1999) Novel prodrug approach for tertiary amines: synthesis and preliminary evaluation of *N*-phosphonooxymethyl prodrugs. *Journal of Medicinal Chemistry*, **42**, 3094.

**66** Krise, J.P., Narisawa, S., and Stella, V.J. (1999) A novel prodrug approach for tertiary amines. 2. Physicochemical and *in vitro* enzymatic evaluation of selected *N*-phosphonooxymethyl prodrugs. *Journal of Pharmaceutical Sciences*, **88**, 922.

**67** Krise, J.P., Charman, W.N., Charman, S.A., and Stella, V.J. (1999) A novel prodrug approach for tertiary amines. 3. *In vivo* evaluation of two *N*-phosphonooxymethyl prodrugs in rats and dogs. *Journal of Pharmaceutical Sciences*, **88**, 928.

**68** Eriksson, U., Liljenvald, A.C., Fager, G., Thuresson, A., and Gabrielsson, M. (2000) The pharmacokinetics, metabolism and elimination of H376/95, a novel direct thrombin inhibitor, in healthy male subjects, after oral and intravenous administration. *Pharmacotherapy*, **20**, 1264.

**69** Gustafsson, D., Nystrom, J.-E., Carlsson, S., Bredberg, U., Eriksson, U., Gyzander, E., Elg, M., Antonsson, T., Hoffmann, K.-J., Ungell, A.-L., Sorensen, H., Nagard, S., Abrahamsson, A., and Bylund, R. (2001) The direct thrombin inhibitor melagatran and its oral prodrug H 376/95: intestinal absorption properties, biochemical and pharmacodynamic effects. *Thrombosis Research*, **101** 171.

**70** Sorbera, L.A., Bayes, M., Castaner, J., and Silvestre, J. (2001) Melagatran and ximelagatran. *Drugs of the Future*, **26**, 1155.

**71** Clement, B. (2002) Reduction of *N*-hydroxylated compounds: amidoximes (*N*-hydroxyamidines) as pro-drugs of amidines. *Drug Metabolism Reviews*, **34**, 565.

**72** Tilley, J.W. (2007) Prodrugs of benzamidines, in *Prodrugs: Challenges and Rewards*, Part 2, AAPS Press/Springer, New York, pp. 189–222.

# 3
# Intellectual Property Primer on Pharmaceutical Patents with a Special Emphasis on Prodrugs and Metabolites

*Eyal H. Barash*

## 3.1
## Introduction

An example of a prodrug on the market today is enalapril, the active ingredient in Merck's Vasotec®. When orally administered, an esterase enzyme metabolizes enalapril hydrolyzing it into the active moiety. FDA approved enalapril, an ACE inhibitor used for the treatment of hypertension, on December 24, 1985. It went generic on August 22, 2000 when Merck's pediatric exclusivity expired. On that date, FDA approved generic versions of Vasotec belonging to nine different generic drug companies.[1)] Nevertheless, Merck enjoyed a nearly 15-year monopoly on sales of this blockbuster drug due to its vigorous patent portfolio. Merck's protection included patents directed to compounds, compositions, methods of treatment, processed of manufacture, and metabolites.

This chapter is divided into two principal sections. Section 3.2 discusses the interface of FDA and patent law, or the Hatch-Waxman Act. Its effect on the pharmaceutical industry cannot be underestimated, and it is a major driver of pharmaceutical patent strategy for both innovators and generic companies. In Section 3.3, several basic concepts of patentability are presented. These concepts focus on pharmaceuticals and discuss the nuances associated with prodrugs and metabolites.

## 3.2
## Patents and FDA Approval Process

FDA has two simple, but arduous, requirements for drug manufacturers to meet in order to legally sell their products in the United States: safety and efficacy. These

1) Data collected from Orange Book located at http://www.accessdata.fda.gov/scripts/cder/ob/default.cfm and by searching for enalapril maleate and tabulating the number of approvals on August 22, 2000.

*Prodrugs and Targeted Delivery: Towards Better ADME Properties.* Edited by Jarkko Rautio

ISBN: 978-3-527-32603-7

deceptively simple standards consume tremendous amounts of resources and more often than not, lead to failure. When a pharmaceutical company embarks upon a development program, it must generate data that the company will use to file a New Drug Application (NDA). The NDA is usually directed to a particular chemical entity and formulation. However, an NDA filer who wishes to protect its product against other innovators must think beyond the commercial product. In other words, it must have "genus" protection so as to include products for which it may have little if any data. Consider, for example, the drug Humira®.

Abbott's Humira drug had sales of about $4.5 billion in 2008.[2] A competing product, Johnson & Johnson's Remicade® had sales of 3.748 billion that same year.[3] Both drugs employ monoclonal antibodies that are specific to TNF-α. Humira is derived solely from human cells using recombinant DNA technology. Remicade, on the other hand, is composed of "human constant and murine variable regions"[4] Humira was approved on December 31, 2002 and Remicade on August 24, 1998. Johnson & Johnson filed suit against Abbott for patent infringement. The act of infringement was not based on Abbott using the same product as Johnson & Johnson, but on a different one that, according to Johnson & Johnson fell within the claims of U.S. Patent 7,070,775. The jury agreed with Johnson & Johnson and awarded damages to the tune of nearly $1.7 billion. Claims 1 and 2 of the patent read as follows:

1) An isolated recombinant anti-TNF-α antibody or antigen-binding fragment thereof, said antibody comprising a human constant region, wherein said antibody or antigen binding fragment (i) competitively inhibits binding of A2 (ATCC Accession No. PTA-7045) to human TNF-α, and (ii) binds to a neutralizing epitope of human TNF-α *in vivo* with an affinity of at least $1 \times 10^8$ liter/mole, measured as an association constant (Ka), as determined by Scatchard analysis.
2) The antibody or antigen-binding fragment of claim 1, wherein the antibody or antigen-binding fragment comprises a human constant region and a human variable region.

Thus, although Johnson & Johnson never made a fully humanized monoclonal antibody product, Claim 2 of its '775 patent was not limited to such an antibody. Rather, the claim language states that the fragment "comprises a human constant region and a human variable region." The jury agreed with Johnson & Johnson that such claim language included within its scope an antibody or fragment thereof, which was fully humanized. In the abstract, the fact that Johnson & Johnson had never made such an antibody is not necessarily fatal to the patent. There is no requirement in patent law that an applicant makes working examples of all species that fall within a genus. However, if a claim is too broad, it may fail if it is determined that the claim encompasses matter that is neither described in the patent nor reproducible. Thus, the question that will certainly be raised on appeal is whether there was sufficient data that include human antibodies in the Johnson & Johnson

2) See Abbott Laboratories 2008 10-K Annual Report, March 3, 2009, p. 61.

3) See Johnson & Johnson 2008 10-K Annual Report, February 20, 2009, p. 36.

4) See Remicade label.

patent application to support such a claim.[5] Nevertheless, if Johnson & Johnson prevails on appeal, it may eliminate a competing innovator product from the marketplace.

The more common foe to the patentee of pharmaceutical drugs is the ANDA filer. The Abbreviated New Drug Application (ANDA) and differs substantially in scope from an NDA. Rather than having to prove safety and efficacy, an ANDA holder needs merely to show that its drug product is "bioequivalent" to the NDA holder's drug product and cite to the NDA for proof of efficacy and safety.[6] Because they do not have to pay for costly research, development, and clinical programs, ANDA holders (typically generic drug companies) spend only a tiny fraction of money of bringing their drug to market compared with the innovator's expenses for their brand-name product.

In order to avoid performing safety and efficacy tests, ANDA filers must have the same active ingredient as the innovator used in its NDA filing. Thus, from a patent perspective, it would appear relatively straightforward to protect against generic competition. One should have what patent practitioners refer to as a "picture" claim, namely, a patent claim covering the chemical entity used in the drug product and nothing more. For example, the drug Abilify® was first marketed in 2002 for the treatment of schizophrenia and has since grown into a blockbuster drug. It is protected by U.S. Patent 5,006,528 that claims the following in Claim 12:

> 12. 7-{4-[4-(2, 3-Dichlorophenyl)-1-piperazinyl]butoxy}-3, 4-dihydrocarbostyril.

This claim simply recites the chemical structure of the active ingredient in Abilify® known as apripazole and nothing more. The claim derives value from the requirement that the generic drug copy the active ingredient of the innovator. The situation is not always so straightforward, however. Often pharmaceutical companies sue over infringement of formulation patents with limitations based on characteristics of the formulation or ingredients. The claim may require, for example, a particular excipient, a particle size distribution, or a release profile. Thus, because the innovator bears burden of proof, it may have to perform tests on the generic formulation to prove infringement.

Effective protection against generic competition also requires a thorough understanding of how patent law and FDA law overlap. While such a comprehensive review is beyond the scope of this chapter, it is worth discussing the basics so that the reader appreciates how prodrugs and metabolites can be used to protect, or to defeat, patent coverage on pharmaceutical products.

5) In order to obtain a patent, there must be sufficient "support" in the patent application to support the patent claim. 35 U.S.C. § 112 ¶1 states that "[t]he specification shall contain a written description of the invention, and of the manner and process of making and using it, in such full, clear, concise, and exact terms as to enable any person skilled in the art to which it pertains, or with which it is most nearly connected, to make and use the same, and shall set forth the best mode contemplated by the inventor of carrying out his invention." There is considerable controversy currently on whether the written description and enablement provisions are separate. This topic is beyond the scope of this chapter.

6) See 21 U.S.C. §355 *et seq.*

A practical place to begin the discussion of brand name and generic drugs is to discuss the case of *Roche v. Bolar.*[7] Roche had developed the drug Dalmane® and brought it onto the market. Bolar wished to develop a generic version of Dalmane and began its research and development program prior to the expiration of the patent covering Dalmane. Roche learned of this program and filed a patent infringement suit against Bolar arguing that this work infringed Roche's patent. The court agreed. Although Bolar attempted to argue that such use was merely research-based and experimental, the court ruled that no such exception to patent infringement was available to Bolar and Roche was able to prevent Bolar from developing a generic version of Dalmane during the term of its patent.

Shortly after deciding this case, Congress enacted the Hatch-Waxman Act that was meant to regulate the tug-of-war between innovator and generic companies. Among the things it attempted to do was to create a balance between the need for patent exclusivity for innovator companies and the access to generic drugs for the public. It struck a compromise that legislatively overturned *Roche v. Bolar,* and among other provisions, established a "safe harbor" from patent infringement whereby the ability to perform research and development on patented pharmaceutical products for the filing of an ANDA was exempt from patent infringement.[8] The Hatch-Waxman Act also created a procedure by which innovators and generics could fight their patent disputes in court prior to the market entry of a generic product.

The disputes begin with the *FDA Orange Book* that lists all approved drug products in the United States. It also lists the patent status associated with each product.[9] Once a generic company decides to launch a product, it must consult the Orange Book to determine the patent status of the product whose NDA it wishes to refer. There are four possible outcomes according to the statute:

(I) There is no patent covering the pharmaceutical product (Paragraph I)
(II) The patents covering the product have expired (Paragraph II)
(III) There are active patents covering the product, but the generic company seeking approval will not launch any drug until the patent covering the product has expired (Paragraph III); or
(IV) A patent covering the product has not expired and a generic believes that it will either not infringe the patent or the patent is invalid and wants the FDA to grant approval the patents notwithstanding (Paragraph IV).

**7)** 733 F.2d 858 (Fed. Cir. 1984).

**8)** The actual language of the statute, 35 U.S.C. § 271(e)(1), reads "It shall not be an act of infringement to make, use, offer to sell, or sell within the United States or import into the United States a patented invention ... solely for uses reasonably related to the development and submission of information under a Federal law which regulates the manufacture, use, or sale of drugs or veterinary biological products." It has been interpreted to be broader than the mere filing of an ANDA (see *Merck KGaA v. Integra Lifesciences I,* Ltd.545 US 193 (2005)) and it is still a matter of debate as to how far the safe harbor extends.

**9)** The Orange Book is publicly available on the FDA Web site www.fda.gov, and is regularly updated.

The first three outcomes involve only the ANDA applicant and the FDA. In certifications involving these first three paragraphs, FDA will approve the application without regard to any patent exclusivity associated with the innovator's product. In a so-called Paragraph IV certification, however, the ANDA applicant is required by law to notify the innovator of its intent to enter the market prior to patent expiry.[10] Upon receipt of the notice, which is supposed to contain the bases for the ANDA applicant's belief that the patent neither will be infringed nor is valid, the innovator has less than 45 days to make a critically important decision – whether to file a patent infringement lawsuit against the ANDA applicant under the assumption that if it were to get FDA approval, its commercial product would infringe the Innovator's patent.[11] If such a suit is filed, a 30-month stay or hold is placed on FDA's approval process and during the time of the stay, although the agency may review the ANDA, it may not approve it absent court intervention. Thus, the filing of a lawsuit in effect puts an automatic delay of 30 months on the market entry of a generic product.[12] It is not hard to appreciate how this stay is of tremendous value to innovators as they plan a strategy to protect their valuable products from generic competition.

A critical caveat to this strategy is that only those patents that the innovator elects to list in the Orange Book are eligible to receive the 30-month stay protection. Thus, failure to list an appropriate patent can have devastating consequences. Unsurprisingly, the law regulates the kinds of patents that may be listed in the Orange Book. Under the Code of Federal Regulations, only the patents such as the following are eligible for listing: drug substance (ingredient) patents, drug product (formulation and composition) patents, and method of use patents. Metabolite patents, for example, are not eligible for listing in the Orange Book.[13] In other words, the Orange Book requires that patents covering the active ingredient prior to patient ingestion may be listed, but transformations upon human consumption, while eligible subject matter for patent protection, generally are not eligible for the added protection afforded by listing in the Orange Book. Accordingly, prodrug patents are eligible for listing in the Orange Book. There is no requirement to identify to FDA that the listed drug is a prodrug.

## 3.3 Obtaining a Patent

Before one can devise an effective patent enforcement strategy, one must go through the patent procurement process. In the United States, the Patent and Trademark Office (PTO) is responsible for issuing patents based on properly prepared patent applications claiming appropriate subject matter. This section explores the requirements of how to obtain such protection with a special emphasis on

10) See 21 U.S.C. § 355(b)(2)(A)(iv).

11) See 21 U.S.C. § 355(c)(3)(C).

12) See *id.* A court may choose to shorten or lengthen the stay although neither is a common occurrence.

13) 21 CFR § 314.53(b)(1).

pharmaceutical products with alerts for special issues that relate to prodrugs and metabolites.

### 3.3.1 Utility

An invention must be useful in order to be patentable. In the pharmaceutical arts, such as for prodrugs and metabolites, this does not mean an invention must be safe or effective as those terms are used by the FDA. This issue arose *In re Brana*[14] where the inventors had filed for a patent application on a class of compounds that they claimed to have antitumor capabilities. The compounds were described as more effective than structurally similar compounds found in the published literature and data were presented in the application showing "good action" against human tumor cells *in vitro*.[15] The examiner rejected the claims arguing that there was insufficient evidence to establish the claimed chemical compounds had a practical utility. Under PTO procedure, when an examiner has rejected a case,[16] the applicant may appeal to a board of administrative law judges who sit at the PTO. In this case, the board agreed with the examiner. Applicants have the right to appeal a board decision to the United States Court of Appeals for the Federal Circuit,[17] which sits in Washington, DC. Upon appeal, the court reversed the board and found that the applicants had met the utility requirement. The court ruled that the standard tumor models, using *in vivo* tests, were sufficient to meet the utility requirement. It may be worth noting, however, that an even stronger case for utility can be made by using art-recognized animal models. Indeed, in prior cases, the courts had ruled that "proof of an alleged pharmaceutical property for a compound by statistically significant tests with standard experimental animals is sufficient to establish utility."[18] However, the *Manual of Patent Examination Procedure*, the MPEP, which is the guide used by examiners in examining patent applications, summarizes case law stating that "[c]ourts have repeatedly found that the mere *identification* of a pharmacological activity of a compound that is relevant to an asserted pharmacological use provides an

**14)** 51 F.3d 1560 (Fed. Cir. 1995).

**15)** *Id.* at 1563.

**16)** In prosecution, after an examiner makes a rejection, the applicants have an opportunity to respond to the examiner. The examiner then reviews the case and arguments a second time and if there is still disagreement, the examiner may issue a "final" rejection. Such a final rejection may be appealed to the PTO Board.

**17)** The Court of Appeals for the Federal Circuit is a subject–matter based court unlike the other courts of appeal. For example, in most cases in the federal system, the disputing parties will choose a trial court based upon geography. The losing side then has the right to appeal the trial court ruling to an appeals court. In most cases, the appeals court which hears the case is based on the location of the lower court. Thus, a lower court's decision in Chicago will be appealed to the Court of Appeals for the Seventh Circuit. A lower court's decision in Los Angeles will be heard by the Court of Appeals for the Ninth Circuit and so on. For patents, however, all appeals, regardless of the location of the lower court are heard by Court of Appeals for the Federal Circuit that also hears appeals from the Patent Office.

**18)** 51 F.3d at 1567.

'immediate benefit to the public' and thus satisfies the utility requirement."[19] The Court in *In re Brana* also noted that structural similarity to known compounds is relevant in the utility inquiry.[20]

### 3.3.2
### Novelty

One cannot obtain a patent on an invention that is not new. Trying to determine whether something is new, however, can be daunting, especially with patents to metabolites. A traditional view of novelty rests with an analysis of what is termed "prior art." Prior art may be such as journal references, patents, sales, and imports that all occur before a particular date. Sometimes, that date is the date before which the applicant filed for a patent application. In other circumstances, the date is that which is before the inventor conceived of the invention. Section 102 of title 35 of the United States Code sets forth the specific requirements of novelty. The two most relevant sections for this chapter are subparts (a) and (b).

Section 102(a) in its entirety reads as follows:

> A person shall be entitled to a patent unless (a) the invention was known or used by others in this country, or patented or described in a printed publication in this or a foreign country, before the invention thereof by the applicant for patent.[21]

Deconstructing section 102(a) reveals that only activities occurring prior to the invention are relevant. Such actions include patents or publications anywhere worldwide whereas knowledge or use is limited to the Untied States. Also note that only actions by third parties may be used as novelty-defeating art under section 102 (a). Actions by the inventors are immune to attach under section 102(a). Thus, it is to the advantage of the inventor to have evidence showing a date of invention that is as early as possible. For this reason, among others, pharmaceutical companies develop laboratory notebook and corroboration evidence policies. Once a third-party publication publishes, even though a patent may not yet be on file, properly kept laboratory notebooks showing a prior date invention date can be used to "antedate" the reference during examination at the PTO.[22]

19) MPEP § 2107.01.

20) 51 F.3d at 1367.

21) 35 U.S.C. § 102(a).

22) The PTO will assume that the date of filing is the date of invention absent evidence to the contrary. Thus, a relevant publication published prior to the filing date will act as section 102(a) prior and will be identified as such in an official communication sent to the applicant termed an "office action." In replying to the office action, the applicant may use laboratory notebook pages with an affidavit showing that the invention occurred prior to the publication. There are other reasons for keeping good laboratory records in a patent context. For example, in an interference, two parties are trying to claim the same invention. With some exceptions, the party who can prove prior invention will be entitled to the patent.

A more nefarious provision of the novelty section of the Patent Act is section 102 b):

> A person shall be entitled to a patent unless (b) the invention was patented or described in a printed publication in this or a foreign country or in public use or on sale in this country, more than one year prior to the date of the application for patent in the United States.[23]

Under section 102(b), novelty is referenced from the date that is exactly one year prior to the filing date of the application (the "critical date"). Like section 102(a), in 102 (b), patents or publications can defeat novelty. Note, however, these actions are not limited to third parties. The applicant's own actions can doom him. For example, suppose the applicant was to publish his or her work in a journal on August 1, 2010, the publication date starts a one-year clock. If the applicant has not filed a patent by August 1, 2011, the patent rights will be forfeited.[24] Section 102(b) also introduces the concepts of public use and "on sale," which are beyond the scope of this chapter.

It is not enough for a reference to meet the timing requirements of section 102; it must also be relevant to the claims of the patent. To anticipate (i.e., render not novel), a reference must teach all of the limitations of the claim at issue. For example, whereas the chemical structure of aspirin is certainly older than any claim currently on file with the PTO, it is hardly relevant to a claim on a new protein drug. Thus, the analysis of the "prior art" is important. Consider the following generic chemical compound:

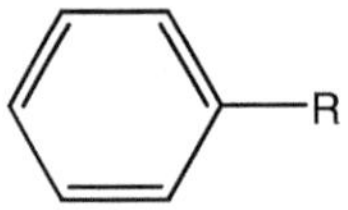


Assume that an applicant has claimed such a structure and defined R as a $C_1-C_6$ alkyl. Thus, the applicant would be defining a genus of compounds as opposed to a single compound. A prior art reference teaching toluene would anticipate that claim for lack of novelty. Suppose there was a second claim in the application to the same structure, but where R is a $C_3-C_6$ alkyl. In that case toluene would not be anticipatory art against this claim. Thus, when preparing a patent application for filing, claim scope becomes a strategic consideration because prior art acts on patent claims, not on the entire patent. Accordingly, patent claims often look like a funnel in terms of scope. Very broad claims are supported by narrower and narrower claims. If it is later determined that a broad claim is held invalid for lack of novelty, a narrower claim might still survive. Therefore, whereas a broad claim captures more intellectual property space than a narrower claim, it also presents a bigger target for prior art attack. Returning to the example where toluene is disclosed in the prior art, practitioners

**23)** 35 U.S.C. §102(b).

**24)** Very few countries have such a grace period. In Europe, for example, there is no grace period. Thus, failure to file a patent application by the publication date results in loss of patent rights. In the era where publications appear on the Internet long before print, pharmaceutical companies must employ vigorous and robust systems for reviewing publications prior to journal submission.

would say that the anticipation is express in that there is a reference that expressly teaches the compound. In some circumstances, however, that teaching is more subtle.

Consider the following claim: Crystalline Form B of Compound I exhibiting X-ray powder diffraction peaks at about 5.7, 7.9, 10.0, and 11.5 degrees two-theta. In this claim, applicants have prepared a purportedly new polymorph of Compound I and wish to obtain patent coverage. As is sometimes the case in the polymorph world, prior art may exist as to the chemical entity. In this case, let us suppose that there is a prior art reference teaching Compound I that fails to teach anything regarding the crystalline form of the compound. Instead, the patent provides a synthetic example with the formation of a "crystalline white powder." Confirmation of structure is given by the usual techniques: NMR, IR, and elemental analysis for instance. Thus, the reference has no express teaching of the crystalline form because there is no indication of which crystalline form was produced. During patent prosecution, the examiner will want to know whether that crystalline form was Form B or another form and will likely reject the claim. If the crystalline material was in fact Form B, it is novelty-defeating prior art. The material that was never analyzed in the prior art is of no concern. The examiner will invite the applicants to reproduce the reference and report the results.[25)]

Inherent anticipation also plays a major role in patents directed to metabolites and prodrugs. In *Schering Corp. v. Geneva Pharmaceuticals*,[26)] Schering had received two patents covering antihistamines: the '233 patent and the '716 patent. The earlier patent, the '233 patent, claimed loratadine, the active ingredient in the blockbuster drug Claritin®. After obtaining the '233 patent, Schering obtained another patent related to loratadine, the '716 patent, which claimed a metabolite of loratadine called descarboethoxyloratadine or DCL.[27)] DCL differs from loratadine in that where loratadine has a carboxyethyl group or a ring nitrogen, DCL has a hydrogen atom (Figure 3.1).[28)] Although the '233 patent did not expressly disclose DCL, the lower court found that "DCL was necessarily formed as a metabolite by carrying out the process disclosed" in the patent.[29)] That ruling was based on teachings within the '233 patent where patients had ingested loratadine. Such ingestion would necessarily form the anticipatory metabolite.[30)] The Federal Circuit agreed with the lower court and invalidated Schering's '716 patent on grounds of inherent anticipation even though at the time the '233 patent was filed, there was no recognition within the reference that DCL would form.[31)]

**25)** This fact pattern is common in the solid-state arts. In not all cases does the examiner succeed in requiring the reproduction of prior art references. See, for example, *Ex Parte Reguri*, Board of Patent Appeals and Interferences Appeal No. 2007-0313 (September 6, 2007).

**26)** 339 F.3d 1373 (2003).

**27)** *Id.* at 1375.

**28)** *Id.*

**29)** *Id.* at 1376. Inherency requires that the anticipated feature "necessarily and inevitably" occur. See *id.* at 1378.

**30)** *Id.* at 1380.

**31)** See *id.* at 1378.

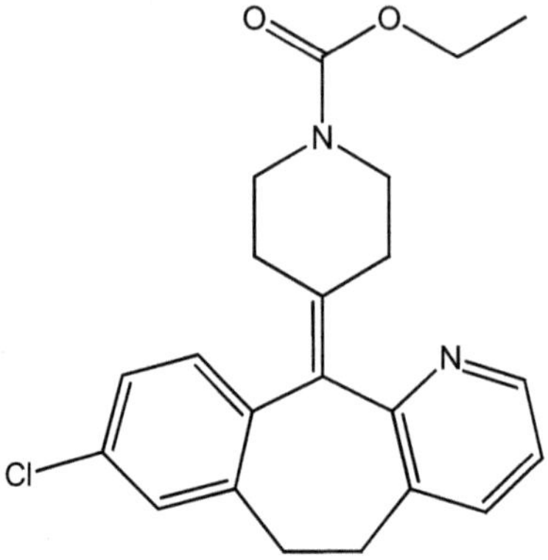

1

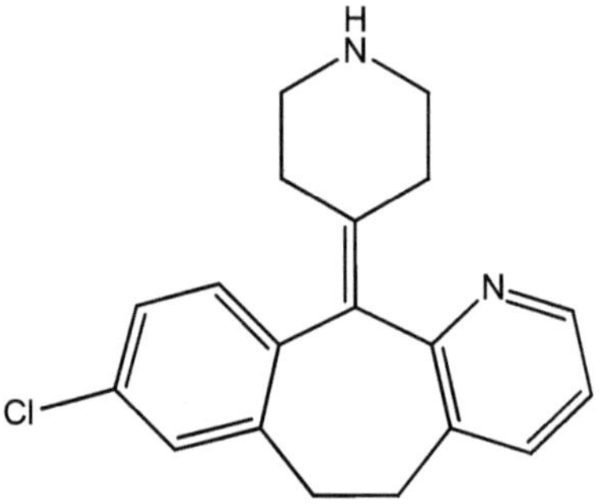

2

**Figure 3.1** Structures of loratadine (**1**) and its metabolite descarboethoxyloratadine (**2**).

Inherent anticipation profoundly affects pharmaceutical patent strategies. Typically, as pharmaceutical companies improve their marketed product, be it by advanced formulations or by better manufacturing practices, they seek to patent those improvements. Under the *Schering* case, a company may have to identify any potentially active metabolites earlier in a drug development process than they would have otherwise. The mere act of disclosing administering a drug to a human might trigger the one-year clock under section 102(b). Many in the pharmaceutical patent community were critical of the *Schering* case. It eliminated the notion that the inherent limitation had to be recognized in the prior art.

In the case of *Continental Can Co. USA, Inc. v. Monsanto,*[32] a patent claimed a container having various technical features that provided it with added strength and impact resistance.[33] Monsanto argued that a prior art reference, the '443 patent, anticipated the claim at issue under section 102(a). The claim at issue required hollow ribs in a container, and according to testimony presented by Monsanto, although the '443 patent did not state that that the ribs were hollow, by practicing the manufacturing process of the '443 patent, one would necessarily obtain hollow ribs. Moreover, the court ruled the following:

> To serve as anticipation when the reference is silent about the asserted inherent characteristic, such gap in the reference may be filled with recourse to extrinsic evidence. Such evidence must make clear that the missing descriptive matter is necessarily present in the thing described in the reference, *and that it would be so recognized by persons of ordinary skill.*[34]

**32)** 948 F.2d 1264 (Fed. Cir. 1991).

**33)** *Id.* at 1266.

**34)** *Id.* at 1268 (emphasis added, citations omitted).

In this case, an article of manufacture contained a characteristic that by inspection could tell it readily possessed. It just so happened that the reference teaching the manufacture was silent on the issue. By comparison, in *Schering*, there was no recognition that the '233 patent could serve as an anticipatory reference because the entire molecule was simply missing from the prior art reference. It was only after Schering spent significant resources isolating and identifying the metabolite that the identity of the molecule was revealed. Nevertheless, the courts have not carved out any exception for cases such as *Schering* and these new lines of inherency cases should be considered in any pharmaceutical patent strategy involving prodrugs or metabolites.

### 3.3.3
### Nonobviousness

The most subjective of the three attributes an invention must possess prior to qualifying for patent protection is that it must be nonobvious. Section 103 of the Patent Act states in part the following:

> A patent may not be obtained though the invention is not identically disclosed or described as set forth in section 102 of this title, if the differences between the subject matter sought to be patented and the prior art are such that the subject matter as a whole would have been obvious at the time the invention was made to a person having ordinary skill in the art to which said subject matter pertains. Patentability shall not be negatived by the manner in which the invention was made.[35]

Imagine Smith is the first person to invent a lamp attached to a reclining chair. Thus, by assumption, it is novel. It is certainly useful since it allows people to read in the dark while reclining. Imagine now that the prior art consists of a substantial amount of chair art and lamp art. Smith is the first person, however, to bring these two disparate arts together into a unitary invention. Is the invention obvious? The statute is of little guidance since it, perhaps ironically, does not define what is meant by obvious. That task has been left to the courts and over the years, several definitions and tests have emerged. In the seminal case of *Graham v. John Deere*, the Supreme Court laid out a four-part test to aid in the determination on whether an invention was obvious over the prior art. Under that test, the following four factors are examined:

1) The scope and content of the prior art
2) Differences between the prior art and the claims at issue
3) The level of ordinary skill in the art
4) Secondary considerations such as commercial success, long felt but unsolved needs, failures of others,[36] and the like.

**35)** 35 U.S.C. § 103(a).

**36)** See *Graham v. John Deere Co.* 383 US 1, 17 (1966).

The so-called *Graham* factors also do not define obviousness but instead describe the criteria to use in an obviousness analysis. The Federal Circuit attempted to clarify by adopting the "TSM" test. TSM stands for "teaching–suggestion–motivation" and under this test, one looks at a combination of prior art and asks whether there is enough of a connection in the art, which would lead one of ordinary skill in the art to connect the art in such a way as to come up with the claimed invention. In other words, it seeks to determine "whether a person of ordinary skill in the art possessed with the general problem facing the inventor, would have been led to make the combination recited in the claims."[37] The TSM test may come explicitly from the prior art or may be implicit.[38]

Under the TSM test, one might, or might not find Smith's invention obvious. What the test would require would be some sort of suggestion, motivation, or teaching which would enable one of ordinary skill in the art to combine the prior art references to achieve Smith's invention at the time Smith filed for his patent. If some sort of TSM could be found, the invention would be obvious. A weakness of this test is that in areas where there is little prior art, it is difficult to find an invention obvious. This criticism was levied against the test in the early days of Internet patents when the paucity of prior art led the PTO to grant many patents despite the feelings of professionals in the industry that the patented inventions would have been obvious to make even without prior art teachings. Perhaps partly in response, in 2007, the Supreme Court revisited the Federal Circuit's obviousness analysis in the case of *KSR v. Teleflex*[39] and although it did not eliminate the TSM test, it did remove it as the sole arbiter of whether an invention is obvious. In a now oft-quoted passage, the Supreme Court ruled the following:

> When there is a design need or market pressure to solve a problem and there are a finite number of identified, predictable solutions, a person of ordinary skill has good reason to pursue the known options within his or her technical grasp. If this leads to the anticipated success, it is likely the product not of innovation but of ordinary skill and common sense. In that instance the fact that a combination was obvious to try might show that it was obvious under § 103.[40]

Turning back to Smith, it is clear that under the *KSR* approach, a patent application directed to the lamp–chair combination would not be valid. Presented with a chair and a lamp, one could readily argue that the combination would be obvious to try with a reasonable expectation of success without having to worry about the teachings or suggestions to combine from the prior art.

**37)** *Alza Corp. v. Mylan Loboratories*, 464 F.3d 1286, 1290 (Fed. Cir. 2006, citations omitted).

**38)** *Id.*

**39)** 550 U.S. 398 (2007).

**40)** *Id.* at 421.

In the pharmaceutical arts, *KSR* lowers the bar for finding an invention obvious. Yet, regardless of which test is employed, whether the prior art or an obvious to try argument prevails, the unpredictability of the claimed invention plays an important role in the analysis. When presented with a new compound to examine, the PTO (and the courts) apply a "lead compound" analysis as it relates to the third *Graham* factor, namely the differences between the claimed invention and the prior art. This analysis "often turns on the structural similarities and differences between the claimed compound and the prior art compounds."[41] The examiner or court compares the claimed invention to the closest prior art compound (the lead compound) and determines whether it would have been obvious, at the time the application was filed, to transform the lead compound into the claimed compound with a reasonable expectation of success. The greater the differences between the lead compounds and the claimed compounds, the harder it is to mount a successful obviousness attack.

This lead compound analysis has particular relevance in the area of prodrugs and metabolites as a recent lower court decision illustrates.

In *Daiichi Sankyo v. Mylan*,[42] a trial court rule that Sankyo's patent covering the active ingredient in Benicar® was not obvious in view of the prior art presented at trial for failing the obviousness prong of patentability. Claim 13 of the 133 page U.S. Patent No. 5,616,599 was directed to olmesartan medoxomil, the active ingredient in Benicar. Benicar is an antihypertensive agent that works by blocking the angiotensin receptor and is within the class of angiotensin converting enzyme inhibitors ("ACE Inhibitors"). Mylan's only challenge to the patent was a lack of obviousness based on several prior art references: DuPont's '069 and '902 patents and 13 scientific articles relating to work done in this field by DuPont.

The first ACE inhibitor introduced to the market was DuPont's losartan (see Figure 3.2) that later was marketed by Merck as Cozaar®

Sankyo's research led it to develop a compound with greater activity than losartan, called olmesartan. Poor oral absorption led Sankyo to form the ester derivative as a prodrug that became known as olmesartan medoxomil (Figure 3.2).

In addition to the '069 patent, DuPont had filed an additional patent application, which matured into the '902 patent, which discloses a number of other related structures with varying lower alkyl substituents at the 4-imidazole position and the 5-position being either an aldehyde or a carboxylic acid.

In a complex trial, Mylan argued that the six compounds disclosed in the '902 patent constitute lead compounds from which it would have been obvious to develop olmesartan medoxomil.[43] "Here, lead compound is defined as a compound with known properties that a medicinal chemist uses as a starting point for drug development."[44] The court, however, disagreed and found that a medicinal chemist would not have used any of the compounds disclosed in the '902 patent as a lead because numerous other second-generation ACE inhibitors existed at the time of

41) *Eisai Co. Ltd. v. Dr. Reddy's Laboratories, Ltd.*, 533 F.3d 1353, 1356-7 (Fed. Cir. 2008).

42) 670 F. Supp. 2d 359 (O. N. J. 2009).

43) *Id.* at 375, −6.

44) *Id* at 375.

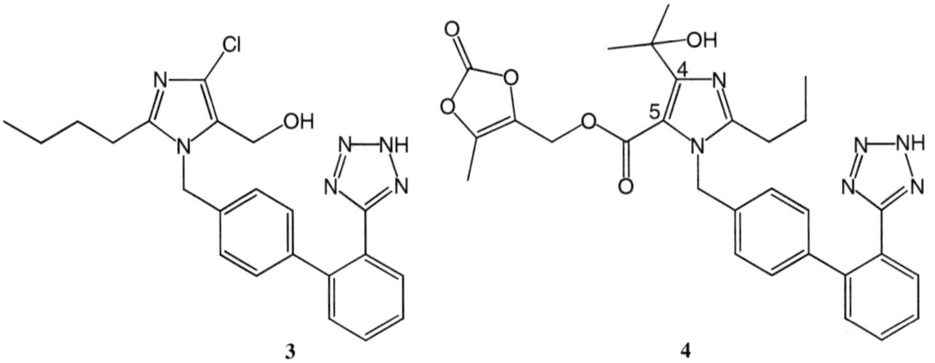


**Figure 3.2** Structures of losartan (**3**) and olmesartan medoxomil (**4**).

filing which exhibited better efficacy than the six compounds identified in the '902 patent.[45] The court further found that even if the compounds disclosed in the '902 patent were considered lead compounds, the structural differences between the purported leads and the claimed compound at the 4 and 5 ring positions of the imidazole ring were substantial. For example, at the 4-position, the court found that olmesartan medoxomil's use of hydrophilic isopropyl alcohol imparted "critical structural differences" on the molecule as compared with the lipophilic small alkyls in the '902 patent. At the 5-position, the court found that the prodrug functionality was key in distinguishing olmesartan medoxomil from the Mylan leads. Turning to documents showing that DuPont had failed to make a successful medoxomil product with one of the examples, the court found that this "highlights the significant differences in overall structure between olmesartan medoxomil and the '902 patent compounds."[46]

The court then looked at whether there was any motivation or suggestion in the prior art to achieve the claimed invention.[47] Finding that a medicinal chemist of ordinary skill would not wish to have a hydrophilic substituent at the 4-position in the ring, the court ruled that there would be no motivation to make that substitution. As for the 5-position in the ring, the court found that Mylan failed to establish that "such a person would have been motivated to transform the '902 patent compounds into a prodrug."[48] Citing trial testimony, the court found that innovators "'avoid prodrugs' because 'there are problems in determining whether the prodrug itself has pharmacology' and 'whether the conversion of the prodrug to the active form is reproducible." Indeed, the court went on to state that as of 1991, the date the

**45)** Mylan presumably argued that the '902 patent compounds were leads most likely because they were closer in structure to olmesartan medoxomil than any other potential leads.

**46)** *Id* at 378.

**47)** Interestingly, the court cites *KSR* earlier in its opinion, but not during this analysis. The Court of Appeals for the Federal Circuit, however, affirmed and explicitly cited *KSR*. See Mylan u. Matrix, 2010 WL 3504 759 at +4 (September 9, 2010 Fed. Cir.)

**48)** *Id.* at 380.

patent application that matured into the '599 patent was filed, "medicinal chemists approached the creation of a prodrug as a 'last resort,' 'a desperation, last-ditch approach' that was unpredictable."[49] Focusing on the facts of the particular case, the court also found that the medoxomil moiety would not have been considered a viable ligand due to failures by DuPont to make medoxomil derivatives of one of the compounds cited in the '902 patent.[50] Thus, the lack of a motivation to make olmesartan medoxomil by combining the prior art references was unable to convince the court that the patent was obvious and should be declared invalid.

The Federal Circuit has carried the lead compound analysis further and applied the *KSR* test in other cases. For example, *Ortho-McNeil Pharmaceutical, Inc. v. Mylan Laboratories Inc.*,[51] the court found in favor of Ortho-McNeil and rejected Mylan's argument that the patent covering Topomax® was invalid for lack of nonobviousness. Mylan advanced the argument that one of ordinary skill in the art when faced with designing an antidiabetes drug would "necessarily design an FBPase inhibitor."[52] Applying the *KSR* test, the court ruled that "contrary to Mylan's characterization, [the invention of Topomax does not present a finite (and small in the context of the art) number of options easily traversed to show obviousness"[53] as indicated by *KSR*. The court cited the numerous decisions and alternative paths a skilled artisan would have to face in the road to developing such a drug and concluded that the range of options is not a "small and finite number of alternatives that *KSR* suggested might support an inference of obviousness."[54] The court ruled that Mylan's expert arrived at his incorrect conclusion by merely retracing the inventor's path with the benefit of hindsight. In doing so, he "discounted the number and complexity of the alternatives."[55] This type of hindsight reasoning runs counter to the clear dictate of section 103 that requires that obviousness be determined "at the time the invention was made."[56] Thus, a way to counter both the TSM test and the more liberal *KSR* standard is to show that the prior art is unpredictable thus making it difficult to state that the invention is obvious.

A further example of this unpredictability was discussed in *Sanofi-Synthelabo v. Apotex, Inc.*[57] In that case, Sanofi asserted the patent covering the active enantiomer in Plavix® against Apotex, who countered that the patent was invalid for several reasons including obviousness. A central theme of Apotex's attack was that as the racemate was known in the prior art, it would have been obvious to separate the racemate, which has only one chiral center, into the two enantiomers. The Federal Circuit, however, relying on testimony and evidence advanced at trial ruled that "the

**49)** *Id.* (citations omitted).
**50)** *Id.*
**51)** 520 F.3d 1358 (Fed. Cir. 2008).
**52)** *Id.* at 1364.
**53)** *Id.*
**54)** *id.*
**55)** *Id.*
**56)** 35 U.S.C. § 103(a); see also *id.*
**57)** 550 F.3d 1075 (Fed. Cir. 2008).

result of this separation of enantiomers was unpredictable"[58] and affirmed the lower court's decision that the patent was not invalid for being obvious.

In an obviousness analysis, a court will determine whether a *prima facie* case of obviousness has been met. The discussions above focus on whether there is enough evidence that, at first glance, appears to suggest that the patented invention may be obvious which, if so, establishes a *prima facie* case. In the chair/lamp analogy, one can readily assume that the rich prior art makes a good case that, under an initial observation, that combination is obvious. Assuming that to be true, it is still possible, however, that the invention survives an obviousness attack. For example, suppose that the chair–lamp combination is a smashing commercial success. Such sales data could be used to rebut the *prima facie* case by suggesting the despite the fact that the invention appears obvious, robust sales suggest that the invention fits a niche or need that was absent in the market. In other words, had it been obvious, someone else should have come up with the invention but failed to do so. Such facts as commercial success and long-felt need are called "secondary consideration of nonobviousness."[59] In addition to these secondary considerations, applicants often rely on unexpected results to rebut a *prima facie* case of obviousness. Patent applications for combination products often get initial obviousness rejections during examination at the PTO. A common way to refute these rejections is to present data that the combination product provides a synergistic rather than an additive effect.[60] The PTO assumes that an additive effect is to be expected whereas a synergistic effect is unexpected and, depending on the magnitude and quality of the data, can be successfully employed to rebut the *prima facie* case of obviousness.

In the *Sankyo* case, the court found that "olmesartan medoxomil exhibits unexpected results as compared to the '901 patent compounds in terms of potency, drug–drug interaction, insurmountable antagonism, inverse agonism, and other rehabilitative properties."[61] The court compared the unexpected results to the '902 patent compounds because "the results must be shown as unexpected compared with the closest prior art."[62] Thus, at trial, the facts supported Sankyo's position that the '599 patent was rightly awarded by the PTO which was confirmed on appeal.[63]

Over the past several years, courts have focused significant energy on evaluating the strengths of pharmaceutical patents from an obviousness perspective. A common thread both from the TSM test and from the less restrictive *KSR* standard is that the more unpredictable the invention, the less likely that the PTO or a court or jury will find the invention obvious. For example, in the area of polymorph patents, a speaker

**58)** *Id.* at 1090.

**59)** See *Graham* 383 U.S. at 17.

**60)** The courts have ruled that in order to be unexpected, the properties or results claimed must show differences in "kind and not merely in degree" from the prior art results. *In re Huang*, 100 F.3d 135, 139 (Federal Circuit 1996).

**61)** 670 F. Supp. 2d at 382.

**62)** *Id.*

**63)** The case was affirmed on September 9, 2010. The opinion currently is available at 2010 WL 3504 759.

representing the PTO gave a presentation recently stating that it would almost never be appropriate to issue an obviousness rejection for a polymorph claim because the art is so unpredictable.[64] It may help to view this as the gold standard for trying to protect prodrug patent claims from inevitable obviousness attacks. A caveat on unpredictability, however, it is not enough to say that the field of prodrugs or pharmaceuticals leads to unpredictable behavior. More specific arguments are necessary. A recent case from the Federal Circuit makes that clear.

In *In re Kubin*,[65] Amgen appealed a ruling by the Patent Office administrative law board[66] (hereafter "Board") that upheld an examiner's determination that a biotechnology patent application sought by Amgen was invalid for failing the nonobviousness requirement. The application at issue claimed DNA molecules encoding Natural Killer Cell Activation Inducing Ligand (NAIL). The court evaluated a representative claim as follows:

> An isolated nucleic acid molecule comprising a polynucleotide encoding a polypeptide at least 80% identical to amino acids 22-221 of SEQ ID NO: 2, wherein the polypeptide binds CD48.[67]

The Board rejected the claim as obvious primarily over two references: U.S. Patent 5,688,690 (Valiante) and a laboratory manual (Sambrook).[68] According to the Board, Valiante taught a receptor protein called "p38" that Amgen agreed is the same protein as NAIL.[69] Valiante also taught that "[t]he DNA and protein sequences for the receptor p38 may be obtained by resort to conventional methodologies known to one of skill in the art."[70] Turning to Sambrook, the Board found that conventional techniques, such as the ones disclosed in Sambrook, were used by Amgen to "isolate and sequence the gene that codes for NAIL."[71] Finally, the Board determined that due to NAIL's important immunochemical role, a scientist of ordinary skill would have been motivated to apply the conventional methodologies of Sambrook and Valiante to isolate NAIL cDNA as required by the claims.[72] Thus, citing *KSR*, the Board ruled that it would have been obvious to isolate NAIL cDNA under the obvious-to-try rubric.[73]

On appeal, the court agreed with the examiner and held the invention to fail for lack of nonobviousness.[74] The court largely followed the reasoning of the Board, and also

**64)** Presentation by PTO at Biotechnology/Chemical/Pharmaceutical Partnership Meeting on September 2, 2009 on Polymorph Patents.

**65)** 561 F.3d 1391 (Fed. Cir. 2009).

**66)** This administrative body is called the Board of Patent Appeals and Interferences and was discussed earlier in this chapter.

**67)** *Id.* at 1353.

**68)** Sambrook J. *et al.* (1989). *Molecular Cloning: A Laboratory Manual*, 2nd ed, pp. 43–84.

**69)** 561 F.3d at 1354.

**70)** *Id.* quoting Valiante at column 7, lines 49–51.

**71)** *Id.* at 1355.

**72)** *Id.*

**73)** See *id.*

**74)** *Id.* at 1361.

held that under *KSR*, no special rules exist for examining biotechnology patent applications.[75] In other words, general arguments about the unpredictability of pharmaceutical or biotechnology applications will not defeat obviousness attacks.

So what kinds of methods exist for attacking obviousness challenges? Common patent claims in the pharmaceutical arts include method of treatment claims in the United States. For example, suppose a prodrug is shown to have a particular effectiveness against a bacterial strain. If the minimum dose is much less than that of a corresponding compound in the prior art, that dosage could be the basis of an unexpected results argument. Even for patent compound claims, *in vivo* tests in animals can be used to show results that are much better than those of the prior art. The concept of a "teaching away" can also be powerful. Suppose a prior art references teaches a potential lead compound and discusses that water solubility is important for the compound to act. In this instance, if the claimed compound has a lower water solubility and is nevertheless effective, however, the prior art teaches away from the claimed invention. Accordingly, one of ordinary skill in the art would not have used the reference in order to try and achieve the invention. This strategy could also be used under an "obvious to try" *KSR* approach by arguing that it would not have been obvious to try if researchers in the field at the time that an application for patent was filed would have not thought that the approach used in the invention was workable.

## 3.4 Conclusion

Strategies for procuring and defending patents in the pharmaceutical arts are by their very nature fact specific. Good patent practitioners rely on solid scientific results to craft a patent strategy. This practitioner believes that it is in the best interest of pharmaceutical companies to have patent attorneys who understand the science driving the company and to have scientists who understand the importance of patent protection and appreciate the rudimentary basics of inventorship, patentability, FDA approval process, and how patent law and FDA intersect under the Hatch-Waxman Act. Prodrug and/or metabolite patents add an extra level of complexity because of scientific and regulatory challenges as well as the inherency niche, discussed above, that acts as a trap for the unwary. As if these challenges were not enough, the recent court decisions in obviousness have made it even more difficult to insulate pharmaceutical patents from attacks. This is not to say it is time to give up. It does mean that scientists and patent attorneys need to work closely together to understand and appreciate the prior art, determine what is and what is not predictable about the invention, and evaluate how and when it is best to protect the invention.

75) *Id.* at 1360.

# Part Two
# Prodrugs Addressing ADMET Issues

*Prodrugs and Targeted Delivery: Towards Better ADME Properties.* Edited by Jarkko Rautio

ISBN: 978-3-527-32603-7

# 4
# Increasing Lipophilicity for Oral Drug Delivery

*Majid Y. Moridani*

## 4.1
## Introduction

Oral drug delivery is an ideal and preferable route of drug administration. When given orally, drugs are generally absorbed in intestinal lumen through passive absorption or carrier-mediated transporters [1]. To be absorbed orally, drugs should have optimum lipid solubility so they can permeate across biological membranes. Often, drug molecules have functional groups that are highly ionizable at physiological pH of intestine hence making them very water soluble and lipid insoluble. They may also possess many nonionizing polar groups such as alcohol functional groups with high solubility in aqueous media preventing the drugs to permeate biological membranes. Prodrug approaches can be attempted to modify these polar nonionizing or ionizing functional groups to enhance their lipid solubility and hence permeability across biological membranes, where they can undergo hydrolysis by esterases present in enterocyte, plasma, and liver [2–5] (Figure 4.1).

When designing prodrugs, a few points should be kept in mind. For instance, an ideal prodrug should be pharmacologically inactive, be stable over a wide range of pH, be water soluble and resistant to hydrolysis in the gastrointestinal tract prior to its absorption, posses a suitable partition coefficient value so that it can permeate across biological membrane, and be readily converted to the parent drug after its absorption. In this chapter, we will limit our discussion to the influence of p$K_a$, degree of ionization, partition coefficient, and distribution coefficient on lipid solubility and membrane permeability of drugs through gastrointestinal tract. We will also discuss about a few successful prodrug strategies with enhanced oral bioavailability of parent drugs in this chapter.

## 4.2
## p$K_a$, Degree of Ionization, Partition Coefficient, and Distribution Coefficient

Drugs can be absorbed by passive absorption process in their unionized form mainly from small intestine due to its larger surface area. Many drug entities have one or

*Prodrugs and Targeted Delivery: Towards Better ADME Properties.* Edited by Jarkko Rautio

ISBN: 978-3-527-32603-7

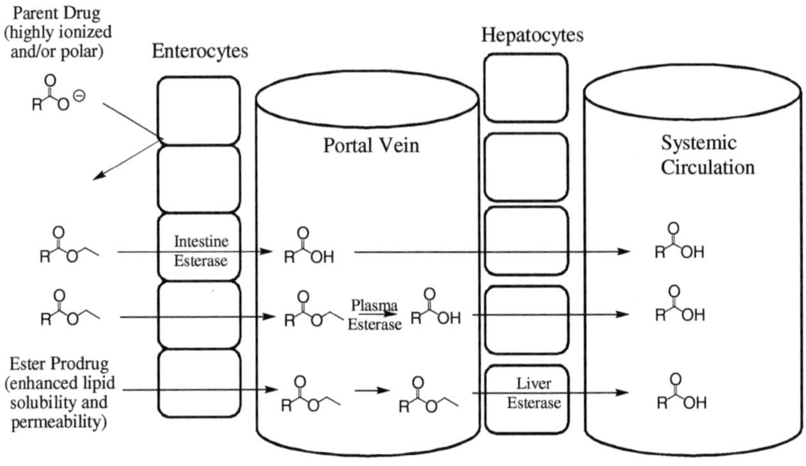


**Figure 4.1** Passive absorption and bioconversion of ester prodrugs through intestinal lumen. In this example, parent drug contains a highly ionizable carboxylate group that limits its absorption whereas its ester prodrug can readily permeate biological membranes due to the absence of ionization. Similarly, ester prodrugs of highly polar molecules with alcohol functional group(s) can be prepared to enhance their biological membrane permeability.

more functional groups that are ionized at the pH of gastrointestinal tract environment that can influence drugs permeability into the biological barrier. Table 4.1 lists the pH range for different parts of gastrointestinal tracts [6]. As can be seen from the data, the intestinal pH varies between 4.7 and 6.5 depending on the location; however, for most part the small intestine has a pH close to 6.5, which will be used in the discussion and log $D$ calculation throughout this chapter [6].

The tendency of a compound to cross biological membrane is generally expressed as partition coefficient or log $P$. A number of methods are used to determine and/or estimate the log $P$ of the drugs [7–11]. One method that is mostly used in pharmaceutical sciences is based on the measure of lipid solubility of the compound at octanol/water interface. However, it should be noted that the distribution

**Table 4.1** pH range of gastrointestinal tract.

| Location | pH range |
|---|---|
| Oral cavity | 5.2–6.8 |
| Stomach | 1.2–3.5 |
| Duodenum | 4.6–6.0 |
| Small intestine | 4.7–6.5 |
| Large intestine | 7.5–8.0 |

Modified from Ref. [6].

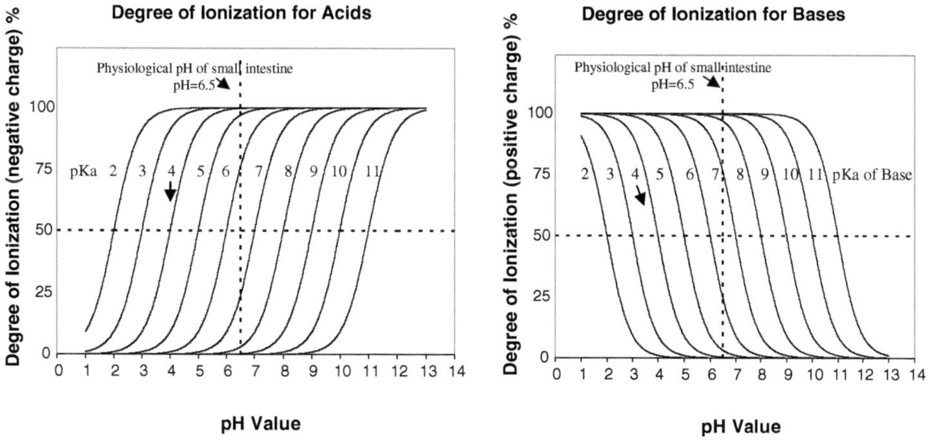


**Figure 4.2** The degree of ionization of acids and bases with $pK_a$ of 2–11 over pH range of 1–13. The vertical line at pH 6.5 highlights the degree of ionization for acids and bases at physiological pH of intestine.

coefficient (log *D*) but not log *P* of a compound determines its tendency to be absorbed by passive absorption via oral route. By definition, distribution coefficient is the partition coefficient of a compound at a given pH. Hence, distribution coefficient takes the degree of ionization into account for measuring the tendency of a compound to permeate across biological membrane at a given pH. The degree of ionization for acidic and basic compounds can be calculated from the following derivative formula using Henderson–Hasselbach equation. The following formulas were used to construct Figure 4.2.

Figure 4.2 shows the degree of ionization for acidic and basic compounds with $pK_a$ of 2–11 over a pH range of 1–13. For instance, a weak acid with $pK_a$ of 4.0 is ionized 99.7% at the physiological pH of 6.5 in small intestine; therefore, only 0.3% of the compound is available in its nonionized form, which can then permeate intestine effectively. However, a weak base with $pK_a$ of 4.0 at intestinal pH of 6.5 is ionized only 0.3% and hence 99.7% of the compound is nonionized, which can readily permeate biological membrane in intestine. A closer examination of Figure 4.2 reveals that generally acids with $pK_a$ of less than 5.0, and bases with $pK_a$ of greater than 8.0, are highly ionized at the pH 6.5 of the small intestine, which can potentially limit the drugs' absorption by oral route.

Because many compounds are ionized at physiological pH and only nonionized fraction of the compound can be available to permeate biological membrane, the distribution coefficient value of a compound is more useful in estimating a drug's tendency to be absorbed via oral route. The distribution coefficient of a drug can be estimated using the following formula in which log *D* is the partition coefficient at a given pH, α (ranging from 0–1) is the degree of ionization at that pH, and log *P* is the partition coefficient at octanol/aqueous interface where the compound is completely in its unionized form. log *D* can also be determined

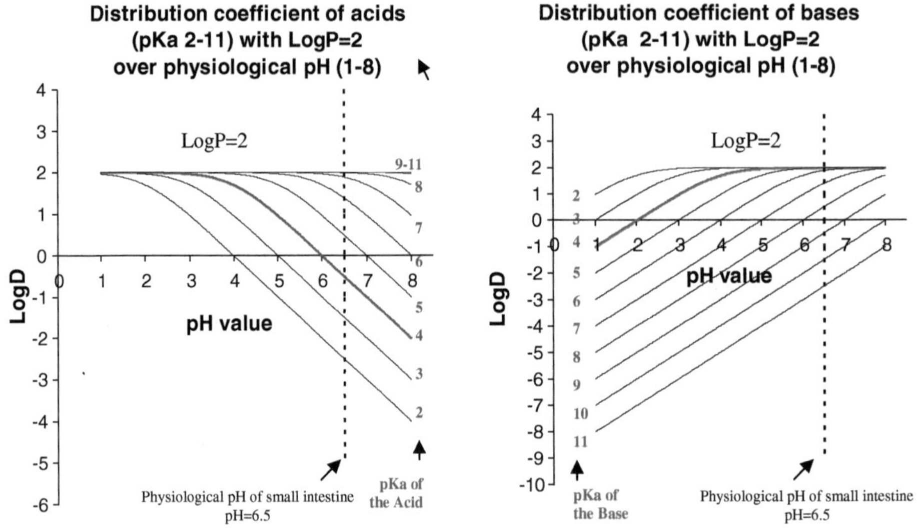


**Figure 4.3** Log $D$ plot of acids and bases containing only one ionizable group with p$K_a$ of 2–11 having a log $P$ value of 2 over a physiological pH range of 1.0–8.0.

experimentally by using a buffer with a desired pH, provided that the drug is stable at the given pH and there is no chemical reaction between the buffer ingredient and the drug.

$$\log D = \log[(1-\alpha)\times P],\quad \alpha = (0-1) \text{ is the degree of ionization at a given pH}$$

The above formula was used to construct Figure 4.3, which illustrates the relationship among pH, log $D$, and log $P$ for acids and bases containing only one ionizable group with p$K_a$ of 2.0–11.0 over a physiological pH range of 1.0–8.0. A log $P$ value of 2.00 was assumed for acids and bases in the calculation. The pH range of 1.0–8.0 represents physiological pH in the gastrointestinal tract (Table 4.1). For instance, for an acid with a p$K_a$ of 4.0, log $P$ of 2.00, the log $D$ value of the compound at pH = 6.5 can be calculated as (−0.52). This is because 99.7% of the drug is ionized at pH 6.5, hence, only 0.3% of the compound is unionized, which can partition by passive process through intestinal tract. On the other hand, for a weak base with p$K_a$ of 4.0, log $P$ of 2.00, the log $D$ value will remain almost equal to log $P$ at pH 6.5 of the intestine because the majority of a basic compound with p$K_a$ of 4.0 is unionized at pH = 6.5.

$\Delta$ (log $P$ − log $D$) is wider for acids with p$K_a$ values <5.0 and for bases with p$K_a$ values >8.0 at pH 6.5 of the intestine. In principle, acids with p$K_a$ >5.0 have log $D$ values closer to their log $P$ at pH 6.5 of intestine. On the other hand, bases with p$K_a$ <8.0 have log $D$ values closer to their log $P$ at pH of 6.5.

The above discussion highlights the influence of ionization on partition coefficient for drugs with one ionizable functional group. However, drugs often have multiple acidic and basic ionizable groups causing the compound to carry multiple positive and negative charges simultaneously at physiological pH preventing the ion from permeating across biological membrane in intestine by passive diffusion. In addition, the fed and the fasting states and the content of food present in gastrointestinal tract can also influence the stability and the permeability of the drugs through biological membrane [12, 13]. For instance, it is suggested that food increases the bioavailability of cefditoren pivoxil [14], a prodrug of cefditoren, by delaying the food and drug transit time in intestinal lumen and by preoccupying the esterases in intestine [15].

## 4.3 Prodrug Strategies to Enhance Lipid Solubility

Various functional groups such as alcohol, carboxylic acid, amine, phenol, amidine, phosphate, phosphinic, and phosphonate are present in the molecular structure of many drugs. Such highly polar compounds are suitable candidates for prodrug development with enhanced lipid solubility for oral administration. Functional groups such as carboxylate, phosphate, and phosphonate are highly ionized at the physiological pH of intestine; hence, only a small fraction of the compound is present in its unionized form, which can essentially permeate biological membrane by passive process. A prodrug moiety that can mask these functional groups can abolish their ionization at the pH of intestine; hence, minimizing the effect of pH on their distribution coefficient and biological membrane permeability. This is readily achievable by esterification of the functional groups by using either (1) a short-chain aliphatic alcohol such as methanol, ethanol, isopropyl alcohol, or butyryl alcohol in the presence and absence of a linker or (2) an acyl group such as acetyl or pivaloyl moieties attached through a spacer such as oxymethyl or oxyethyl (Figure 4.4).

Short-chain alcohol and acyl groups are used in prodrug design to enhance oral absorption of the drug. Long-chain aliphatic alcohol or acyl groups are used mostly in the preparation of prodrugs for slow release formulations such as IM injection (e.g., haloperidol decanoate) and are generally not used for the purpose of

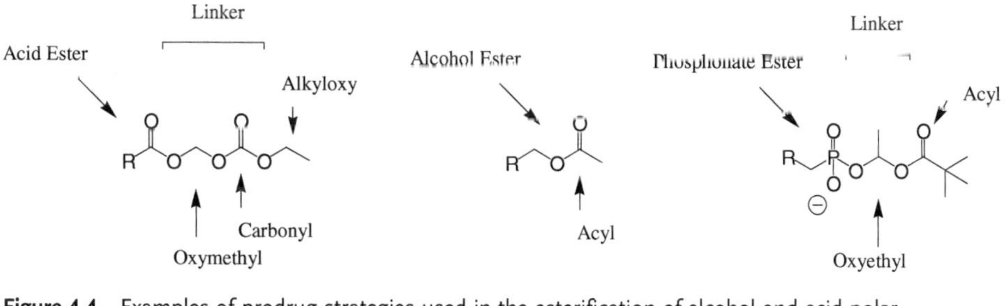


**Figure 4.4** Examples of prodrug strategies used in the esterification of alcohol and acid polar groups with or without a linker.

enhancing lipid solubility of a drug in oral administration. In addition to short-chain aliphatic alkyloxy and acyl groups, a few aromatic acids have also found limited uses as masking moiety in prodrug design to enhance lipid solubility and oral bioavailability of parent drugs.

Spacers such as carbonyl, oxymethyl, and oxyethyl are generally used to facilitate the hydrolysis of the masking prodrug moiety (Figure 4.4). The use of a spacer is especially important when a bulky group is present in the molecule that can potentially hinder hydrolysis of the ester group. Spacers generally undergo spontaneous decomposition after esterases act upon the masking moiety of the prodrug.

Similar esterification strategies can also be employed for polar alcohol-based drugs with no ionizable functional groups. Nucleotide-based drugs with an alcohol side chain or acidic functional groups are also suitable candidates for prodrug preparation. In another approach, the alcohol analogue can be used as the prodrug of carboxylic acid if the alcohol functional group can be rapidly metabolized/oxidized to the corresponding carboxylic acid. One such example is losartan [16]. Generally, the alcohol analogue has a better partition coefficient than carboxylic acid derivative mainly because it is not ionized at physiological pH 1.0–8.0 of gastrointestinal tract (Table 4.1) [6]. However, this strategy is mostly avoided in prodrug design due to polymorphisms in cytochrome P450 (CYP) enzymes and variability in oxidation of alcohol moiety to carboxylic acid group. One should also note that some publications do not regard losartan as a prodrug because it has a weak pharmacological activity in comparison to its metabolite. However, in this chapter, we regard losartan as a prodrug since its pharmacological activity is negligible in comparison to the metabolite.

Alcohol Functional Group
Carboxylate
Ionizable Functional Group
pKa =3.20
OH
N–NH
N
N
Cl
O
O⊖
Oxidation
E3174
(Pharmacologically
20 times more active)
Calculated LogP = 4.8
Calculated LogD(pH = 6.5) = 1.5
Losartan (a prodrug)
(Enhanced oral absorption)
Experimental LogP = 6.1
Calculated LogD(pH = 6.5) = 6.1

In the following, using some of the above prodrug strategies, we shall discuss a few successful examples of prodrug design with enhanced lipid solubility for oral absorption. The log $P$ values were predicted using ACD/ChemSketch software from Advanced Chemistry Development www.acdlabs.com. The p$K_a$ values were estimated using ALOGPS 2.1 program available from Virtual Computational Chemistry Laboratory at http://www.vcclab.org/lab/alogps/.

Log *D* was calculated at pH = 6.5 using formulas discussed in Section 4.2. If a compound possessed more than one ionizable group, all the p$K_a$ values were used to calculate the log *D* value at pH 6.5. For instance, oseltamivir carboxylate has two ionizable functional groups with p$K_a$ values of 4.60 and 7.90. If the degree of ionization for carboxylic acid functional group is used in calculation, the calculated log *D* will be (−1.46) at pH 6.5. However, if the degree of ionization for both functional groups is taken into account, the calculated log *D* will be (−2.88) at pH 6.5, which is far less than the log *P* value of oseltamivir carboxylate at 1.35.

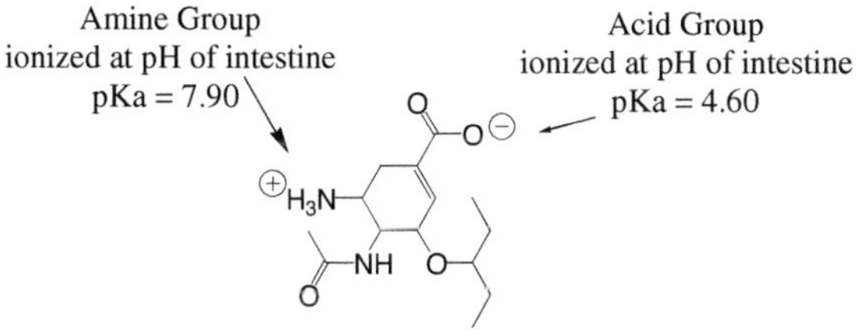


**Oseltamivir carboxylate**
**cannot be absorbed orally (<5% is absorbed)**
**Predicted LogP = 0.45**
**Calculated LogD$_{(pH = 6.5)}$ = - 2.88**

## 4.4 Prodrug Examples for Antibiotics

### 4.4.1 Bacampicillin

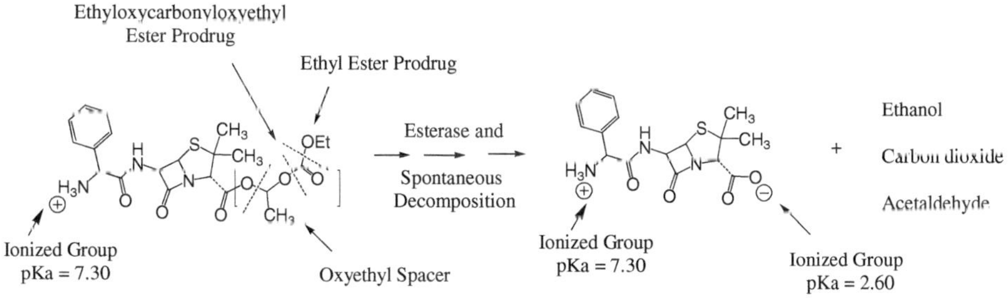


**Bacampicillin prodrug**
**(80-98% oral absorption)**
**Predicted LogP = 2.08**
**Calculated LogD$_{(pH = 6.5)}$ = 1.22**

**Ampicillin**
**(30-55% oral absorption)**
**Predicted LogP = 1.35**
**Calculated LogD$_{(pH = 6.5)}$ = - 3.41**

Bacampicillin is a prodrug of ampicillin. Although ampicillin has a reasonable absorption of 30–55% via oral route, its oral bioavailability can be significantly enhanced using a prodrug approach. After its absorption, bacampicillin ester prodrug is first hydrolyzed by esterase to produce ethanol and carbon dioxide, followed by spontaneous hydrolysis to release ampicillin and acetaldehyde. Ampicillin has lower lipid solubility than bacampicillin because of the presence of a carboxylic functional group in its chemical structure, which is significantly ionized at intestinal pH. One should also note that ampicillin is present in zwitterion form, which further limits its oral absorption. The esterification of carboxylic functional group can prevent the ionization of the group as a result of which the prodrug will no longer be a zwitterion. In addition to preventing the ionization, the esterification of carboxylic acid moiety of ampicillin increases the prodrug log *P* value. This enhances its membrane permeability and hence contributes to its nearly complete absorption when administrated orally. The comparison of their log *D* values at pH 6.5 reveals that the distribution coefficient value of bacampicillin prodrug is 4.6 orders of magnitude greater than ampicillin. The nearly complete absorption of the prodrug prevents excess of unabsorbed ampicillin from remaining in intestinal lumen, which can affect the natural microflora of the gastrointestinal tract and hence causing diarrhea [17].

### 4.4.2
### Carindacillin

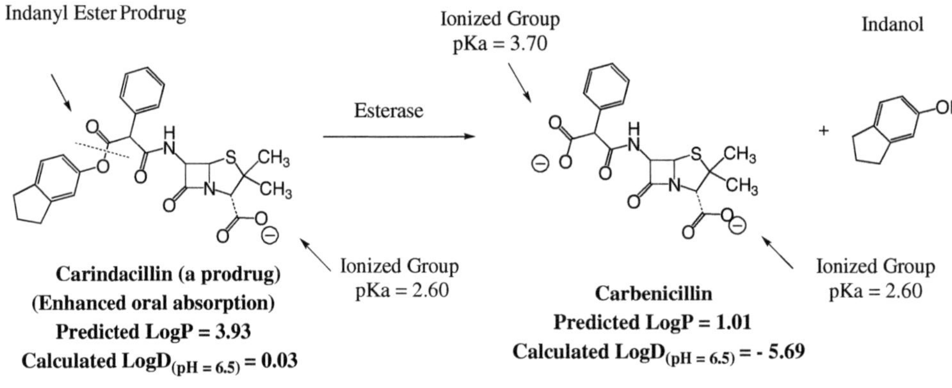


Carindacillin is one of the few examples of ester prodrugs that use an aryl moiety instead of an aliphatic moiety to mask a carboxylic acid functional group. The majority of protecting groups used in the preparation of ester prodrugs are short-chain aliphatic moieties. Carindacillin is an oral bioavailable indanyl ester prodrug of carbenicillin [18]. Antibiotic carbenicillin possesses two ionizing carboxylic acids one of which is masked by 5-indanol moiety. As a result of indanol esterification of carbenicillin, the log *P* value of the prodrug increases by three orders of magnitude to 3.93. However, the comparison of their log *D* values at pH 6.5 reveals that the distribution coefficient value of carindacillin prodrug is 5.7 orders of magnitude greater than carbenicillin. The esterification also reduces the number of ionizable group to one carboxylic acid group, which makes carindacillin a suitable substrate for monocarboxylic acid transporters [19]. Approximately 30–40% of carbenicillin indanyl is rapidly absorbed following oral administration [20, 21]. After absorption, carbenicillin indanyl is hydrolyzed to carbenicillin and indanol.

### 4.4.3 Cefditoren Pivoxil

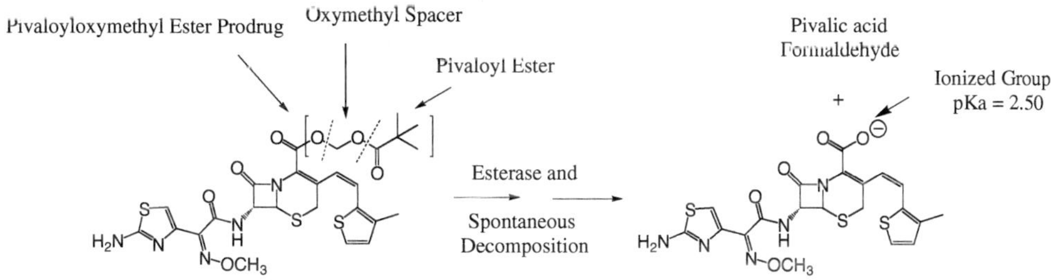


**Cefditoren Pivoxil**
**(inactive prodrug)**
**Predicted LogP = 4.33**
**Calculated LogD$_{(pH = 6.5)}$ = 4.33**

**Cefditoren**
**Predicted LogP = 3.07**
**Calculated LogD$_{(pH = 6.5)}$ = - 0.93**

Cefditoren pivoxil is an orally active cephalosporin broad-spectrum antibiotic [22]. The parent drug cefditoren is not orally active and is ionized greater than 99% at physiological pH 6.5 of intestine. Cefditoren pivoxil is a pivaloyloxymethyl ester prodrug of cefditoren [23]. The comparison of their log *D* values at pH 6.5 reveals that the distribution coefficient value of cefditoren pivoxil prodrug is 5.2 orders of magnitude greater than cefditoren. Generally, Δlog *D* value provides a better explanation why prodrugs are better absorbed from oral route than Δlog *P* value.

Pivaloyloxymethyl ester is one of the acyloxymethyl ester derivatives that are widely used to enhance lipid solubility of drugs with low oral bioavailability. The oxymethyl spacer group permits the ester group to readily undergo hydrolysis by enterocyte esterases. Pivalic acid by-product is relatively nontoxic because only a negligible amount is produced during the bioconversion of cefditoren pivoxil to cefditoren.

However, a large quantity of pivalic acid may lead to carnitine depletion and associated toxicity [24].

### 4.4.4
### Cefuroxime Axetil

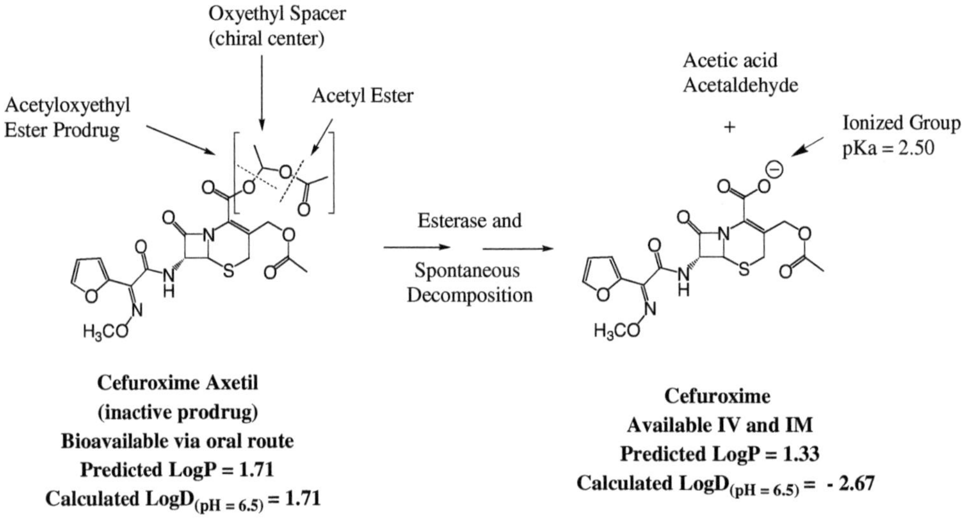


Cefuroxime axetil is an orally bioavailable ester prodrug of the cefuroxime. The parent active drug is not orally bioavailable and is given IV or IM [25]. Because of a highly ionizable carboxylic functional group in its chemical structure, cefuroxime is present only in its ionized form in intestinal lumen and hence it cannot permeate biological membranes. About 1% of cefuroxime is absorbed via oral route [26] whereas 25–45% of cefuroxime axetil is bioavailable via oral route [27]. The comparison of their log $D$ values at pH 6.5 reveals that the distribution coefficient value of cefuroxime axetil prodrug is 4.4 orders of magnitude greater than cefuroxime. Acetyloxyethyl ester prodrug of cefuroxime is not active biologically. The ester bond needs to be hydrolyzed by esterases to release cefuroxime as the active drug, acetic acid, and acetaldehyde as nontoxic by-products. The use of oxyethyl as a spacer has an advantage over oxymethyl because the latter forms formaldehyde, which is potentially more toxic than acetaldehyde. However, when oxymethyl is used as a spacer the amount of formaldehyde released is not large enough to cause a concern regarding toxicity [28]. One disadvantage in using an oxyethyl linker is the introduction of a new chiral center to cefuroxime, which is not a major concern in this case.

### 4.4.5
### Cefpodoxime Proxetil

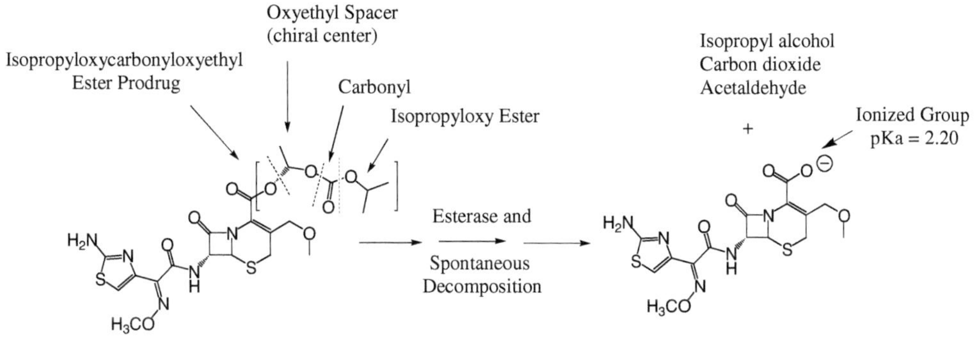


**Cefpodoxime Proxetil**
**(inactive prodrug)**
**can be absorbed via oral route**
**Predicted LogP = 2.17**
**Calculated $LogD_{(pH = 6.5)}$ = 2.17**

**Cefpodoxime**
**is not absorbed via oral route**
**Predicted LogP = 0.94**
**Calculated $LogD_{(pH = 6.5)}$ = - 3.36**

Cefpodoxime proxetil is used as an oral active antibiotic with a bioavailability of 50% [29]. Cefpodoxime proxetil is an isopropyloxycarbonyloxyethyl ester prodrug of cefpodoxime [30]. Cefpodoxime is not orally active because it is extensively ionized at intestinal pH. Isopropyloxycarbonyloxyethyl ester masks the ionizable carboxylic functional group and increases the lipid solubility of the prodrug for one order of magnitude to a log *P* value of 2.17. The comparison of their log *D* values at pH 6.5 reveals that the distribution coefficient value of cefpodoxime proxetil prodrug is 5.5 orders of magnitude greater than cefpodoxime parent drug. Cefpodoxime proxetil can permeate through biological membrane and is hydrolyzed by intracellular enterocyte esterases followed by spontaneous decomposition to active cefpodoxime drug, and isopropyl alcohol, carbon dioxide, and acetaldehyde as by-products, which are not toxic at quantities formed. One advantage of isopropyloxycarbonyl over pivaloyl ester is that the former moiety produces isopropyl alcohol that is nontoxic and is rapidly metabolized to acetone in the body, whereas pivaloyl ester prodrugs can potentially lead to carnitine depletion, an important entity involved in coenzyme A and β-oxidation of fatty acids [31].

## 4.5
## Antiviral Related Prodrugs

### 4.5.1
### Oseltamivir

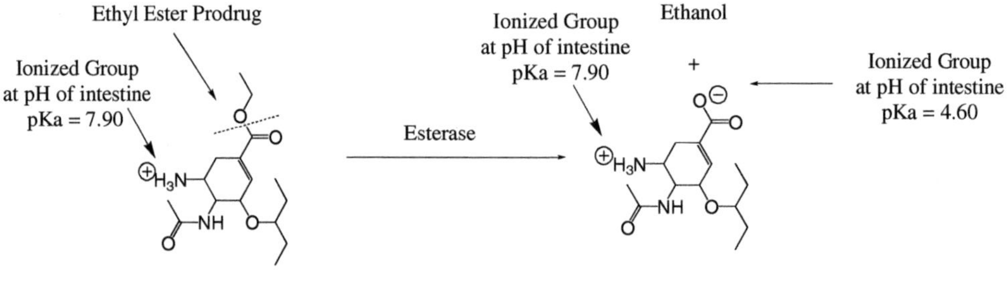


**Oseltamivir (a prodrug)**
**can be absorbed orally (80%)**
**Predicted LogP = 1.49**
**Calculated $\mathrm{LogD}_{(pH = 6.5)} = 0.07$**

**Oseltamivir carboxylate**
**cannot be absorbed orally (<5% is absorbed)**
**Predicted LogP = 0.45**
**Calculated $\mathrm{LogD}_{(pH = 6.5)} = -2.88$**

Oseltamivir is an ethyl ester prodrug of oseltamivir carboxylate. 80% of oseltamivir is orally bioavailable [37]. Oseltamivir carboxylate is highly ionized at physiological pH of intestine; hence, it is absorbed less than 5% when administered orally. The ethyl ester prodrug prevents the ionization of carboxylic acid group on oseltamivir carboxylate and significantly increases the partition coefficient of prodrug for one order of magnitude leading to an improvement in oseltamivir oral bioavailability. The comparison of their log *D* values at pH 6.5 reveals that the distribution coefficient value of oseltamivir prodrug is nearly three orders of magnitude greater than oseltamivir carboxylate drug. Oseltamivir is hydrolyzed by carboxylesterases to oseltamivir carboxylate drug and ethanol, which is a nontoxic by-product.

### 4.5.2
### Famciclovir

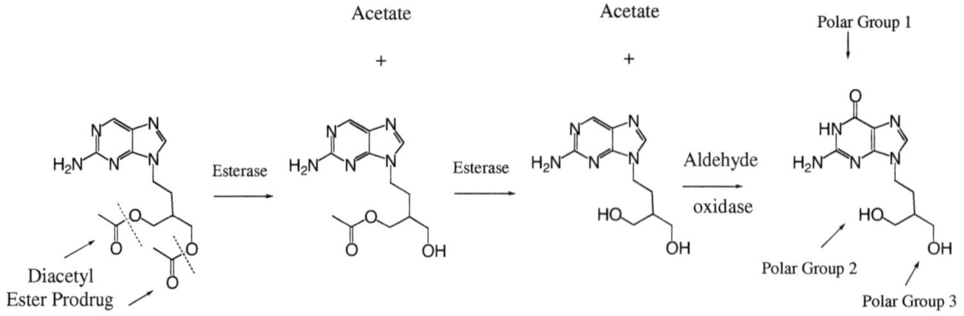


**Famciclovir (a prodrug)**
**can be absorbed orally (77% in man)**
**Predicted LogP = - 0.67**

**Deoxy Penciclovir**
**10% absorbed in rats**

**Penciclovir**
**is not orally active**
**(4% absorbed in man)**
**Predicted LogP = - 2.03**

Famciclovir is an orally bioavailable diacetyl ester prodrug of antiviral agent penciclovir [35]. Penciclovir is a nucleoside-based antiviral agent that is not orally active and can be absorbed through oral route for 4%. Although penciclovir lacks ionizable groups, it has many polar groups capable of forming hydrogen bonds with water molecules hindering penciclovir permeating biological membranes. Famciclovir design is focused on masking three polar groups present in penciclovir chemical structure as shown by arrows in the scheme. The acetylation of the two alcohol groups of penciclovir and removing the carbonyl oxygen group in the ring increases the lipid solubility of the prodrug famciclovir for 1.5 orders of magnitude and hence its bioavailability to 77% in man. After its absorption, famciclovir undergoes hydrolysis by esterases present in intestine and liver to form 6-deoxy penciclovir, which further is metabolized to penciclovir by liver aldehyde oxidase [36]. The acetate by-product is not toxic at the quantity it is formed.

## 4.5.3
## Adefovir Dipivoxil

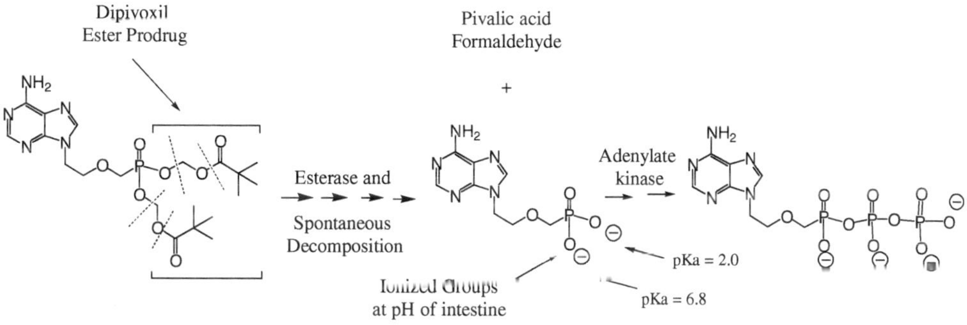


**Adefovir Dipivoxil (a preprodrug)**
**can be absorbed orally**
**Predicted LogP = 2.45**
**Calculated LogD$_{(pH = 6.5)}$ = 2.45**

**Adefovir (a prodrug)**
**cannot be absorbed orally**
**Predicted LogP = - 2.06**
**Calculated LogD$_{(pH = 6.5)}$ = - 6.74**

**Adefovir diphosphate**
**active drug**

Adefovir dipivoxil is an orally active bis-pivaloyloxymethyl ester prodrug of anti-hepatitis B drug adefovir. About 60% of adefovir dipivoxil prodrug is absorbed via oral route [32] whereas adefovir drug is not orally active due to the presence of a polar phosphonate moiety in its chemical structure [33]. The p$K_a$ values of phosphonate group of adefovir are 2.0 and 6.8 because of which phosphonate group is highly ionized at physiological pH of intestine hindering adefovir to permeate effectively through biological membrane. The esterification of phosphonate group of adefovir significantly increases the lipid solubility of adefovir dipivoxil prodrug by preventing the ionization of phosphonate group. The log *P* value and distribution coefficient value of adefovir dipivoxil prodrug is several orders of magnitude greater than adefovir. After oral administration and its absorption, adefovir dipivoxil is rapidly bioactivated by esterase followed by spontaneous decomposition to release adefovir, pivalic acid, and formaldehyde. The amounts of pivalic acid and formaldehyde formed are insignificant and hence nontoxic. Subsequent to hydrolysis, adefovir undergoes phosphorylation by kinases to form the active adefovir diphosphate metabolite [34].

### 4.5.4
### Tenofovir Disoproxil

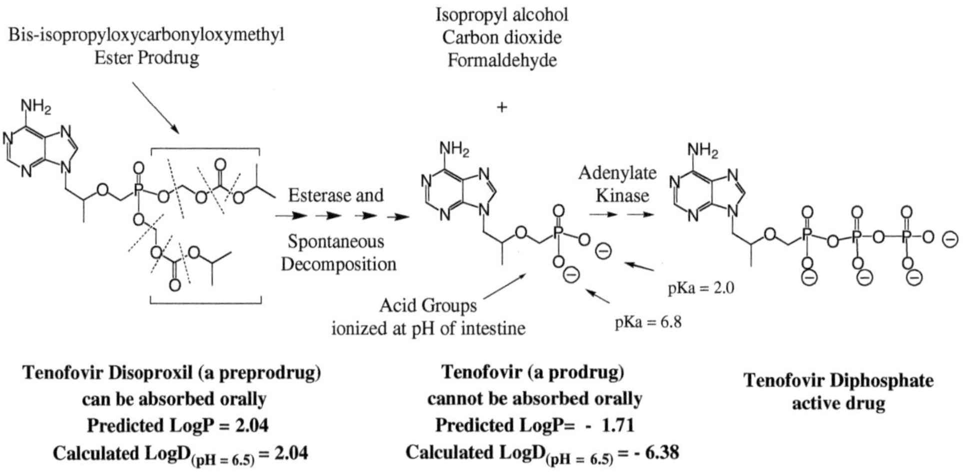


Tenofovir disoproxil is an orally active prodrug of antiviral agent tenofovir, which belongs to the class of nucleoside phosphonate with p$K_a$ of 2.0 and 6.8. Tenofovir is highly ionized at physiological pH of intestine with limited lipid solubility [38]. Tenofovir disoproxil is bis-isopropyloxycarbonyloxymethyl ester of tenofovir. The ester modification of tenofovir enhances the log $P$ value and log $D_{(\mathrm{pH}\,=\,6.5)}$ value of the prodrug tenofovir disoproxil for 3.7 and 8.4 orders of magnitudes, respectively. The prodrug is not ionized at physiological pH. Upon its absorption, tenofovir disoproxil prodrug is hydrolyzed by esterases and then by spontaneous decomposition to tenofovir parent drug [39]. During the process of hydrolysis, isopropyl alcohol, carbon dioxide, and formaldehyde are produced in nontoxic amounts. Oxycarbonyloxymethyl linker provides some space between the ester group and the parent drug to facilitate the action of esterase on tenofovir disoproxil prodrug. Oxycarbonyloxymethyl linker undergoes spontaneous decomposition to form tenofovir, which subsequently undergoes phosphorylation to form the active drug tenofovir diphosphate.

## 4.6 Cardiovascular Related Prodrugs

### 4.6.1 Enalapril

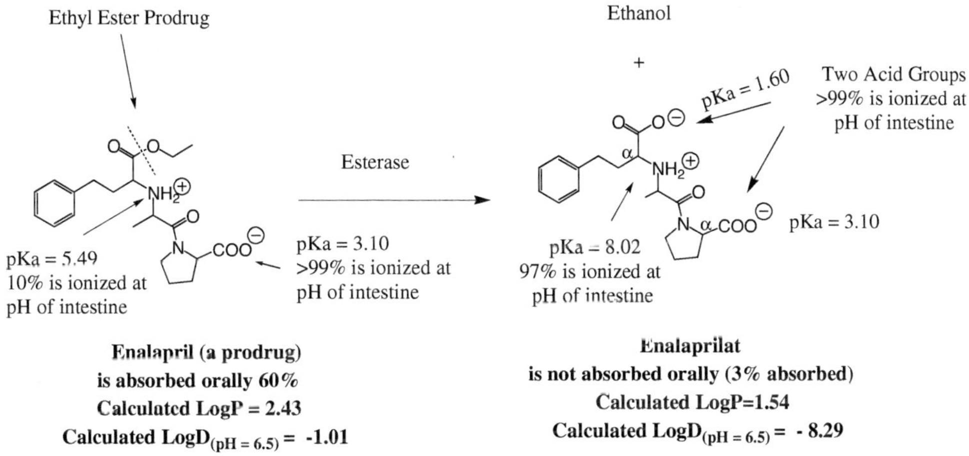


Enalapril is an ethyl ester prodrug of ACE inhibitor enalaprilat. Because of the presence of two carboxylic acids and an amine group in its chemical structure, enalaprilat is highly ionized at physiological pH of intestine and hence only 3% is absorbed via oral administration [40, 41]. The esterification of the carboxylic acid enhances the lipid solubility of the prodrug, abolishes the ionization of one of the carboxylic acid groups. The peptide like structure of enalapril provides a suitable substrate for intestinal peptide transporter. The p$K_a$ value of the amine group in enalaprilat is calculated to be 8.02, which is highly ionized at pH 6.5, whereas the p$K_a$ value of the amine group in enalapril prodrug is calculated to be 5.49, which is minimally ionized at pH 6.5.

Generally, the p$K_a$ values of carboxylic acids are considered to be around 4.5; however, the p$K_a$ values of carboxylic acid groups in enalaprilat are significantly lower due to the presence of an amine/amide group at alpha positions and the ability of one of the carboxylic acid group (p$K_a = 1.60$) to form an intramolecular hydrogen bond with amine group at alpha position. The higher p$K_a$ value for amine group of enalaprilat drug leads to a zwitterion formation, which contributes to the low oral bioavailability of enalaprilat. On the other hand, the amine group of enalapril is ionized only less than 10% at physiological pH of intestine (pH = 6.5). The comparison of their log $D$ values at pH 6.5 reveals that the distribution coefficient value of enalapril prodrug is nearly 7.3 orders of magnitude greater than enalaprilat.

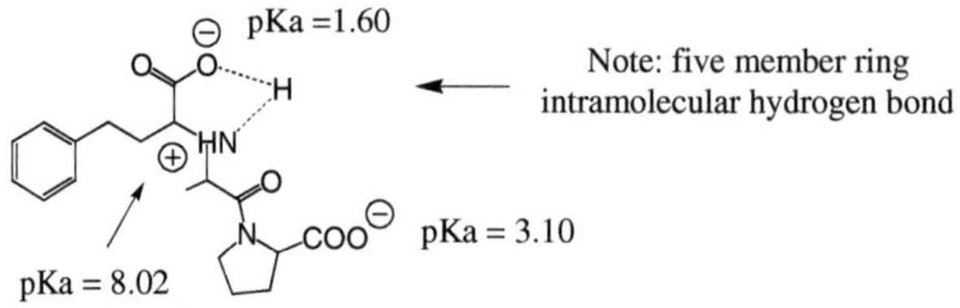


**Enalaprilat**

After its absorption from intestine, enalapril prodrug undergoes hydrolysis by liver carboxylesterase to enalaprilat and ethanol as a nontoxic by-product [40, 41]. The presence of both carboxylic acids groups and proline is needed for the inhibition of ACE enzyme by enalaprilat. Other examples of ethyl ester prodrugs of ACE inhibitors include moexipril, perindopril, quinapril, ramipril, spirapril, and trandolapril, which undergo a similar bioconversion [42].

### 4.6.2
### Fosinopril

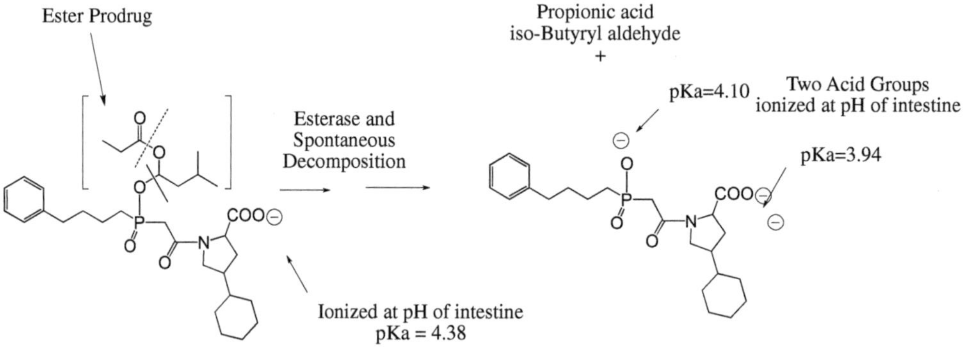


**Fosinopril (prodrug)**
**is absorbed orally (36%)**
**Calculated LogP = 6.32**
**Calculated LogD$_{(pH=6.5)}$= 4.20**

**Fosinoprilat**
**is not absorbed orally**
**Calculated LogP=4.58**
**Calculated LogD$_{(pH=6.5)}$= - 0.38**

Fosinopril is an orally active propanoyloxyisobutyl ester prodrug of ACE inhibitor fosinoprilat. Because it contains two acidic groups that are significantly ionized at physiological pH of intestine, fosinoprilat is not orally active [43–45]. Propanoyloxyisobutyl ester group masks the highly ionizable phosphinic group of fosinoprilat and hence makes the prodrug more lipid soluble and a suitable substrate for peptide transporter [46]. The $\Delta \log D$ values at pH 6.5 reveals that the distribution coefficient value of fosinopril prodrug is 4.6 orders of magnitude greater than fosinoprilat. Upon its absorption, fosinopril undergoes hydrolysis by esterases present in intestine and liver followed by spontaneous decomposition to active drug fosinoprilat, and propionic acid and isobutyl alcohol as by-products. Both by-products are safe because they can be metabolized in the body and are nontoxic in the quantities produced.

### 4.6.3
### Olmesartan Medoxomil

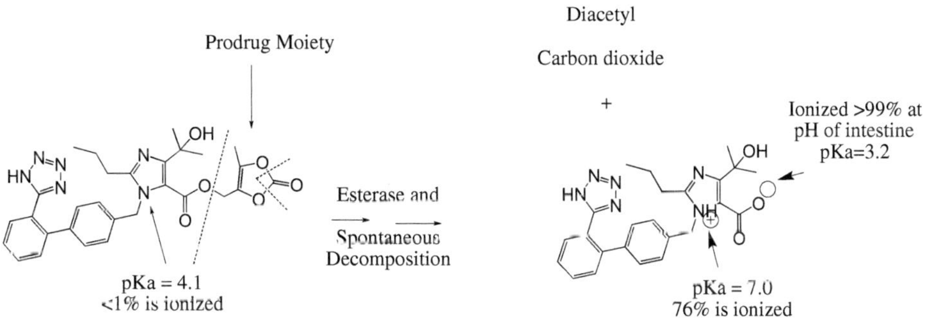


**Olmesartan Medoxomil (prodrug)**
**is absorbed orally**
**Calculated LogP = 4.70**
**Calculated $LogD_{(pH=6.5)}$= 4.69**

**Olmesartan**
**is not absorbed orally**
**Calculated LogP=3.19**
**Calculated $LogD_{(pH=6.5)}$= - 0.73**

Olmesartan medoxomil is an angiotensin II receptor blocker. Olmesartan medoxomil prodrug has a superior oral bioavailability to that of olmesartan. Due to significant ionization of carboxylic group present in its chemical structure, olmesartan has a limited oral bioavailability. Carboxylic acid groups generally have a p$K_a$ value of about 4.5. However, the p$K_a$ value of carboxylic acid in olmesartan is 3.2, which is significantly lower than 4.5. This is because olmesartan carboxylic acid group can form an intramolecular hydrogen bond with nitrogen atom in nearby imidazole group, which can lead to the formation of a zwitterion at pH 6.5. The esterification of carboxylate group not only completely abolishes the ionization of the carboxylic acid entity but also lowers the p$K_a$ value for the imidazole ring preventing the formation of a zwitterion. Hence, 99% of olmesartan medoxomil prodrug is in nonionized form. The Δlog *D* values at pH 6.5 reveals that the distribution coefficient value of olmesartan medoxomil prodrug is 5.4 orders of magnitude greater than the drug itself. Olmesartan medoxomil undergoes esterase hydrolysis [47–49] followed by spontaneous decomposition of masking group to form active parent drug olmesartan and nontoxic carbon dioxide and diacetyl by-products. Olmesartan medoxomil is an interesting ester prodrug because it was designed to be labile to plasma paraoxonase enzymes to avoid nonproductive metabolism by cellular esterases.

## 4.7 Lipophilic Prodrugs of Benzamidine Drugs

Lipophilic prodrugs of benzamidine-based drugs represent another important class of drugs amenable for lipophilic prodrug approach, and in these cases, the linkage would not be an ester type. In this chapter, we discuss two lipophilic prodrug examples of benzamidine-based drugs, namely, ximelagatran and dabigatran. Although the former was withdrawn from the market, the latter is marketed in Europe and Canada. Both ximelagatran and dabigatran are known as double prodrugs. This is because their designs are based on the modification of two highly ionizable groups present in the molecular structures of the parent drugs. Upon absorption, the prodrugs undergo hydrolysis and/or reduction in two-step processes to release the drugs.

### 4.7.1 Ximelagatran

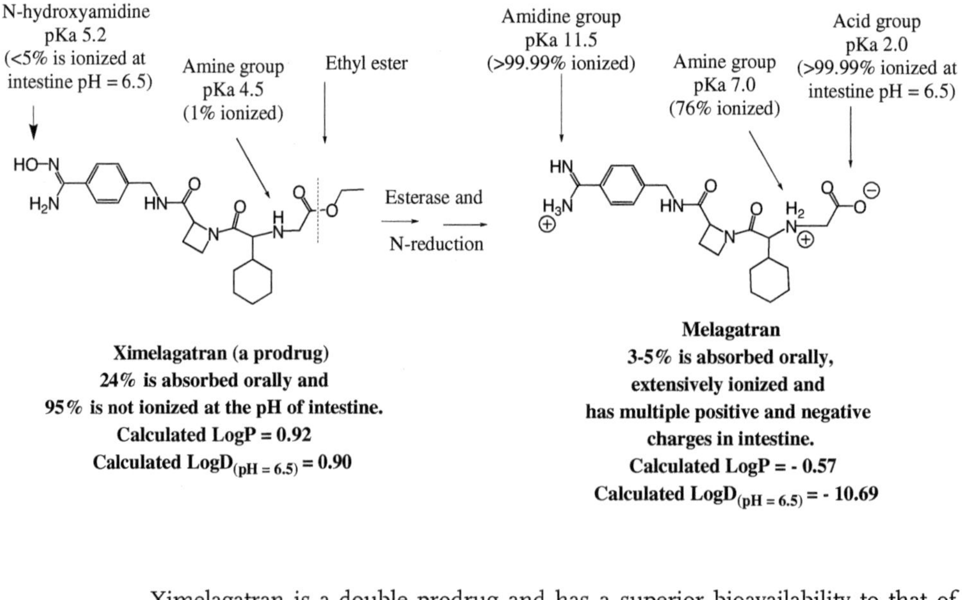


Ximelagatran is a double prodrug and has a superior bioavailability to that of melagatran [50, 51]. The double prodrugs mask two of the highly ionized groups of melagatran namely carboxylate and benzamidine groups. These modifications also reduces the p$K_a$ value of the amine group in the ximelagatran prodrug to 4.5; hence, preventing its ionization at pH 6.5. More than 95% of ximelagatran is in unionized form at pH 6.5 of intestine. In contrast, the parent drug melagatran not only is ionized more than 99.99% but also carries multiple positive and negative charges at physiological pH of 6.5 in intestine. Upon its absorption from intestine, ximelagatran undergoes esterase cleavage and N-reduction to release melagatran, a potent thrombin inhibitor. The $\Delta$log $D$ values at pH 6.5 reveals that the distribution coefficient value of ximelagatran prodrug is nearly 11.7 orders of magnitude greater than the melagatran itself.

## 4.7.2
## Dabigatran Etexilate

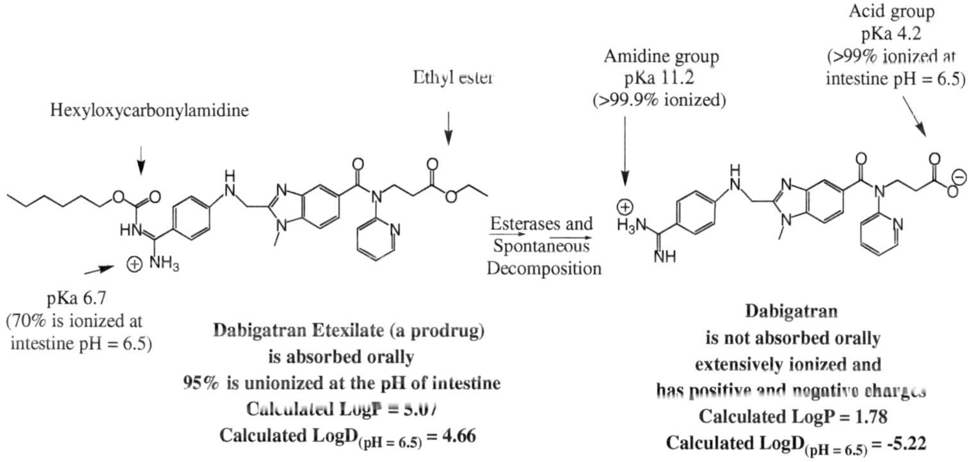


Dabigatran is a reversible, competitive, direct thrombin inhibitor that has been shown to be an effective antithrombotic agent and to be efficacious and safe in the prevention of thrombosis. However, it is not orally bioavailable. Dabigatran etexilate is an $n$-hexyloxycarbonyl (carbamylated) prodrug that is orally bioavailable. Dabigatran etexilate is rapidly absorbed from intestine [52], undergoes esterase enzymatic hydrolysis followed by spontaneous decomposition to release $n$-hexanol, carbon dioxide, and ethanol as nontoxic by-products and dabigatran as the parent drug. Dabigatran etexilate prodrug possesses higher lipid solubility than dabigatran [53]. The $\Delta$log $D$ values at pH 6.5 reveals that the distribution coefficient value of dabigatran etexilate prodrug is nearly 10 orders of magnitude greater than dabigatran itself.

## 4.8 Miscellaneous Examples

### 4.8.1 Capecitabine

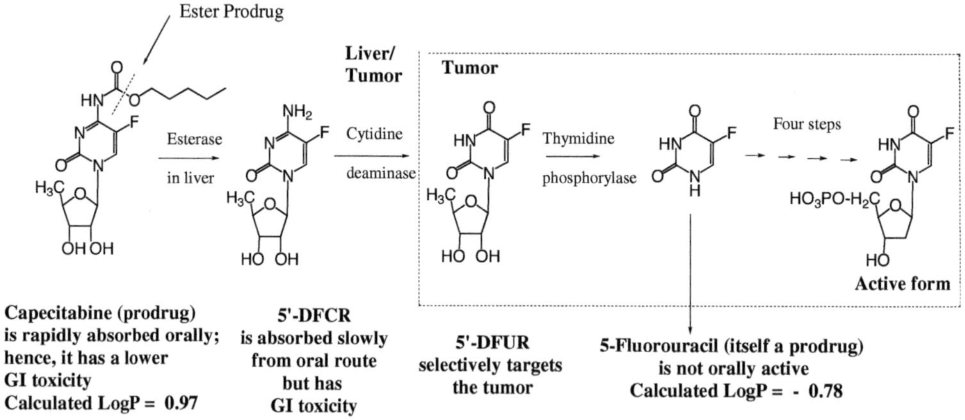


Capecitabine is an excellent example of successful prodrug design fulfilling multiple goals such as enhanced lipid solubility, enhanced oral bioavailability, reduced gastrointestinal toxicity, and tumor targeted prodrug bioactivation for treatment of metastatic breast and colorectal cancer. Capecitabine is an *n*-pentyloxycarbonyl (carbamylated) prodrug that is orally bioavailable. After absorption in intestine, capecitabine undergoes enzymatic hydrolysis by liver carboxylesterase followed by spontaneous decomposition to release *n*-pentanol, carbon dioxide, and 5′-DFCR. Then 5′-DFCR undergoes deamination to 5′-DFUR by thymidine deaminase present in liver and tumor. 5′-DFUR is selectively converted to 5-fluorouracil by thymidine phosphorylase present in tumors; hence, limiting toxicity in other organs [54, 55]. A higher log *P* value of 0.97 makes it possible for capecitabine to be orally bioavailable whereas 5-fluorouracil has a negative log *P* (−0.78), lacks oral bioavailability and is administered by infusion due to its higher rate of clearance.

### 4.8.2
### Mycophenolate Mofetil

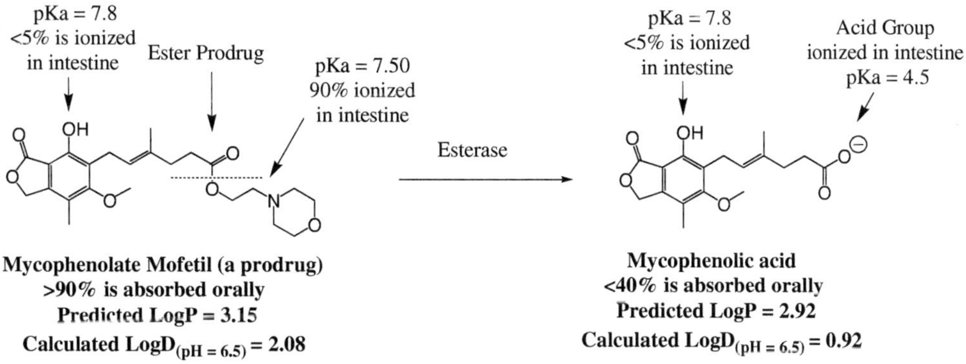


Mycophenolate mofetil is an oral prodrug of immunosuppressive agent mycophenolic acid [56, 57]. The mycophenolate mofetil prodrug is hydrolyzed by liver and enterocyte esterases to its active form mycophenolic acid. Its oral bioavailability is more than 90% in comparison to the active drug mycophenolic acid, which is less than 40% bioavailable when administered via oral route. In addition to a greater oral bioavailability, the variability in the plasma concentration range is significantly less for mycophenolate mofetil than for parent drug mycophenolic acid, suggesting that mycophenolate mofetil is a safer drug from a dosing perspective.

Mycophenolic acid is ionized >99% at the pH of intestine, which limits its absorption when administered orally. 4-(2-Hydroxyethyl)morpholine ester prodrug derivative has enhanced the oral bioavailability of the prodrug. About 10% of mycophenolate mofetil is not ionized at pH 6.5 of intestine, which makes it readily permeate across biological membranes. The Δlog *P* values at pH 6.5 reveals that the distribution coefficient value of mycophenolate mofetil prodrug is one order of magnitude greater than mycophenolic acid itself. Mycophenolate mofetil is a good example of the fact that limiting the ionization of a molecule can significantly increase the oral bioavailability of a prodrug without significantly changing its log *P* value [58].

### 4.8.3
### Misoprostol

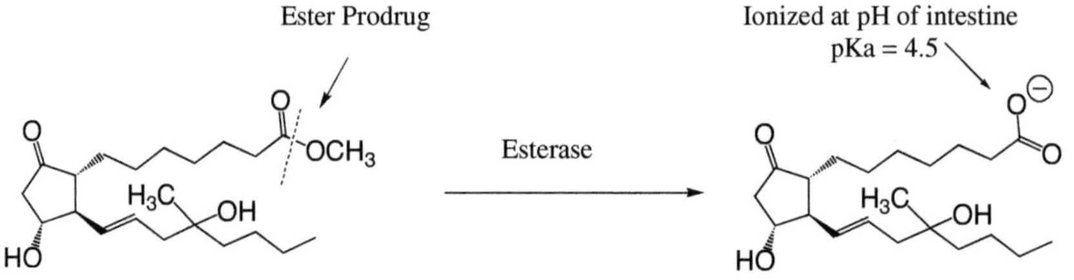


**Misoprostol is absorbed orally**
**Predicted LogP = 2.91**
**Calculated LogD$_{(pH = 6.5)}$ = 2.91**

**PGE1 analogue**
**Predicted LogP = 2.45**
**Calculated LogD$_{(pH = 6.5)}$ = 0.44**

Misoprostol is a methyl ester prostaglandin prodrug that is orally bioavailable and is used in the treatment of NSAID-induced gastrointestinal toxicity [59–61]. NSAIDs are one of the most commonly used therapeutic agents. Almost all of the current nonselective COX 1 and COX 2 inhibitors NSAIDs share the undesirable property of damaging gastric and intestinal mucosa, which can result in ulcers and gastrointestinal bleeding. The primary mechanism of action for NSAIDs is the inhibition of prostaglandins biosynthesis at cyclooxygenase step, which results in the inhibition of biosynthesis of protective prostaglandins in gastric mucosa. The use of PGE1 to reduce NSAID-induced damage to gastrointestinal tract is limited by its oral absorption whereas misoprostol, a prostaglandin methyl ester prodrug, is orally active and is used for the prevention of NSAID-induced gastric ulcers in patients at high risk. The esterification of PGE1 carboxylic acid group not only completely abolishes its ionization but also improves the log *P* and log *D* values of the misoprostol prodrug. The Δlog *D* values at pH 6.5 reveals that the distribution coefficient value of misoprostol prodrug is 2.5 orders of magnitude greater than PGE1.

### 4.8.4
### Additional Examples

Attempts are also made to increase lipid solubility of other drugs such as NSAIDs that are already orally bioavailable. The main reason behind this strategy is to increase lipid solubility of the drug so that the ester prodrugs can be absorbed more rapidly; hence, reducing gastrointestinal side effects of NSAIDs [62].

Other examples of orally bioavailable ester prodrugs include lovastatin, simvastatin, fenofibrate, and diphenoxylate [31]. Although their corresponding active drugs are also orally bioavailable only the prodrugs lovastatin and simvastatin are available on the market. On the other hand, both drugs fenofibric acid and difenoxin and their respective prodrugs fenofibrate and diphenoxylate are commercially available for prescription.

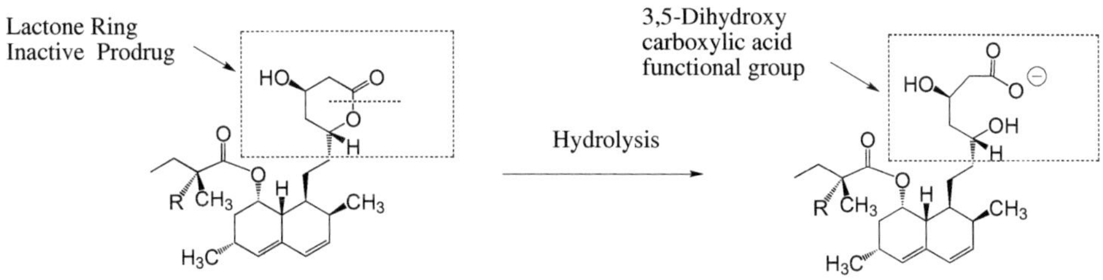


**Lovastatin (R=H), Predicted LogP = 4.07**
**Simvastatin (R=CH$_3$), Predicted LogP = 4.42**
**(Prodrugs)**

**(R=H or CH$_3$)**
**(Pharmacologically Active From)**

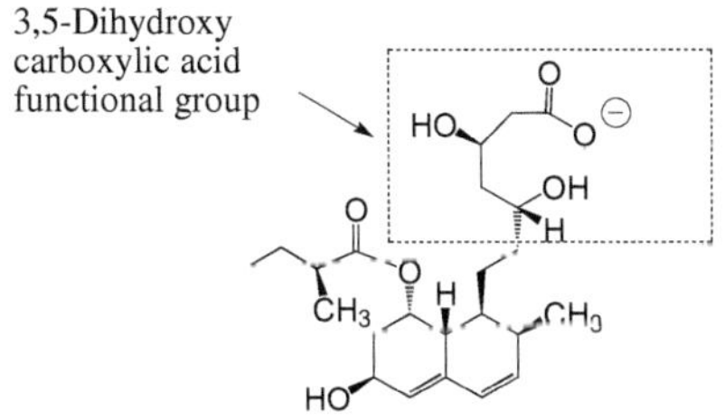


**Pravastatin**
**(Pharmacologically Active From)**
**17% orally bioavailable**
**Predicted LogP = 1.44**

Lovastatin (R = H) and simvastatin (R = CH$_3$) are available on the market as HMG-CoA reductase inhibitors for treatment of hypercholesterolemia [63–65]. Lovastatin and simvastatin are not active and first they need to be hydrolyzed to active forms that contain an opened ring with a dihydroxy acid functional group. Lovastatin hydrolysis produces the active metabolite. The prodrugs have higher lipophilicity than the active form that can penetrate lipophilic membranes including peripheral cells with higher degree of side effects. The metabolites, however, have better selectivity to the liver with minimal penetration to peripheral tissue [66, 67]. Lovastatin then served as a lead compound in further development of HMG-CoA reductase inhibitors. Minor modification of the bicyclic ring and side chain ester of lovastatin produced pravastatin, which is an active drug. Pravastatin, a ring opened dihydroxy acid with a hydroxy group on the bicyclic ring, is much more hydrophilic than either lovastatin or simvastatin, orally active and selectively target the liver with minimal distribution to peripheral tissues.

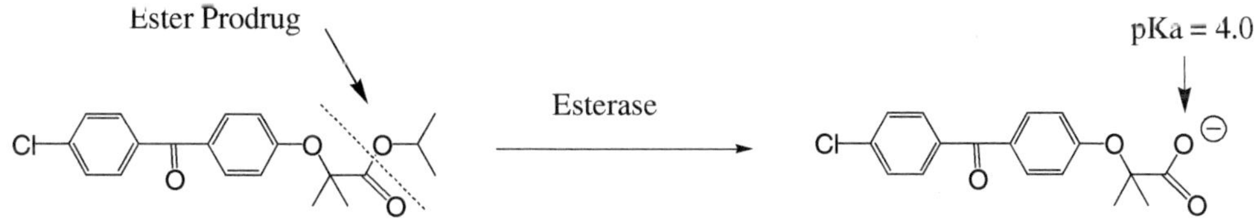


**Fenofibrate**
**LogP = 5.3**

**Fenofibric acid**
**LogP = 3.85**
**LogD$_{(pH = 6.5)}$ =1.34**

Fenofibrate is an ethyl ester prodrug of fenofibric acid. Both are used in the treatment of hypertriglyceridemia, both are available on the market as prescription drugs [32], and both are orally bioavailable despite the fact that fenofibric acid has a carboxylic acid with a p$K_a$ of 4.0, which is highly ionizable at the pH of intestine. This could be because the predicted log $D$ value of fenofibric acid has a positive value of 1.34 at pH 6.5. The kinetic profiles and dosing of fenofibrate and fenofibric acid are also similar.

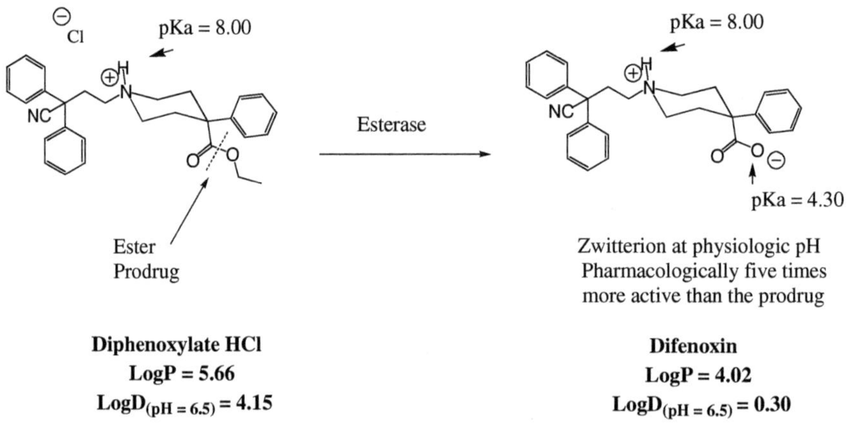


Diphenoxylate is used in combination with atropine for controlling diarrhea. Diphenoxylate itself has a low μ-opioid activity. It is rapidly metabolized by ester hydrolysis to difenoxin. The latter is pharmacologically fivefold more active when given orally. This is because difenoxin has a free zwitterionic carboxylate group that is essential for its activity. Diphenoxylate is an ethyl ester prodrug of difenoxin. Both drugs are orally bioavailable and available on the market as prescription drugs [32, 42]. Diphenoxylate is not a prodrug in the strict definition because it has a low μ-opioid activity on its own. However, because diphenoxylate is very rapidly hydrolyzed to its active metabolite, difenoxin, diphenoxylate is widely considered as a prodrug rather than a drug.

## 4.9 Summary and Conclusion

Oral administration of drugs is the preferable route in systemic drug therapy unless a rapid therapeutic response is needed in which case IV and IM formulations are more appropriate. Often, pharmacological entities are significantly ionized at physiological pH of intestine or have numerous polar nonionizable functional groups that prevent the drug entities to be absorbed through biological membranes in the intestine. Using prodrug approaches to enhance drugs' oral bioavailability, these ionizable and polar groups can be readily masked by ester derivatives with or without a linker separating the masking group from the drug entity. Examples of the functional groups that are suitable for esterification and carbamylation include carboxylic acid, phosphonate, phosphinic, phosphate, nucleotide, and alcohol groups and amidine groups, respectively. The ester and carbamylated prodrugs then undergo hydrolysis by esterases that are abundantly present in enterocytes, plasma, and liver to release the active drug. Examples of protecting masking groups and linkers that are used successfully in the design of prodrugs with enhanced lipid solubility are summarized in Table 4.2. Linkers are generally used to facilitate hydrolysis of ester functional group by esterases.

Although ester prodrugs are the most common type of prodrugs in clinical use, there are also disadvantages in using them. Premature hydrolysis in enterocytes can account for less than perfect bioavailability for esters. This behavior is also responsible for side effects such as diarrhea for beta-lactam antibiotics. Other disadvantages include chemical instability and nonproductive hydrolysis. One should also note species differences in esterase activities when studying prodrug hydrolysis and chemical stability in cell cultures, plasma, liver, and intestinal homogenates obtained from animals, and in *in vivo* preclinical studies as the esterase activities may differ from those in humans [68–72].

In conclusion, it is now possible to use prodrug approaches to enhance lipid solubility and oral bioavailability of the drugs and/or reduce drugs' toxicity to gastrointestinal tract. Many examples of successful prodrug approaches have reached the market.

**Table 4.2** General structure of prodrugs, examples of functional groups, linker, and ester moieties suitable for enhancing lipid solubility for oral delivery.

| Functional group of the parent drug | General Structure of Prodrugs | | | | |
|---|---|---|---|---|---|
| | Linker | | Ester moiety | | |
| | Oxyalkyl[a)] | Carbonyl | Alkyloxy[b)] | Acyl[c)] | Alkyl[d)] |
| Carboxylate | — | — | — | — | Yes |
| Phosphonate | Yes | Yes | Yes | | — |
| Phosphate | Yes | — | — | Yes | — |
| Alcohol | — | — | — | Yes | — |
| $NH_2$ | — | Yes | Yes | — | — |

*Note:* For examples of chemical structure, see Figure 4.4.

a) Examples of oxyalkyl group: oxymethyl, oxyethyl, and oxyisobutyl.
b) Examples of alkyloxy groups: methyloxy, ethyloxy, and isopropyloxy.
c) Examples of acyl groups: acetyl, propanoyl, and pivaloyl.
d) Examples of alkyl groups: methyl, ethyl, propyl, and morpholine.

## References


1 Lennernäs, H. (2007) Intestinal permeability and its relevance for absorption and elimination. *Xenobiotica: The Fate of Foreign Compounds in Biological Systems*, **37** (10–11), 1015–1051.

2 Peterson, L.W. and McKenna, C.E. (2009) Prodrug approaches to improving the oral absorption of antiviral nucleotide analogues. *Expert Opinion on Drug Delivery*, **6** (4), 405–420.

3 Li, F., Maag, H., and Alfredson, T. (2008) Prodrugs of nucleoside analogues for improved oral absorption and tissue targeting. *Journal of Pharmaceutical Sciences*, **97** (3), 1109–1134.

4 Gomez-Orellana, I. (2005) Strategies to improve oral drug bioavailability. *Expert Opinion on Drug Delivery*, **2** (3), 419–433.

5 Beaumont, K., Webster, R., Gardner, I., and Dack, K. (2003) Design of ester prodrugs to enhance oral absorption of poorly permeable compounds: challenges to the discovery scientist. *Current Drug Metabolism*, **4** (6), 461–485.

6 Gupta, P.K. and Robinson, J.R. (1991) Oral control release delivery, in *Treatise on Controlled Drug Delivery: Fundamentals, Optimization, Applications* (ed. A.F. Kydonieus), Taylor & Francis, Inc., pp. 255–314.

7 Dressman F J.B., Thelen, K., and Jantratid, E. (2008) Towards quantitative prediction of oral drug absorption. *Clinical Pharmacokinetics*, **47** (10), 655–667.

8 Allen, L.V. Jr. (2008) Dosage form design and development. *Clinical Therapeutics*, **30** (11), 2102–2111.

9 Kah, M. and Brown, C.D. (2008) Log *D*: lipophilicity for ionisable compounds. *Chemosphere*, **72** (10), 1401–1408.

10 Valkó, K. (2004) Application of high-performance liquid chromatography based measurements of lipophilicity to model biological distribution. *Journal of Chromatography A*, **1037** (1–2), 299–310.

11 Buchwald, P. and Bodor, N. (1998) Octanol–water partition: searching for predictive models. *Current Medicinal Chemistry*, **5** (5), 353–380.

12 Lentz, K.A. (2008) Current methods for predicting human food effect. *AAPS Journal*, **10** (2), 282–288.

13 Genser, D. (2008) Food and drug interaction: consequences for the nutrition/health status. *Annals of Nutrition and Metabolism*, **52** (Suppl. 1), 29–32.

14 Li, J.T., Hou, F., Lu, H., Li, T.Y., and Li, H. (1997) Phase I clinical trial of cefditoren pivoxil (ME 1207): pharmacokinetics in healthy volunteers. *Drugs Under Experimental and Clinical Research*, **23** (5–6), 145–150.

15 Ruiz-Balaguer, N., Nacher, A., Casabo, V.G., and Merino Sanjuan, M. (2002) Intestinal transport of cefuroxime axetil in rats: absorption and hydrolysis processes. *International Journal of Pharmaceutics*, **234** (1–2), 101–111.

16 Sica, D.A., Gehr, T.W., and Ghosh, S. (2005) Clinical pharmacokinetics of losartan. *Clinical Pharmacokinetics*, **44** (8), 797–814.

17 Sjövall, J., Magni, L., and Bergan, T. (1978) Pharmacokinetics of bacampicillin compared with those of ampicillin, pivampicillin, and amoxycillin. *Antimicrobial Agents and Chemotherapy*, **13** (1), 90–96.

18 Modr, Z., Dvovácek, K., Janků, I., and Krebs, V. (1977) Pharmacokinetics of carfecillin and carindacillin. *International Journal of Clinical Pharmacokinetics and Biopharmaceutics*, **15** (2), 81–83.

19 Li, Y.H., Tanno, M., Itoh, T., and Yamada, H. (1999) Role of the monocarboxylic acid transport system in the intestinal absorption of an orally active beta-lactam prodrug: carindacillin as a model. *International Journal of Pharmaceutics*, **191** (2), 151–159.

20 Barza, M. (1977) Antimicrobial spectrum, pharmacology and therapeutic use of antibiotics. Part 2. Penicillins. *American Journal of Hospital Pharmacy*, **34**, 57–67.

21 Barza, M. and Weinstein, L. (1976) Pharmacokinetics of the penicillins in man. *Clinical Pharmacokinetics*, **1**, 297–308.

22 Sakagami, K., Atsumi, K., Tamura, A., Yoshida, T., Nishihata, K., and Fukatsu, S.

(1990) Synthesis and oral activity of ME1207, a new orally active cephalosporin. *The Journal of Antibiotics*, **43** (8), 1047–1050.

23 Kees, F. and Grobecker, H. (1995) Systematics of beta-lactams: chemical properties and structure activity relationship of oral cephalosporins. *The Journal of Antimicrobial Chemotherapy*, **47**, 1–7.

24 Brass, E.P. (2002) Pivalate-generating prodrugs and carnitine homeostasis in man. *Pharmacological Reviews*, **54** (4), 589–598.

25 O'Callaghan, C.H., Sykes, R.B., Ryan, D.M., Foord, R.D., and Muggleton, P.W. (1976) Cefuroxime: a new cephalosporin antibiotic. *The Journal of Antibiotics*, **29** (1), 29–37.

26 Foord, R.D. (1976) Cefuroxime: human pharmacokinetics. *Antimicrobial Agents and Chemotherapy*, **9** (5), 741–747.

27 Williams, P.E. and Harding, S.M. (1984) The absolute bioavailability of oral cefuroxime axetil in male and female volunteers after fasting and after food. *The Journal of Antimicrobial Chemotherapy*, **13** (2), 191–196.

28 Dhareshwar, S.S. and Stella, V.J. (2008) Your prodrug releases formaldehyde: should you be concerned? No! *Journal of Pharmaceutical Sciences*, **97** (10), 4184–4193.

29 Tremblay, D., Dupront, A., Ho, C., Coussediere, D., and Lenfant, B. (1990) Pharmacokinetics of cefpodoxime in young and elderly volunteers after single doses. *The Journal of Antimicrobial Chemotherapy*, **26** (Suppl. E), 21–28.

30 Fujimoto, K., Ishihara, S., Yanagisawa, H., Ide, J., Nakayama, E., Nakao, H., Sugawara, S., and Iwata, M. (1987) Studies on orally active cephalosporin esters. *The Journal of Antibiotics*, **40** (3), 370–384.

31 Brass, E.P. (2002) Pivalate-generating prodrugs and carnitine homeostasis in man. *Pharmacological Reviews*, **54** (4), 589–598.

32 online.lexi.com March 8, 2010.

33 Naesens, L., Balzarini, J., Bischofberger, N., and De Clercq, E. (1996) Antiretroviral activity and pharmacokinetics in mice of oral bis(pivaloyloxymethyl)-9-(2-phosphonylmethoxyethyl)adenine, the bis (pivaloyloxymethyl) ester prodrug of 9-(2-phosphonylmethoxyethyl)adenine. *Antimicrobial Agents and Chemotherapy*, **40** (1), 22–28.

34 Qaqish, R.B., Mattes, K.A., and Ritchie, D.J. (2003) Adefovir dipivoxil: a new antiviral agent for the treatment of hepatitis B virus infection. *Clinical Therapeutics*, **25** (12), 3084–3099.

35 Boyd, M.R., Bacon, T.H., Sutton, D., and Cole, M. (1987) Antiherpesvirus activity of 9-(4-hydroxy-3-hydroxy-methylbut-1-yl) guanine (BRL 39123) in cell culture. *Antimicrobial Agents and Chemotherapy*, **31** (8), 1238–1242.

36 Jarvest, R.L., Sutton, D., and Vere Hodge, R.A. (1998) Famciclovir. Discovery and development of a novel antiherpes virus agent. *Pharmaceutical Biotechnology*, **11**, 313–343.

37 He, G., Massarella, J., and Ward, P. (1999) Clinical pharmacokinetics of the prodrug oseltamivir and its active metabolite Ro 64-0802. *Clinical Pharmacokinetics*, **37** (6), 471–484.

38 Cundy, K.C., Sue, I.L., Visor, G.C., Marshburn, J., Nakamura, C., Lee, W.A., and Shaw, J.P. (1997) Oral formulations of adefovir dipivoxil: *in vitro* dissolution and *in vivo* bioavailability in dogs. *Journal of Pharmaceutical Sciences*, **86** (12), 1334–1338.

39 Shaw, J.P., Sueoka, C.M., Oliyai, R., Lee, W.A., Arimilli, M.N., Kim, C.U., and Cundy, K.C. (1997) Metabolism and pharmacokinetics of novel oral prodrugs of 9-[(*R*)-2-(phosphonomethoxy)propyl] adenine (PMPA) in dogs. *Pharmaceutical Research*, **14** (12), 1824–1829.

40 Kubo, S.H. and Cody, R.J. (1985) Clinical pharmacokinetics of the angiotensin converting enzyme inhibitors. A review. *Clinical Pharmacokinetics*, **10** (5), 377–391.

41 Morrison, R.A., Chong, S., Marino, A.M., Wasserman, M.A., Timmins, P., Moore, V.A., and Irwin, W.J. (1996) Suitability of enalapril as a probe of the dipeptide transporter system: *in vitro* and *in vivo* studies. *Pharmaceutical Research*, **13** (7), 1078–1082.

42 Harrold, M.W (2008), Angiotensin converting enzyme inhibitors, antagonists and calcium blockers, in *Foye's Principles of Medicinal Chemistry*, 6th edn, (eds T.L.

Lemke, D.A. Williams, V.F. Roche, S.W. Zito), Lippincott Williams & Wilkins, Baltimore, pp. 738–768.

43 Morrison, R.A., Singhvi, S.M., Peterson, A.E., Pocetti, D.A., and Migdalof, B.H. (1990) Relative contribution of the gut, liver, and lung to the first-pass hydrolysis (bioactivation) of orally administered $^{14}$C-fosinopril sodium in dogs. *In vivo* and *in vitro* studies. *Drug Metabolism and Disposition*, **18** (2), 253–257.

44 DeForrest, J.M., Waldron, T.L., Harvey, C., Scalese, B., Rubin, B., Powell, J.R., Petrillo, E.W., and Cushman, D.W. (1989) Fosinopril, a phosphinic acid inhibitor of angiotensin I converting enzyme: *in vitro* and preclinical *in vivo* pharmacology. *Journal of Cardiovascular Pharmacology*, **14** (5), 730–736.

45 Singhvi, S.M., Duchin, K.L., Morrison, R.A., Willard, D.A., Everett, D.W., and Frantz, M. (1988) Disposition of fosinopril sodium in healthy subjects. *British Journal of Clinical Pharmacology*, **25** (1), 9–15.

46 Friedman, D.I. and Amidon, G.L. (1989) Passive and carrier-mediated intestinal absorption components of two angiotensin converting enzyme (ACE) inhibitor prodrugs in rats: enalapril and fosinopril. *Pharmaceutical Research*, **6** (12), 1043–1047.

47 Schwocho, L.R. and Masonson, H.N. (2001) Pharmacokinetics of CS-866, a new angiotensin II receptor blocker, in healthy subjects. *Journal of Clinical Pharmacology*, **41** (5), 515–527.

48 Laeis, P., Püchler, K., and Kirch, W. (2001) The pharmacokinetic and metabolic profile of olmesartan medoxomil limits the risk of clinically relevant drug interaction. *Journal of Hypertension*, **19** (Suppl. 1), S21–S32.

49 Koike, H., Sada, T., and Mizuno, M. (2001) *In vitro* and *in vivo* pharmacology of olmesartan medoxomil, an angiotensin II type AT1 receptor antagonist. *Journal of Hypertension*, **19** (Suppl. 1), S3–14.

50 Gustafsson, D. and Elg, M. (2003) The pharmacodynamics and pharmacokinetics of the oral direct thrombin inhibitor ximelagatran and its active metabolite melagatran: a mini-review. *Thrombosis Research*, **109** (Suppl. 1), S9–S15.

51 Gustafsson, D., Nyström, J., Carlsson, S., Bredberg, U., Eriksson, U., Gyzander, E., Elg, M., Antonsson, T., Hoffmann, K., Ungell, A., Sörensen, H., Nägård, S., Abrahamsson, A., and Bylund, R. (2001) The direct thrombin inhibitor melagatran and its oral prodrug H 376/95: intestinal absorption properties, biochemical and pharmacodynamic effects. *Thrombosis Research*, **101** (3), 171–181.

52 Blech, S., Ebner, T., Ludwig-Schwellinger, E., Stangier, J., and Roth, W. (2008) The metabolism and disposition of the oral direct thrombin inhibitor, dabigatran, in humans. *Drug Metabolism and Disposition*, **36** (2), 386–399.

53 Remko, M. (2009) Molecular structure, lipophilicity, solubility, absorption, and polar surface area of novel anticoagulant agents. *Journal of Molecular Structure*, **916** (1–3), 76–85.

54 Pentheroudakis, G. and Twelves, C. (2002) Capecitabine (Xeloda): from the laboratory to the patient's home. *Clinical Colorectal Cancer*, **2** (1), 16–23.

55 Pentheroudakis, G. and Twelves, C. (2002) The rational development of capecitabine from the laboratory to the clinic. *Anticancer Research*, **22** (6B), 3589–3596.

56 Fulton, B. and Markham, A. (1996) Mycophenolate mofetil. A review of its pharmacodynamic and pharmacokinetic properties and clinical efficacy in renal transplantation. *Drugs*, **51** (2), 278–298.

57 Hood, K.A. and Zarembski, D.G. (1971) Mycophenolate mofetil: a unique immunosuppressive agent. *American Journal of Health-System Pharmacy*, **54** (3), 285–294.

58 Lee, W.A., Gu, L., Miksztal, A.R., Chu, N., Leung, K., and Nelson, P.H. (1990) Bioavailability improvement of mycophenolic acid through amino ester derivatization. *Pharmaceutical Research*, **7** (2), 161–166.

59 Lanza, F.L., Chan, F.K., Quigley, E.M., and Practice Parameters Committee of the American College of Gastroenterology. (2009) Guidelines for prevention of NSAID-related ulcer complications. *The American Journal of Gastroenterology*, **104** (3), 728–738.

**60** Helsper, C.W., Smeets, H.M., Numans, M.E., Knol, M.J., Hoes, A.W., and de Wit, N.J. (2009) Trends and determinants of adequate gastroprotection in patients chronically using NSAIDs. *Pharmacoepidemiology and Drug Safety*, **18** (9), 800–806.

**61** Freston, J.W. (1990) Overview of medical therapy of peptic ulcer disease. *Gastroenterology Clinics of North America*, **19** (1), 121–140.

**62** Halen, P.K., Murumkar, P.R., Giridhar, R., and Yadav, M.R. (2009) Prodrug designing of NSAIDs. *Mini-Reviews in Medicinal Chemistry*, **9** (1), 124–139.

**63** Mauro, V.F. (1993) Clinical pharmacokinetics and practical applications of simvastatin. *Clinical Pharmacokinetics*, **24** (3), 195–202; Erratum in Mauro, V.F. (1993) *Clinical Pharmacokinetics*, **24** (6), 518.

**64** Pentikainen, P.J., Saraheimo, M., Schwartz, J.I., Amin, R.D., Schwartz, M.S., Brunner-Ferber, F., and Rogers, J.D. (1992) Comparative pharmacokinetics of lovastatin, simvastatin and pravastatin in humans. *Journal of Clinical Pharmacology*, **32** (2), 136–140.

**65** Serajuddin, A.T., Ranadive, S.A., and Mahoney, E.M. (1991) Relative lipophilicities, solubilities, and structure–pharmacological considerations of 3-hydroxy-3-methylglutaryl-coenzyme A (HMG-CoA) reductase inhibitors pravastatin, lovastatin, mevastatin, and simvastatin. *Journal of Pharmaceutical Sciences*, **80** (9), 830–834.

**66** Sliskovic, D.R., Blankley, C.J., Krause, B.R., Newton, R.S., Picard, J.A., Roark, W.H., Roth, B.D., Sekerke, C., Shaw, M.K., and Stanfield, R.L. (1992) Inhibitors of cholesterol biosynthesis. 6. *trans*-6-[2-(2-*N*-Heteroaryl-3,5-disubstituted-pyrazol-4-yl)ethyl/ethenyl] tetrahydro-4-hydroxy-2*H*-pyran-2-ones. *Journal of Medicinal Chemistry*, **35** (11), 2095–2103.

**67** Bone, E.A., Davidson, A.H., Lewis, C.N., and Todd, R.S. (1992) Synthesis and biological evaluation of dihydroeptastatin, a novel inhibitor of 3-hydroxy-3-methylglutaryl coenzyme A reductase. *Journal of Medicinal Chemistry*, **35** (18), 3388–3393.

**68** Taketani, M., Shii, M., Ohura, K., Ninomiya, S., and Imai, T. (2007) Carboxylesterase in the liver and small intestine of experimental animals and human. *Life Sciences*, **81** (11), 924–932.

**69** Imai, T. (2006) Human carboxylesterase isozymes: catalytic properties and rational drug design. *Drug Metabolism and Pharmacokinetics*, **21** (3), 173–185.

**70** Imai, T. (2007) Hydrolysis by carboxylesterase and disposition of prodrug with ester moiety. *Yakugaku Zasshi*, **127** (4), 611–619.

**71** Imai, T., Imoto, M., Sakamoto, H., and Hashimoto, M. (2005) Identification of esterases expressed in Caco-2 cells and effects of their hydrolyzing activity in predicting human intestinal absorption. *Drug Metabolism and Disposition*, **33** (8), 1185–1190.

**72** Yoshigae, Y., Imai, T., Taketani, M., and Otagiri, M. (1999) Characterization of esterases involved in the stereoselective hydrolysis of ester-type prodrugs of propranolol in rat liver and plasma. *Chirality*, **11** (1), 10–13.

# 5
# Modulating Solubility Through Prodrugs for Oral and IV Drug Delivery

*Victor R. Guarino*

## 5.1
## Introduction

While "good" aqueous solubility can greatly simplify delivery strategies, the ultimate goal in drug discovery is to select a suitable *drug* candidate, not necessarily a highly soluble molecule. A balance is sought between multiple attributes typically including a selective activity at the desired biological target(s) (e.g., enzyme, receptor, DNA, etc.), a suitable safety profile, and a reasonable physicochemical and pharmacokinetic profile to allow adequate exposure of the drug to the chosen biological target(s). Given the cost and time estimates of US$ 1.3 billion[1)] [1] and 12–15 years [2, 3], respectively, that it takes to produce an approved new molecular entity drug product, there is a continual driving force to quickly select drug candidates with an efficient use of resources in an attempt to reduce some of these time and cost-related risks. The more attributes (including solubility) that a team is trying to balance into one drug candidate, the more time and resources are likely required to select that candidate, which could translate to diminished market potential for the therapeutic concept. While in some cases, designing improved solubility into the drug candidate would just involve more time and resource expenditure (which carries its own level of risk), in other cases, it might simply not be a reasonable expectation, possibly due to the biological target demanding a set of physicochemical properties that are not compatible with high aqueous solubility. In this latter scenario, it could be a complete waste of time and resources if the team does not face this reality.

Having viable drug delivery technologies to overcome solubility limitations can allow faster and less costly candidate selection at the very least, and in regard to the latter scenario above, can potentially enable a candidate selection that would otherwise not be possible. The prodrug technology [4–7] can successfully modulate solubility [8] to enable oral and parenteral drug delivery, and the focus of this chapter is to illustrate both potential applications and some advantages and challenges of employing prodrugs for this purpose. The intent of writing this chapter is not to provide an extensive review of solubility-modulating literature examples; rather the

1) Cost estimate is in 2005 dollars.

*Prodrugs and Targeted Delivery: Towards Better ADME Properties.* Edited by Jarkko Rautio

ISBN: 978-3-527-32603-7

goal is to provide an appreciation to the reader, utilizing *representative* examples, for the potential usefulness of solubility-modulating prodrugs in enabling a faster and less costly drug discovery and development process. While this chapter's emphasis is on solubility modulation, solubility is certainly not the only property that can be altered using the prodrug concept, as illustrated in other chapters of this book, as well as recently summarized elsewhere [4]. The remainder of this chapter is divided into five primary sections, listed as follows:

1) Basics of solubility and oral/IV drug delivery
2) Prodrug applications for enhanced aqueous solubility
3) Challenges with solubilizing prodrugs of insoluble drugs
4) Additional applications of prodrugs for modulating solubility
5) Parallel exploration of analogues and prodrugs in drug discovery (commentary)

## 5.2
## Basics of Solubility and Oral/IV Drug Delivery

To set up later prodrug-oriented discussions, this section covers some basic principles and considerations regarding solubility as well as oral and intravenous (IV) drug delivery while avoiding too much detail as an extensive treatment of solubility [9] and oral/IV drug delivery [10] is beyond the scope of this chapter. Readers already well versed in these areas are encouraged to skip ahead to Section 5.3.

### 5.2.1
### Some Basic Fundamentals of Solubility

In pharmaceutical applications, the term solubility often refers to some concentration of solute (e.g., a drug) present in a dissolved state that is in *equilibrium* with some solid state of that same material. The dissolution of a molecule from the solid state into the solution state can be envisioned as occurring in three separate steps, and this simple model can be useful for recognizing some important factors involved in the solubility of a compound (Figure 5.1). In the first step, the molecule is separated from its solid state where it previously participated in intermolecular cohesive interactions, and therefore this separation requires the expenditure of work to disrupt these interactions. The second step involves the creation of a "pocket" in the solvent for the separated solute molecule to occupy, and the creation of this space also requires the expenditure of work to disrupt the intermolecular cohesive interactions within the solvent. The third step involves the insertion of the solute molecule into the created solvent cavity that should be favorable (work gained) due to the new adhesive interactions established between solute and solvent. An equilibrium between the solid and the solution state is achieved once the chemical potential of the drug becomes equivalent in both the dissolved state and the solid state, and at this point the *net* transfer of the drug molecule from one phase to another ceases, assuming no further changes are made to the system. The solubility is defined at this equilibrium

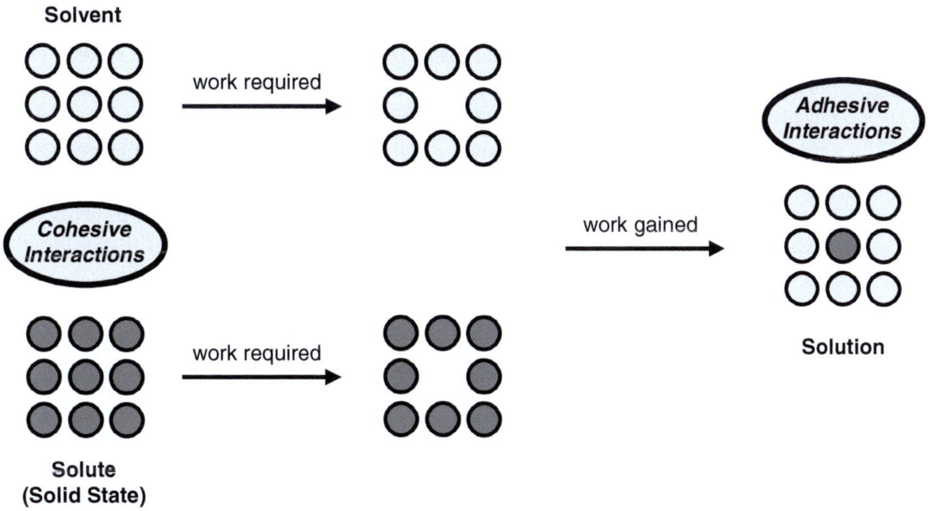


**Figure 5.1** Simplified depiction of solubility illustrating cohesive and adhesive interactions.

point as the concentration of the drug molecules in the solution state. If the drug happens to be in solution at a concentration above its solubility, it will be in a supersaturated state, and if it is below the solubility, it will be in a subsaturated state; in either case, there will be a thermodynamic driving force toward the equilibrium solubility concentration that will encourage precipitation or dissolution, respectively.

The equilibrium solubility can be manipulated by altering the chemical potential of the drug in either of the two states, and by doing so, would provide a new thermodynamic driving force for *net* transfer of drug molecules from higher chemical potential to lower chemical potential. For instance, if a nonpolar drug with low aqueous solubility is at its equilibrium water solubility with respect to a defined solid state, then instantaneously switching the water to a less polar medium (e.g., ethanol) would lower the chemical potential of the dissolved drug due to the more favorable solubilization afforded by ethanol thereby establishing a driving force for more drug molecules to transfer from the solid state to the solution state. Again, this net transfer would happen until the chemical potential of the drug in the solution state is raised enough to match the chemical potential in the solid state. It is useful to note that while the solubility would be higher in ethanol compared to water, the final chemical potential of the drug in ethanol and water would be the same, assuming that the chemical potential of the drug in the solid state did not change. Finally, an alternative way to disturb the equilibrium would be to keep the solvent the same and instead perturb the solid phase. For instance, if the solid phase in the original aqueous scenario was instantaneously destabilized to a higher energy metastable form, such as an amorphous solid, then a chemical potential differential would again result causing a net transfer of molecules from the solid state to the solution state. It is useful to note that in this scenario, because the solid state was altered to a higher energy form, both the final chemical potential of the drug in solution and the solubility would increase despite the solvent staying the same. These hypothetical scenarios illustrate why a measured solubility of a substance in a solvent is tied to the particular solid form of that substance *present at equilibrium* and why it is often possible to obtain multiple solubilities for the same molecule in the same solvent. One well-known and very unfortunate example illustrating the potential impact of solid form on solubility is the experience with the antiviral drug ritonavir, where a new and less soluble polymorph form of the drug appeared after manufacturing had already been established, which translated to detrimental effects on the product's ability to release the drug [11].

For simplicity, the above hypothetical scenarios implied that the "solution state" was composed of dissolved drug molecules existing in just one "form" totally surrounded by solvent molecules. However, depending on the nature of the drug molecule, there can often be more than one form of the drug present in solution. For example, if the drug contains a weakly basic moiety, then it will exist in two states when dissolved in water – a neutral and a protonated state. The ratio of these states will depend on the $pK_a$ for the conjugate acid of the basic moiety and the pH of the aqueous solvent. The protonated state is typically far more soluble than the neutral state because of the favorable solubilization from the water interacting with the ionization center. Everything else being equal, the additional equilibrium between the dissolved neutral form and the dissolved protonated form will drive more drug into solution from the solid state until the drug's chemical potential in the solid state (assuming neutral form in this example) and two solution states (neutral and ionized) are equal. The solubility in this case will be equal to the total amount of drug in the solution state (neutral plus ionized) at equilibrium, and this solubility will be pH dependent. Figure 5.2 shows how the total solubility of a weakly basic drug (intrinsic solubility assumed to be 1 $\mu$g/ml) is related to both the $pK_a$ of the ionizable moiety and the pH of the surrounding aqueous solvent. Besides ionization approaches, other common ways to increase solubility by introducing additional solution-state equilibria are complexation (e.g., cyclodextrins) and micelle formation through the addition of surfactant excipients. Some drugs can also complex with themselves in solution and each complex (dimer, trimer, etc.) is a new form, introducing an additional solution-state equilibrium serving to drive more total drug into solution until equilibrium is reached among all available forms including the solid state. This drug–drug intermolecular complexation has been observed to arise in the use of solubilizing prodrugs since the prodrugs can often solubilize both themselves and the parent drug [12–14]. Finally, ionization equilibrium is particularly emphasized above because many of the solubilizing prodrug techniques rely on introducing ionization potential into the poorly soluble molecule through the attachment of an ionizable promoiety (e.g., a phosphate moiety).

### 5.2.2
### Some General Comments on IV Drug Delivery

A typical goal in drug delivery is to introduce the drug into systemic circulation where the drug is either active or, at least, can be easily transported to various sites of action.

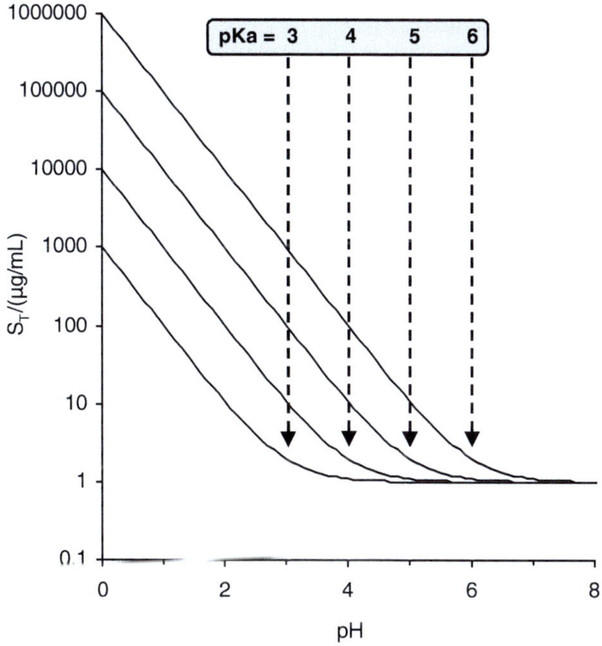


**Figure 5.2** Total aqueous solubility of a weakly basic drug as a function of pH and p$K_a$ (intrinsic solubility is 1 µg/ml).

Although quite invasive, IV administration is certainly the most straightforward method of achieving this goal since the drug is forced into circulation through a needle and should therefore result in 100% bioavailability of any drug, as defined by the fraction of administered dose that reaches systemic circulation. Other advantages that it brings include the ability to *immediately* introduce drug into systemic circulation to achieve a rapid onset of drug action (important for emergency conditions) and bypass physicochemical and biochemical barriers to enter the circulation from other routes of administration. However, regarding this latter advantage, it is useful to note that while certainly being a very efficient delivery route, the IV route does bypass many natural defenses that keep foreign substances out of circulation, and therefore extra care must be taken to ensure the formulation is safe (e.g., no bacterial growth, no unacceptable particulate matter, tolerable excipient levels, etc.).

Generally, IV formulations are solutions[2] that are either ready to use (i.e., stored as a solution) or produced as a powder to be reconstituted into a solution prior to administration. From the patient's perspective, the ready-to-use solution formulation

2) *Note:* There are IV formulations that contain nanoparticulates of the active ingredient, but they would not be emphasized in this chapter.

is convenient since it avoids reconstitution steps that carry the potential for errors. The solution aspect of IV formulations makes significant physicochemical demands on the drug candidate, such as suitable solubility and stability in the IV formulation to allow manufacturing, sterilization, and shelf life; furthermore, because the entire formulation is injected into the systemic circulation, the levels and types of excipients that can be used to aid solubilization and/or stabilization can be limited compared to other routes of delivery. However, while there might be less flexibility in formulation options, one advantage is that the formulator has a high level of control over the conditions that the drug product will experience prior to reaching systemic circulation, and it is ensured that the drug will have 100% bioavailability upon administration. For instance, if the drug has a physicochemical obstacle at a particular pH (e.g., a problem with stability or solubility), the formulator might avoid this issue by using a buffering system adjusted away from that problematic pH. Also, the absolute impact of solubility on the success of the IV drug product is better defined versus an oral product since the required solubility, as well as the nature of the relevant solvent medium (in this case the formulation), is defined and controlled by the formulator. Because of the obvious need for solubility in solution-based IV products, solubilizing prodrugs have found significant utility in enabling poorly soluble compounds to be formulated into IV products using very tolerable formulations, as illustrated through specific examples later in the chapter.

### 5.2.3
### Some General Comments on Oral Drug Delivery

In stark contrast to the IV route of administration, the oral route is less invasive with regard to the body's natural defense mechanisms against foreign substances entering the systemic circulation. It is also a more convenient and tolerable route of administration for many patients and therefore can encourage patient compliance. However, given its less invasive nature, there are very different challenges associated with this route of administration. The first main difference is that the formulator has far less control over, and understanding of, *exactly* what the drug will experience prior to reaching systemic circulation; furthermore, there can be high variability in the different drug delivery barriers that the compound will face in different individuals, and even within the same individual at different time periods. Some common sources of this variability can be eating habits, disease states, genetic differences, age, sex, and other coadministered medications. Unlike IV administration, there is an "absorption phase" of systemic drug levels following oral administration since time is involved as the drug transits from the mouth to the small intestine before being absorbed. During this transit, the drug molecules encounter a wide pH gradient, digestive enzymes, and other intestinal contents including food and bile contents; furthermore, even after arriving intact in the small intestine, the drug must have sufficient access to the solution state in the intestinal media and possess the right hydrophilic/lipophilic balance to allow efficient passage through enterocytes, all the while possessing a sufficient biochemical profile to avoid major elimination by transporters and/or metabolic enzymes in both enterocytes and hepatocytes. Only after surviving the liver is the drug molecule considered to have reached systemic circulation such that it can arrive at its site of action, and because of the various physical and biochemical barriers existing prior to this point, the bioavailability following oral administration is often less than 100%; however, as long as a reliable systemic exposure can be attained with acceptable levels of variability, the oral route is often preferred. Some advantages inherent to the oral route of administration are that the drug can be formulated as a solid, which can make it convenient for both the patient and the manufacturer, and there is more flexibility in the excipient types and levels that can be used since many of these excipients do not reach the systemic circulation in dangerous levels; furthermore, the drug does not necessarily have to be highly soluble relative to most IV examples since solids can be administered and there are greater formulation options which can provide sufficient solution levels of drug at the site of absorption. However, modulating solubility through prodrugs can still be a useful and sometimes even essential technique to enable sufficient systemic exposure from a viable formulation.

Determining exactly what absolute solubility is necessary, and even in what media to evaluate solubility [15], is less straightforward when considering the oral delivery route. Reaching systemic circulation from the oral route depends on a set of *kinetic* processes that typically include dissolution, precipitation, GI transit, and absorptive flux; furthermore in this highly *kinetic* situation, the drug can sometimes become supersaturated at the site of absorption which can be very beneficial for driving absorptive flux as long as it does not result in significant precipitation. So in short, the effects of "solubility" on oral drug delivery are not as straightforward as in IV drug delivery; however, it is generally appreciated that solubility can play an important role in the kinetics of both dissolution/precipitation and absorptive flux.

## 5.3 Prodrug Applications for Enhanced Aqueous Solubility

The purpose of this section is to highlight some successful examples demonstrating the potential enhanced drug delivery offered through the solubilizing prodrug approach [8]. The information will be divided into IV and oral routes of administration due to the different aspects inherent to each delivery route. But, first, some general comments on the prodrug concept are included in the following section.

### 5.3.1 Prodrug Concept

The prodrug approach [4–7] is a chemically oriented drug delivery tool where a parent drug's intrinsic physicochemical properties are modulated through a temporary chemical change that is often accomplished through the covalent attachment of a chemical moiety (promoiety) to the drug to create the prodrug. Due to the prodrug being a totally new chemical, a different physicochemical property profile should exist intended to allow easier drug delivery. Once the prodrug has overcome the barrier that existed for the parent drug, it must reconvert by enzymatic or chemical means to release the parent drug such that it can exert its therapeutic action. As illustrated in Figure 2.1, while the prodrug does not face the drug delivery barrier present for the parent drug, it often encounters an eventual therapeutic barrier due to its different chemical nature from the parent drug, and therefore reconversion to the parent drug must take place at some appropriate point "postdelivery" in order for efficacy to be realized. Therefore, the chemical modifications used in prodrug design must be reversible, and any by-product from reconversion should not raise significant safety concerns within the context of the therapeutic target and area.

### 5.3.2
### Examples of Prodrugs to Enhance Aqueous Solubility for IV Administration

High aqueous solubility is a very advantageous characteristic to have in a drug candidate for IV administration since it can allow the formulator to choose a more tolerable formulation vehicle. Because many active compounds do not possess high aqueous solubility, the use of the prodrug approach to enhance solubility is an obvious choice. Particularly for IV administration, the prodrug concept works well since the formulator has a high level of control over the conditions that the prodrug encounters prior to reaching systemic circulation, so essentially the only question that remains is whether the prodrug will actually reconvert in the expected manner. In general, phosphate monoester prodrugs have shown great promise as prodrugs for IV administration because they tend to possess a relatively good chemical stability, the potential for dramatic solubilization, and an established reconversion pathway once in systemic circulation that is attributed to reaction with alkaline phosphatase. In order to emphasize this particular promise of phosphate monoesters, two of the three examples included in this section utilize this design approach.

#### 5.3.2.1 Fosphenytoin
Fosphenytoin has been extensively reviewed [16, 17] and is a very successful prodrug example illustrating the great utility of the phosphate monoester design approach to enable IV and other parenteral drug delivery of poorly soluble parent drugs. Fosphenytoin (**1**, Cerebyx®) is a highly water-soluble prodrug of the anticonvulsant drug phenytoin (**2**), an imide-based NH-acidic compound with a p$K_a$ of 8.3 and an intrinsic solubility of ~20–30 µg/ml at 25 °C. Scheme 5.1 illustrates the proposed bioreconversion mechanism for fosphenytoin that involves initial reaction with alkaline phosphatase to form the *N*-hydroxymethyl intermediate that subsequently undergoes rapid unimolecular degradation to release phenytoin and one equivalent of formaldehyde [18]. Fosphenytoin's water solubility of 142 mg/ml (25 °C; pH ~9) is equivalent to 88.2 mg/ml of phenytoin, allowing fosphenytoin to be formulated in an aqueous vehicle at a final pH ~8.5. Phenytoin, on the other hand, is formulated for IV delivery as the sodium salt in a 10% ethanol, 40% propylene glycol, 50% aqueous cosolvent-based vehicle adjusted to a final pH of ~12 due to the relatively weak acidity of this imide-based NH acid. This sodium phenytoin formulation introduces some significant safety concerns that range from irritation/pain at the injection site to

potential death if administered too quickly. Fosphenytoin, being orders of magnitude more soluble at neutral pH, is able to be formulated without cosolvents or very alkaline pH, and can even be administered more quickly than sodium phenytoin. An additional advantage of fosphenytoin is that it can be administered intramuscularly (IM) and still deliver 100% bioavailability of phenytoin in systemic circulation in a reasonable time frame, which can be an advantage for patients who cannot be given an IV infusion. In contrast, an IM administration of the sodium phenytoin formulation is not a viable strategy as it leads to precipitation of the phenytoin free acid at the site of injection resulting in highly variable and prolonged, incomplete systemic exposures.

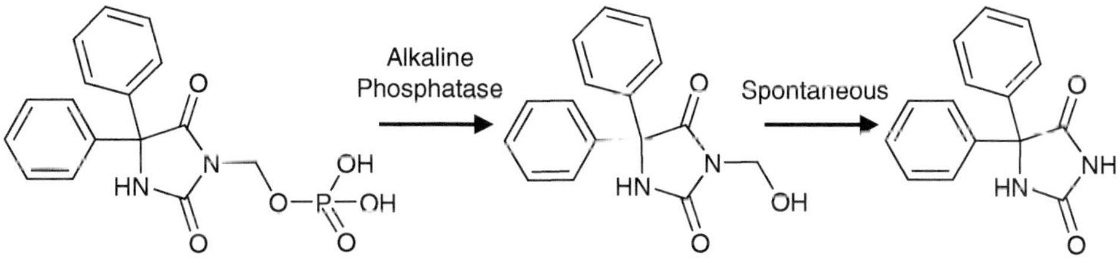


1 2

**Scheme 5.1** Proposed reconversion of fosphenytoin to phenytoin.

5.3.2.2 **Fospropofol**

Fospropofol (**3**, Lusedra®) was recently approved by the FDA for monitored anesthesia care and is administered through IV bolus injection. Fospropofol, being a phosphoryloxymethyl prodrug of the anesthetic propofol (**4**), is a second successful example displaying the promise in the phosphate monoester prodrug approach for making highly soluble, chemically stable prodrugs for IV administration. Scheme 5.2 illustrates the proposed *in vivo* reconversion mechanism for fospropofol. Similar to the fosphenytoin example above, there was already a commercial formulation of propofol that in this case is an oil-in-water emulsion that can be prone to bacterial growth and can cause concerns regarding the effective lipid load if administered over prolonged periods (e.g., to aid in keeping a patient in a coma). In comparison, fospropofol does not require the oil-in-water emulsion due to its greatly enhanced aqueous solubility (~500 mg/ml) compared to propofol (0.150 mg/ml) [7]. A very interesting aspect of fospropofol is that it appears to cause less pain at the injection site compared to propofol, presumably because the tissues at the local injection site do not experience high solution concentrations of propofol since the prodrug has not fully converted at that initial point of injection [8]. This point is certainly something to keep in mind as another potential promise in the prodrug approach to drug delivery that directly stems from a prodrug being a totally different, and often inactive, molecule from the parent drug.

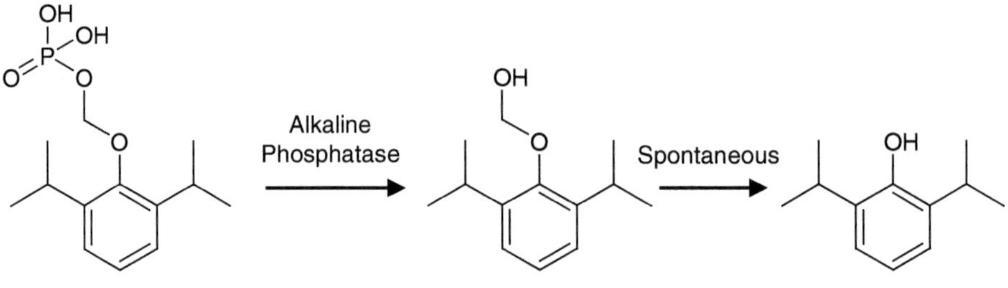


3 4

**Scheme 5.2** Proposed reconversion of fospropofol to propofol.

#### 5.3.2.3 **Parecoxib**

The above two examples illustrated the phosphate monoester design approach, but there are certainly other approaches that can be used to design water-soluble prodrugs suitable for parenteral delivery [7, 8]. A good example is parecoxib (**5**, Dynastat®), a prodrug of valdecoxib (**6**, Bextra®) [19]. The unique aspect in this prodrug design is that a water-soluble prodrug was created through the attachment of a *neutral* promoiety, which created a more acidic moiety in the *parent drug* that afforded enhanced water solubility suitable for a parenteral formulation. This is in contrast to the more common design strategy of introducing the ionization site as part of the promoiety. While parecoxib is not approved for use by the FDA, it is approved in other countries and represents a water-soluble prodrug that enabled a commercial IV product of a COX-2 inhibitor.

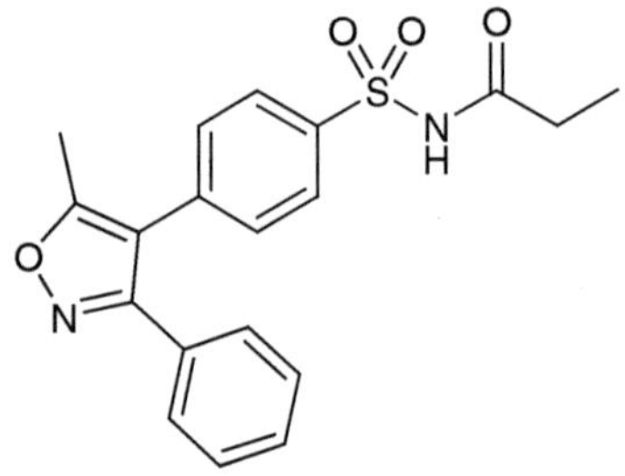

5

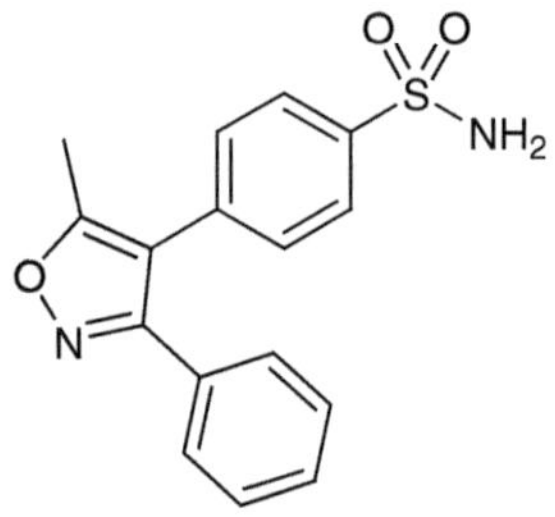

6

#### 5.3.2.4 **Irinotecan**

A second commercial example utilizing a nonphosphate solubilizing strategy for parenteral delivery is irinotecan (**7**, Camptosar®), a prodrug of the antineoplastic agent SN-38 (**8**), whose amine-based promoiety is attached to the phenol of **8** through a carbamate linkage. As described in Section 2.3.1.4, the carbamate linkage attaching the promoiety to the parent drug is relatively stable resulting in an extended exposure of the prodrug and prolonged release of the parent drug [20].

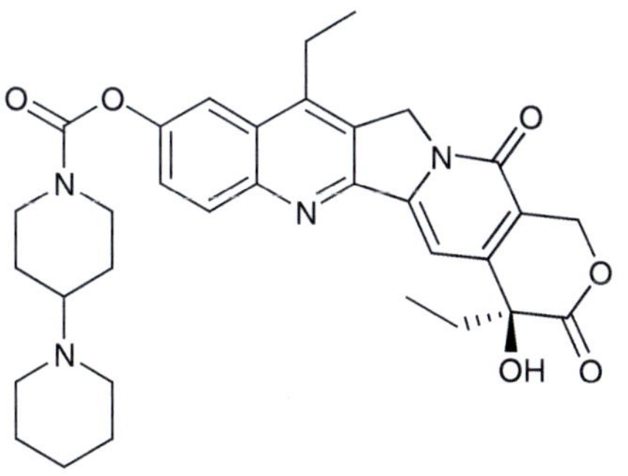

7

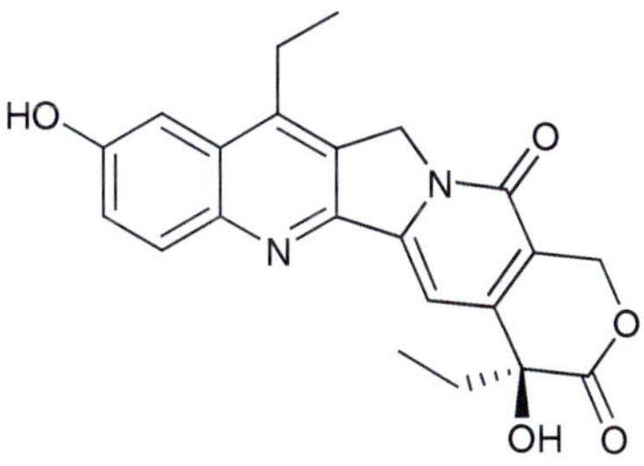

8

### 5.3.3
### Prodrugs to Enhance Aqueous Solubility for Oral Administration

Designing solubilizing prodrugs for oral administration can potentially be more straightforward than designing oral prodrugs to enhance either permeability or metabolic stability since quite frequently the solubilizing prodrug is purposely designed to reconvert at some point along the GI tract to release the parent drug into solution, and therefore the prodrug is not required to survive the enterocytes intact. From this point of view, phosphate monoesters again have great promise due to their typically favorable chemical stability combined with the expression of alkaline phosphatase on the surface of the enterocytes. This expression of alkaline phosphatase can serve to release the parent drug from a phosphate monoester prodrug in proximity to the primary site of absorption; furthermore, because the phosphate monoester prodrug is expected to have poor passive permeability, this design strategy can help ensure that minimal, if any, prodrug will actually reach circulation, which can greatly simplify the analytical and toxicological evaluations of these prodrugs.

#### 5.3.3.1 Fosamprenavir

A very successful example illustrating the promise in the phosphate monoester approach is fosamprenavir (**9**, Lexiva®) [21–23], the phosphate monoester prodrug of the HIV protease inhibitor amprenavir (**10**, Agenerase®), whose proposed bioreconversion is through the action of alkaline phosphatase. Similar to fosphenytoin and fospropofol, amprenavir was actually marketed before fosamprenavir as a solubilized formulation in a vehicle containing propylene glycol, polyethylene glycol 400, and vitamin E TPGS. Soft gelatin capsules were used containing 150 mg of amprenavir in each capsule. Because the desired dose was 1200 mg taken twice daily, the patient was required to take 16 capsules per day (8 capsules at each dosing period), which is a very inconvenient dosing regimen to maintain. Fosamprenavir, due to its enhanced aqueous solubility can actually be formulated in a solid tablet that contains the molar equivalent of 600 mg of amprenavir (i.e., four times as much active drug as the solubilized soft gelatin capsule formulation). The significantly greater drug loading per dosage unit allowed the patient to need only 4 tablets per day (instead of 16) to achieve the desired 1200 mg dose while also avoiding the continual ingestion of cosolvents such as propylene glycol. Therefore, fosamprenavir is clearly a successful example displaying the potential for dramatic improvements in both commercial viability and patient convenience afforded by solubilizing prodrugs for oral administration.

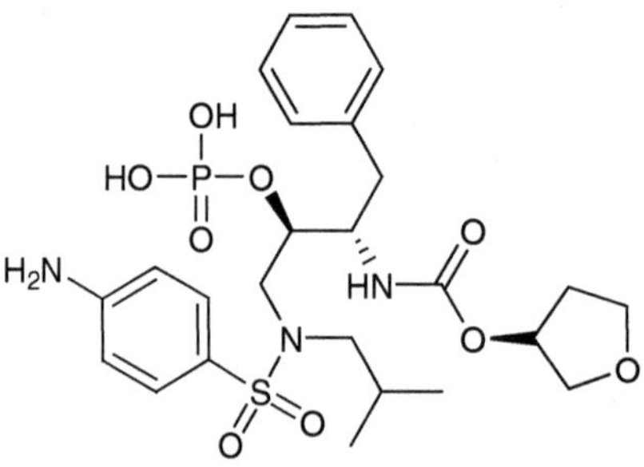

**9**

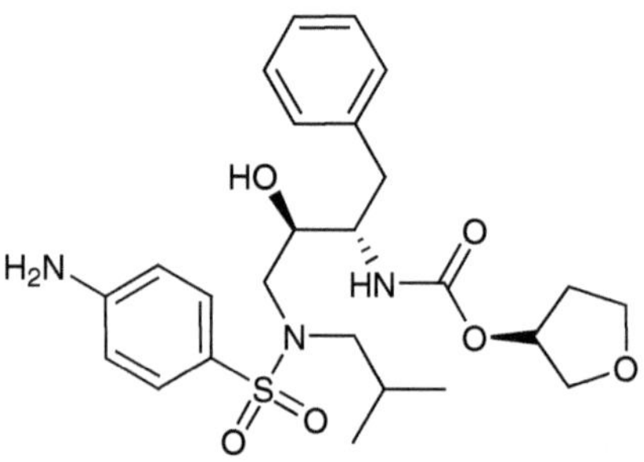

**10**

5.3.3.2 **Valganciclovir**

Nonphosphate solubilizing approaches have also found commercial success for enhancing oral delivery. One approach is to introduce an ionizable amine, and a common strategy to do this is through the attachment of amino acids, although sometimes other properties can be simultaneously altered in a way that affects drug delivery. For example, while valganciclovir (**11**, Valcyte®), the valine-based prodrug of the antiviral drug ganciclovir (**12**, Cytovene®), contains an ionizable amine that might typically be envisioned as a solubility altering approach, it was found that the promoiety enabled the prodrug to be recognized by an intestinal influx peptide transporter PEPT1 that aids drug delivery [24] (described in Section 2.3.1.3). This example illustrates some potentially distinguishing features of amino acid promoieties versus phosphate promoieties stemming from their different structures and ionization behavior along the GI tract. More specifically, phosphate promoieties greatly discourage systemic exposure of the prodrug because of the low passive permeability of the predominantly ionized structure combined with the alkaline phosphatase activity at the brush border membrane; in contrast, amino acid prodrugs that possess suitable stability can have a relatively higher potential to cross enterocytes and reach systemic circulation through passive permeation of the neutral species and/or recognition by influx transporters.

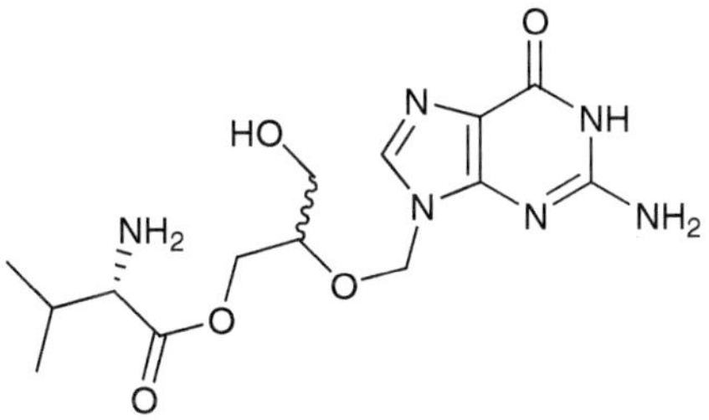

11

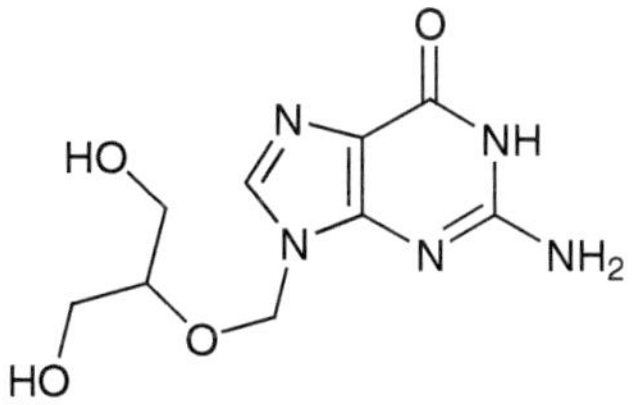

12

## 5.4
## Challenges with Solubilizing Prodrugs of Insoluble Drugs

The previous sections illustrated four very successful examples supporting the design of solubilizing prodrugs to enable the delivery of poorly soluble parent drugs. However, there are certainly challenges that are useful to recognize. The purpose of this section will be to highlight some common challenges in using solubilizing prodrugs to enable parenteral and oral delivery of poorly soluble parent drugs.

### 5.4.1
### Challenges with Solubilizing Prodrug Strategies for IV Administration

Chemical stability is generally a very important factor in IV formulations, and can become an even more significant factor when formulating ready-to-use solutions of solubilizing prodrugs, particularly when the chemical degradation of the prodrug leads to the formation of either the poorly soluble parent drug or other poorly soluble degradant. The typically large solubility differential between the prodrug and the parent drug means that a relatively small amount of prodrug degradation will result in enough poorly soluble parent drug for precipitation to occur, creating particulate matter in the parenteral formulation. An often generically stated shelf-life specification for pharmaceutical products is the time for 10% degradation, and a common aim is to have a shelf life of 2 years. However, this 90% remaining rule-of-thumb for shelf life assumes that the 10% degradation does not introduce any safety concerns for the drug product, such as toxic degradants. For an IV product, particulate formation would typically be considered a safety issue, and if these particulates form before reaching a 10% loss of product, then the effective shelf life would instead be based on the time for producing particulate matter, making the shelf-life goal of 2 years even tougher to obtain.

Fosphenytoin [16, 17] is a good example to illustrate some of these challenges. The first aspect worth noting is that the phenytoin IV product[3] itself also has significant

3) Formulation vehicle is 10% ethanol, 40% propylene glycol, and 50% aqueous adjusted to a pH of ~12.

challenges associated with precipitation, but in this case the challenge is primarily an avoidance of pH shift caused by either carbon dioxide absorption or too much predilution. In fact, the sodium phenytoin formulation is typically administered with little or no predilution to avoid precipitation issues. If the pH does shift toward the acidic direction, phenytoin has a risk of precipitating, and the cosolvents are present to help prevent that precipitation. Fosphenytoin, on the other hand, can be formulated in an aqueous vehicle that is far better for the patient; however, chemical degradation to the poorly soluble phenytoin parent drug would cause an immediate precipitation issue since there are no cosolvents to help with solubilization. It is interesting to note that fosphenytoin is actually formulated at a pH that is slightly more alkaline (pH ~8.5) than its pH of maximum chemical stability (pH 7.5–8.0). The reason for this is the known stability profile of fosphenytoin; more specifically, while the degradation of fosphenytoin at its pH of maximum stability primarily produces phenytoin, at pH 8.5 and above, the main degradants are more soluble ring-opened degradants that do not carry the same risk of precipitation in the aqueous formulation. So in this case, a pH corresponding to a faster degradation of fosphenytoin is chosen since the degradants formed are actually more soluble and therefore easier to manage. This is a great example showing the importance of chemical stability as a significant determinant in the design and formulation of solubilizing prodrugs; moreover, it nicely illustrates an earlier point that one advantage in IV formulations is the high level of control that the formulator has over choosing the conditions that the drug product will experience prior to reaching systemic circulation. The formulator not only can choose an appropriate pH to modulate degradation rates and/or degradation products but also can consider adding excipients to help solubilize the degradants. For instance, it has been shown that by incorporating a parenterally safe sulfobutyl ether cyclodextrin ($SBE_{7M}$-β-CD), which serves to solubilize phenytoin and therefore greatly slow down particulate formation, the pH of the formulation can be lowered to pH 7.4–8.0 to enable a ready-to-use solution formulation for storage at 25 °C (Cerebyx® requires refrigerated storage) [25]. It is also useful to note that solubilizing prodrugs can potentially help solubilize their poorly soluble parent drugs to some extent, presumably by the formation of associative complexes between prodrug and parent drug molecules, which can also slow down particulate formation in an IV product [12–14]. Finally, some of these stability challenges can often be alleviated through the formulation of powders of the prodrug (not ready-to-use solutions) that are formulated to allow rapid reconstitution into a solution just prior to dosing by the addition of a blank vehicle; however, these types of reconstitution strategies are not as convenient for emergency situations and other scenarios where reconstitution is not a viable option.

### 5.4.2
### Challenges with Solubilizing Prodrug Strategies for Oral Administration

As previously mentioned, a significant challenge for oral drug delivery stems from the formulator's loss of control over what happens to the drug product between administration and exposure to systemic circulation. Residing between those points are many variables as alluded to earlier and extensively covered elsewhere [10]. Therefore, choosing a prodrug design strategy is more challenging in some ways depending on the desired target site for reconversion, which is in turn related to where the actual barrier to parent drug delivery exists. As mentioned previously, one fortunate aspect with solubilizing prodrugs is that the goal is often just to deliver the parent drug into the solution state *within the GI tract* so that the parent drug can then be absorbed, and there are multiple design strategies that can allow this; in contrast, prodrugs designed to enhance permeability and/or metabolic stability often need to not only arrive at the site of absorption but also survive passage at least into, if not through, the enterocytes and liver.

Another potential challenge, or potential advantage for that matter, can stem from the significant solubility differential between the prodrug and the parent. More specifically, when a highly soluble prodrug reconverts in the GI tract to form the insoluble parent, a convoluted kinetic relationship begins between the following: (1) transit time of the parent drug to the site of absorption, (2) transit time away from the site of absorption, (3) precipitation kinetics, and (4) absorptive flux kinetics through the enterocytes; furthermore, if precipitation of the parent drug actually occurs, then a fifth kinetic process pertaining to dissolution of the parent drug is introduced. Because the solubilizing prodrug can typically achieve much higher solution concentrations than the parent drug, the reconversion process has the potential to produce a supersaturated concentration of the parent drug, which can provide a greater driving force for both absorptive flux through the enterocytes and precipitation in the GI tract. One advantage with the phosphate monoester prodrug approaches is that these prodrugs are likely to convert to form the parent drug at the surface of the enterocytes, which is commonly the main site of absorption. By converting at this surface, potentially supersaturated solutions of parent drug can be created with a minimal transit time necessary to reach the absorption site. Therefore, with any decent permeability in the parent drug, there should be a good chance to have the supersaturated conditions work favorably toward driving absorptive flux instead of precipitation [26]. Finally, it is useful to note that even if precipitation of a parent drug does occur, this precipitate can frequently be amorphous, which should have faster dissolution than crystalline drug; therefore, in this latter case, the "solubilizing" prodrug might enhance oral exposure indirectly through the delivery of amorphous parent drug.

## 5.5
## Additional Applications of Prodrugs for Modulating Solubility

The purpose behind many solubilizing prodrug efforts is to generically increase aqueous solubility, and that can certainly be a useful strategy; however, there are other drug delivery enhancements that can stem from alternative forms of solubility modulation. The following sections are intended to introduce alternative applications for solubility-modulating prodrugs.

### 5.5.1
### Alleviating pH-Dependent Oral Bioavailability of Weakly Basic Drugs

As shown in Figure 5.2, the aqueous solubility of a weakly basic drug typically depends on pH and dramatically increases as the pH drops below the p$K_a$ of the conjugate acid for the weakly basic moiety [9]. One can easily appreciate from Figure 5.2 that when the pH drops below the inflection region surrounding the p$K_a$, the total solubility of the compound begins to increase approximately 10-fold for every further pH unit drop. This trend will continue until the solubility of the first available salt is reached (not included on the plot). Because the GI tract, in its fasted state, can be very acidic in the stomach (pH 1–2) and fairly neutral in the small intestine (pH 6.5) [10], there can be dramatic solubility differences for a weak base as it transits to the small intestine. For example, a hypothetical weakly basic drug with an intrinsic solubility of 1 μg/ml and a p$K_a$ of 5 will have an expected aqueous solubility of 1 μg/ml at pH 6.5 (small intestine pH) and 1–10 mg/ml at pH 1–2 (stomach pH) that introduces a potential solubility differential up to a 10 000-fold. This increased solubility in the stomach can be very advantageous for dissolving the drug for later absorption and can sometimes be the sole contributor allowing the parent to reach suitable solution-state concentrations, given that gross precipitation does not occur during further GI transit. However, this potential solubilization advantage offered by the acidity of the stomach will not be present for patients taking medication to reduce acid secretions (i.e., raise the pH of the stomach), which can translate into very low and/or variable systemic exposures of the weakly basic drug, commonly referred to as pH-dependent bioavailability. There are certainly formulation strategies that can help alleviate this effect, but sometimes those formulation strategies are not compatible with the intrinsic properties of the parent drug. In these latter cases, a prodrug strategy could be used to temporarily modulate the pH–solubility characteristics of the parent drug. For example, by introducing a weakly acidic ionization center present in the attached promoiety (e.g., a phosphate), a zwitterionic species could be created that would have a very different pH–solubility profile from the parent drug, which should translate into a very different pH dependence for oral bioavailability. Also, one could directly remove or at least alter the weakly basic p$K_a$ by derivatization of that ionization site. Some examples of this latter approach might include *N*-Mannich base approaches [27] or quaternary derivatives in the case of tertiary amines [28–30] (refer to Chapter 2 for more details on these approaches). No matter which design approach is taken, the emphasis of this section is to point out that modulating pH–solubility relationships is one additional way by which solubilizing prodrugs can enhance drug delivery other than just simply increasing aqueous solubility in a generic manner.

### 5.5.2
### Aligning pH-Solubility and pH-Stability Relationships for IV Products

It is very convenient for the formulator of an IV product if the pH of maximum solubility happens to coincide with the pH of maximum chemical stability, but this is not always the case. Using the same ability to modulate pH–solubility relationships as described above, the prodrug approach could also address this latter formulation challenge such that the pH of adequate solubility is better aligned with the pH of adequate stability. Modulating pH–solubility profiles not only can make IV formulations possible but also can allow a wider pH tolerance for the formulation during storage (shelf-life consideration). For instance, if a parent drug formulation is required to be at a pH where the solubility is highly sensitive to small pH variations (steep pH–solubility relationship), then being able to flatten that pH–solubility relationship through a prodrug approach could allow a more robust formulation that does not require a tight pH control in order to meet specifications. This could translate into an easier product to develop, which might therefore require less time and costs to bring to market. Again, in both this section and the previous section, the strategy is toward modulating pH–solubility relationships, not necessarily absolute solubilities at any given pH.

### 5.5.3 Modulating Solubility In Negative Direction

With the previous sections discussing applications for increasing aqueous solubility in general and/or modulating the pH dependence of aqueous solubility, this section illustrates how sometimes the dramatic *lowering* of solubility can be an advantage for enhancing drug delivery. Some orally administered drugs are formulated as suspensions instead of solid tablets or capsules, and in designing these oral suspension formulations, it is useful to recognize that some amount of drug will be in solution in the mouth and therefore available to interact with taste receptors, which can be an issue for marketability and patient compliance if the drug has a foul taste. The bad taste can be potentially alleviated through a temporary modification in the drug's physicochemical properties. For instance, if solubility can be temporarily lowered, there will be far less compound in solution to actually taste; furthermore, the chemical modification of the drug could intrinsically change its interaction with the taste receptors. Both of these alterations can be created using a solubility-modulating prodrug approach and one example where this approach was taken is with the palmitate ester prodrug of chloramphenicol (**13**), which enabled a pediatric oral suspension product. The palmitate ester alleviates the foul taste [31] of the parent drug chloramphenicol (**14**), and the palmitate ester is later hydrolyzed to release the active chloramphenicol so that it can exert its therapeutic action. So it is interesting to note that in this case, the barrier to effective drug delivery was actually taste, and to alleviate this issue, a temporary bioreversible modification was made that actually resulted in the *reduction* of solubility, pointing out that the parent drug's solubility (combined with its chemical structure) was actually too high in this case for its intended route of administration.

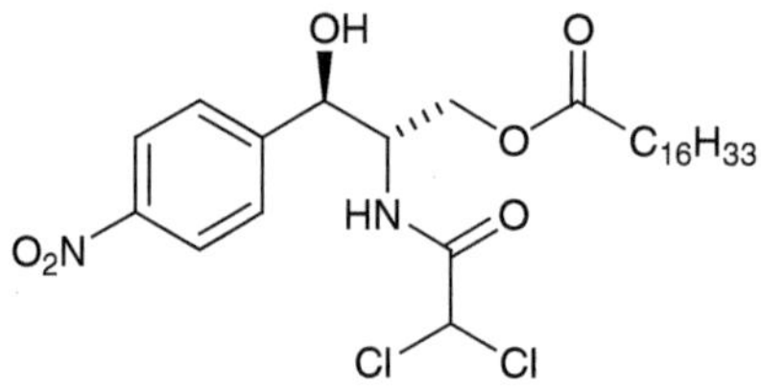

13

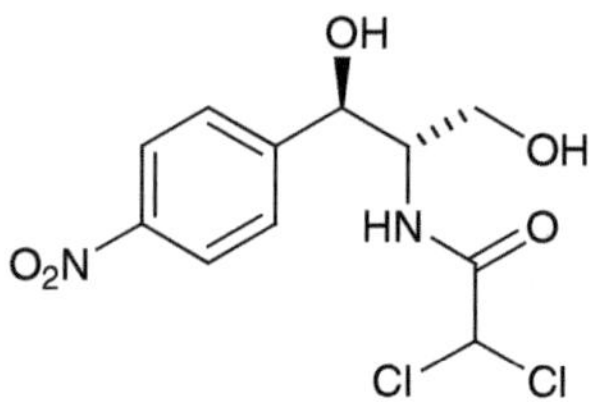

14

## 5.6
## Parallel Exploration of Analogues and Prodrugs in Drug Discovery (Commentary)

The purpose of this last section is to provide some commentary for the potential value of considering prodrugs as an integral part of the drug discovery effort. Regarding the three phosphate prodrug examples included earlier in this chapter, it is worth noting that not only did these three prodrugs utilize very straightforward and reliable design strategies but also certainly appear as the more advantageous candidates to market compared to their parent drugs. With the ever increasing multidisciplinary nature of drug candidate design and selection, hopefully it will continually become easier to recognize these opportunities in drug discovery (before candidate selection), so as to potentially select the prodrug the first time through and actually avoid spending resources on developing the problematic parent drug altogether.

Another potential advantage of bringing the prodrug concept into discovery can stem from using them as molecular probes to help answer questions regarding bioavailability limitations. For example, it is common to have poorly soluble molecules that also display poor oral bioavailability, but it can be difficult sometimes to determine whether poor solubility is the actual cause of poor bioavailability. Because the common *in vitro* assays for evaluating passive permeability, active transport, and metabolic stability all require some minimum amount of aqueous solubility, poorly soluble molecules can give highly ambiguous results due to precipitation and nonspecific binding events. In these scenarios, a common tendency is to blame poor solubility for the lack of *in vivo* performance, which might not be a correct assessment, and could greatly mislead the subsequent SAR (structure–activity relationship) efforts. If the molecule possesses an appropriate structural feature to make a very straightforward solubilizing prodrug, this prodrug could be dosed to determine if the enhanced solubility translates into better bioavailability relative to dosing the parent drug *per se*. If the same poor bioavailability is witnessed between dosing the prodrug and the parent drug, one should at least strongly question whether poor solubility is actually the only limiting factor. On the other hand, if the bioavailability is dramatically increased through dosing the prodrug, the team will have potentially established a drug delivery approach for driving exposure, and arguments could even be made toward keeping that same structural feature in subsequent analogues to allow a similar prodrug design on the final candidate if needed.

Finally, prodrugs could have utility even earlier in drug discovery than lead optimization, such as in enabling an early proof-of-principle study to justify spending more resources on the program. In these cases, the goal might be to simply demonstrate a biological effect *in vivo* with any suitable molecule in the shortest time frame possible. If a prodrug can enable the exposure of a tool molecule for this purpose, it seems very reasonable to take that approach, as opposed to spending additional resources to find another suitable molecule. It can be useful to recognize that any resource a given team uses is potentially a resource that could be employed by another team. So if a prodrug can enable a molecule for the above purpose for one team, it might not only help that team move forward but also can potentially free a resource to be used to help another team move forward.

However, if prodrug and analogue efforts are truly considered in parallel as part of the drug discovery process, it is likely valuable to keep the prodrug efforts highly focused in many of the cases. Given their synthetic efficiency, it can be easy for medicinal chemists to become "distracted" toward synthesizing a great number of potential prodrugs, and an argument could be made that a better use of resources would be to discover a new analogue. So it is at least this author's opinion that when blending prodrug and analogue philosophies into one unified effort, one should be careful not to let either approach become too dominating but instead strive to use them in a complementary fashion. With the correct balance struck, the availability of more design philosophies should enable faster candidate selection and even potentially higher quality candidate selection.

## 5.7 Conclusions

The purpose of this chapter was to discuss and provide examples of the potential applications of prodrugs in modulating solubility properties to enhance oral and parenteral drug delivery. While this chapter is not intended as a comprehensive review of the literature, it is hoped that the selected examples will illustrate important aspects to consider when developing solubilizing prodrugs; furthermore, it is hoped that the included discussion will be helpful to the reader for generating new ideas toward potential applications of solubilizing prodrugs and prodrugs in general.

## References

1 DiMasi, J.A. and Grabowski, H.G. (2007) The cost of biopharmaceutical R&D: is biotech different? *Managerial and Decision Economics*, **28**, 469.

2 From molecule to medicine, 2008, http://www.jnjpharmarnd.com/jnjpharmarnd/molMedVideo.html.

3 PhRMA (2008) What goes into the cost of prescription drugs, http://www.phrma.org/files/Cost_of_Prescription_Drugs.pdf.

4 Stella V.J., Borchardt, R.T., Hageman M.J., Oliyai, R., Maag, H. and Tilley, J.W. (eds.) (2007) *Prodrugs: Challenges and*

*Rewards*, AAPS Press/Springer, New York.

**5** Testa, B. and Mayer, J.M. (2003) *Hydrolysis in Drug and Prodrug Metabolism*, Wiley-VCH Verlag GmbH, Weinheim.

**6** Bundgaard, H. (ed.) (1985) *Design of Prodrugs*, Elsevier, Amsterdam.

**7** Rautio, J., Kumpulainen, H., Heimbach, T., Oliyai, R., Oh, D., Jarvinen, T., and Savolainen, J. (2008) Prodrugs: design and clinical applications. *Nature Reviews. Drug Discovery*, **7**, 255.

**8** Stella, V.J. and Nti-Addae, K.W. (2007) Prodrug strategies to overcome poor water solubility. *Advanced Drug Delivery Reviews*, **59**, 677.

**9** Yalkowsky, S.H. (1999) *Solubility and Solubilization in Aqueous Media*, ACS/Oxford, Washington.

**10** Washington, N., Washington, C., and Wilson, C.G. (2001) *Physiological Pharmaceutics: Barriers to Drug Absorption*, 2nd edn, Taylor & Francis, New York.

**11** Bauer, J., Spanton, S., Henry, R., Quick, J., Dziki, W., Porter, W., and Morris, J. (2001) Ritonavir: an extraordinary example of conformational polymorphism. *Pharmaceutical Research*, **18**, 859.

**12** Anderson, B.D., Conradi, R.A., Knuth, K.E., and Nail, S.L. (1985) Strategies in the design of solution-stable, water-soluble prodrugs. II: properties of micellar prodrugs of methylprednisolone. *Journal of Pharmaceutical Sciences*, **74**, 375.

**13** Muller, D.G., Stella, V.J., and Lotter, A.P. (1991) Factors influencing the precipitation time of phenytoin in the presence of DDMS, one of its prodrugs. *International Journal of Pharmaceutics*, **75**, 201.

**14** Muller, D.G., Stella, V.J., and Lotter, A.P. (1994) Determination of the position of the ester bond in a micellar prodrug of phenytoin. *International Journal of Pharmaceutics*, **102**, 109.

**15** Dressman, J.B., Vertzoni, M., Goumas, K., and Reppas, C. (2007) Estimating drug solubility in the gastrointestinal tract. *Advanced Drug Delivery Reviews*, **59**, 591.

**16** Stella, V.J. (1996) A case for prodrugs: fosphenytoin. *Advanced Drug Delivery Reviews*, **19**, 311.

**17** Stella, V.J. (2007) Case study: fosphenytoin, a prodrug of phenytoin, in: *Prodrugs: Challenges and Rewards*, Part 2, AAPS Press/Springer, New York, pp. 559–567.

**18** Dhareshwar, S.S. and Stella, V.J. (2008) Your prodrug releases formaldehyde: should you be concerned? No!. *Journal of Pharmaceutical Sciences*, **97**, 4184.

**19** Talley, J.J., Bertenshaw, S.R., Brown, D.L., Carter, J.S., Graneto, M.J., Kellogg, M.S., Koboldt, C.M., Yuan, J.H., Zhang, Y.Y., and Seibert, K. (2000) *N*-(5-Methyl-3-phenylisoxazol-4-yl)-phenyl sulfonyl propanamide, sodium salt, parecoxib sodium: a potent and selective inhibitor of COX-2 for parenteral administration. *Journal of Medicinal Chemistry*, **43**, 1661.

**20** Slatter, J.G., Schaaf, L.J., Sams, J.P., Feenstra, K.L., Johnson, M.G., Bombardt, P.A., Cathcart, K.S., Verburg, M.T., Pearson, L.K., Compton, L.D., Miller, L.L., Baker, D.S., Pesheck, C.V., and Lord, R.S. (2000) Pharmacokinetics, metabolism, and excretion of irinotecan (CPT-11) following I.V. infusion of [$^{14}$C] CPT-11 in cancer patients. *Drug Metabolism and Disposition*, **28** 423.

**21** GlaxoSmithKline and Vertex (2009) Lexiva (fosamprenavir calcium): prescribing information http://us.gsk.com/products/assets/us_lexiva.pdf, p. 45.

**22** Furfine, E.S., Baker, C.T., Hale, M.R., Reynolds, D.J., Salisbury, J.A., Searle, A.D., Studenberg, S.D., Todd, D., Tung, R.D., and Spaltenstein, A. (2004) Preclinical pharmacology and pharmacokinetics of GW433908, a water-soluble prodrug of the human immunodeficiency virus protease inhibitor amprenavir. *Antimicrobial Agents and Chemotherapy*, **48**, 791.

**23** Wire, M.B., Shelton, M.J., and Studenberg, S. (2006) Fosamprenavir: clinical pharmacokinetics and drug interactions of the amprenavir prodrug. *Clinical Pharmacokinetics*, **45**, 137.

**24** Sugawara, M., Huang, W., Fei, Y., Leibach, F., Ganapathy, V., and Ganapathy, M. (2000) Transport of valganciclovir, a ganciclovir prodrug, via peptide transporters PEPT1 and PEPT2. *Journal of Pharmaceutical Sciences*, **89**, 781.

25 Narisawa, S. and Stella, V.J. (1998) Increased shelf-life of fosphenytoin: solubilization of a degradant, phenytoin, through complexation with $(SBE)_{7M}$-β-CD. *Journal of Pharmaceutical Sciences*, **87**, 926.

26 Fleisher, D., Stewart, B.H., and Amidon, G.L. (1985) Design of prodrugs for improved gastrointestinal absorption by intestinal enzyme targeting. *Methods in Enzymology*, **112**, 360.

27 Bundgaard, H. and Johansen, M. (1980) Pro-drugs as drug delivery systems. X. *N*-Mannich bases as novel pro-drug candidates for amides, imides, urea derivatives, amines and other NH-acidic compounds. Kinetics and mechanisms of decomposition and structure–reactivity relationships. *Archiv for Pharmaciog Chemi, Scientific Edition*, **8**, 29.

28 Krise, J.P., Zygmunt, J., Georg, G.I., and Stella, V.J. (1999) Novel prodrug approach for tertiary amines: synthesis and preliminary evaluation of *N*-phosphonooxymethyl prodrugs. *Journal of Medicinal Chemistry*, **42**, 3094.

29 Krise, J.P., Narisawa, S., and Stella, V.J. (1999) A novel prodrug approach for tertiary amines. 2. Physicochemical and *in vitro* enzymatic evaluation of selected *N*-phosphonooxymethyl prodrugs. *Journal of Pharmaceutical Sciences*, **88**, 922.

30 Krise, J.P., Charman, W.N., Charman, S.A., and Stella, V.J. (1999) A novel prodrug approach for tertiary amines. 3. *In vivo* evaluation of two *N*-phosphonooxymethyl prodrugs in rats and dogs. *Journal of Pharmaceutical Sciences*, **88**, 928.

31 Glazko, A.J., Edgerton, W.H., Dill, W.A., and Lenz, W.R. (1952) Chloromycetin palmitate: a synthetic ester of chloromycetin. *Antibiotics and Chemotherapy*, **2**, 234.

# 6
# Prodrugs Designed to Target Transporters for Oral Drug Delivery

*Mark S. Warren and Jarkko Rautio*

## 6.1
## Introduction

In drug discovery, many drug candidates show effective therapeutic promise but are dropped prior to development because they do not possess the optimal physiochemical properties needed to overcome biological barriers. For orally administered drugs, the intestinal epithelial cells constitute the principal barrier that limits uptake and bioavailability (Figure 6.1). These cells form tight junctions that limit the paracellular flux of drug molecules. In addition, a variety of efflux pumps, such as P-glycoprotein and several multidrug-resistance proteins in the ABC transporter family, are expressed on the apical side of these epithelial cells, limiting uptake into these epithelial cells. In order for a drug to be well absorbed from the gastrointestinal tract, researchers have traditionally focused on optimizing the physiochemical properties that allow it to permeate the epithelial cells by transcellular diffusion [1]. One way this can be accomplished is by masking polar and/or ionizable functional groups with lipophilic moieties, increasing passive diffusion while trying to avoid recognition by biological processes such as metabolizing enzymes and efflux transporters [61]. However, the pharmacokinetic properties of drugs are also partly determined by their interaction with transporters, both efflux pumps that remove them from cells and solute carriers that expedite their transport into cells. Many nutrients are recognized and absorbed by membrane transporters expressed by the epithelial cells of the GI tract [2]. Instead of trying to avoid recognition by these transporters, one may be able to take advantage of them. Drug analogues or prodrugs that are targeted toward these transporters may be able to significantly enhance the absorption of poorly permeating therapeutic agents.

## 6.2
## Serendipity: An Actively Transported Prodrug

The antiviral drug acyclovir (2) was approved as an oral medication in 1985, although it suffered from limited and variable oral bioavailability due to its high polarity. In

*Prodrugs and Targeted Delivery: Towards Better ADME Properties.* Edited by Jarkko Rautio

ISBN: 978-3-527-32603-7

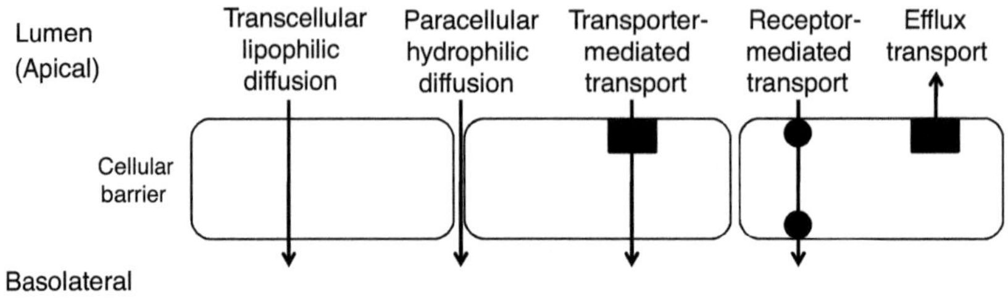


**Figure 6.1** Drug transport routes across the intestinal epithelial cell monolayer.

order to circumvent these problems, Beauchamp *et al.* synthesized and tested 18 amino acid esters of acyclovir as potential prodrugs [3]. None of these esters showed more activity than the parent compound using *in vitro* antiviral assays against herpes simplex virus type 1. However, when orally administered to rats, 10 of the compounds produced greater amounts of acyclovir in rat urine than the parent compound itself. Their quest to create a prodrug was thus successful: 10 compounds that had no or limited activity until they had been absorbed and converted to the active phosphorylated species *in vivo*. The L-valyl ester (**1**) was shown to be the best prodrug of the group, with 63% of the administered dose excreted as acyclovir in the urine – a considerable improvement over the 19% observed for acyclovir itself. Since this L-valyl ester prodrug of acyclovir was shown to be stable in aqueous solutions, the authors concluded that the conversion of acyclovir was likely enzyme catalyzed. Clinical evaluation showed that this prodrug (valacyclovir) also had three to five times higher systemic availability compared to acyclovir in humans [4]. After clinical evaluation, valacyclovir was approved as an oral medication and is used for the treatment of several viral infections. Although the original goal of this study was most likely to simply improve the bioavailability of acyclovir by creating a prodrug with greater passive permeability, these researchers had, by serendipity, created a prodrug that was actively absorbed in the intestine.

Further evaluation of the amino acid esters of acyclovir showed that the L-amino acids were better prodrugs than either the D-amino acids or mixtures of the D- and L-isomers, suggesting the involvement of a stereoselective transporter [3]. It was later suggested that human peptide transporter 1 (hPEPT1)-mediated uptake of valacyclovir into intestinal cells could be the underlying mechanism for this elevated absorption [5]. Other reports suggested that multiple membrane transporters, including PEPT1, could be involved in valacyclovir uptake [6], and the transport kinetics of valacyclovir were concentration dependent and saturable [7]. However, these studies used rat tissue or Caco-2 cells, where numerous transporters potentially involved in valacyclovir transport are found. More definitive studies using Chinese hamster ovary (CHO) cells transfected with hPEPT1 followed, providing direct evidence that (1) valacyclovir uptake was higher in hPEPT1-transfected CHO cells than in control cells; (2) valacyclovir uptake was concentration dependent and saturable with a Michaelis–Menten constant around 1 mM; and (3) known PEPT1 substrates, such as various dipeptides and β-lactam antibiotics, could block valacyclovir uptake [8, 9]. After absorption, valacyclovir is then hydrolyzed to acyclovir by "human valacyclovirase," an alpha-amino acid ester hydrolase capable of activating valacyclovir and other prodrugs [10, 11]. Furthermore, acyclovir is converted to its active phosphorylated form (**3**) by various kinases, thus being a prodrug in its own right.

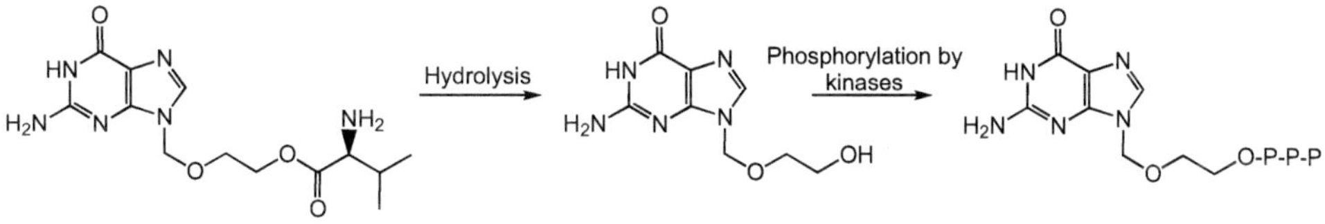


Valacyclovir (**1**)
Substrate of PEPT1
Oral bioavailability 3-5 fold higher than acyclovir

Acyclovir (**2**)
Not substrate of PEPT1

Active triphosphorylated form (**3**)

## 6.3
## Requirements for Actively Transported Prodrugs

Although valacyclovir was not necessarily designed to take advantage of active transport mechanisms, it did raise the possibility of using such mechanisms in drug design. Indeed, it has been shown in many cases that it is possible to improve oral absorption substantially by chemically modifying the drug to form a prodrug that can act as a substrate for a known transport system. This is particularly important for polar or charged drugs that may have negligible passive absorption.

Obviously, not every transporter is suitable for prodrug uptake. Transporters that are optimal for prodrug uptake have several properties: First, transporters used for orally administered prodrugs must be expressed in the gastrointestinal tract. Second, the transporter must not be too specific in its recognition of substrates; otherwise it would be very difficult to design prodrugs that could be recognized. In addition, the transporter should be expressed at relatively high levels in order to facilitate rapid drug uptake. Finally, the candidate transporter should have a relatively high capacity in order to avoid being inhibited by an excess of prodrug molecules, which could block uptake of the normal nutrients recognized by that transporter. Fortunately, several different classes of transporters appear to satisfy all of these criteria and many of them have successfully been used (either by design or by serendipity) to enhance the uptake of prodrugs. Examples of uptake transporters found in the intestine are provided in Table 6.1.

In this chapter, only uptake transporters that have been active prodrug targets, for example, peptide, monocarboxylate, and bile acid transporters, are discussed in more detail.

## 6.4
## Peptide Transporters: PEPT1 and PEPT2

Members of the oligopeptide transporter family (SLC15) mediate proton-coupled cotransport of many diverse peptide and peptidomimetic substrates. Well-characterized family members are PEPT1 (SLC15A1) and PEPT2 (SLC15A2). PEPT1

**Table 6.1** Uptake transporters affecting intestinal absorption of drugs and their representative drug substrates.

| Transporter | Examples of drugs with active uptake transport |
|---|---|
| Oligopeptide transporter (PEPT1) | ACE inhibitors (e.g., captopril, enalapril, and fosinopril), β-lactam antibiotics (e.g., penicillins and cephalosporins), valacyclovir, valganciclovir |
| Monocarboxylate transporters | Salicylic acid, β-lactam antibiotics, statins |
| Bile acid transporters (ASBT/IBAT) | Various drugs conjugated to bile salts |
| Organic anion transporter polypeptide (OATP1) | Fexofenadine |

is highly expressed in the absorptive cells of the intestinal epithelium, whereas cells of the renal epithelium express predominantly PEPT2 and also PEPT1. Both transporters have been cloned in mammals [12, 13], but their three-dimensional structure has not been elucidated due to the difficulty in purifying and crystallizing membrane proteins. Therefore, the structural requirements for molecular recognition have been based both on uptake or transport studies and on computational modeling. Both transporters differ in their substrate specificity, affinity, and transport capacity.

The intestinal PEPT1 is perhaps the drug transporter that has captured the most recent attention in oral drug delivery. The expression of PEPT1 increases from the duodenum to the ileum [14], and at the villus level is more abundant at the tip. Almost all 400 dipeptides and 8000 tripeptides derived from the common protein-forming amino acids, but not free amino acids or peptides with more than 3 amino acid residues, are substrates for PEPT1. A detailed characterization of its substrates has been performed [15], demonstrating that it has a particular affinity for molecules in which the amino and carboxylic acid groups are separated by about 6 Å, even in nonpeptidic substrates. The PEPT1 substrate recognition site is proposed to have the following characteristics: (1) a strong binding site for N-terminal $NH_3^+$, (2) a hydrogen bond to the carbonyl group of the first peptide bond, (3) a carboxylate binding site, and (4) a hydrophobic pocket for the side chain of an amino acid (Figure 6.2). Moreover, PEPT1 is stereospecific and it prefers L-L-di- and L-L-L-tripeptides over their D-enantiomers.

Comparatively, PEPT1 is considered a low-affinity ($K_m$ of 200 μM–10 mM), high-capacity transporter, while PEPT2 has higher substrate affinity ($K_m$ of 5–500 μM) and lower transport capacity. Taken together, peptide transporters are capable of mediating the transport of a huge variety of molecules, from endogenous peptides to various therapeutic drugs, including nonpeptidyl drugs, with a large diversity of physicochemical properties (Figure 6.3). The substrates of peptide transporters include several β-lactam antibiotics, angiotensin-converting enzyme inhibitors such as captopril, enalapril, and fosinopril, as well as bestatin and antibacterial peptide analogues such as alafosfalin. Even compounds without an obvious peptide bond,

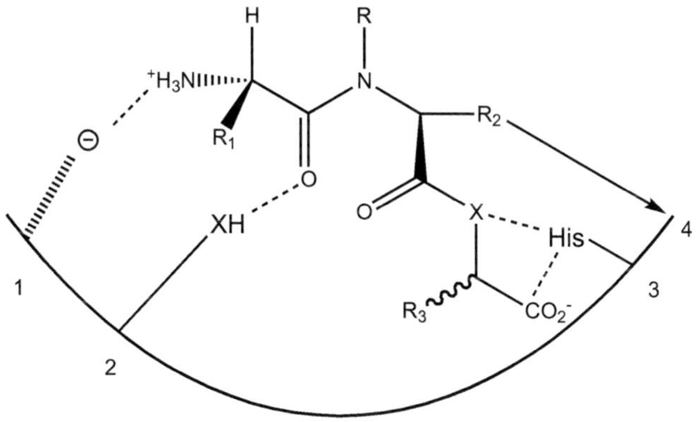


**Figure 6.2** PEPT1 substrate recognition site contains four key structural characteristics (modified from Ref. [15]).

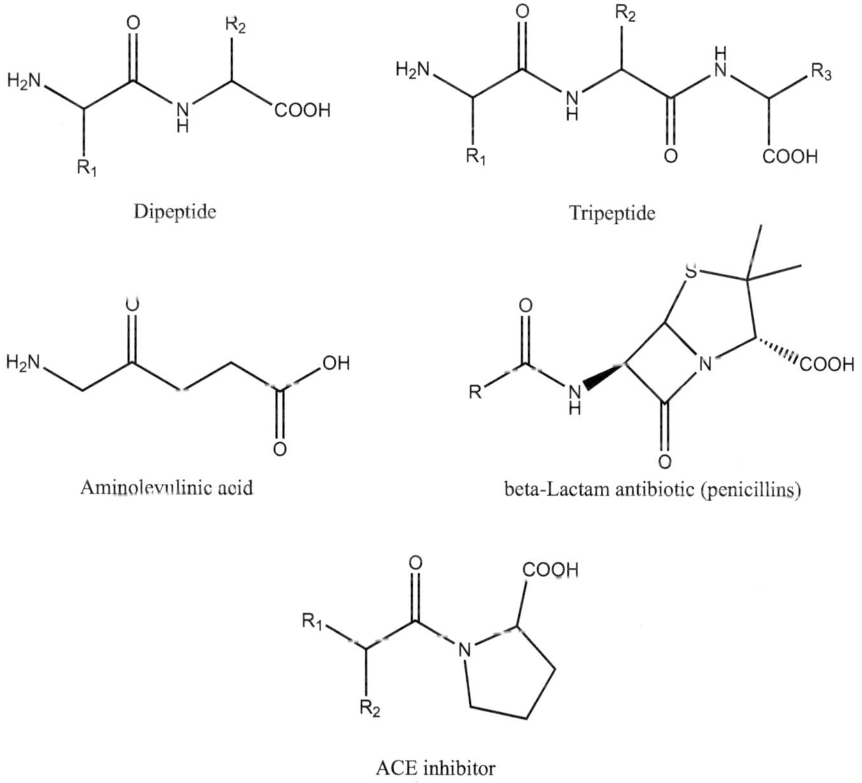


**Figure 6.3** Substrates of peptide transporters.

such as δ-aminolevulinic acid, possessing a ketomethylene group, are transported by peptide transporters.

Its broad substrate specificity, reasonable high capacity, and high level of expression in the intestinal epithelium make PEPT1 an attractive target for prodrug design. As seen earlier in the case of valacyclovir, by engineering the prodrug to be recognized by PEPT1, a low permeability drug can obtain significantly higher oral absorption. Like valacyclovir, a valine ester prodrug of ganciclovir (**4**), namely, valganciclovir (**5**), is actively transported by PEPT1, which results in approximately 60% oral bioavailability of ganciclovir in humans, while the oral bioavailability of ganciclovir itself is less than 10% [16]. The transport mechanism was confirmed in studies using Caco-2 cell monolayers where the transport of valganciclovir was inhibited by a dipeptide, Gly-Phe [17]. In the same transport studies, the bis-valine ester of ganciclovir and ganciclovir itself proved not to be PEPT1 substrates. Valganciclovir has also been shown to be a substrate of the PEPT2 transporter, which is mainly present in the kidney [17], and the amino acid transporter $ATB^{0,+}$, expressed primarily in the colon, lung, and eye [18]. Only very low levels of the prodrug can be detected in the systemic circulation after oral administration, suggesting a rapid and complete hydrolysis to ganciclovir *in vivo*. Recently, it has been demonstrated that conversion of valganciclovir is due to the biphenyl hydrolase-like protein, valacyclovirase [10]. Valganciclovir has been approved as an oral prodrug for the treatment of cytomegalovirus (CMV).

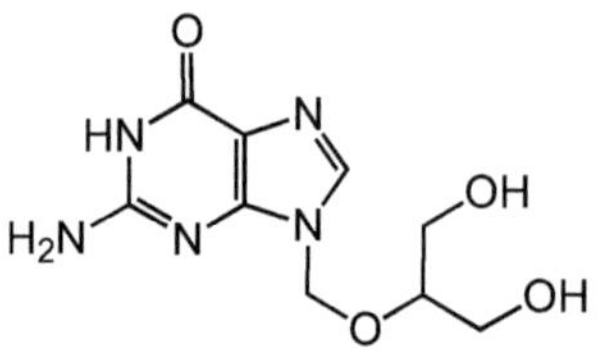

Ganciclovir (**4**)
Oral bioavailability 6%
Not substrate of PEPT1

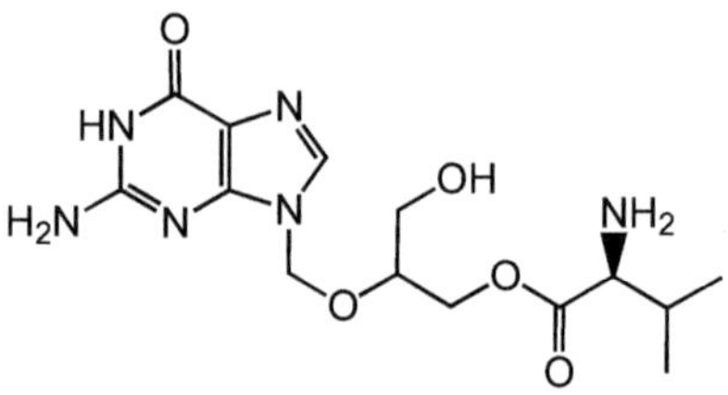

Valganciclovir (**5**)
Oral bioavailability 60%
Substrate of PEPT1

The pioneering success with valacyclovir and valganciclovir in the clinic paved the way for the development of several L-valine prodrugs of other poorly absorbed drugs, especially various nucleoside analogues. Levovirin valinate (**6**), valopicitabine (**7**), and valtorcitabine (**8**) are prodrugs of levovirin, 2′-*C*-methylcytidine and 2′-deoxy-β-L-cytidine, respectively, and their improved oral absorption may be attributed to the involvement of PEPT1-mediated transport. All these L-valine prodrugs, including valomaciclovir stearate (**9**), which is a valyl/stearyl diester prodrug of H2G (omaciclovir), are undergoing clinical trials. Therefore, the L-valine monoester concept has proved to be an important landmark in the development of PEPT1-targeted oral prodrugs.

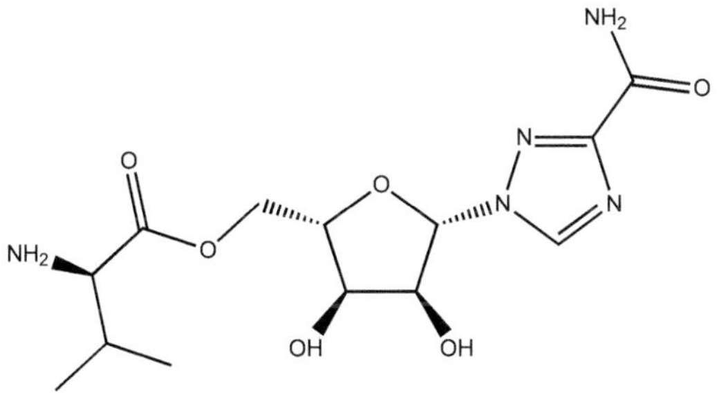

Levovirin valinate (**6**)

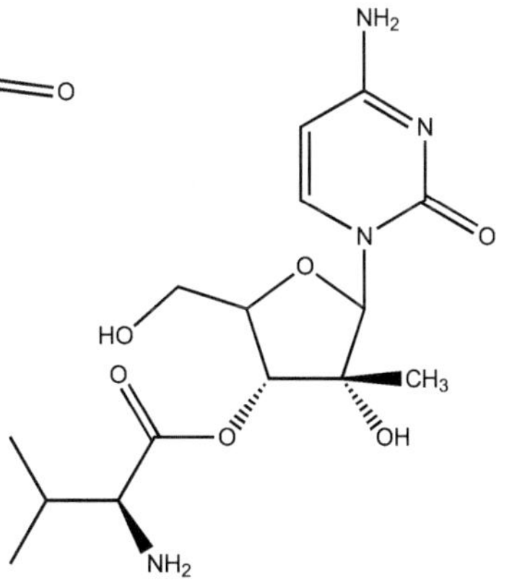

Valopitacitabine (**7**)

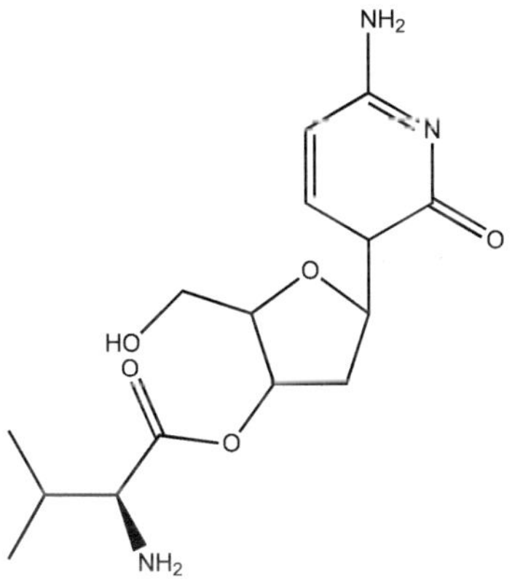

Valtorcitabine (**8**)

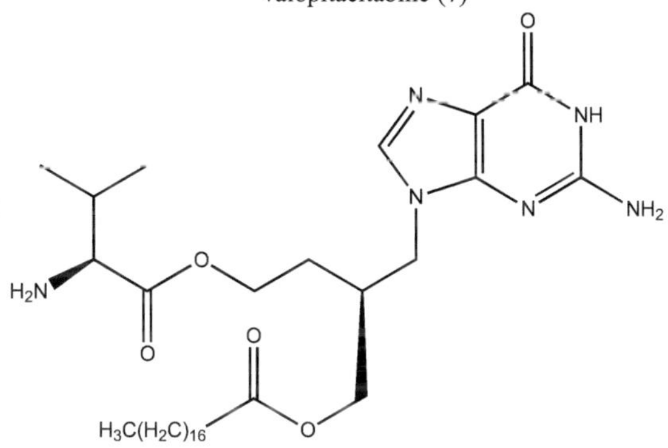

Valomaciclovir stearate (**9**)

The prodrug strategy targeting PEPT1 has also been effective in improving oral absorption of polar parent drugs using amino acids other than valine. The peptidyl prodrugs such as L-α-methyldopa-L-Phe, L-Phe-L-α-methyldopa, and L-α-methyldopa-L-Pro achieved 4–20 times higher intestinal wall permeability than α-methyldopa itself in a rat ileum perfusion model [19, 20]. While α-methyldopa is itself a relatively poor substrate for the L-aromatic amino acid transporter, the uptake of the α-methyldopa prodrugs was inhibited by known PEPT1 substrates, thus demonstrating peptide transporter-mediated absorption. Similarly, L-dopa-L-Phe showed peptide transporter-mediated uptake that was 40-fold higher than that of L-dopa across Caco-2 cell monolayers [21].

Recently, an L-alanylamide prodrug (LY544344 or talaglumetad, **11**) emerged from a series of C-2, C-6, and N peptides derived from an agonist of the metabolic glutamate receptor 2 (LY354740, **10**), with a variety of amino acids and dipeptides as promoieties. The prodrug was selected on the basis of its effective active transport [22]. In subsequent assays, this prodrug not only showed high affinity to PEPT1 in Caco-2 cells and hPEPT1-transfected CHO cells but also significantly reduced permeability in the presence of the known PEPT1 substrate Gly-Sar in *in situ* rat intestinal perfusion studies [22, 23]. The prodrug also underwent extensive presystemic intestinal activation, with more than 97% of prodrug hydrolysis occurring before its appearance in the hepatic portal vein [24]. In clinical studies, the prodrug has been shown to increase systemic LY354740 exposure by approximately 13-fold compared to equivalent LY544344 doses.

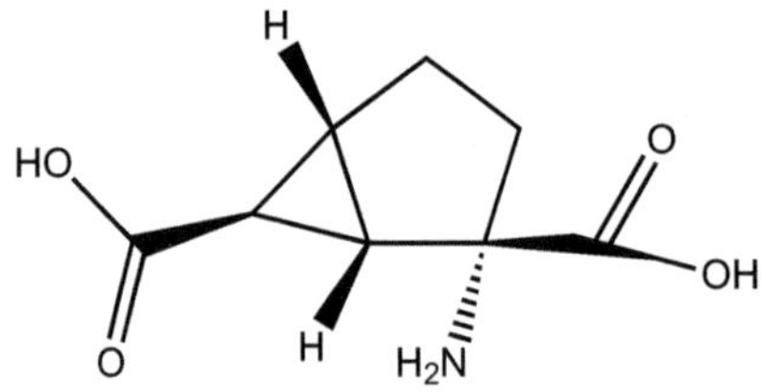


LY354740 (**10**)

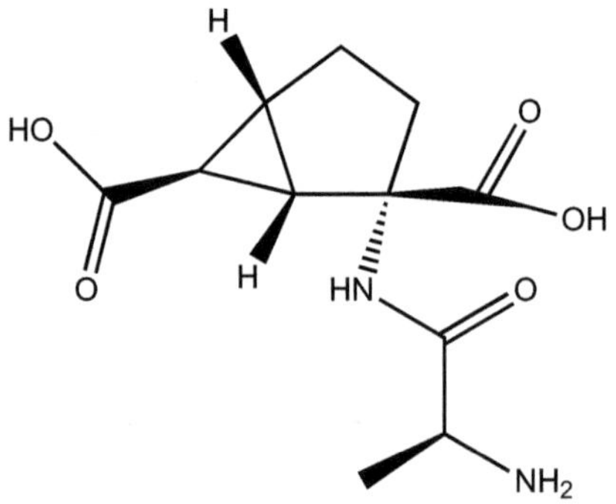


LY544344 (**11**)

## 6.5 Monocarboxylate Transporters

The monocarboxylate transporter (MCT) family (SLC16) is comprised of 14 members, although only the first 4 members have been shown to transport monocarboxylates [25, 26]. These four transporters, MCT1 (SLC16A1), MCT2 (SLC16A7), MCT3 (SLC16A8), and MCT4 (SLC16A3), have been shown to transport a diverse group of aliphatic monocarboxylates in a process that does not require ATP, but is instead controlled by proton and substrate gradients [26]. For proper localization and functional expression of these transporters in the membrane, coexpression of an accessory protein is also required. CD147, also known as basigin, has been shown to serve this role for MCT1, MCT3, and MCT4 [27], while gp70, also known as embigin, is used by MCT2 [28].

Of these four MCT transporters, only MCT3 has relatively restricted tissue expression, primarily being expressed in the retinal pigment epithelium and choroid plexus epithelium [29]. The other MCTs are expressed in a variety of tissues, demonstrating high expression in the gastrointestinal tract [26], with MCT1 and MCT4 being the predominant isoforms expressed in the human colon [30]. Since the transit time is longer in the colon than in the rest of the gastrointestinal tract, MCT1 and MCT4 may be ideal candidates for use as prodrug transporters.

Using immunoblotting studies on purified apical and basolateral membranes isolated from different regions of the small and large intestines, Gill *et al.* reported that MCT1 was localized apically, with increasing abundance along the gastrointestinal tract and predominant expression in the colon [30]. In addition, they performed immunohistochemical studies on colonic crypts obtained from human biopsy samples to confirm that MCT1 was predominantly confined to the apical membranes. Similar studies by Iwanaga *et al.* using mouse, rat, and human tissues confirmed the broad expression of MCT1 throughout the gastrointestinal tract, with greater expression in the large intestine than in the stomach or small intestine; however, in contrast to the results obtained by Gill *et al.*, they showed MCT1 expression to be on the basolateral cell membranes [31]. In addition, they used immunoelectron microscopy to confirm the subcellular localization of MCT1 in the cecum of mice, showing that MCT1 was present only in the basolateral membranes of enterocytes and not in the microvillous region. The differences reported by these two groups may be a result of differences in the antibody recognition sites, which could indicate that MCT1 is actually expressed on both sides of the membrane.

Immunoblotting studies of MCT4 demonstrated that this transporter is localized to the basolateral colonic membranes [30], with highest expression in the distal colon, followed by the proximal colon, and followed by the ileum. The MCT4 antibody was unsuitable for immunohistochemical studies [30], and other studies also failed to detect any visible signals for MCT4 in the digestive tract of mice [31].

Lactate (**12**) and pyruvate (**13**) are natural substrates for MCT1 and MCT4. In addition, both MCT1 and MCT4 transport the short-chain fatty acids acetate, propionate, and butyrate, which collectively represent the most abundant anions in the colon [30]. However, the specificity of MCT1 and MCT4 is not limited to these molecules. Both proteins have been shown to transport a variety of small carboxylates, such as chloropropionate, hydroxybutyrate, alpha-ketoisocaproate, and alpha-ketoisovalerate [32, 33]. In fact, when MCT1 was first cloned, it was identified as "MEV," a protein facilitating high uptake of the cholesterol precursor mevalonic acid [34].

MCT1 and MCT4 can also transport pharmaceutical agents. Gamma-hydroxybutyrate (GHB, **14**), a naturally occurring metabolite of gamma-aminobutyric acid, is found in mammalian brain, heart, liver, and kidney [35]. While GHB is used therapeutically for treating narcolepsy [36] and alcohol and heroin withdrawal [37], it is also widely abused by body builders for its growth hormone releasing properties [38], as well as drug abusers for its euphoric effects and for drug-facilitated sexual assault [39, 40].

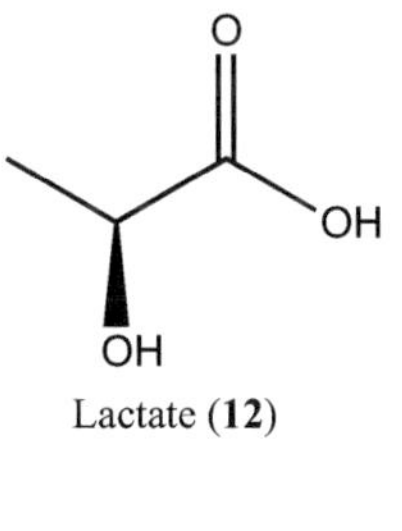

Lactate (**12**)

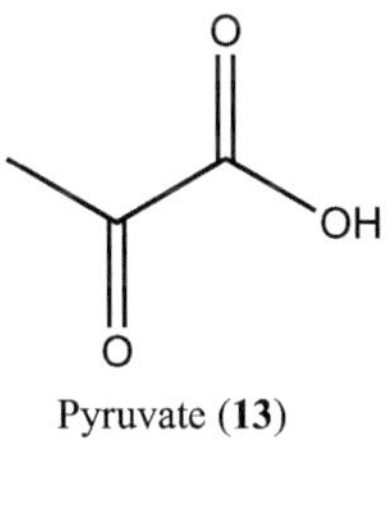

Pyruvate (**13**)

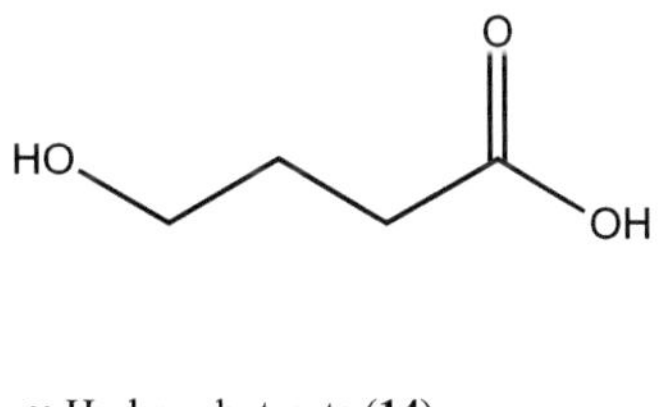

γ-Hydroxybutyrate (**14**)

In addition to endogenous substrates, MCT1 has also been shown to transport a variety of xenobiotic compounds. Using tissue-specific cell lines, membrane vesicles, Caco-2 cells, NBL-2 cells, MDCK cells, or *in vivo* investigations, MCTs have been demonstrated to transport compounds as diverse as β-lactam antibiotics carindacillin [41, 42] and cefdinir [43], valproic acid [44, 45], salicylic acid [46], fluorescein [47], ferulic acid [48], pravastatin [49], simvastatin [50], and atorvastatin [51]. However, while the statins are substrates of MCT1, they are also inhibitors of MCT4, with the more lipophilic statins demonstrating the strongest inhibition [52].

With the wide variety of structures recognized by MCT1, as well as the high expression in the gastrointestinal tract, it should be possible to design prodrugs to take advantage of MCT1. One such first prodrug was the β-lactam antibiotic prodrug carindacillin (**15**), which is converted to carbenicillin (**16**) [53], although it was not specifically designed to take advantage of MCT1 (which itself would not be described for another 20 years). However, the role of MCT1 in the intestinal uptake of carindacillin has been confirmed in rat intestinal brush border membrane vesicles, and this MCT1-dependent uptake is believed to contribute to improved exposure to carbenicillin [41, 42].

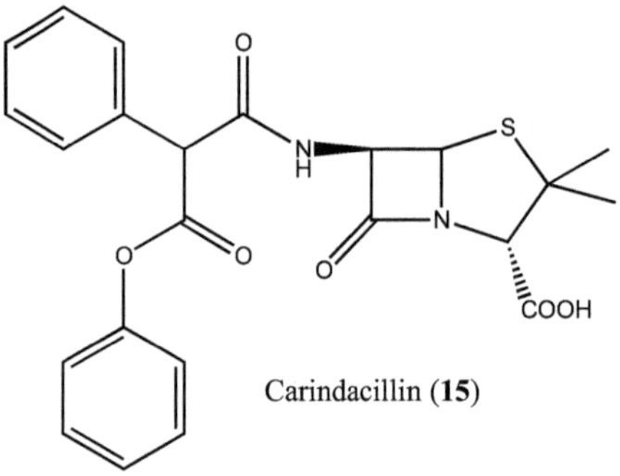

Carindacillin (**15**)

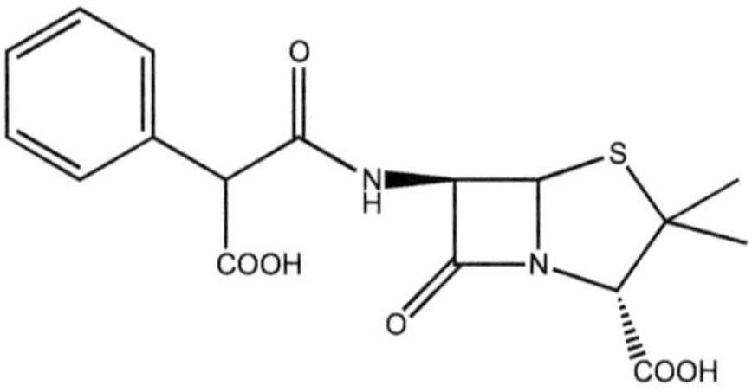

Carbenicillin (**16**)

This concept has also been used in the design of a gabapentin prodrug, XP13512 (or gabapentin enacarbil, **17**), which was designed to overcome the poor intestinal absorption of gabapentin in part by taking advantage of MCT1 and another transporter, the sodium-dependent multivitamin transporter SMVT. The uptake of XP13512 was shown to be MCT1 mediated both in HEK-derived cells and in MCT1-expressing oocytes [54]. While gabapentin (**18**) absorption occurs in only a limited region of the small intestine and saturates at doses used clinically, resulting in dose-dependent pharmacokinetics, high interpatient variability, and potentially ineffective drug exposure, XP13512 is absorbed throughout the entire length of the intestine. *In vivo* studies on XP13512 demonstrated predictable dose-proportional bioavailability of gabapentin from XP13512 compared to that resulting from gabapentin itself, as well as improved colonic absorption [55–58].

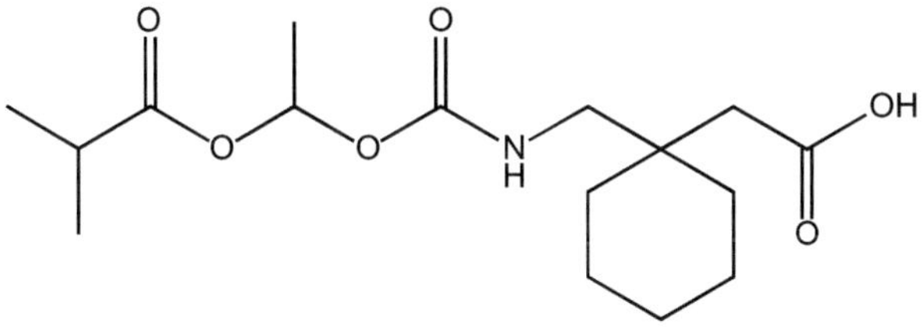


XP13512 (**17**)

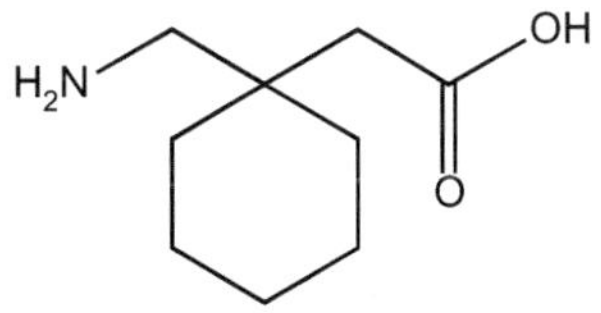


Gabapentin (**18**)

A prodrug of *R*-baclofen, arbaclofen placarbil (**19**), has also been designed to take advantage of MCT1 [57, 58]. The prodrug was shown to compete with the natural MCT1 substrate lactate in LLC-PK1-derived cells expressing high levels of MCT1 and demonstrated increased uptake in MCT1-expressing oocytes compared to control oocytes. In contrast, *R*-baclofen (**20**) itself did not show any significant interaction with MCT1 [57, 58]. Arbaclofen placarbil has demonstrated enhanced colonic absorption with 5-fold higher *R*-baclofen exposure in rats and 12-fold higher in monkeys compared to intracolonic administration of *R*-baclofen. Sustained release formulations of arbaclofen placarbil demonstrated sustained *R*-baclofen exposure in dogs with bioavailability up to 68%.

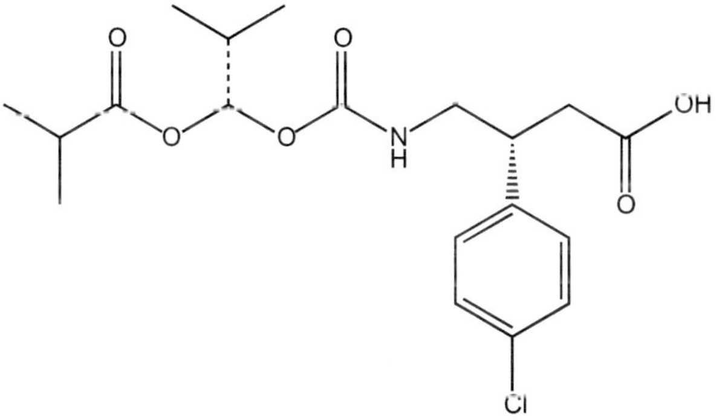


Arbaclofen placarbil (**19**)

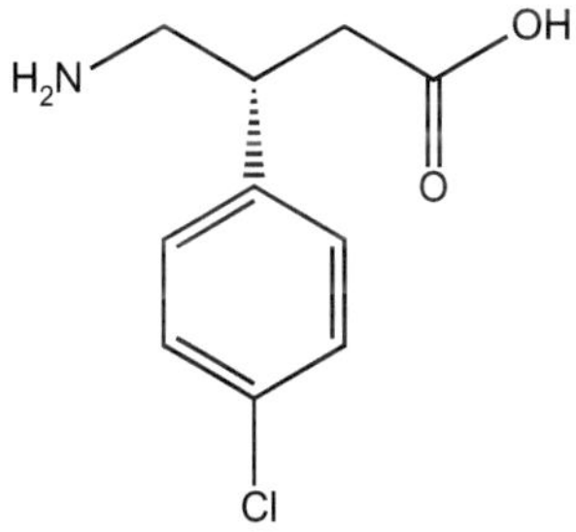


R-Baclofen (**20**)

With numerous endogenous and exogenous compounds, including prodrugs, already known to be recognized by MCT1, this transporter shows considerable promise as a target for future prodrugs that can be designed to take advantage of its broad substrate recognition, high capacity, and high colonic expression.

## 6.6
## Bile Acid Transporters

Bile, consisting of bile acids, phospholipids, cholesterol, biliary pigments, and proteins, is concentrated and stored in the gall bladder. During digestion, bile is secreted into the small intestine. As they travel through the gastrointestinal tract, the bile acids are nearly completely reabsorbed by both active and passive mechanisms. Bile acids then recirculate to the liver via the portal vein.

In humans, the primary bile acids, cholate and chenodeoxycholate, are synthesized in hepatocytes from cholesterol, while secondary bile acids (such as deoxycholate and lithocholate) are formed via bacterial metabolism in the small intestine [59]. The principal bile acids in human bile are mainly conjugated cholic acid and chenodeoxycholic acid [60]. Conjugation increases bile acid polarity and lowers passive transport, resulting in most bile acid reabsorption being controlled by the human apical sodium-dependent bile acid transporter hASBT (SLC10A2, also known as IBAT for ileal/intestinal bile acid transporter). This situation facilitates high intraluminal bile acid concentration to aid in lipid absorption. Conjugation also improves bile acid solubility, helping to decrease any precipitation in the presence of high calcium ion concentrations found in the gall bladder [61].

The enterohepatic circulation of bile acids occurs repeatedly (6–15 times/day) [62]. The bile acid pool in humans is about 3–5 g, resulting in a turnover of 12–18 g of bile acid each day [60]. In spite of this repeated cycling, the loss of bile acid in the feces is less than 0.5 g/day, reflecting the tremendous capacity and efficiency of hASBT [63].

ASBT is expressed on the apical membrane of enterocytes in the terminal ileum, and mediates the reabsorption of bile acids into the ileum. The second bile acid transporter, the sodium-dependent hepatocyte bile salt uptake transporter (NTCP, SLC10A1, also known as LBAT for liver bile acid transporter), is expressed in hepatocytes and localized on the basolateral (sinusoidal) domain to reabsorb bile salts from the portal circulation. These two transporters have broad substrate specificity, high affinity for efficient absorption, and very high capacity, making them excellent targets for designing prodrugs [59].

Bile acids are versatile building blocks. Drug substances may be attached to different positions of the steroidal skeleton or to the side chain using different chemical bonds, or by linkers with different structures, lengths, stereochemistries, polarities, and functional groups. The carboxylic acid group of the bile acid molecule may be esterified, amidated, or reduced, while the steroidal hydroxyl groups can be used to make esters and ethers, or can be oxidized or reduced [62].

Pioneering work in developing bile acid-derived prodrugs came from the research group of Kramer and Wess, who synthesized conjugates of bile acids containing drugs such as chlorambucil, oxaprolyl peptide, HR780, and lovastatin (Figure 6.4) [64–71]. Their work on chlorambucil–bile acid conjugates showed that these compounds were absorbed from the ileum and secreted by the liver, as demonstrated by *in situ* perfusion experiments of rat liver and ileal segments. In contrast, chlorambucil itself is cleared by the kidney. These intact bile acid conjugates retain the alkylating activity of chlorambucil. Later studies showed that human hepatocellular carcinomas were capable of mediating the uptake of a chlorambucil–taurocholate conjugate with high affinity, demonstrating the feasibility of bile acid–drug conjugates in liver-specific drug targeting [70].

A prime target for a liver-specific drug would be the statins, which are widely used in efforts to lower plasma cholesterol levels. Drugs such as pravastatin, lovastatin, and simvastatin inhibit the activity of HMG-CoA reductase, which is responsible for the

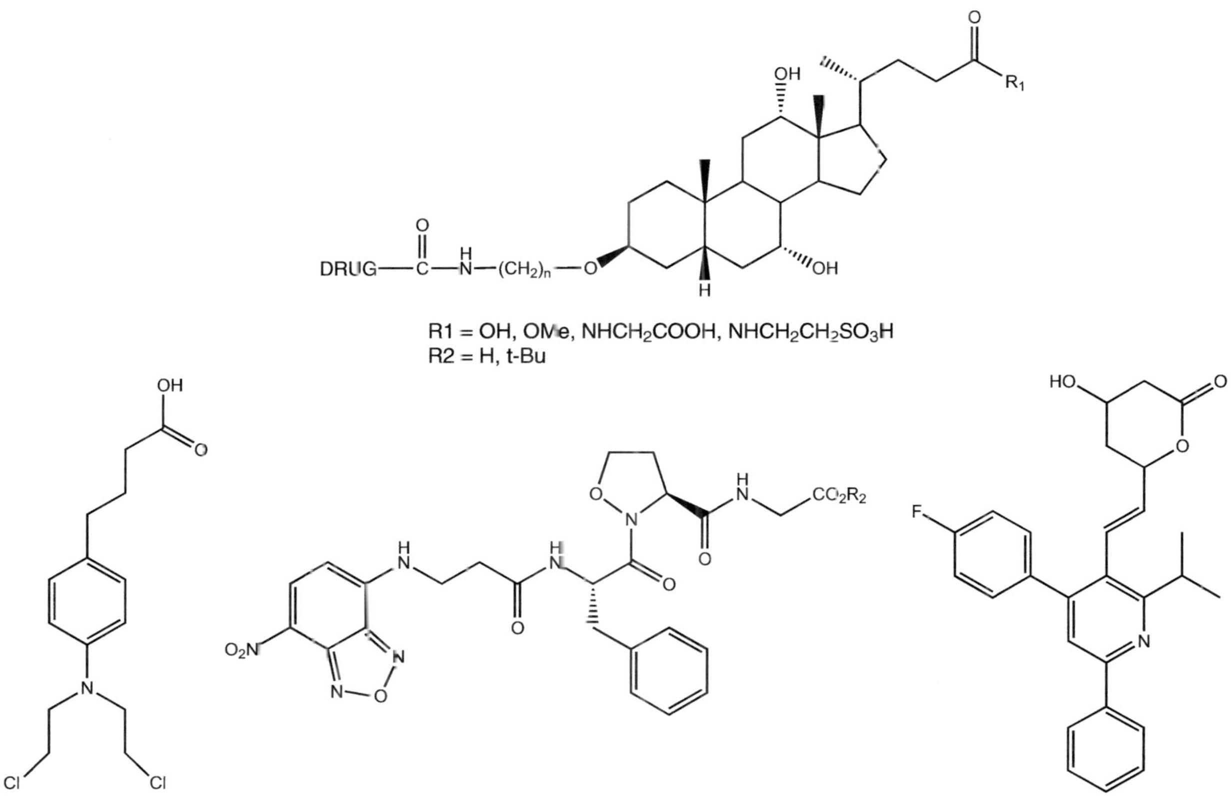


Chlorambucil

Oxaproline peptide

HR780

**Figure 6.4** Bile acid-derived prodrugs.

rate-limiting step in cholesterol biosynthesis, the transformation of β-hydroxy-β-methylglutaryl-CoA (HMG-CoA) to mevalonate [65, 66]. Since bile acids undergo enterohepatic circulation restricting them to the liver and small intestine, a statin-bile acid prodrug that specifically targeted cholesterol biosynthesis in the liver and intestines could reduce potential side effects due to cholesterol biosynthesis in other tissues.

Kramer *et al.* utilized two approaches: combining structural features of HMG-CoA reductase inhibitors with bile acids to create hybrid molecules (**22**) and creation of prodrugs by conjugation of the HMG-CoA reductase inhibitors to the bile acid (**21**) [65, 66]. The hybrid molecules were able to inhibit HMG-CoA reductase, while the prodrugs, prior to hydrolysis from the bile acid promoiety, could not. However, the prodrugs did release the active inhibitor, as evident by the presence of a major metabolite, and the concentration of the conjugated drug in extrahepatic tissues in rats was considerably lower than the concentration in liver, demonstrating tissue selectivity. *In vivo* experiments also showed an inhibition of hepatic cholesterol biosynthesis after oral dosage of the prodrugs, whereas the hybrid molecules were inactive after oral dosing [65, 66].

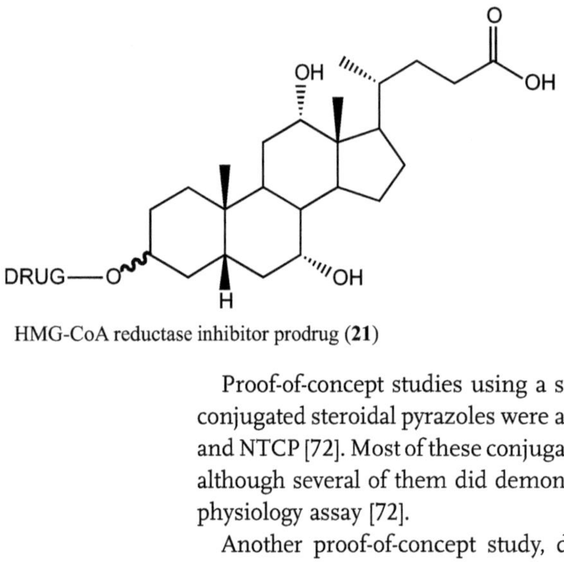


HMG-CoA reductase inhibitor prodrug (**21**)

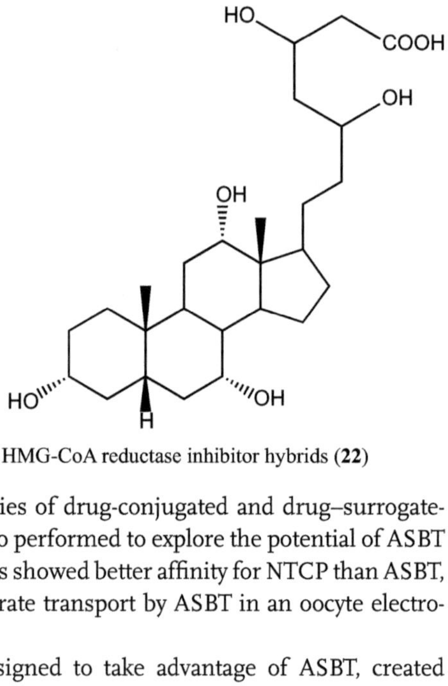


HMG-CoA reductase inhibitor hybrids (**22**)

Proof-of-concept studies using a series of drug-conjugated and drug–surrogate-conjugated steroidal pyrazoles were also performed to explore the potential of ASBT and NTCP [72]. Most of these conjugates showed better affinity for NTCP than ASBT, although several of them did demonstrate transport by ASBT in an oocyte electrophysiology assay [72].

Another proof-of-concept study, designed to take advantage of ASBT, created acyclovir prodrugs by conjugation to a variety of bile acids [73]. Affinities were assessed by measuring inhibition of taurocholate uptake in ASBT-transfected COS-7 cells, and the prodrug with the highest affinity was further evaluated *in vitro* and *in vivo*. This prodrug, acyclovir valylchenodeoxycholate (**23**), was cleaved by an esterase to release acyclovir, and resulted in greater acyclovir accumulation from the prodrug than could be obtained from the drug alone due to a combination of active uptake by ASBT and increased passive permeability. Oral administration of the prodrug in rats resulted in a twofold increase in acyclovir bioavailability compared to acyclovir itself, demonstrating that a bile acid prodrug strategy could be useful in improving the oral bioavailability of compounds with limited intestinal permeability [73].

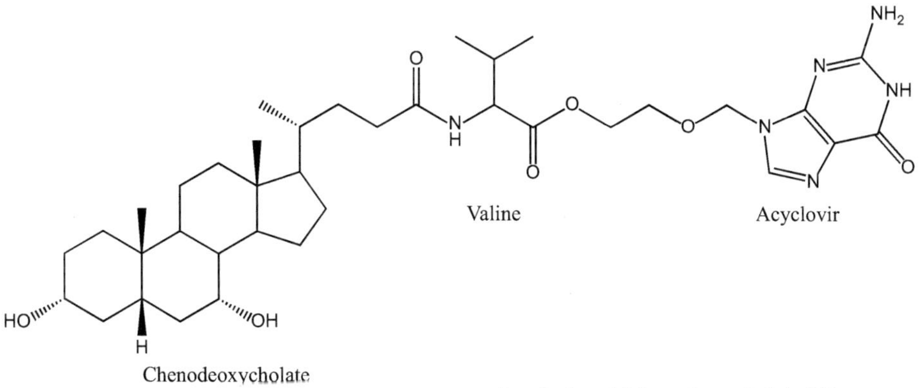


**Acyclovir valylchenodeoxycholate (23)**

## 6.7 Conclusions

Drug uptake transporters in the intestinal tract play a major role in the absorption and disposition of some drugs. They also offer an intriguing target in designing prodrugs with a view to improving intestinal absorption of poorly absorbed drugs, as can be seen from successful prodrug examples discussed in this chapter. Moreover, in some cases, membrane transporters may also enable selective drug uptake to the target organ or tissue, or utilize the genetic polymorphism of drug transporters by designing drugs toward a specific portion of the patient population. Challenges with relying on drug transporters in drug absorption include transport capacity becoming rate limiting or saturable, susceptibility to drug–drug and drug–endogenous ligand interactions, and genetic variability in a population. The prodrug approach targeting intestinal uptake transporters is now widely exploited as demonstrated by the many novel prodrugs that are under investigation and development.

## References

1 Martinez, M.N. and Amidon, G.L. (2002) A mechanistic approach to understanding the factors affecting drug absorption: a review of fundamentals. *Journal of Clinical Pharmacology*, **42** (6), 620–643.

2 Dobson, P.D. and Kell, D.B. (2008) Carrier-mediated cellular uptake of pharmaceutical drugs: an exception or the rule? *Nature Reviews. Drug Discovery*, **7** (3), 205–220.

3 Beauchamp, L.M., Orr, G.F., De Miranda, P., Burnette, T., and Krenitsky, T.A. (1992) Amino acid ester prodrugs of acyclovir. *Antiviral Chemistry and Chemotherapy*, **3** (3), 157–164.
4 Weller, S., Blum, M.R. *et al.* (1993) Pharmacokinetics of the acyclovir prodrug valaciclovir after escalating single- and multiple-dose administration to normal volunteers. *Clinical Pharmacology and Therapeutics*, **54** (6), 595–605.
5 Lee, C.-P., De Vrueh, R. L. A., and Smith, P. L. (1996) Transport of a prodrug of Acyclovir, L-val-acyclovir, via the oligopeptide transporter. *Proc. Int. Symp. Control. Release. Bioact. Mater.*, **23**, 47–48.
6 Sinko, P.J. and Balimane, P.V. (1998) Carrier-mediated intestinal absorption of valacyclovir, the L-valyl ester prodrug of acyclovir: 1. Interactions with peptides, organic anions and organic cations in rats. *Biopharmaceutics & Drug Disposition*, **19** (4), 209–217.
7 de Vrueh, R.L., Smith, P.L. *et al.* (1998) Transport of L-valine-acyclovir via the oligopeptide transporter in the human intestinal cell line, Caco-2. *The Journal of Pharmacology and Experimental Therapeutics*, **286** (3), 1166–1170.
8 Han, H., de Vrueh, R.L. *et al.* (1998) 5′-Amino acid esters of antiviral nucleosides, acyclovir, and AZT are absorbed by the intestinal PEPT1 peptide transporter. *Pharmaceutical Research*, **15** (8), 1154–1159.
9 Guo, A., Hu, P. *et al.* (1999) Interactions of a nonpeptidic drug, valacyclovir, with the human intestinal peptide transporter (hPEPT1) expressed in a mammalian cell line. *The Journal of Pharmacology and Experimental Therapeutics*, **289** (1), 448–454.
10 Kim, I., Chu, X.Y. *et al.* (2003) Identification of a human valacyclovirase: biphenyl hydrolase-like protein as valacyclovir hydrolase. *The Journal of Biological Chemistry*, **278** (28), 25348–25356.
11 Lai, L., Xu, Z. *et al.* (2008) Molecular basis of prodrug activation by human valacyclovirase, an alpha-amino acid ester hydrolase. *The Journal of Biological Chemistry*, **283** (14), 9318–9327.
12 Fei, Y.J., Kanai, Y. *et al.* (1994) Expression cloning of a mammalian proton-coupled oligopeptide transporter. *Nature*, **368** (6471), 563–566.
13 Liu, W., Liang, R. *et al.* (1995) Molecular cloning of PEPT 2, a new member of the $H^+$/peptide cotransporter family, from human kidney. *Biochimica et Biophysica Acta*, **1235** (2), 461–466.
14 Tanaka, H., Miyamoto, K.I. *et al.* (1998) Regulation of the PEPT1 peptide transporter in the rat small intestine in response to 5-fluorouracil-induced injury. *Gastroenterology*, **114** (4), 714–723.
15 Bailey, P.D., Boyd, C.A. *et al.* (2000) How to make drugs orally active: a substrate template for peptide transporter PEPT1. *Angewandte Chemie. International Edition in English*, **39** (3), 505–508.
16 Brown, F., Banken, L. *et al.* (1999) Pharmacokinetics of valganciclovir and ganciclovir following multiple oral dosages of valganciclovir in HIV- and CMV-seropositive volunteers. *Clinical Pharmacokinetics*, **37** (2), 167–176.
17 Sugawara, M., Huang, W. *et al.* (2000) Transport of valganciclovir, a ganciclovir prodrug, via peptide transporters PEPT1 and PEPT2. *Journal of Pharmaceutical Sciences*, **89** (6), 781–789.
18 Umapathy, N.S., Ganapathy, V. *et al.* (2004) Transport of amino acid esters and the amino-acid-based prodrug valganciclovir by the amino acid transporter ATB(0, +). *Pharmaceutical Research*, **21** (7), 1303–1310.
19 Hu, M., Subramanian, P. *et al.* (1989) Use of the peptide carrier system to improve the intestinal absorption of L-alpha-methyldopa: carrier kinetics, intestinal permeabilities, and *in vitro* hydrolysis of dipeptidyl derivatives of L-alpha-methyldopa. *Pharmaceutical Research*, **6** (1), 66–70.
20 Bai, J.P., Hu, M. *et al.* (1992) Utilization of peptide carrier system to improve intestinal absorption: targeting prolidase as a prodrug-converting enzyme. *Journal of Pharmaceutical Sciences*, **81** (2), 113–116.

21 Tamai, I., Nakanishi, T. *et al.* (1998) Improvement of L-dopa absorption by dipeptidyl derivation, utilizing peptide transporter PEPT1. *Journal of Pharmaceutical Sciences*, **87** (12), 1542–1546.

22 Bueno, A.B., Collado, I. *et al.* (2005) Dipeptides as effective prodrugs of the unnatural amino acid (+)-2-aminobicyclo [3.1.0]hexane-2,6-dicarboxylic acid (LY354740), a selective group II metabotropic glutamate receptor agonist. *Journal of Medicinal Chemistry*, **48** (16), 5305–5320.

23 Eriksson, A.H., Varma, M.V. *et al.* (2010) The intestinal absorption of a prodrug of the mGlu2/3 receptor agonist LY354740 is mediated by PEPT1: *in situ* rat intestinal perfusion studies. *Journal of Pharmaceutical Sciences*, **99** (3), 1574–1581.

24 Perkins, E.J. and Abraham, T. (2007) Pharmacokinetics, metabolism, and excretion of the intestinal peptide transporter 1 (SLC15A1)-targeted prodrug (1S,2S,5R,6S)-2-[(2′S)-(2-amino) propionyl]aminobicyclo[3.1.0.]hexen-2, 6-di carboxylic acid (LY544344) in rats and dogs: assessment of first-pass bioactivation and dose linearity. *Drug Metabolism and Disposition: The Biological Fate of Chemicals*, **35** (10), 1903–1909.

25 Meredith, D. and Christian, H.C. (2008) The SLC16 monocaboxylate transporter family. *Xenobiotica; The Fate of Foreign Compounds in Biological Systems*, **38** (7–8), 1072–1106.

26 Merezhinskaya, N. and Fishbein, W.N. (2009) Monocarboxylate transporters: past, present, and future. *Histology and Histopathology*, **24** (2), 243–264.

27 Kirk, P., Wilson, M.C. *et al.* (2000) CD147 is tightly associated with lactate transporters MCT1 and MCT4 and facilitates their cell surface expression. *EMBO Journal*, **19** (15), 3896–3904.

28 Wilson, M.C., Meredith, D. *et al.* (2005) Basigin (CD147) is the target for organomercurial inhibition of monocarboxylate transporter isoforms 1 and 4: the ancillary protein for the insensitive MCT2 is EMBIGIN (gp70). *The Journal of Biological Chemistry*, **280** (29), 27213–27221.

29 Yoon, H., Fanelli, A. *et al.* (1997) Identification of a unique monocarboxylate transporter (MCT3) in retinal pigment epithelium. *Biochemical and Biophysical Research Communications*, **234** (1), 90–94.

30 Gill, R.K., Saksena, S. *et al.* (2005) Expression and membrane localization of MCT isoforms along the length of the human intestine. *American Journal of Physiology. Cell Physiology*, **289** (4), C846–C852.

31 Iwanaga, T., Takebe, K. *et al.* (2006) Cellular expression of monocarboxylate transporters (MCT) in the digestive tract of the mouse, rat, and humans, with special reference to SLC5A8. *Biomedical Research (Tokyo, Japan)*, **27** (5), 243–254.

32 Manning Fox, J.E., Meredith, D. *et al.* (2000) Characterisation of human monocarboxylate transporter 4 substantiates its role in lactic acid efflux from skeletal muscle. *The Journal of Physiology*, **529** (Pt 2), 285–293.

33 Morris, M.E. and Felmlee, M.A. (2008) Overview of the proton-coupled MCT (SLC16A) family of transporters: characterization, function and role in the transport of the drug of abuse gamma-hydroxybutyric acid. *AAPS Journal*, **10** (2), 311–321.

34 Kim, C.M., Goldstein, J.L. *et al.* (1992) cDNA cloning of MEV, a mutant protein that facilitates cellular uptake of mevalonate, and identification of the point mutation responsible for its gain of function. *The Journal of Biological Chemistry*, **267** (32), 23113–23121.

35 Maitre, M. (1997) The gamma-hydroxybutyrate signalling system in brain: organization and functional implications. *Progress in Neurobiology*, **51** (3), 337–361.

36 Mamelak, M., Scharf, M.B. *et al.* (1986) Treatment of narcolepsy with gamma-hydroxybutyrate. A review of clinical and sleep laboratory findings. *Sleep*, **91** Pt (2), 285–289.

37 Gallimberti, L., Spella, M.R. *et al.* (2000) Gamma-hydroxybutyric acid in the treatment of alcohol and heroin

dependence. *Alcohol (Fayetteville, NY)*, **20** (3), 257–262.
38 Okun, M.S., Boothby, L.A. et al. (2001) GHB: an important pharmacologic and clinical update. *Journal of Pharmacy & Pharmaceutical Sciences: A Publication of the Canadian Society for Pharmaceutical Sciences*, **4** (2), 167–175.
39 Schwartz, R.H., Milteer, R. *et al.* (2000) Drug-facilitated sexual assault ('date rape'). *Southern Medical Journal*, **93** (6), 558–561.
40 Wong, C.G., Chan, K.F. *et al.* (2004) Gamma-hydroxybutyric acid: neurobiology and toxicology of a recreational drug. *Toxicology Review*, **23** (1), 3–20.
41 Li, Y.H., Ito, K. *et al.* (1999) Mechanism of intestinal absorption of an orally active beta-lactam prodrug: uptake and transport of carindacillin in Caco-2 cells. *The Journal of Pharmacology and Experimental Therapeutics*, **290** (3), 958–964.
42 Li, Y.H., Tanno, M. *et al.* (1999) Role of the monocarboxylic acid transport system in the intestinal absorption of an orally active beta-lactam prodrug: carindacillin as a model. *International Journal of Pharmaceutics*, **191** (2), 151–159.
43 Tsuji, A., Tamai, I. *et al.* (1993) Intestinal brush-border transport of the oral cephalosporin antibiotic, cefdinir, mediated by dipeptide and monocarboxylic acid transport systems in rabbits. *The Journal of Pharmacy and Pharmacology*, **45** (11), 996–998.
44 Utoguchi, N. and Audus, K.L. (2000) Carrier-mediated transport of valproic acid in BeWo cells, a human trophoblast cell line. *International Journal of Pharmaceutics*, **195** (1–2), 115–124.
45 Hosoya, K. and Kondo, T. *et al.* (2001) MCT1-mediated transport of L-lactic acid at the inner blood–retinal barrier: a possible route for delivery of monocarboxylic acid drugs to the retina. *Pharmaceutical Research*, **18** (12), 1669–1676.
46 Neuhoff, S., Ungell, A.L. *et al.* (2005) pH-Dependent passive and active transport of acidic drugs across Caco-2 cell monolayers. *European Journal of Pharmaceutical Sciences*, **25** (2–3), 211–220.
47 Konishi, Y., Hagiwara, K. *et al.* (2002) Transepithelial transport of fluorescein in Caco-2 cell monolayers and use of such transport in *in vitro* evaluation of phenolic acid availability. *Bioscience, Biotechnology, and Biochemistry*, **66** (11), 2449–2457.
48 Konishi, Y. and Shimizu, M. (2003) Transepithelial transport of ferulic acid by monocarboxylic acid transporter in Caco-2 cell monolayers. *Bioscience, Biotechnology, and Biochemistry*, **67** (4), 856–862.
49 Tamai, I., Takanaga, H. *et al.* (1995) Proton-cotransport of pravastatin across intestinal brush-border membrane. *Pharmaceutical Research*, **12** (11), 1727–1732.
50 Tsuji, A., Saheki, A. *et al.* (1993) Transport mechanism of 3-hydroxy-3-methylglutaryl coenzyme A reductase inhibitors at the blood–brain barrier. *The Journal of Pharmacology and Experimental Therapeutics*, **267** (3), 1085–1090.
51 Wu, X., Whitfield, L.R. *et al.* (2000) Atorvastatin transport in the Caco-2 cell model: contributions of P-glycoprotein and the proton-monocarboxylic acid co-transporter. *Pharmaceutical Research*, **17** (2), 209–215.
52 Kobayashi, M., Otsuka, Y. *et al.* (2006) Inhibitory effects of statins on human monocarboxylate transporter 4. *International Journal of Pharmaceutics*, **317** (1), 19–25.
53 English, A.R., Retsema, J.A. *et al.* (1972) Carbenicillin indanyl sodium, an orally active derivative of carbenicillin. *Antimicrobial Agents and Chemotherapy*, **1** (3), 185–191.
54 Cundy, K.C., Branch, R. *et al.* (2004) XP13512 [(+/−)-1-([(alpha-isobutanoyloxyethoxy)carbonyl] aminomethyl)-1-cyclohexane acetic acid], a novel gabapentin prodrug: I. Design, synthesis, enzymatic conversion to gabapentin, and transport by intestinal solute transporters. *The Journal of Pharmacology and Experimental Therapeutics*, **311** (1), 315–323.
55 Cundy, K.C., Annamalai, T. *et al.* (2004) XP13512 [(+/−)-1-([(alpha-isobutanoyloxyethoxy)carbonyl]

aminomethyl)-1-cyclohexane acetic acid], a novel gabapentin prodrug: II. Improved oral bioavailability, dose proportionality, and colonic absorption compared with gabapentin in rats and monkeys. *The Journal of Pharmacology and Experimental Therapeutics*, **311** (1), 324–333.

56 Cundy, K.C., Sastry, S. *et al.* (2008) Clinical pharmacokinetics of XP13512, a novel transported prodrug of gabapentin. *Journal of Clinical Pharmacology*, **48** (12), 1378–1388.

57 Lal, R., Sukbuntherng, J. *et al.* (2009) Pharmacokinetics and tolerability of single escalating doses of gabapentin enacarbil: a randomized-sequence, double-blind, placebo-controlled crossover study in healthy volunteers. *Clinical Therapeutics*, **31** (8), 1776–1786.

58 Lal, R., Sukbuntherng, J. *et al.* (2009) Arbaclofen placarbil, a novel R-baclofen prodrug: improved absorption, distribution, metabolism, and elimination properties compared with R-baclofen. *The Journal of Pharmacology and Experimental Therapeutics*, **330** (3), 911–921.

59 Balakrishnan, A. and Polli, J.E. (2006) Apical sodium dependent bile acid transporter (ASBT, SLC10A2): a potential prodrug target. *Molecular Pharmacology*, **3** (3), 223–230.

60 Hofmann, A.F. (1999) The continuing importance of bile acids in liver and intestinal disease. *Archives of Internal Medicine*, **159** (22), 2647–2658.

61 Hofmann, A.F. and Mysels, K.J. (1992) Bile acid solubility and precipitation *in vitro* and *in vivo*: the role of conjugation, pH, and $Ca_2^+$ ions. *Journal of Lipid Research*, **33** (5), 617–626.

62 Sievanen, E. (2007) Exploitation of bile acid transport systems in prodrug design. *Molecules*, **12** (8), 1859–1889.

63 St-Pierre, M.V., Kullak-Ublick, G.A. *et al.* (2001) Transport of bile acids in hepatic and non-hepatic tissues. *The Journal of Experimental Biology*, **204** (Pt 10), 1673–1686.

64 Kramer, W., Wess, G. *et al.* (1992) Liver-specific drug targeting by coupling to bile acids. *The Journal of Biological Chemistry*, **267** (26), 18598–18604.

65 Kramer, W., Wess, G. *et al.* (1994) Bile acid derived HMG-CoA reductase inhibitors. *Biochimica et Biophysica Acta*, **1227** (3), 137–154.

66 Kramer, W., Wess, G. *et al.* (1994) Intestinal absorption of peptides by coupling to bile acids. *The Journal of Biological Chemistry*, **269** (14), 10621–10627.

67 Wess, G., Kramer, W. *et al.* (1994) Specific inhibitors of ileal bile acid transport. *Journal of Medicinal Chemistry*, **37** (7), 873–875.

68 Wess, G., Kramer, W. *et al.* (1994) Synthesis and biological activity of bile acid-derived HMG-CoA reductase inhibitors. The role of 21-methyl in recognition of HMG-CoA reductase and the ileal bile acid transport system. *Journal of Medicinal Chemistry*, **37** (20), 3240–3246.

69 Kramer, W. and Wess, G. (1996) Bile acid transport systems as pharmaceutical targets. *European Journal of Clinical Investigation*, **26** (9), 715–732.

70 Kullak-Ublick, G.A., Glasa, J. *et al.* (1997) Chlorambucil-taurocholate is transported by bile acid carriers expressed in human hepatocellular carcinomas. *Gastroenterology*, **113** (4), 1295–1305.

71 Starke, D., Lischka, K. *et al.* (2001) Bile acid-oligodeoxynucleotide conjugates: synthesis and liver excretion in rats. *Bioorganic & Medicinal Chemistry Letters*, **11** (7), 945–949.

72 Bhat, L., Jandeleit, B. *et al.* (2005) Synthesis and biological evaluation of novel steroidal pyrazoles as substrates for bile acid transporters. *Bioorganic & Medicinal Chemistry Letters*, **15** (1), 85–87.

73 Tolle Sander, S., Lentz, K.A. *et al.* (2004) Increased acyclovir oral bioavailability via a bile acid conjugate. *Molecular Pharmacology*, **1** (1), 40–48.

# 7
# Topical and Transdermal Delivery Using Prodrugs: Mechanism of Enhancement

*Kenneth Sloan, Scott C. Wasdo, and Susruta Majumdar*

## 7.1
## Introduction

Topical delivery of drugs either for local or systemic effects offers numerous advantages. It also presents one major disadvantage that is that not many drugs exhibit the requisite physicochemical properties to passively diffuse across the barrier to permeation into (dermal delivery) and through the skin (transdermal delivery). For skin, this barrier to passive diffusion is generally accepted to reside in the stratum corneum (SC) [1, 2]. According to Fick's law [3, 4], since passive diffusion is driven by differences in concentration between the first and the last layers of a membrane (the SC in this case), and since the higher the concentration is in the first layer the greater the driving force for passive diffusion will be across the membrane, low passive diffusion is the result of low solubility of the permeant in the first few layers of the SC [5, 6].

There are three ways to overcome the low solubility of the permeant in the SC. The first approach is to change the physicochemical properties of the SC to match those of the drug (permeant) by a formulation approach. A chemical entity (penetration enhancer) is added to the vehicle in which the drug is applied. The penetration enhancer diffuses into the SC and changes the physicochemical properties of the SC to more closely match those of the drug: like dissolves like. The second approach is to change the physicochemical properties of the drug to more closely match those of the SC. A chemical entity (promoiety) is added reversibly to the drug to give a prodrug. The prodrug's physicochemical properties now match those of the SC: again, like dissolves like. The prodrug approach has the potential advantage that the reversibly added promoiety and the drug are present in a one-to-one ratio compared to the formulation approach where the penetration enhancer is present in excess of the drug and the penetration enhancer has its own toxicity profile [6, 7]. The third approach is to use a mechanical/electrical device to reversibly bypass the barrier to passive diffusion. An example of this approach is to use a microneedle array that reversibly introduces holes in the barrier through which drug is delivered to the systemic circulation. Compared to the third approach, the prodrug or the penetration enhancer approach is much less invasive.

*Prodrugs and Targeted Delivery: Towards Better ADME Properties.* Edited by Jarkko Rautio

ISBN: 978-3-527-32603-7

Here, we focus only on the prodrug approach, provide some insight into the physicochemical properties of the SC that affect the solubility of drugs (and prodrugs) in the SC, and compare the relative effectiveness of acyl- and soft alkyl-type prodrug approaches to enhancing transdermal delivery based on their solubility properties. Initially, the macroscopic solubility properties exhibited by the barrier to diffusion were identified indirectly from correlations of the solubility properties of drugs (and prodrugs) with their abilities to diffuse across the barrier to diffusion and affect transdermal delivery. Over 25 years ago, the observation was made that, in addition to increasing the lipid solubility of a prodrug, increasing the water solubility of a prodrug compared to its parent drug was also important to optimize the transdermal delivery of the parent drug [8]. The simplistic rationale for this correlation between transdermal delivery (flux) of the parent drug and the solubility of the prodrug both in water and in lipid was that skin, like other "biological membranes presents lipid–water (biphasic) barriers" [8] that must be traversed in series to give effective transdermal delivery of the drug. Thus, the prodrug must be sufficiently soluble in both lipid and aqueous phases to cross the barrier to diffusion. For a homologous series of prodrugs that are more lipophilic, the members of the series that are more water soluble will generally give the higher flux values [9]. However, the member with the highest water solubility will not necessarily give the highest flux: a balance of lipid and aqueous solubilities is important to optimize flux [7, 9].

This correlation between a balance of lipid and aqueous solubilities and flux holds both for homologous series of nonprodrugs and for prodrugs. In fact, although it is not generally recognized, the earliest illustration of this correlation is the classic study of the diffusion of a homologous series of alcohols from saturated water solutions or from the pure liquids across human skin *in vitro* [10]. For those alcohols that were not miscible with water (starting with butanol), the more water-soluble members of the series gave the higher fluxes regardless of whether they were applied as a saturated water solution or as a pure liquid.

Although the correlation is quite clear, the exact position and arrangement of these aqueous and lipid (biphasic) barriers in the overall barrier to diffusion has been the subject of much discussion. Initially, it was assumed that the material occupying the space between the corneocytes of the SC, through which the drug/prodrugs must diffuse, presented a solubility-based resistance that was purely lipoidal in nature [3, 4, 11]. Thus, it was assumed that in order to change the physicochemical properties of the drug to match those of the material occupying the space between the corneocytes, the drug only needed to be made more lipid soluble. In fact, the solubility parameter of the diffusion barrier to transdermal delivery in the skin was estimated to be between 9.7 and 10.0 $cal^{0.5}\ cm^{-1.5}$ based on the correlation between the fluxes and the solubility parameters of a homologous series of alkanoic acids [12]. This estimated solubility parameter of skin is essentially the same as that of the well-known lipid, octanol (10.3 $cal^{0.5}\ cm^{-1.5}$). Any dependence of flux on the water solubility of the drug/prodrug was attributed to (1) the stagnant water layer at the interface between an aqueous vehicle and the SC surface [13] or to (2) the primarily aqueous epidermis and dermis that underlie the SC [14]. In each case, an extra aqueous solubility-based resistance to diffusion was presented to poorly water-soluble drugs/prodrugs that was external to the SC.

However, these attributions were not consistent with existing data. First, even the earliest data from Scheuplein and Blank's study of the transdermal delivery of alcohols showed that the same correlation between flux and a balance of lipid and aqueous solubility obtained regardless of whether the vehicle was water or the alcohol itself [10]: there can be no stagnant water layer if there is no water in the case of the flux of the pure alcohols. Also, the correlation between flux of prodrugs from a lipid vehicle (isopropyl myristate, IPM) and a balance of lipid and aqueous solubilities is well established [7, 9, 15]. Second, highly lipid-soluble prodrugs (compared to the parent drug) exhibiting very low water solubilities (compared to the parent drug) that hydrolyze very rapidly in the skin ($t_{1/2}$ less than 5 min) give much lower fluxes than the parent drug or those prodrugs in the same series that exhibit water solubility at least comparable to the parent drug [16]. The decreased fluxes compared to the parent drug by more lipid prodrugs that are less water soluble than the parent drug but hydrolyze very rapidly to the more water-soluble parent drug cannot be attributed to an extra water solubility-based resistance in the viable epidermis/dermis because only the more water-soluble parent drug would be presented to the viable epidermis/dermis. It is the initial poor balance of lipid and aqueous solubilities exhibited by the intact prodrug that leads to its decreased solubility in the SC and subsequent poor flux.

## 7.2
## Arrangement of Water in the Stratum Corneum

If the water phase that contributes to the solubility-based barrier to diffusion is not in the vehicle or not in the lower strata of the skin, where is it? It has to exist in the same compartment as the lipid phase that contributes to the solubility-based barrier to diffusion: it has to exist in the material occupying the space between the corneocytes through which the drug/prodrug diffuses. Although an extensive amount of research has been committed to elucidate the exact composition, conformation, and arrangement of the lipid phase of the barrier to diffusion because of its obvious importance and complexity [17–21], very little has been done to identify the exact arrangement of the water phase component of the space between the corneocytes. The general assumption is that only the lipid phase contributed to the resistance to diffusion so the water phase, even if it existed, was not sufficiently important to study.

What has been determined is that the stratum corneum can absorb water up to 40% w/w of the weight of the hydrated SC ($SC_{HYD}$) without affecting the presence of the approximately 13.4 nm repeat distance in the bilayer organization: 0.40 g of water plus 0.60 g of dry SC ($SC_{DRY}$) [19]. The presence of the 13.4 nm long periodicity phase (LPP) observed from small-angle X-ray scattering (SAXS) analysis of the SC is considered to be essential to the maintenance of a complete barrier to diffusion through the SC [20]. It has also been determined that up to 0.30 g of water can be absorbed by 1.00 g of $SC_{DRY}$ before an endotherm due to the melting of unbound water appears in the differential scanning calorimetry (DSC) trace of frozen, hydrated SC [22]. The 0.30 g of bound water per 1.00 g of $SC_{DRY}$ corresponds to 0.18 g of bound water per 0.60 g of $SC_{DRY}$. Thus, $SC_{DRY}$ can absorb 0.18 g of bound water and 0.22 g of unbound water per 0.60 g of $SC_{DRY}$ before the important 13.4 nm LPP is lost.

Where is the 0.22 g of unbound water located in the 1.00 g of $SC_{HYD}$? The bound water is assumed to be located in the corneocytes bound to protein; the unbound water is assumed to be uniformly distributed through the $SC_{HYD}$. Neutron diffraction studies of a mixture of ceramide CER 6 (AP), cholesterol (Ch), palmitic acid (PA), and cholesterol sulfate (ChS) [23] showed that there was very little water between the polar head groups of opposing bilayer leafs (0.08 nm thick), that water molecules penetrated 0.38 nm deep into the region of the hydrocarbon chains of AP and PA past the polar head group, and that water was associated with but not necessarily hydrogen bonded to the 0.35 nm deep polar head group region. Thus, the total hydrophilic region of one leaf of the bilayer was about 0.73 nm. The total depth of one leaf of the bilayer was about 2.27 nm (a repeat distance of 4.54 nm) meaning that 1.54 nm of one leaf of the bilayer was hydrophobic. Since ceramide CER1 (a linoleic acid linked to the omega-hydroxy groups on one of the alkyl chains of the ceramide) was not present in the mixture, no 13.4 nm LPP was observed [20]. However, the absence of the 13.4 nm LPP should not affect the arrangement of water around the polar head groups of the bilayers.

Since the nominal surface area of ceramides is about 0.40–0.50 $nm^2$ [24], the minimum total volume in the bilayer occupied by a ceramide is 0.91 $nm^3$ and the volume of the ceramide occupied by water is 0.29 $nm^3$. If the weight of unbound water in 1.00 g of hydrated SC ($SC_{HYD}$) is 0.22 g and if it is assumed that 1.00 g of $SC_{HYD}$ occupies 1.00 $cm^3$, then the concentration of water molecules in the $SC_{HYD}$ is 12.22 mol/l or 7.36 molecules of water/$nm^3$. Since the volume of an individual ceramide is 0.91 $nm^3$, there are 6.7 molecules of water per ceramide and they are localized in 0.29 $nm^3$ of the polar end of the ceramide. It is assumed that PA and Ch in this mixture have approximately the same number of water molecules associated with their polar head groups for the same surface area that the ceramide occupies. It is also assumed that the 6–7 water molecules associated with the polar portion of the bilayers occupy void space between adjacent head groups and do not increase the total volume of the lipid or the bilayer thickness. For phospholipids, it was found that 10–14 water molecules per lipid could occupy that void space without affecting the total volume or thickness of the bilayer [25].

## 7.3
## A New Model for Diffusion Through the Stratum Corneum: The Biphasic Solubility Model

Taking into account the fact that multiple bilayers form the material that occupies the space between corneocytes and the fact that the bilayers run parallel to the horizontal arrangement of the corneocytes in the SC, Figure 7.1 provides a cartoon representation of the path that a drug/prodrug takes in its diffusion through the bilayers and

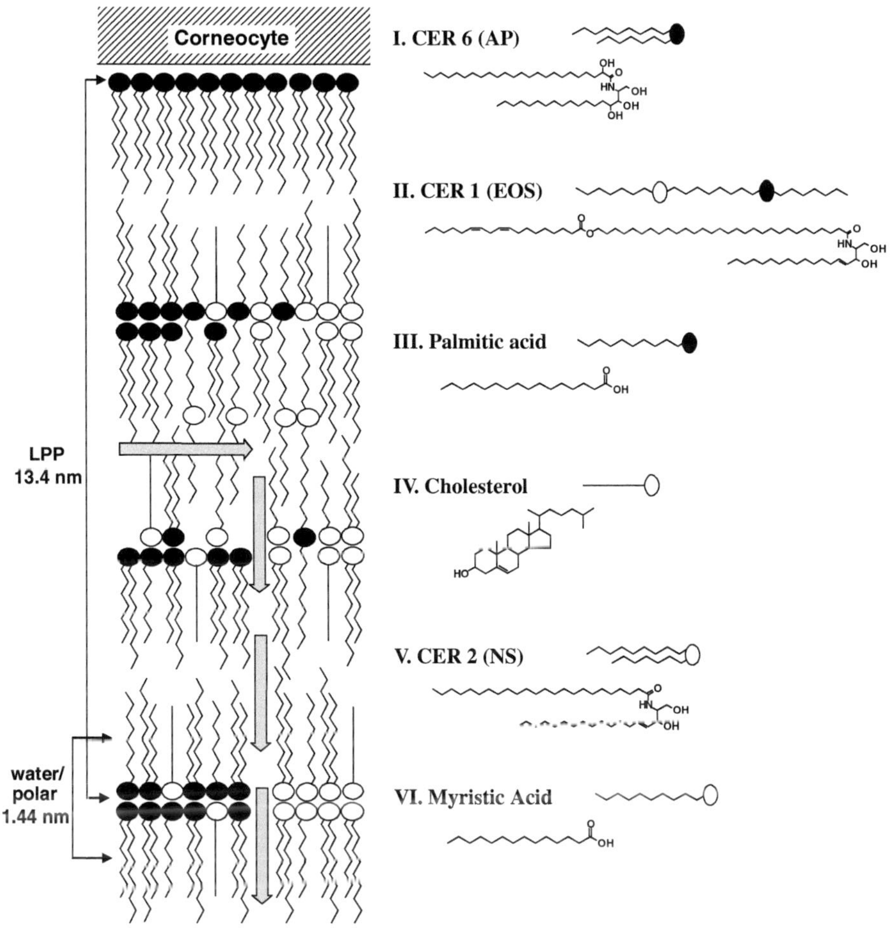


**Figure 7.1** Pathway for diffusion through the stratum corneum based on the biphasic solubility model.

around the corneocytes. The structures of the lipid components of the barrier to diffusion are identified in the figure as I–VI: I represents a ceramide such as CER6 (AP), II represents a ceramide such as CER1 (EOS), III represents the long-chain fatty acid palmitic acid ($C_{16}$), IV represents cholesterol, V represents a ceramide such as CER 2 (NS), and VI represents the long-chain fatty acid myristic acid ($C_{14}$) that has a different chain length from III. The lipid components of the barrier have been arranged (1) to show a 13.4-nm LPP as in the sandwich model [20, 21, 26], (2) to show the EOS ceramide in an extended conformation with the linoleic acid portion bridging the space between two broad, crystalline layers to give a more fluid narrow layer in the middle, and (3) to show separate domain mosaics [21, 27, 28] formed by ceramides with a different polar head group (V) from I combined with fatty acids of different chain length (VI) from III.

The path of least resistance to diffusion by the drug/prodrug is through the more fluid center of the 13.4 nm LPP (sandwich model) for the lipid part of the diffusion path. However, in order for the diffusion process to be productive (get to the other side of the bilayer and ultimately to the other side of the SC), it has to diffuse through the boundaries between the separate domains caused by chain length mismatches (domain mosaic model) and across a polar layer containing a high concentration of water. Thus, in order to cross the SC, a drug/prodrug permeant must exhibit a balance of lipid and aqueous solubilities because it has to dissolve in and diffuse through a series of lipid and aqueous phases in the spaces between the corneocytes (the biphasic solubility model) to achieve transdermal delivery [8, 28]. Hence the mechanism for increasing transdermal delivery of a parent drug by its prodrugs is to increase the lipid and aqueous solubilities of the prodrugs compared to their parent drug.

## 7.4 Equations for Quantifying Effects of Solubility on Diffusion Through the Stratum Corneum

The cartoon representation of the path of the diffusion of permeants is easy to see, and the conclusion that a balanced increase in lipid and aqueous solubilities is necessary to increase the flux of a drug by a prodrug approach is easy to reach on the basis of the experimental results. However, it is important for the design of prodrugs to develop a model equation that predicts these results and to put the design of prodrugs on a quantitative basis [5]. Although Fick's law itself does not contain separate parameters for lipid and aqueous solubilities, it is straightforward to derive a model equation starting with Fick's law that does. From Fick's law equation (7.1) [29], the driving force for the diffusion of a permeant across any membrane acting as a barrier to flux, $J$, is the difference in the concentration of the permeant in the first few layers of the membrane, $C_{\mathrm{M1}}$, and in the last few layers of the membrane, $C_{\mathrm{M}n}$ (units of $\mu$ mol/cm$^3$). In Eq. (7.1), $J$ is in units of $\mu$ mol/(cm$^2$ h), $D$ is the diffusion coefficient (units of cm$^2$/h), and $L$ is the thickness of the SC membrane (units of cm).

$$J = (D/L)(C_{\mathrm{M1}} - C_{\mathrm{M}n}) \tag{7.1}$$

It is assumed that $C_{\mathrm{M}n}$ approaches zero concentration because the permeant is continually removed from the interface between the last layer of the SC and the viable epidermis. It is also assumed that $C_{\mathrm{M1}}$ is the concentration of the permeant in the first multilamellar bilayers that occupy the space between the corneocytes in the SC and that $J$ is proportional to $C_{\mathrm{M1}}$: a concept that is not new [3, 4, 30]. However, it is difficult to experimentally measure $C_{\mathrm{M1}}$ accurately. Thus, $C_{\mathrm{M1}}$ is usually estimated from the product of the partition coefficient of the permeant between the aggregate components of the multilamellar bilayers in the SC and the vehicle, $K_{\mathrm{M1:VEH}}$, and the concentration of the permeant in the vehicle, $C_{\mathrm{VEH}}$: $C_{\mathrm{M1}} = (K_{\mathrm{M1:VEH}})(C_{\mathrm{VEH}})$ or $C_{\mathrm{M1}} = (C_{\mathrm{M1}}/C_{\mathrm{VEH}})(C_{\mathrm{VEH}})$ [4, 29] in Eq. (7.2).

$$J_{VEH} = (D/L)(C_{VEH})(K_{\mathrm{M1:VEH}}) \tag{7.2}$$

### 7.4.1 The Roberts–Sloan Equation When the Vehicle is Water

However, it is also difficult to measure $K_{M1:VEH}$. So a surrogate for $K_{M1:VEH}$ is measured and substituted for it. The concentration of the permeant in a lipid ($C_{LIPID}$) is substituted for $C_{M1}$ [4] and the concentration in the vehicle is assumed to be the concentration in water ($C_{AQ}$) or a buffer (pH 7.4 or $C_{7.4}$) because water is frequently a major component of topical formulations. Thus, $K_{LIPID:AQ}$ becomes the surrogate for $K_{M1:VEH}$. In addition, the lipid surrogate for M1 that is frequently used is octanol (OCT) because there are large data bases of the resulting $K_{OCT:AQ}$ and numerous programs are available to estimate $K_{OCT:AQ}$ on a theoretical basis. Furthermore, $C_{OCT}$ cannot accurately represent the anistropic nature of the solubility properties of M1 so $K_{M1:VEH} = K_{OCT:AQ}$ becomes $K_{M1:VEH} = (K_{OCT:AQ})^y c$, where "$c$" is a constant and "$y$" accounts for the differences between the solubility properties of M1 and OCT [5]. Thus, Eq. (7.2) becomes Eq. (7.3).

$$J_{AQ} = (D/L)(C_{AQ})(K_{OCT:AQ})^y\, c \tag{7.3}$$

The diffusion coefficient, $D$, can be estimated from $D = D_0\, e\,(-\beta MV)$ [31, 32] where $\beta$ is a constant and MV is molecular volume that can be conveniently substituted by molecular weight (MW), and $D_0$ is the diffusivity of a hypothetic molecule of zero molecular volume [4, 33]. Assuming $L$ is a constant for a specific type of membrane, taking the logs of the parameters, and combining log $(D_0)/(L)$ with the constant "log $c$" from $y$ log $K_{OCT:AQ}$ + log $c$ to give another constant "$x$" gives Eq. (7.4) [34].

$$\log J_{AQ} = x - (\beta/2.303)MW + y \log K_{OCT:AQ} + \log C_{AQ} \tag{7.4}$$

If a saturated solution of a permeant in the aqueous vehicle is used, then $J_{AQ}$ becomes the maximum flux, $J_{MAQ}$ and $C_{AQ}$ becomes $S_{AQ}$. In addition, because a saturated solution of the permeant is used, $C_{M1}$ becomes $S_{M1}$ and $K_{OCT:AQ}$ becomes ($S_{OCT}/S_{AQ}$). Substitutions for $y$ log $K_{OCT:AQ}$ by the equivalent solubilities gives $y$ log $S_{OCT} - y$ log $S_{AQ}$ and Eq. (7.4) becomes Eq. (7.5) [34].

$$\log J_{MAQ} = x - (\beta/2.303)MW + y \log S_{OCT} - y \log S_{AQ} + \log S_{AQ} \tag{7.5}$$

When $\beta/2.303$ is $z$ and the solubility terms are combined, the Roberts–Sloan equation (7.6) for flux from an aqueous vehicle results [34],

$$\log J_{MAQ} = x - z\,MW + y \log S_{OCT} + (1 - y) \log S_{AQ} \tag{7.6}$$

which is a model equation developed from Fick's law that includes terms for solubility in lipid and in water, in addition to MW, as descriptors for maximum flux.

An important contributor to the development of Eq. (7.6) and to establishing a theoretical basis for the observed dependence of flux on solubilities both in water and in lipids is the use of saturated solutions of the permeant in diffusion cell experiments that generate the flux data [3, 4, 8, 35, 36]. Although the driving force for diffusion is the difference between the concentration of the permeant in the first few and the last few layers of the membrane in Fick's law equation (7.1), the fact that the actual driving force is the difference in the thermodynamic activities (or chemical potentials) of the permeant in those layers was established almost 50 years ago [37].

The maximum thermodynamic activity of a drug/prodrug permeant, $\alpha_i$, is exhibited by the pure permeant: $\alpha_i = 1$. When excess permeant is in equilibrium with a saturated solution of the permeant in a vehicle (a suspension), the activity of the permeant in that saturated solution, $\alpha_{i,\mathrm{VEH}}$, is also equal to 1. Furthermore, when that saturated solution of the permeant in a vehicle is in equilibrium with the material, M1, occupying the space between the corneocytes through which the permeant must diffuse to achieve transdermal delivery, the activity of the permeant in M1, $\alpha_{i,\mathrm{M1}}$, is also equal to 1. So regardless of the vehicle, if a saturated solution of the permeant is applied, the same solubility of the permeant in M1 will be achieved ($S_{\mathrm{M1}}$) irrespective of $S_{\mathrm{VEH}}$ and the same thermodynamic activity of the permeant will be achieved ($\alpha_{i,\mathrm{M1}} = 1$). This assumes that the vehicle does not interact with M1 to change its solubility properties. If the vehicle does interact, the coefficients to the parameters in Eq. (7.6) will change but they will be a constant for that vehicle [5].

For different permeants in a specific vehicle, the solubility of each permeant, $S_{\mathrm{VEH}}$, will be different. However, if each permeant is at saturation, its thermodynamic activity in the vehicle and in M1, and hence its chemical potential in each, will be at its maximum. For different permeants in a specific vehicle, $S_{\mathrm{M1}}$ for each will be different but their chemical potentials will be the same and each permeant will be evaluated at the same chemical potential in diffusion cells [5]. Since $S_{\mathrm{VEH}}$ has been eliminated as a variable, $S_{\mathrm{M1}}$ is the only solubility-related variable predicting maximum flux from Eq. (7.6) [5]. Nonetheless, $S_{\mathrm{VEH}}$ remains important from the practical point of view of estimating $S_{\mathrm{M1}}$ from $(K_{\mathrm{M1:VEH}})(S_{\mathrm{VEH}})$ [5].

### 7.4.2
### The Roberts–Sloan Equation When the Vehicle is a Lipid

Although reference has been made to "vehicles" in the discussion above, it was assumed that water or aqueous vehicles were used. If a lipid vehicle is used, a different derivation must be used [15] because, since it is assumed that the barrier to diffusion is at least partially lipoidal in nature, it is difficult to establish a standard partitioning system where both phases are lipid: they would tend to dissolve in each other since like dissolves like. In order to overcome this problem, the following identity, Eq. (7.7), can be used [38]:

$$K_{\mathrm{M1:LIPID}} = (K_{\mathrm{M1:AQ}})/(K_{\mathrm{LIPID:AQ}}) \tag{7.7}$$

In this identity, two different partition coefficients are used where the lipids phases are different but where each is not miscible with water, which is the other phase in the two partition coefficients. Then, since we can substitute a different lipid for M1 in Eq. (7.7) to give $K_{\mathrm{M1:AQ}} = (K_{\mathrm{LIPID:AQ}})^{y}c$, we obtain Eq. (7.8).

$$K_{\mathrm{M1:LIPID}} = (K_{\mathrm{LIPID:AQ}})^{y}\, c/(K_{\mathrm{LIPID:AQ}}) \tag{7.8}$$

Although different lipids can be used in the two partition coefficients in Eq. (7.8), the equation can be simplified by using the same lipid that was used as the vehicle in both partition coefficients. Substitution of Eq. (7.8) where LIPID = isopropyl myristate (IPM) into Eq. (7.3) for $(K_{OCT:AQ})^y c$, $J_{IPM}$ for $J_{AQ}$, and $C_{IPM}$ for $C_{AQ}$ gives Eq. (7.9) [15].

$$J_{IPM} = (D/L)(C_{IPM})(K_{IPM:AQ})^y c/(K_{IPM:AQ}) \tag{7.9}$$

Assuming that saturated solutions of drug/prodrug permeants in IPM are applied to the membranes, by analogy to the development of Eqs. (7.5) and (7.6) from (7.3), Eq. (7.9) becomes Eq. (7.10) [15].

$$\begin{aligned} \log J_{MIPM} &= x - (\beta/2.303)\mathrm{MW} + y \log S_{IPM} - y \log S_{AQ} - \log S_{IPM} + \log S_{AQ} + \log S_{IPM} \\ &= x - zMW + y \log S_{IPM} + (1-y) \log S_{AQ} \end{aligned} \tag{7.10}$$

Thus, if a lipid vehicle is used, the same dependence of maximum flux on the solubility of the permeant in lipid and in water obtains. The form of Eqs. (7.6) and (7.10) are the same except that a different lipid surrogate for the lipid phase of the biphasic resistance to diffusion is used and a different vehicle is used in each. The result is that there are different values for the coefficients $x$, $y$, and $z$ in each equation, but the value for $y$ remains about 0.5–0.6 regardless of the lipid surrogate or the vehicle, confirming the importance of both the water and the lipid solubility of the permeant in enabling its effective transdermal delivery [8]. The importance of $S_{AQ}$ in Eq. (7.10), which describes flux from a lipid vehicle, IPM, establishes that the cause of the water solubility-based resistance to flux cannot be due to a stagnant water layer at the interface between the vehicle and the SC: there cannot be a stagnant water layer if there is no water in the applied phase.

### 7.4.3
### The Series/Parallel Equation When the Vehicle is a Lipid

The Roberts–Sloan equations (7.6) [34] and (7.10) [15] based on Fick's law are simple, straightforward equations with which to work. However, it does not include the concept that permeants have to cross a series of lipid–water phases (alternating lipophilic and hydrophilic layers) to achieve transdermal delivery as originally proposed [8] to explain the dependence of flux on the lipid and aqueous solubilities of the permeant. A more complex equation that includes this concept has also been developed that not only allows the existence of a path through the material between the corneocytes in the SC, which crosses alternating lipid and aqueous phases (series), but also parallel paths across lipid-only and aqueous-only phases [30]. The basic form of this series/parallel equation that depends on solubility-based resistances to maximum flux is Eq. (7.11), where diffusion through the aqueous phases is inversely proportional to the square root of MW and diffusion through the lipid phases is proportional to the product of the exponent of a negative parameter, Φ, and MW.

$$\begin{aligned} \log J_{MIPM} = \log \{&1/[1/(aS_{IPM}10^{\Phi MW}) + 1/(bS_{AQ}/\mathrm{MW}^{0.5})] \\ &+ cS_{IPM}10^{\Phi MW} + dS_{AQ}/\mathrm{MW}^{0.5}\} \end{aligned} \tag{7.11}$$

When the same experimental data (log $J_{MMIPM}$, log $S_{IPM}$, log $S_{AQ}$, and MW, Table 7.1) that were fitted to Eq. (7.10) were fitted to Eq. (7.11) [30], it was found that a path across aqueous-only phases was not necessary to adequately explain the data. In addition, it was found that the highest capacity path (highest flux) was by the path through the series of alternating lipid and aqueous phases. But as the prodrug became more lipid soluble, the parallel path through the lipid-only phases becomes the higher capacity path. However, the capacity of the lipid-only path was never as high as that of the lipid–aqueous series path. For example, the most water-soluble member of the alkyloxycarbonyl-5-fluorouracil (1-AOC-5-FU) homologous series of prodrugs (see Table 7.1) was the C2 member. Based on the solubility properties and MW of the C2 member, the flux through the series path was 27 times greater than the flux through the lipid-only path, when calculated from Eq. (7.11), while the experimental flux of the C2 member was 27 times greater than the experimental flux of 5-FU itself from the same vehicle. On the other hand, the most lipid-soluble member of the series, the C6 member, gave experimental flux only five times the experimental flux of 5-FU itself, and the flux of prodrug through the series path was only about 0.5 times its flux through the lipid-only path when calculated from Eq. (7.11). Thus, for this homologous series of prodrugs (and for most other series of molecules), the more water-soluble member of a more lipophilic series of prodrugs will give the higher flux, and the path for diffusion for those more water-soluble members of a more lipophilic series of prodrugs, based on calculations from Eq. (7.11), will be primarily by a high-capacity path across alternating lipid and aqueous phases. Prodrugs exhibiting only improved lipid solubility compared to their parent drugs may also give higher flux values than their parent drugs, but they will not give the highest flux values possible from that series of prodrugs because they will diffuse through a low-capacity lipid-solubility-only path [30].

## 7.5
## Design of Prodrugs for Topical and Transdermal Delivery Based on the Biphasic Solubility Model

The use of prodrugs to enhance topical (dermal and transdermal) delivery has advantages over the use of penetration enhancers in vehicles or the use of mechanical/electrical devices to enhance topical delivery [5–7]. In addition, a mechanistic model (biphasic solubility model) has been developed to correlate the experimental flux values with the experimental physicochemical properties of prodrugs such as solubilities in lipid and water (as well as MW) that provides the basis for designing prodrugs that enhance the delivery of the parent drug. Furthermore, two equations (Roberts–Sloan [15, 34] and the series/parallel [30] equations) have been developed to provide a quantitative basis for predicting the maximum flux values of other prodrugs from their solubility properties. Thus, there is a solubility-based paradigm for designing better prodrugs/drugs for topical delivery [5]. The fact that these solubility-based design concepts are underutilized arises from the pervasive reliance of prodrug/drug designers on partition coefficients ($K_{OCT:AQ}$) and their direct

**Table 7.1** Physicochemical properties: melting point, log solubility in IPM (log $S_{IPM}$), log solubility in water (log $S_{AQ}$), log partition coefficients between IPM and water (log $K_{IPM:AQ}$), log flux from IPM through hairless mice skins ($J_{MMIPM}$), and log permeability coefficients through hairless mice skins from IPM (log $P_{MIPM}$).

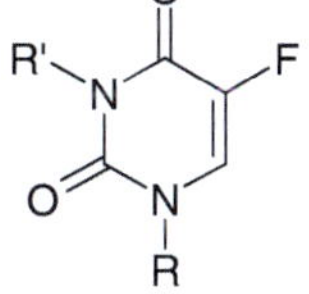

| Compound[a] | mp °C[b] | log $S_{IPM}$[c] | log $S_{AQ}$[c),d] | log $K_{IPM:AQ}$ | log $J_{MMIPM}$[e] | log $P_{MIPM}$[f] |
|---|---|---|---|---|---|---|
| 1-AC-5FU | | | | | | |
| **1**, R′ = H, R = COC1 | 130 | 1.34 | 2.08 | −0.73 | 0.97 | −0.37 |
| **2**, R′ = H, R = COC2 | 131 | 1.56 | 1.68 | −0.12 | 0.63 | −0.93 |
| **3**, R′ = H, R = COC3 | 146 | 1.24 | 0.81 | 0.43 | 0.11 | −1.13 |
| **4**, R′ = H, R = COC4 | 121 | 1.59 | 0.54 | 1.05 | 0.00 | 1.59 |
| **5**, R′ = H, R = COC5 | 102 | 2.05 | 0.47 | 1.58 | 0.04 | −2.01 |
| **6**, R′ = H, R = COC7 | 84 | 2.04 | −0.84 | 2.88 | 0.22 | −2.26 |
| 5-FU | 282 | −1.30 | 1.98 | −3.28 | −0.62 | 0.68 |
| 1-AOC-5FU | | | | | | |
| **7**, R′ = H, R = $CO_2$C1 | 160 | 0.33 | 2.05 | −1.72 | 0.42 | 0.09 |
| **8**, R′ = H, R = $CO_2$C2 | 128 | 1.12 | 2.24 | −1.12 | 0.77 | −0.35 |
| **9**, R′ = H, R = $CO_2$C3 | 126 | 1.18 | 1.63 | −0.45 | 0.36 | −0.82 |
| **10**, R′ = H, R = $CO_2$C4 | 98 | 1.53 | 1.37 | 0.16 | 0.35 | −1.18 |
| **11**, R′ = H, R = $CO_2$C6 | 67 | 2.19 | 0.70 | 1.48 | 0.19 | −2.00 |
| **12**, R′ = H, R = $CO_2$C8 | 98 | 1.56 | −0.89 | 2.46 | −0.53 | −2.09 |
| 5-FU | 282 | −1.30 | 1.98 | −3.28 | −0.62 | 0.68 |
| 1-ACOM-5FU | | | | | | |
| **13**, R′ = H, R = $CH_2$OCOC1 | 124 | 0.52 | 2.26 | −1.74 | 0.46 | −0.06 |
| **14**, R′ = H, R = $CH_2$OCOC2 | 102 | 0.99 | 2.22 | −1.23 | 0.58 | −0.41 |
| **15**, R′ = H, R = $CH_2$OCOC3 | 91 | 1.16 | 1.63 | −0.47 | 0.41 | −0.75 |
| **16**, R′ = H, R = $CH_2$OCOC4 | 88 | 1.17 | 1.10 | 0.08 | 0.11 | −1.06 |
| **17**, R′ = H, R = $CH_2$OCOC5 | 91 | 1.17 | 0.35 | 0.82 | −0.25 | −1.42 |
| **18**, R′ = H, R = $CH_2$OCOC7 | 108 | 1.00 | −0.77 | 1.77 | −0.92 | −1.92 |
| **19**, R′ = H, R = $CH_2$OCOC9 | 115 | 0.63 | −2.51 | 3.14 | −1.82 | −2.45 |
| 5-FU | 282 | −1.30 | 1.98 | −3.28 | −0.62 | 0.68 |
| 3-AC-5FU | | | | | | |
| **20**, R = H, R′ = COC1 | 117 | 0.63 | 2.22 | −1.39 | 0.64 | 0.01 |
| **21**, R = H, R′ = COC2 | 103 | 1.15 | 2.30 | −0.97 | 0.71 | −0.44 |
| **22**, R = H, R′ = COC3 | 112 | 1.34 | 1.72 | −0.01 | 0.34 | −1.00 |
| **23**, R = H, R′ = COC4 | 111 | 0.96 | 0.70 | 0.22 | −0.26 | −1.22 |
| 5-FU | 282 | −1.30 | 1.98 | −3.28 | −0.62 | 0.68 |
| 3-ACOM-5FU | | | | | | |
| **24**, R = H, R′ = $CH_2$OCOC1 | 161 | 0.09 | 1.80 | −1.62 | −0.22 | −0.31 |
| **25**, R = H, R′ = $CH_2$OCOC2 | 95.5 | 1.20 | 2.25 | −1.03 | 0.34 | −0.86 |
| **26**, R = H, R′ = $CH_2$OCOC3 | 76 | 1.42 | 1.92 | −0.45 | 0.46 | −0.96 |

(Continued)

**Table 7.1** (*Continued*)

| Compound[a)] | mp °C[b)] | log $S_{IPM}$[c)] | log $S_{AQ}$[c),d)] | log $K_{IPM:AQ}$ | log $J_{MMIPM}$[e)] | log $P_{MIPM}$[f)] |
|---|---|---|---|---|---|---|
| 27, R = H, R′ = $CH_2OCOC4$ | 94 | 1.47 | 1.32 | 0.13 | 0.12 | −1.35 |
| 28, R = H, R′ = $CH_2OCOC5$ | 71 | 1.63 | 0.92 | 0.74 | 0.00 | −1.63 |
| 29, R = H, R′ = $CH_2OCOC7$ | 70 | 1.60 | −0.25 | 1.90 | −0.77 | −2.37 |
| 5-FU | 282 | −1.30 | 1.98 | −3.28 | −0.62 | 0.68 |

a) C1, C2, and so on indicate the number of carbons in the alkyl chain.
b) Only the last number of the melting point is given.
c) Units of mM.
d) Experimental solubility in water or estimated solubility in pH 4.0 buffer.
e) Units of $\mu mol/(cm^2\ h)$.
f) Units of cm/h.

relationship with permeability coefficients ($P = J/C_{VEH} = (D/L)(K_{OCT:AQ})$) [33, 39]. However, $K_{OCT:AQ}$ is merely a ratio and does not give any information about absolute lipid or aqueous solubilities, and $P$ is in units of, for example, cm/h that does not give any information about the amount that has diffused. Since knowledge of the amount delivered is essential for assessing a therapeutic response [5], $P$ is not a useful quantity and $K$ is not a useful quantity except for estimating $S_{M1}$.

The final component to the logical development of a prodrug approach to enhancing the topical delivery of a parent drug is the choice of the chemical entity that is to be reversibly attached to the drug: the promoiety. There are two considerations for making a choice. First, by definition the promoiety must be reversible; it must revert in a controlled and predictable manner to the parent drug. Second, since this is a solubility-based design paradigm [5], the promoiety must improve the solubility properties (lipid and aqueous solubilities) of the parent drug by subtracting a problematic functional group in the drug (by masking it) and/or by adding a solubility enhancing functional group in the promoiety [7]. In reality, it is difficult to separate these two considerations because the choice of a reversible promoiety sufficiently stable to formulate will dictate the choice of available approaches to manipulate the solubility of the prodrug. Here, we will discuss several simple examples of these interactions and the results from the application of two general chemical approaches (acyl and soft alkyl derivatives) to satisfying both considerations at the same time.

### 7.5.1
### 5-Fluorouracil Prodrugs

The reason that many drugs do not exhibit the requisite physicochemical properties for adequate transdermal delivery (a balance of lipid and aqueous solubilities) is that they contain functional groups that either are too polar to easily dissolve in a lipid phase or are too lipid-like to dissolve in a water phase [7, 9, 40]. An example of a drug that is too polar to easily dissolve in a lipid phase is 5-fluorouracil (5-FU). The high melting point (mp) and the poor physicochemical properties exhibited by 5-FU, and other uracil-type molecules, is primarily due to the highly polarized imide (O=C–NH–C=O) and vinylogous imide (O=C–CH=CH–NH–C=O) functional groups where the NH group forms strong intermolecular hydrogen bonds in the crystal lattice with C=O groups [7, 40]. Regardless that 5-FU contains polar functional groups, 5-FU is only moderately soluble in water because of those same strong intermolecular hydrogen bonds that form in the crystal lattice [7, 40].

#### 7.5.1.1 *N*-Acyl 5-FU Prodrugs

If those NH groups in 5-FU are reacted with alkylcarbonyl chlorides or alkyloxycarbonyl chlorides to mask the problem NH groups and to give N-acylated derivatives, some of the derivatives (1-AC-5FU) hydrolyze with a half-life ($t_{1/2}$) of 2.5–4.8 min at pH 7.1 and 32 °C [41], while others (1-AOC-5FU) hydrolyze with a $t_{1/2}$ of 190–550 min at pH 7.4 and 37 °C [42]. Although *N*-acyl derivatives are generally considered to be very stable under those conditions, in the hydrolysis of the 5-FU acyl derivatives the leaving group is a good nucleofuge with a $pK_a$ of about 8–9 while in the hydrolysis of a normal amide, such as acetamide, the leaving group in the breakdown of the tetrahydral intermediate is a very poor nucleofuge with a $pK_a$ of about 39 [40].

The *N*-acyl derivatives (**1–6** and **7–12**, Table 7.1) [43, 44] exhibit a decrease in melting point and an increase in lipid solubility (log $S_{IPM}$) and partition coefficient between IPM and water (log $K_{IPM:AQ}$) compared to 5-FU. The biggest improvement in the physicochemical properties of the prodrugs compared to 5-FU was in the large increase in log $S_{IPM}$ values obtained by masking a polar NH group in 5-FU with an acyl group (400–3000 times 5-FU $S_{IPM}$). In addition, the log $S_{AQ}$ values, estimated from log $S_{IPM}$–log $K_{IPM:AQ}$, for the first few members of each series, were higher than the log $S_{AQ}$ of 5-FU itself. However, the increase in log $S_{AQ}$ values of the *N*-acyl derivatives was not substantial (1.2–2.0 times 5-FU $S_{AQ}$) compared to the increase in log $S_{IPM}$ values. Thus, it is possible to not only increase lipid but also aqueous solubilities for the shorter alkyl chain members of the series by masking the polar NH groups with acyl groups and hence decreasing those intermolecular hydrogen bonds in the crystal lattice of 5-FU. Most importantly, the more water-soluble member of each series of more lipid-soluble prodrugs gave the highest flux values for the delivery of 5-FU from IPM through hairless mouse skin *in vitro*, log $J_{MMIPM}$. While these results support a biphasic solubility model, the Roberts–Sloan [15] and series/parallel equations [30] both give accurate calculated log $J_{MMIPM}$ values for each member of each of these series.

The 3-AC-5FU derivatives (**20–23**) exhibited similar decreases in melting points and increases in log $S_{IPM}$ and log $K_{IPM:AQ}$ compared to 5-FU [45]. The estimated log $S_{AQ}$ values for the first two members of the series were also higher than that of 5-FU, and again the derivative that exhibited the higher log $S_{AQ}$ value also gave the higher log $J_{MMIPM}$ value. The hydrolysis of the 3-AC-5FU derivatives (**20–23**) follows a more complicated mechanism than the 1-AC (**1–6**) or 1-AOC (**7–12**) derivatives: an O-acylated intermediate is formed that then hydrolyzes [46]. Regardless of the mechanism, the 3-AC-5FU derivatives are readily reversible: $t_{1/2}$ = 200–300 min [46].

All three *N*-acyl series exhibit the same trends in their physicochemical properties. Although log $S_{IPM}$ values increase initially, as the alkyl chain length continues to increase, log $S_{IPM}$ values eventually decrease. On the other hand, log $K_{IPM:AQ}$ values continue to increase monotonically as alkyl chain length increases: log $K_{IPM:AQ}$ is not a good surrogate for log $S_{IPM}$. Log $S_{AQ}$ values within a series peak for the first or second member of the series and then decline, and log $J_{MMIPM}$ values generally mirror the trend in log $S_{AQ}$ values. In these experiments where a lipid vehicle is used, log $P_{MIPM}$ values mirror the trend in log $J_{MMIPM}$ values and not log $K_{IPM:AQ}$ values. Thus, the direct relationship between log $P_{MIPM}$ and log $K_{IPM:AQ}$ suggested by others [33, 39] does not exist if the vehicle is a lipid where log $J_{MMIPM}$ values decrease as log $S_{IPM}$ values increase.

#### 7.5.1.2 **N-Soft Alkyl 5-FU Prodrugs**

If those NH groups in uracil itself are replaced by a methyl alkyl group to mask the hydrogen-bonding NH group, the melting points decrease [47], the partition coefficients between chloroform ($CHCl_3$) and water ($K_{CHCl3:AQ}$) increase [48], and the lipid solubilities calculated from ($K_{CHCl3:AQ}$)($S_{AQ}$) increase. Thus, it is possible not only to increase lipid solubility by adding an alkyl group that masks a polar NH functional group but also to increase the water solubility, analogous to the results obtained by adding an acyl group.

The problem with this approach is that an *N*-alkyl derivative is not as readily reversible as an *N*-acyl derivative. It is known that a cytochrome P-450 monooxygenase can oxidize a $N-CH_3$ group [49] to an intermediate $N-CH_2OH$ group that will then rapidly hydrolyze chemically back to the NH group, but this first oxidation step is generally not a reaction that can be assumed to go to completion. For example, a similar oxidation of the $O-CH_3$ group in codeine to give an intermediate $O-CH_2OH$ group that rapidly hydrolyzes chemically to the OH group, converts codeine to morphine that binds several thousand times more tightly to opioid receptors than codeine. However, this conversion is highly variable and on average only about 10% of codeine is converted to morphine [50].

In order to retain the desired stability of an alkyl derivative for formulation purposes, yet bypass the inefficient and unpredictable cytochrome P-450 oxidation step that makes it reversible, soft alkyl derivatives have been developed [7, 51, 52]. Essentially, the soft alkyl derivative is the acyl derivative of the intermediate $N-CH_2OH$: $N-CH_2O(C=O)R$. $N-CH_2OH$ is stabilized to rapid chemical hydrolysis so that the resulting $N-CH_2O(C=O)R$ is not only more easily formulated but it also contains a "soft" ester functional group ($CH_2O(C=O)R$) that can be readily hydrolyzed (enabling group) by esterases *in vivo* to give the chemically unstable $N-CH_2OH$ group. Although most embodiments of this type of soft alkyl derivative are based on ester or carbonate enabling groups that require esterase-catalyzed hydrolysis to release the parent drug, soft alkyl derivatives based on amide, imide, and carbamate enabling groups, which undergo chemical hydrolysis, have also been developed [53–55]. These soft alkyl derivatives can be obtained from the reaction of $ZCH_2X(C=O)R$ with NH, SH, OH, or even CH (if they are sufficiently acidic) groups in drug molecules where Z = Cl, Br, or I; X = O, S, or $NR^1$; R = alkyl, aryl, alkylX, or arylX; and $R^1$ = alkyl or aryl. The possibility of creating so many different combinations of X, R, and $R^1$ exhibiting so many different physicochemical properties makes the soft alkyl derivative approach much more flexible than the acyl derivative approach in terms of fine-tuning the stability of the prodrug in its formulation and its ease of hydrolysis *in vivo* [7].

Two different series of soft alkyl derivatives of 5-FU were synthesized: the 1-N [56] and the 3-N [57] series. When the 1-NH or 3-NH groups were alkylated with $ZCH_2O$ (C=O)-alkyl reagents, the resulting 1-alkylcarbonyloxymethyl derivatives (**13–19**, 1-ACOM) and 3-alkylcarbonyloxymethyl derivatives (**24–29**, 3-ACOM) exhibited trends in melting point, solubilities, partition coefficients, fluxes for the delivery of 5-FU through hairless mouse skin from an IPM vehicle, and permeability coefficients that were very similar to the trends exhibited by the simple *N*-acyl derivatives. All of the members of both soft alkyl series exhibited lower melting points and higher log $S_{IPM}$ values than 5-FU. The log $S_{IPM}$ values initially increased with increasing alkyl chain length but then decreased after about C5 (**17** and **28**). The biggest improvement in the physicochemical properties of 5-FU was in the large increase in log $S_{IPM}$ values obtained by masking a polar NH group in 5-FU with an ACOM group (200 and 500 times 5-FU $S_{IPM}$). The log $S_{AQ}$ values peaked for the first or second member of each series and then decreased with increasing chain length. However, the increase in log $S_{AQ}$ values of the *N*-ACOM derivatives was not substantial (1.65 and 1.78 times 5-FU $S_{AQ}$) compared to the increase in log $S_{IPM}$. The log $K_{IPM:AQ}$ values increased monotonically with increasing chain length, but the log $P_{MIPM}$ values decreased with increasing chain length. The log $J_{MMIPM}$ values peaked at the second and third member of the 1-N and 3-N series, respectively, then decreased with increasing chain length. Both log $P_{MIPM}$ and log $J_{MMIPM}$ trended in the opposite direction of log $K_{IPM:AQ}$ and log $S_{IPM}$, but in the same direction as log $S_{AQ}$, trends that were the same as observed for the *N*-acyl derivatives. Except for the first member of the series, the members of the 3-N ACOM series generally exhibited lower melting points, higher log $S_{IPM}$, and log $S_{AQ}$ values than the 1-N series analogous to the trends observed while comparing the 1-$NCH_3$ with 3-$NCH_3$ uracil derivatives. Four of the six 3-N ACOM derivatives also exhibited higher log $J_{MMIPM}$ values than the corresponding members of the 1-N ACOM series. In the case of **24** versus **13**, the lower $J_{MMIPM}$ values of **24** would be expected on the basis of its lower log $S_{IPM}$ and log $S_{AQ}$ values. On the other hand, **25** is an anomaly since it exhibits somewhat higher log $S_{IPM}$ and log $S_{AQ}$ values than **14**. The performance of **25** appears to be an outlier to the trends in the ACOM series.

### 7.5.2
### Acetaminophen (APAP) Prodrugs

An example of a drug that exhibits a lower melting point and higher log $S_{IPM}$ value than 5-FU (38-fold) but about the same log $S_{AQ}$ value is acetaminophen (APAP) [58]. However, the large increase in the log $S_{IPM}$ value results only in a twofold increase in $J_{MMIPM}$ for a molecule that is roughly the same size as 5-FU. On the other hand, the log $S_{IPM}$ values for the best performing prodrug in each 5-FU series are 200–500 times greater than that of 5-FU itself or 5–13 times greater than that of APAP. In addition, the log $S_{AQ}$ values for the best performing prodrugs in each 5-FU series are 1.2–2 times greater than 5-FU or APAP. So, in order to obtain improvement in the flux of APAP similar to that obtained in the flux of 5-FU, both log $S_{IPM}$ and log $S_{AQ}$ need to be substantially improved.

In the example of 5-FU, the polar NH groups were an obvious target for derivatization to decrease intermolecular hydrogen bonds in the crystal lattice and increase lipid solubility especially. In the APAP example, the intermolecular hydrogen bonds in the crystal lattice are not nearly as strong as evidenced by the lower mp exhibited by APAP compared to 5-FU [58]. There is an amide NH in APAP but it is involved only in one hydrogen bond and it is not easily derivatized because of steric crowding. On the other hand, there are two intermolecular hydrogen bonds in the crystal lattice that involve the phenolic OH group, either as a donor (C=O ··· H−O−) or as an acceptor (N−H ··· O(H)−) [59]. In addition, although the acidic p$K_a$ value of the phenol is 9.5 [53], and hence not highly ionized at the nominal pH of the skin (pH = 5), the phenolic OH group is the most polar functional group in APAP and hence an obvious target for derivatization.

#### 7.5.2.1 *O*-Acyl APAP Prodrugs

Analogous to the 5-FU example, the *O*-acyl and *O*-soft alkyl derivatives of APAP have been evaluated. In the *O*-acyl series the enabling functional group is a carbonate [58]. The five members of the simple alkyloxycarbonyl prodrugs (**30–34**, Table 7.2) all exhibit higher log $S_{IPM}$ values than APAP (and comparable to the log $S_{IPM}$ values exhibited by the best 5-FU prodrugs), but there was no consistent trend in log $S_{IPM}$ values with increasing alkyl chain length and little variation: 4.9–12.3 times APAP $S_{IPM}$. On the other hand, log $S_{AQ}$ values decreased with increasing alkyl chain length as did log $J_{MMIPM}$ (except the log $J_{MMIPM}$ of **32**) and log $P_{MIPM}$. The lower mp exhibited by **32** compared to the mp of the contiguous members of the series resulted in higher log $S_{IPM}$ values for **32** and higher than expected log $S_{AQ}$ values. Since the log $S_{IPM}$ and log $S_{AQ}$ values of **32** are higher than the contiguous members, the higher log $J_{MMIPM}$ values of **32** compared to those exhibited by the contiguous members is to be expected based on the expectations implicit in the biphasic solubility model and the Roberts–Sloan equation. Also, as expected on the basis of the biphasic solubility model and the Roberts–Sloan equation, the prodrug that gave the highest log $J_{MMIPM}$ value was the most water-soluble member (**30**) of the more lipid-soluble series. Unfortunately, even though **30** contained the shortest alkyl chain (C1), it only exhibited one-sixth the $S_{AQ}$ value of APAP. This decrease in $S_{AQ}$ was balanced by only a sixfold increase in $S_{IPM}$, so it was not surprising, according to the Roberts–Sloan equation, that $J_{MMIPM}$ for **30** was only twice that of APAP.

In an attempt to increase the log $S_{AQ}$ values of the 4-AOC derivatives without decreasing log $S_{IPM}$ values, two AOC derivatives that incorporated methoxy ethyleneoxy (C2OM, **35**) and methoxy propyleneoxy (C3iOM, **36**) groups in place of the simple alkyl groups were evaluated [58]. The methoxy ethyleneoxy prodrug **35** exhibited a higher log $S_{AQ}$ value than the best simple alkyl AOC derivative (**30**), but it was one-fifth that of APAP. Moreover, the log $S_{IPM}$ value for **35** was only five times that of APAP so there was no substantial improvement in log $J_{MMIPM}$ (only one

**Table 7.2** Physicochemical properties: melting point, log solubility in IPM (log $S_{IPM}$), log solubility in water (log $S_{AQ}$), log partition coefficients between IPM and water (log $K_{IPM:AQ}$), log flux from IPM through hairless mice skins ($J_{MMIPM}$), and log permeability coefficients through hairless mice skins from IPM (log $P_{MIPM}$).

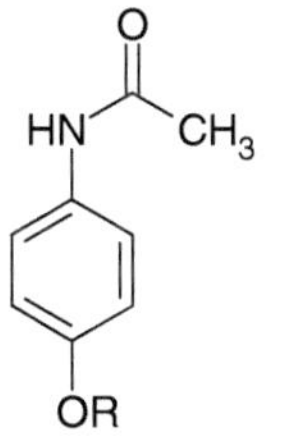


| Compound[a)] | mp °C[b)] | log $S_{IPM}$[c)] | log $S_{AQ}$[c),d)] | log $K_{IPM:AQ}$ | log $J_{MMIPM}$[e)] | log $P_{MIPM}$[f)] |
|---|---|---|---|---|---|---|
| 4-AOC-APAP | | | | | | |
| **30**, R = $CO_2C1$ | 115 | 1.08 | 1.23 | −0.16 | 0.00 | −1.08 |
| **31**, R = $CO_2C2$ | 122 | 0.97 | 0.65 | 0.32 | −0.76 | −1.73 |
| **32**, R = $CO_2C3$ | 106 | 1.37 | 0.48 | 0.90 | −0.45 | −1.82 |
| **33**, R = $CO_2C4$ | 120 | 1.14 | −0.35 | 1.50 | −1.01 | −2.15 |
| **34**, R = $CO_2C6$ | 110 | 1.22 | −1.49 | 2.71 | −1.49 | −2.71 |
| **35**, R = $CO_2C2OM$ | 81 | 1.01 | 1.31 | −0.30 | −0.11 | −1.12 |
| **36**, R = $CO_2C3iOM$ | 123 | 0.53 | 0.39 | 0.13 | −1.06 | −1.59 |
| APAP | 170 | 0.28 | 2.00 | −1.72 | −0.29 | 0.57 |
| 4-ACOM-APAP | | | | | | |
| **37**, R = $CH_2OCOC1$ | 95 | 0.92 | 1.21 | −0.29 | −0.14 | −1.06 |
| **38**, R = $CH_2OCOC2$ | 59 | 1.79 | 1.42 | 0.37 | 0.27 | −1.52 |
| **39**, R = $CH_2OCOC3$ | 58 | 1.87 | 0.92 | 0.95 | −0.11 | −1.98 |
| **41**, R = $CH_2OCOC7$ | 54 | 1.99 | −1.32 | 3.32 | −0.96 | −2.95 |
| APAP | 170 | 0.28 | 2.00 | −1.72 | −0.29 | −0.57 |
| 4-AOCOM-APAP | | | | | | |
| **42**, R = $CH_2OCO_2C1$ | 106 | 0.90 | 0.86 | −0.02 | −0.35 | −1.25 |
| **43**, R = $CH_2OCO_2C2$ | 85 | 1.32 | 0.89 | 0.44 | −0.18 | −1.50 |
| **44**, R = $CH_2OCO_2C3$ | 69 | 1.66 | 0.30 | 0.96 | −0.55 | −2.21 |
| **45**, R = $CH_2OCO_2C8$ | 65 | 1.82 | −2.40 | 3.43 | −1.68 | −3.50 |
| **46**, R = $CH_2OCO_2C10$ | 56 | 2.11 | −3.25 | 4.42 | −2.13 | −4.24 |
| APAP | 170 | 0.28 | 2.00 | −1.72 | −0.29 | −0.57 |
| 4-NANAOCAM-APAP | | | | | | |
| **47**, R = $CH_2(NCH_3)CO_2C1$ | 88 | 1.15 | 1.66 | −0.45 | 0.04 | −1.10 |
| **48**, R = $CH_2(NCH_3)CO_2C2$ | 77 | 1.30 | 1.20 | 0.08 | −0.21 | −1.50 |
| **49**, R = $CH_2(NCH_3)CO_2C3$ | 60 | 1.61 | 0.95 | 0.69 | −0.29 | −1.90 |
| **50**, R = $CH_2(NCH_3)CO_2C4$ | oil | 1.83 | 0.56 | 1.27 | −0.37 | −2.19 |
| **51**, R = $CH_2(NCH_3)CO_2C6$ | oil | 2.12 | −0.16 | 2.28 | −0.66 | −2.78 |
| APAP | 170 | 0.28 | 2.00 | −1.72 | −0.29 | −0.57 |

a) C1, C2, and so on indicate the number of carbons in the alkyl chain.
b) Only the last number of the melting point is given.
c) Units of mM.
d) Experimental solubility in water or estimated solubility in pH 4.0 buffer.
e) Units of μmol/(cm² h).
f) Units of cm/h.

and a half times the $J_{MMIPM}$ of APAP) as the effect of the changes in the two solubilities canceled each other.

#### 7.5.2.2 *O*-Soft Alkyl APAP Prodrugs

In the three *O*-soft alkyl prodrug series, three different types of enabling groups were evaluated as part of the promoieties [60–62]. The first *O*-soft alkyl prodrug series used an ester as the enabling group (**37–41**, Table 7.2) [60] and the second series used a carbonate functional group as the enabling group (**42–46**, Table 7.2) [61]. In both series, the initial step in their conversion to APAP involved an enzymatically catalyzed hydrolysis to give a very short-lived $O-CH_2-OH$ intermediate that chemically hydrolyzed to the OH group. The third *O*-soft alkyl prodrug series used a carbamate enabling group (**47–51**, Table 7.2) [62] that chemically hydrolyzed by an $S_N1$-type mechanism without biological mediation.

In each series, the melting point decreased while the log $S_{IPM}$ and log $K_{IPM:AQ}$ values increased with increasing alkyl chain length. The log $S_{IPM}$ values for the *O*-soft alkyl derivatives were all greater than the log $S_{IPM}$ value for APAP and somewhat greater than the log $S_{IPM}$ values for the *O*-acyl derivatives of comparable alkyl chain length. The log $S_{AQ}$ values for the *O*-soft alkyl derivatives were, like the *O*-acyl derivatives, all less than those of APAP. They peaked for the first or second member of the series and then decreased with increasing alkyl chain length. The trend in the log $J_{MMIPM}$ and log $P_{MIPM}$ values followed the trend in the log $S_{AQ}$ values and not the trend in log $S_{IPM}$ or log $K_{IPM:AQ}$ values. As expected, based on the biphasic solubility model, those members of these more lipophilic series of prodrugs that exhibited the higher log $S_{AQ}$ values exhibited the higher log $J_{MMIPM}$ values: **38**, **43**, and **47**. Also, when the data for the series were fitted to the Roberts–Sloan equation, the calculated values for log $J_{MMIPM}$ identified **38**, **43**, and **47** as giving the highest log $J_{MMIPM}$ in each of their respective series.

### 7.5.3
### *S*-Soft Alkyl Prodrugs of 6-Mercaptopurine

There are numerous other examples of acyl or soft alkyl prodrug derivatives of drugs containing OH- or NH-type functional groups that have been characterized and evaluated for their abilities to deliver their parent drugs through hairless mouse skin from IPM. The trends in mp, log $S_{IPM}$, log $S_{AQ}$, log $K_{IPM:AQ}$, and log $J_{MMIPM}$ are generally the same. There are, however, only a few examples of derivatives of drugs containing a SH group. In Table 7.3, data for the *S*-soft alkyl derivatives of 6-mercaptopurine (6-MP) are given [63]. The trends in the physicochemical characteristics are the same as for the *O*- and *N*-soft alkyl derivatives. The mp decreases with increasing alkyl chain length until the C5 derivative, **56**, and then increases slightly, while log $S_{IPM}$ values follow the inverse of that trend. Log $S_{AQ}$ and log $P_{MIPM}$ decrease while log $K_{IPM:AQ}$ increases with increasing alkyl chain length. The trend for log $J_{MMIPM}$ is not clear. Since the balances between log $S_{IPM}$ and log $S_{AQ}$ for the first four members of the series are quite similar, the log $J_{MMIPM}$ values are not significantly different from each other. However, it is quite clear that the 150 times increase in $S_{IPM}$

**Table 7.3** Physicochemical properties: melting point, log solubility in IPM (log $S_{IPM}$), log solubility in water (log $S_{AQ}$), log partition coefficients between IPM and water (log $K_{IPM:AQ}$), log flux from IPM through hairless mice skins ($J_{MMIPM}$), and log permeability coefficients through hairless mice skins from IPM (log $P_{MIPM}$).

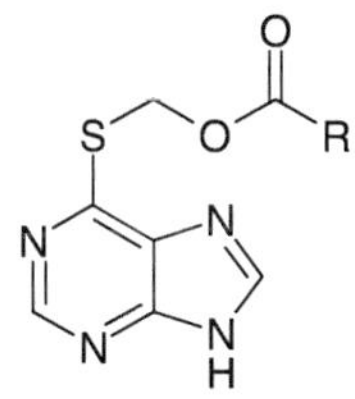

| Compound[a)] | mp °C[b)] | log $S_{IPM}$[c)] | log $S_{AQ}$[c),d)] | log $K_{IPM:AQ}$ | log $J_{MMIPM}$[e)] | log $P_{MIPM}$[f)] |
|---|---|---|---|---|---|---|
| 6-ACOM-6MP | | | | | | |
| 52, R = C1 | 194.5 | 0.02 | 0.86 | −0.84 | −0.69 | −0.71 |
| 53, R = C2 | 165 | 0.36 | 0.61 | −0.25 | −0.67 | −1.03 |
| 54, R = C3 | 154 | 0.52 | 0.31 | 0.21 | −0.58 | −1.10 |
| 55, R = C4 | 148.5 | 0.62 | −0.10 | 0.72 | −0.66 | −1.28 |
| 56, R = C5 | 151 | 0.57 | −0.63 | 1.20 | −1.26 | −1.83 |
| 6MP | >300 | −1.65 | 0.05 | −1.70 | −2.42 | −0.77 |

a) C1, C2, and so on indicate the number of carbons in the alkyl chain.
b) Only the last number of the melting point is given.
c) Units of mM.
d) Experimental solubility in water or estimated solubility in pH 4.0 buffer.
e) Units of μmol/(cm$^2$ h).
f) Units of cm/h.

and 2 times increase in $S_{AQ}$ exhibited by **54** was responsible for its 69 times increase in $J_{MMIPM}$ compared to that of 6-MP. It is also quite clear that when both $S_{IPM}$ and $S_{AQ}$ decrease, the log $J_{MMIPM}$ value decreases substantially: **56**. Thus, for acyl derivatives of OH and NH groups, and soft alkyl derivatives of OH, NH, and SH groups, the same trends in log $S_{IPM}$ and log $S_{AQ}$ lead to optimization of log $J_{MMIPM}$ and confirmation of the biphasic solubility model.

#### 7.5.3.1 Effect of Vehicles on Topical and Transdermal Delivery

The effect of vehicles on the absolute values for flux can be quite substantial. However, the earliest studies on the effect of vehicles on the ability of prodrugs to enhance transdermal delivery showed that regardless of the absolute values of maximum flux, the trends were the same: those members of a more lipophilic series of prodrugs that exhibited the higher $S_{AQ}$ value gave the higher flux value [64]. More recently, the evaluation of the ability of prodrugs to deliver their parent drugs through mouse skin from water, log $J_{MMAQ}$, has been expanded from a single 6-MP series ($n = 4$) [64] to two 6-MP series and one 5-FU series ($n = 18$) [65] to $n = 32$ including parabens and APAP prodrugs [66]. A much better fit of the $n = 32$ database to the Roberts–Sloan equation than the equations that only included parameters for lipid solubility and MW or for MW alone was obtained [66]. In Table 7.4, we show the

**Table 7.4** Comparison of log flux values from water through hairless mice skins ($\log J_{MMAQ}$) and their corresponding log permeability coefficients ($\log P_{MAQ}$) for three representative prodrug series from Tables 7.1 to 7.3.

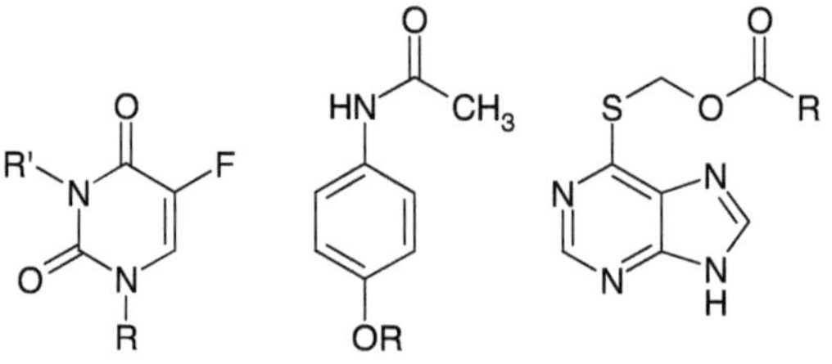

**24-29** **30-34** **52-56**

| Compound | $\log J_{MMAQ}$ [a)] | $\log P_{MAQ}$ [b)] | Compound | $\log J_{MMAQ}$ [a)] | $\log P_{MAQ}$ [b)] | Compound | $\log J_{MMAQ}$ [a)] | $\log P_{MAQ}$ [b)] |
|---|---|---|---|---|---|---|---|---|
| 24 | −1.77 | −3.57 | 30 | −1.50 | −2.81 | 52 | −2.55 | −3.41 |
| 25 | −1.41 | −3.66 | 31 | −1.69 | −2.27 | 53 | −2.19 | −2.80 |
| 26 | −1.13 | −3.06 | 32 | −1.66 | −2.09 | 54 | −2.00 | −2.31 |
| 27 | −1.43 | −2.75 | 33 | −2.15 | −1.78 | 55 | −2.18 | −2.08 |
| 28 | −1.41 | −2.33 | 34 | −2.28 | −0.96 | 56 | −2.37 | −1.74 |
| 29 | −1.85 | −1.60 | | | | | | |

a) Units of $\mu mol/(cm^2\ h)$.
b) Units of cm/h.

$\log J_{MMAQ}$ and the corresponding log permeability coefficients, $\log P_{MAQ}$, for three of the series presented in Tables 7.1–7.3. The trend (Figure 7.2) in the $\log J_{MMAQ}$ values is the same as in the $\log J_{MMIPM}$ values, but the absolute values are much less because IPM has a flux enhancing effect on mouse skin [65]. So, regardless of water being the vehicle, for the same types of prodrugs the more water-soluble members of a more lipophilic series of prodrugs give the higher maximum flux values, and the biphasic solubility model is confirmed whether the polar vehicle, water, or the lipid vehicle, IPM, is used. Another important trend is that $\log P_{MAQ}$ now trends in the opposite direction of $\log J_{MMAQ}$ and in the same direction as $\log K_{IPM:AQ}$ (Figure 7.2). This is because, although $J_{MMAQ}$ values are decreasing (just like $J_{MMIPM}$ values), $S_{AQ}$ values are decreasing even faster (while $S_{IPM}$ vehicle values were increasing) so that the net effect is that $J_{MMAQ}/S_{AQ} = P_{MAQ}$ increases (while $P_{MIPM}$ values were decreasing). Finally, both $\log J_{MMIPM}$ and $\log J_{MMAQ}$ trend in the opposite direction as $\log K_{IPM:AQ}$.

## 7.6
## Comparison of Human and Mouse Skin Experiments

Although the evidence that the biphasic solubility model provides a mechanism for the diffusion of permeants through the SC and that the Roberts–Sloan equation

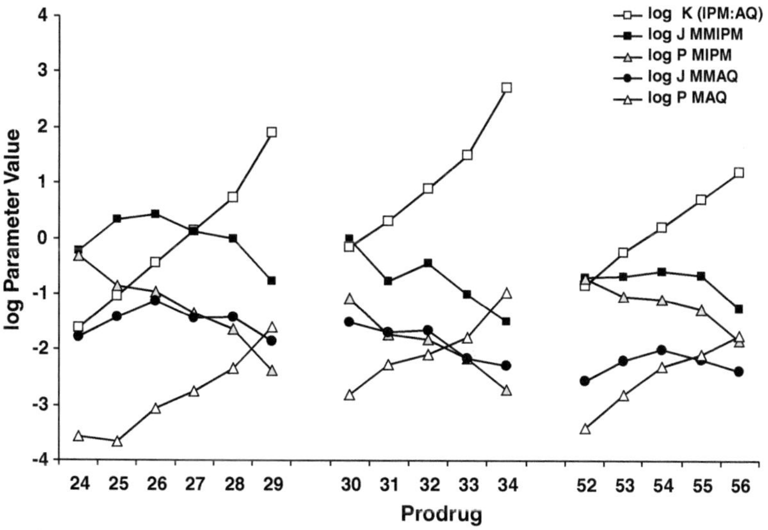


**Figure 7.2** Trends in fluxes and permeability coefficients from a lipid vehicle versus an aqueous vehicle ($\log J_{MMIPM}$ and $\log P_{MIPM}$ versus $\log J_{MMAQ}$ and $\log P_{MAQ}$, respectively) for prodrugs compared to their partition coefficients ($\log K_{IPM:AQ}$).

provides a mathematical basis for quantifying the contributions of solubility and MW to maximum flux from the *in vitro* studies with mouse skin is compelling, evidence from *in vitro* studies with human skin is equally compelling. The fit of the latest compilation of data for the transdermal delivery of drugs and prodrugs through human skin from water, $J_{MHAQ}$, to the Roberts–Sloan equation gives Eq. (7.12) [67]:

$$\log J_{MHAQ} = -2.506 + 0.538 \log S_{OCT} + 0.462 \log S_{AQ} - 0.00402\,\mathrm{MW} \quad (7.12)$$

where $n = 185$, $r^2 = 0.839$, and the average of the absolute values for the differences between the experimental $\log J_{MHAQ}$ and $\log J_{MHAQ}$ calculated from Eq. (7.12), $\Delta \log J_{MHAQ}$, was 0.474 log units. Only 25 of the $n = 185$ were prodrugs.

For comparison, fitting the latest data for the transdermal delivery of prodrugs through mouse skin from water, $J_{MMAQ}$, to the Roberts–Sloan equation gives Eq. (7.13) [66]:

$$\log J_{MMAQ} = -2.30 + 0.575 \log S_{IPM} + 0.425 \log S_{AQ} - 0.00248\,\mathrm{MW} \quad (7.13)$$

where $n = 32$, $r^2 = 0.904$, and $\Delta \log J_{MMAQ} = 0.141$ log units. The values for the $x$ and $y$ coefficients are very similar but the value for $z$ from the human skin data is much larger than that from the mouse skin data. This suggests that although human skin and mouse skin are quite similar to each other in their dependence on lipid and aqueous solubilities, the human skin is thicker so the inverse dependence of its diffusion on MW should be greater.

Also for comparison, fitting the latest data for the transdermal delivery of prodrugs through mouse skin from IPM, $J_{MMIPM}$, to the Roberts–Sloan equation gives Eq. (7.14) [61]:

$$\log J_{\mathrm{MMIPM}} = -0.562 + 0.501 \log S_{\mathrm{IPM}} + 0.499 \log S_{\mathrm{AQ}} - 0.00248\,\mathrm{MW} \quad (7.14)$$

where $n = 71$, $r^2 = 0.923$, and $\Delta \log J_{\mathrm{MMIPM}} = 0.156$ log units. Thus, for *in vitro* studies the dependence of maximum flux on solubilities in both lipid and water obtains regardless of whether the skin is human or mouse and regardless of whether the vehicle itself is a lipid or water.

Although the majority of studies that form the basis for the biphasic solubility model and the Roberts–Sloan equation are from *in vitro* studies, there are two *in vivo* studies that also support them. When data from the *in vivo* delivery of nonsteroidal anti-inflammatory drug through human skin from mineral oil (MO) [68] was fitted to the Roberts–Sloan equation, Eq. (7.15) was obtained for $n = 10$ ($r^2 = 0.934$) [69].

$$\log J_{\mathrm{MHMO}} = -1.46 + 0.72 \log S_{\mathrm{MO}} + 0.28 \log S_{\mathrm{AQ}} - 0.00013\,\mathrm{MW} \quad (7.15)$$

Similarly, when data from the *in vivo* delivery of various sunscreens, antioxidants, antimicrobial agents, and plasticizers through human skin from propylene glycol: water (30:70) was fitted to the Roberts–Sloan equation, Eq. (7.16) was obtained for $n = 10$ ($r^2 = 0.97$) [70].

$$\log J_{\mathrm{MHPG:AQ}} = -2.12 + 0.45 \log S_{\mathrm{OCT}} + 00.55 \log S_{\mathrm{AQ}} - 0.00048\,\mathrm{MW} \quad (7.16)$$

## 7.7 Summary

A new model has been proposed that combines concepts embodied in previous models of the physicochemical mechanism of transdermal permeation with the concept that permeants diffusing perpendicular to the skin surface through the multilamellar space between corneocytes have to diffuse not only through a lipid lamellar phase but also through an aqueous lamellar phase. The result is that the permeant must exhibit adequate solubility in both lipid and water phases to effectively cross the stratum corneum: the biphasic solubility model. Thus, the mechanism for enhancing the topical/transdermal delivery of parent drugs by their prodrugs is to increase the aqueous and lipid solubilities of the prodrugs compared to their parent drug.

The mathematical basis for the biphasic solubility model derives from Fick's law for diffusion where maximum flux across a membrane, $J_{\mathrm{M}}$, depends on the solubility of the permeant in the first few layers of the membrane: $S_{\mathrm{M1}}$. Since $S_{\mathrm{M1}}$ can be estimated from the sum of $y \log S_{\mathrm{LIPID}}$, $(1-y) \log S_{\mathrm{AQ}}$, and $\log c$, Fick's law can be restated as $\log J_{\mathrm{M}} = x + y \log S_{\mathrm{LIPID}} + (1-y) \log S_{\mathrm{AQ}} - z\,\mathrm{MW}$: the Roberts–Sloan equation. When data for $J_{\mathrm{M}}$, solubilities, and MW for prodrugs and drugs are fitted to the Roberts–Sloan equation, the coefficients for the solubility-based parameters are almost equal, as expected on the basis of the biphasic solubility model. The $J_{\mathrm{M}}$ values calculated from Eqs. (7.6) and (7.10) are in good agreement with the experimental $J_{\mathrm{M}}$.

Analysis of the $S_{\mathrm{LIPID}}$ and $S_{\mathrm{AQ}}$ data from a series of simple alkyl acyl and soft alkyl prodrug derivatives of drugs containing NH, OH, and SH functional groups show that unless the prodrug modification is capable of causing a dramatic decrease in intermolecular hydrogen bonding, the increases in $S_{LIPID}$ and $S_{AQ}$ are not dramatic, and neither are the increases in $J_M$. Although the incorporation of methoxy ethyleneoxy groups for simple alkyl groups to increase $S_{AQ}$, and hence $J_M$, has been explored, the results have not been dramatic either [58]. One promising approach that has not been exhaustively explored is to incorporate amino groups into the simple alkyl groups to increase $S_{AQ}$, and hence $J_M$. Preliminary results suggest that this approach may have the best chance for eliciting dramatic increases in $J_M$ [71–74].

## References


1 Scheuplein, R.J. (1965) Mechanism of percutaneous absorption. I. Routes of penetration and the influence of solubility. *The Journal of Investigative Dermatology*, **45**, 334–346.

2 Scheuplein, R.J. (1967) Mechanism of percutaneous absorption. II. Transient diffusion and the relative importance of various routes of skin penetration. *The Journal of Investigative Dermatology*, **48**, 79–88.

3 Michaels, A.S., Chandrasekaran, S.K., and Shaw, J.E. (1975) Drug permeation through human skin: theory and *in vitro* experimental measurement. *AIChE Journal*, **21**, 985–996.

4 Kasting, G.B., Smith, R.L., and Cooper, E.R. (1987) Effect of lipid solubilities and molecular size on percutaneous absorption, in *Skin Pharmacokinetics*, (eds B. Shroot and H. Schaefer) Karger, Basel, pp. 138–153.

5 Sloan, K.B., Wasdo, S.C., and Rautio, J. (2006) Design for optimized topical delivery: prodrugs and a paradigm change. *Pharmaceutical Research*, **23**, 2729–2747.

6 Sloan, K.B. and Wasdo, S.C. (2008) The role of prodrugs in penetration enhancement, in *Dermal Absorption and Toxicity Assessment* (eds M. Roberts and K. Walters), Marcel Dekker, New York, pp. 605–622.

7 Sloan, K.B. (1992) Functional group considerations in the development of prodrug approaches to solving topical delivery problems, in *Prodrugs: Topical and Ocular Drug Delivery* (ed. K.B. Sloan), Marcel Dekker, New York, pp. 11–116.

8 Sloan, K.B., Koch, S.A.M., and Siver, K.B. (1984) Mannich base derivatives of theophylline and 5-fluorouracil: syntheses, properties and topical delivery characteristics. *International Journal of Pharmaceutics*, **21**, 251–264.

9 Sloan, K.B. (1989) Prodrugs for Dermal delivery. *Advanced Drug Delivery Reviews*, **3**, 67–101.

10 Scheuplein, R. and Blank, I. (1973) Mechanism of percutaneous absorption. IV. Penetration of nonelectrolytes (alcohols) from aqueous solutions and pure liquids. *The Journal of Investigative Dermatology*, **60**, 286–296.

11 Johnson, M.E., Blankschtein, D., and Langer, R. (1997) Evaluation of solute permeation through the stratum corneum: lateral diffusion as the primary transport mechanism. *Journal of Pharmaceutical Sciences*, **86**, 1162–1172.

12 Liron, Z. and Cohen, S. (1984) Percutaneous absorption of alkanoic acids II: application of regular solution theory. *Journal of Pharmaceutical Sciences*, **73**, 538–542.

13 Flynn, G.L. and Yalkowsky, S.H. (1972) Correlation and prediction of mass transport across membranes. I. Influence of alkyl chain length on flux determining properties of barrier and diffusant. *Journal of Pharmaceutical Sciences*, **61**, 838–852.

14 Scheuplein, R.J. and Blank, I.H. (1971) Permeability of the skin. *Physiological Reviews*, **51**, 702–747.

15 Roberts, W.J. and Sloan, K.B. (1999) Correlation of aqueous and lipid solubilities with flux for prodrugs of 5-fluorouracil, theophylline and

6-mercaptopurine: a Potts–Guy approach. *Journal of Pharmaceutical Sciences*, **88**, 515–522.

**16** Beall, H.D. and Sloan, K.B. (1996) Transdermal delivery of 5-fluorouracil (5-FU) by 1-alkylcarbonyl-5-FU prodrugs. *International Journal of Pharmaceutics*, **129**, 203–210.

**17** Elias, P.M. and Friend, D.S. (1975) The permeability barrier in mammalian epidermis. *The Journal of Cell Biology*, **65**, 180–191.

**18** Swartzendruber, D.C., Wertz, P.W., Kitko, D.J., Madison, K.C., and Downing, D.T. (1989) Molecular models of the intercellular lipid lamellae in mammalian stratum corneum. *The Journal of Investigative Dermatology*, **92**, 251–257.

**19** Bouwstra, J.A., Gooris, G.S., van der Spek, J.A., and Bras, W. (1991) Structural investigations of human stratum corneum by small angle X-ray scattering. *The Journal of Investigative Dermatology*, **97**, 1005–1012.

**20** Bouwstra, J.A., Gooris, G.S., Dubbelaar, F.E.R., and Ponec, M. (2002) Phase behavior of stratum corneum lipid mixtures based on human ceramides: the role of natural and synthetic ceramide 1. *The Journal of Investigative Dermatology*, **118**, 606–617.

**21** Kessner, D., Ruettinger, A., Kiselev, M.A., Wartewig, S., and Neubert, R.H.H. (2008) Properties of ceramides and their impact on the stratum corneum structure: a review. *Skin Pharmacology and Physiology*, **21**, 58–74.

**22** Walkley, K. (1972) Bound water in stratum corneum measured by differential scanning calorimetry. *The Journal of Investigative Dermatology*, **59**, 225–227.

**23** Kiselev, M.A., Ryabova, N.Y., Balagurov, A.M., Dante, S., Hauss, T., Zbytovska, J., Wartewig, S., and Neubert, R.H.H. (2005) New insights into the structure and hydration of a stratum corneum lipid model membrane by neutron diffraction. *European Biophysics Journal*, **34**, 1030–1040.

**24** Lofgren, H. and Pascher, I. (1977) Molecular arrangements of sphingolipids. The monolayer behavior of ceramides. *Chemistry and Physics of Lipids*, **20**, 273–284.

**25** Scherer, J.R. (1987) The partial molar volume of water in biological membranes. *Proceedings of National Academy of Science USA*, **84**, 7938–7942.

**26** Bouwstra, J.A., Gooris, G.S., Dubblelaar, F.E.R., and Ponec, M. (2000) The lipid organization in the skin barrier. *Acta Dermato-Venereologica*, **208**, 23–30.

**27** Forslind, B. (1994) A domain mosaic model of the skin barrier. *Acta Dermato-Venereologica*, **74**, 1–6.

**28** Forslind, B., Engstrom, S., Engblom, J., and Norlen, L. (1997) A novel approach to the understanding of human skin barrier function. *Journal of Dermatological Science*, **14**, 115–125.

**29** Martin, A., Swarbrick, J., and Cammarata, A. (eds) (1983) *Physical Pharmacy*, 3rd edn, Lea and Febiger, Philadelphia, p. 402.

**30** Roberts, W.J. and Sloan, K.B. (2000) Prediction of transdermal flux of prodrugs of 5-fluorouracil, theophylline and 6-mercaptopurine with a series/parallel model. *Journal of Pharmaceutical Sciences*, **89**, 1415–1431.

**31** Lieb, W.R. and Stein, W.D. (1969) Biological membranes behave as non-porous polymer sheets with respect to diffusion of non-electrolytes. *Nature*, **224**, 240–243.

**32** Cohen, M.H. and Turnbull, D. (1959) Molecular transport in liquids and gases. *Journal of Chemical Physics*, **31**, 1164–1165.

**33** Potts, R.O. and Guy, R.H. (1992) Predicting skin permeability. *Pharmaceutical Research*, **9**, 663–669.

**34** Majumdar, S., Thomas, J., Wasdo, S., and Sloan, K.B. (2007) The effect of water solubility of solutes on their flux through human skin *in vitro*. *International Journal of Pharmaceutics*, **329**, 25–36.

**35** Poulson, B.J., Young, E., Coquilla, V., and Katz, M. (1968) Effect of vehicle composition on the *in vitro* release of fluocinolone acetonide and its acetate ester. *Journal of Pharmaceutical Sciences*, **57**, 928–933.

**36** Sloan, K.B., Koch, S.A.M., Siver, K.G., and Flowers, F.P. (1986) Use of solubility parameters of drug and vehicle to predict flux through skin. *The Journal* *of Investigative Dermatology*, **87**, 244–252.

37 Higuchi, T. (1960) Physical chemical analysis of percutaneous absorption process from creams and ointments. *Journal of the Society of Cosmetic Chemists*, **11**, 85–97.

38 Surber, C., Wilhelm, K.P., Hori, M., Maibach, H.I., and Guy, R. (1990) Optimization of topical therapy: partitioning of drugs into the stratum corneum. *Pharmaceutical Research*, **7**, 1320–1324.

39 Flynn, G.L. (1990) Physicochemical determinates of skin absorption, in *Principles of Route-to-Route Extrapolation for Risk Assessment* (eds J.R. Gerrity and C.J. Henry), Elsevier, Amsterdam, pp. 93–127.

40 Sloan, K.B. and Wasdo, S.C. (2003) Designing for topical delivery: prodrugs can make the difference. *Medicinal Research Reviews*, **23**, 763–793.

41 Beall, H.D., Prankerd, R.J., and Sloan, K.B. (1996) 1-Alkylcarbonyl-5-fluorouracil prodrugs: synthesis, thermal and hydrolytic stability. *Drug Development and Industrial Pharmacy*, **22**, 85–90.

42 Buur, A. and Bundgaard, H. (1986) Prodrugs of 5-fluorouracil: V. 1-Alkyloxycarbonyl derivatives as potential prodrug forms for improved rectal or oral delivery of 5-fluorouracil. *Journal of Pharmaceutical Sciences*, **74**, 522–527.

43 Beall, H.D. and Sloan, K.B. (1996) Transdermal delivery of 5-fluorouracil (5-FU) by 1-alkylcarbonyl-5-FU prodrugs. *International Journal of Pharmaceutics*, **129**, 203–210.

44 Beall, H.D., Prankerd, R., and Sloan, K.B. (1994) Transdermal delivery of 5-fluorouracil (5-FU) through hairless mouse skin by 1-alkyloxycarbonyl-5-FU prodrugs: physicochemical characterization of prodrugs and correlations with transdermal delivery. *International Journal of Pharmaceutics*, **111**, 223–233.

45 Beall, H.D. and Sloan, K.B. (2001) Topical delivery of 5-fluorouracil (5-FU) by 3-alkylcarbonyl-5-FU prodrugs. *International Journal of Pharmaceutics*, **217**, 127–137.

46 Beall, H.D., Prankerd, R.J., Todaro, L.J., and Sloan, K.B. (1993) Structure of 3-acetyl-5-fluorouracil: implications for its rearrangement during hydrolysis and upon heating. *Pharmaceutical Research*, **10**, 905–912.

47 Bansal, P.C., Pitman, I.H., Tam, J.N.S., Mertes, M., and Kamiski, J.J. (1981) *N*-Hydroxymethyl derivatives of nitrogen heterocycles as possible prodrugs I: *N*-hydroxymethylation of uracils. *Journal of Pharmaceutical Sciences*, **70**, 850–854.

48 Shih, P., Pedersen, L.G., Gibbs, P.R., and Wolfenden, R. (1998) Hydrophobicities of the nucleic acid bases: distribution coefficients from water to cyclohexane. *Journal of Molecular Biology*, **280**, 421–430.

49 Williams, D.A. (2008) Drug metabolism, in *Foye's Principles of Medicinal Chemistry*, 6th edn (eds T.L. Lemke and D.A. Williams), Lippincott Williams and Wilkins, Baltimore, pp. 253–326.

50 Lemke, T.L. and Williams, D.A. (eds) (2008) *Foye's Principles of Medicinal Chemistry*, 6th edn, Lippincott Williams and Wilkins, Baltimore, p. 666.

51 Sloan, K.B. and Bodor, N. (1982) Hydroxymethyl and acyloxymethyl prodrugs of theophylline: enhanced delivery of polar drugs through skin. *International Journal of Pharmaceutics*, **12**, 299–313.

52 Sloan, K.B., Hashida, M., Alexander, J., Bodor, N., and Higuchi, T. (1983) Prodrugs of 6-thiopurines: enhanced delivery through the skin. *Journal of Pharmaceutical Sciences*, **72**, 372–378.

53 Getz, J.J., Prankerd, R.J., and Sloan, K.B. (1992) Mechanism of hydrolysis of benzamidomethyl derivatives of phenols and its implication for prodrug design. *The Journal of Organic Chemistry*, **57**, 1702–1706.

54 Getz, J.J., Prankerd, R.J., and Sloan, K.B. (1993) Mechanism of hydrolysis of *O*-imidomethyl derivatives of phenols. *The Journal of Organic Chemistry*, **58**, 4913–4918.

55 Majumdar, S. and Sloan, K.B. (2006) Synthesis, hydrolysis and dermal delivery of *N*-alkyl-*N*-alkyloxycarbonylaminomethyl (NANAOCAM) derivatives of phenol,

imide and thio containing drugs. *Bioorganic & Medicinal Chemistry Letters*, **16**, 3590–3594.

56 Taylor, H.E. and Sloan, K.B. (1998) 1-Alkylcarbonyloxymethyl prodrugs of 5-fluorouracil (5FU): synthesis, physicochemical properties and topical delivery of 5FU. *Journal of Pharmaceutical Sciences*, **87**, 15–20.

57 Roberts, W.J. and Sloan, K.B. (2003) Topical delivery of 5-fluorouracil (5-FU) by 3-alkylcarbonyloxymethyl-5-FU prodrugs. *Journal of Pharmaceutical Sciences*, **92**, 1028–1036.

58 Wasdo, S.C. and Sloan, K.B. (2004) Topical delivery of a model phenolic drug: alkyloxycarbonyl prodrugs of acetaminophen. *Pharmaceutical Research*, **21**, 940–946.

59 Wang, S.-L., Lin, S.-Y., and Wei, Y.-S. (2002) Transformation of metastable forms of acetaminophen studied by thermal Fourier transform infrared (FT-IR) microscopy. *Chemical & Pharmaceutical Bulletin*, **50**, 153–156.

60 Thomas, J. and Sloan, K.B. (2007) *In vitro* evaluation of alkylcarbonyloxymethyl (ACOM) ethers as novel prodrugs of phenols for topical delivery: ACOM prodrugs of acetaminophen. *International Journal of Pharmaceutics*, **346**, 80–88.

61 Thomas, J. and Sloan, K.B. (2009) Evaluation of alkyloxycarbonyloxymethyl (AOCOM) ethers as novel prodrugs of phenols for topical delivery: AOCOM prodrugs of acetaminophen. *International Journal of Pharmaceutics*, **371**, 25–32.

62 Majumdar, S. and Sloan, K.B. (2007) Synthesis and topical delivery of *N*-alkyl-*N*-alkyloxycarbonylaminomethyl prodrugs of a model phenolic drug: acetaminophen. *International Journal of Pharmaceutics*, **337**, 48–55.

63 Waranis, R.P. and Sloan, K.B. (1988) Effects of vehicles and prodrug properties and their interaction on the delivery of 6-mercaptopurine through skin: S6-acyloxymethyl-6-mercaptopurine prodrugs. *Journal of Pharmaceutical Sciences*, **77**, 210–215.

64 Waranis, R.P. and Sloan, K.B. (1987) Effects of vehicles and prodrug properties and their interactions on the delivery of 6-mercaptopurine through skin: bisacyloxymethyl-6-mercaptopurine prodrugs. *Journal of Pharmaceutical Sciences*, **76**, 587–595.

65 Sloan, K.B., Wasdo, S., Ezike-Mkparu, U., Murray, T., Nickels, D., Singh, S., Shanks, T., Tovar, J., Ulmer, K., and Waranis, R. (2003) Topical delivery of 5-fluorouracil and 6-mercaptopurine by their alkylcarbonyloxymethyl prodrugs from water: vehicle effects on design of prodrugs. *Pharmaceutical Research*, **20**, 639–645.

66 Wasdo, S., Juntunen, J., Devarajan, H., and Sloan, K.B. (2009) A comparison of the fit of flux through hairless mouse skin from water to three model equations. *International Journal of Pharmaceutics*, **366**, 65–73.

67 Juntunen, J., Majumdar, S., and Sloan, K.B. (2008) The effect of water solubility of solutes on their flux through human skin *in vitro*: a prodrug database integrated into the extended Flynn database. *International Journal of Pharmaceutics*, **351**, 92–103.

68 Wenkers, B.P. and Lippold, B.C. (1999) Skin penetration of nonsteroidal anti-inflammatory drugs out of a lipophilic vehicle: influence of the viable epidermis. *Journal of Pharmaceutical Sciences*, **88**, 1326–1331.

69 Roberts, W.J. and Sloan, K.B. (2001) Application of the transformed Potts–Guy equation to *in vivo* human skin data. *Journal of Pharmaceutical Sciences*, **90**, 1318–1323.

70 Majumdar, S. and Sloan, K. (2005) Prediction of the flux of sunscreens and other compounds from PG/water through human skin *in vivo* using the Roberts–Sloan (RS) equation. *AAPS Journal*, **8** (S2), M1139.

71 Milosovich, S., Hussain, A., Dittert, L., Aungst, B., and Hussain, M. (1993) Testosteronyl-4-dimethylbutyrate HCl: a prodrug with improved skin penetration rate. *Journal of Pharmaceutical Sciences*, **82**, 227–228.

72 Jona, J.A., Dittert, L.W., Crooks, P.A., Milosovich, S.M., and Hussain, A.A. (1995) Design of novel prodrugs for the enhancement of the transdermal delivery

of indomethacin. *International Journal of Pharmaceutics*, **123**, 127–136.

73 Rautio, J., Nevalainen, T., Taipale, H., Vepsalainen, J., Gynther, J., Laine, K., and Jarvinen, T. (2000) Piperazinylalkyl prodrugs of naproxen improve *in vivo* skin permeation. *European Journal of Pharmaceutical Sciences*, **11**, 157–163.

74 Rautio, J., Nevalainen, T., Taipale, H., Vepsalainen, J., Gynther, J., Laine, K., and Jarvinen, T. (2000) Synthesis and *in vitro* evaluation of novel morpholinyl and methylpiperazinylacyloxyalkyl prodrugs of 2-(6-methoxy-2-naphthyl) propionic acid (naproxen) for topical delivery. *Journal of Medicinal Chemistry*, **43**, 1489–1494.

# 8
# Ocular Delivery Using Prodrugs

*Deep Kwatra, Ravi Vaishya, Ripal Gaudana, Jwala Jwala, and Ashim K. Mitra*

## 8.1
## Introduction

The term prodrug can be applied to compounds that undergo biotransformation before exhibiting their pharmacological action. These compounds are inactive derivatives of parent drugs, which upon chemical or enzymatic transformations generate the active parent compound. Prodrug modification has been considered as a viable strategy to overcome a variety of delivery-related problems. Enhancement of drug solubility, stability, targeting, efflux pump evasion, and decrease in toxicity are some of the advantages associated with a prodrug strategy.

## 8.2
## Criteria for an Ideal Ophthalmic Prodrug

As stated earlier, the primary reason behind designing a prodrug is to overcome any physical, chemical, and/or biopharmaceutical problems of a drug. Multiple formulation or drug delivery-related issues associated with a therapeutic agent can be solved using prodrug strategy, which would otherwise limit the clinical use of drug. Following are the ideal properties of an ophthalmic prodrug to be clinically effective:

1) **Chemical stability**: The prodrug must possess adequate shelf life in aqueous solutions. This will help in formulating topical eye drop solutions and suspensions.
2) **Aqueous solubility**: As most of the ophthalmic formulations are liquid (eye drops), aqueous solubility of a prodrug molecule will determine the doses that can be administered in a 30 μl eye drop. Aqueous solubility is also important when it is necessary to deliver a water insoluble or lipophilic molecule such as steroids via periocular route.
3) **Partition coefficient**: Prodrug should have optimal lipophilicity depending upon the cellular barrier it needs to cross in ocular delivery. For example, a prodrug

*Prodrugs and Targeted Delivery: Towards Better ADME Properties*. Edited by Jarkko Rautio

ISBN: 978-3-527-32603-7

must have optimal log *P* (log *P*: 2–3) so as to achieve maximal permeation across the cornea.

4) **Bioreversion**: These chemical entities must undergo bioconversion to the parent drug. The rate of bioconversion should be optimized so as to avoid elimination before it reaches target site as well as to prolong duration of action.
5) **Toxicity**: Ideally both the parent drug and the prodrug should not possess any cytotoxicity or irritability. The promoiety attached also should not have any toxicity of its own. Systemic absorption of ocular drugs can result in side effects and hence the prodrugs should exhibit high affinity for the target site as well as low uptake by the blood capillaries and lymphatic vessels.

Thus, such compounds should be designed by considering not only the physiochemical and formulation parameters but also the enzymatic bioconversion of the prodrug back to the drug. To better understand the fate of a prodrug upon dosing, the anatomy and the physiology of the eye must be thoroughly studied.

## 8.3 Anatomy and Physiology of the Eye

The eye can be broadly divided into two parts: (i) anterior chamber and (ii) posterior chamber (Figure 8.1). The anterior chamber encompasses the cornea, conjunctiva,

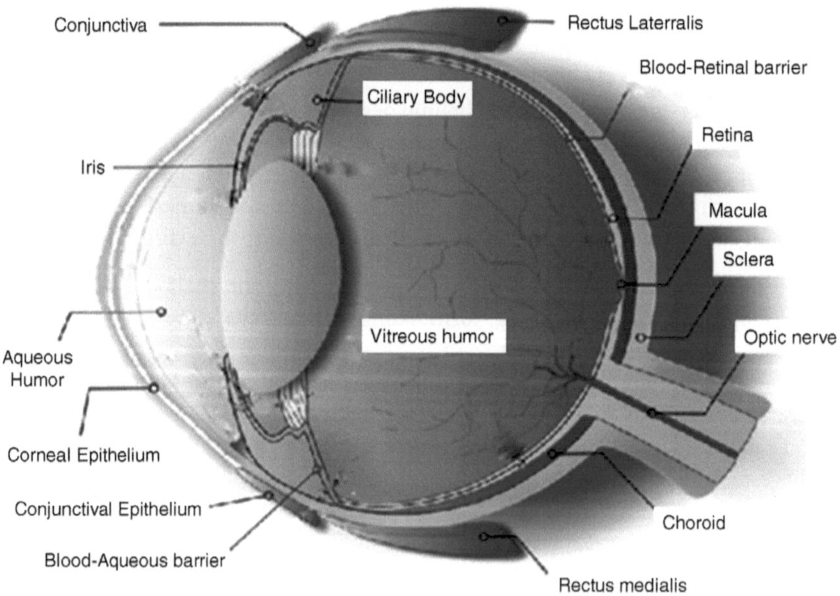


**Figure 8.1** Anatomy of the eye.

iris, ciliary body, aqueous humor, and lens while the posterior chamber consists of sclera, choroid, retina, and vitreous humor.

### 8.3.1 Anterior Chamber

Cornea is the avascular, outermost transparent multilayered membrane of the eye, which comprises of five layers, that is, corneal epithelium, Bowman's membrane, stroma, Descemet's membrane, and endothelium (arranged in the order of outermost to innermost) [1]. The epithelial layer comprises of five to six layers of columnar cells. The first layer is composed of nonkeratinized squamous cells. These cells have intercellular tight junctions. Bowman's layer and stroma (substantia propria) are mostly composed of collagen fibrils. Descemet's membrane is a thick basal lamina sandwiched between stroma and endothelium. The endothelium represents a monolayer of squamous cells [1]. Iris consists of pigmented epithelial cells and circular muscles (constrictor iridial sphincter muscles). It also contains the dilator muscles, responsible for dilation of the pupils upon sympathetic stimulation [2]. Ciliary body is produced by ciliary muscles and processes. Nonpigmented epithelial cells form the blood–aqueous barrier (BAB), which restricts the movement of proteins and colloids into the aqueous humor [2]. Conjunctiva consists of a clear mucous membrane lines inside the eyelids and spreads from the anterior surface of sclera up to the limbus. It is composed of nonkeratinized stratified columnar epithelial cells that play significant role in lubrication of the eye [2].

### 8.3.2 Posterior Chamber

Sclera represents a matrix above the choroid, which principally shields the internal organs of the eye. It mainly consists of collagen bundles with dispersed melanocytes and elastic fibers [3]. Choroid is a sandwiched and highly vascularized tissue between retina and sclera. It is further subdivided into vessel layer, choriocapillaris, and Bruch's membrane. The vessel layer comprises of arteries and veins, whereas choriocapillaries, as the name suggests is a dense network of capillaries. Bruch's membrane is situated between choroid and retinal pigmented epithelium (RPE). It is composed of basal lamellae of RPE and the endothelial cells of choroid [4]. Retina is a light-sensitive tissue comprising of two major layers that is, RPE and neurosensory retina. RPE is directly in contact with the light-sensing neural cells rods and cones. RPE functions as a nutrient source to the retina via the choroid. Inner part of the neurosensory retina mainly obtains its blood supply from the retinal artery, whereas the outer portions fulfill their nutritional requirements by the choriocapillaris. RPE forms tight junctions flanked by the choroid and retina [4]. Finally, vitreous humor – a hydrogel matrix (98 to 99.7% water) is localized between retina and lens. It also consists of hyaluronic acid and collagen fibrils [5]. Thinning of vitreous has been noted with age.

## 8.4
## Barriers to Ocular Drug Delivery

### 8.4.1
### Tear Film

It is maintained by ocular surface epithelial secretions and orbital glands. The film contains lipids, proteins, electrolytes, mucin, and other basic nutrients [6]. Upon instillation of an eye drop, a large fraction of the instilled dose is washed away within 2–5 min due to rapid dilution and tear turnover resulting in poor overall bioavailability of the drug (normally 1–5%) [7].

### 8.4.2
### Corneal Epithelium

The cornea is a multilayered clear and avascular tissue [8]. The corneal epithelium acts as a barrier to the traverse absorption of hydrophilic drugs. The epithelial cells express tight junctions and high transepithelial electrical resistance (TEER). Stroma that lies beneath the cornea and consists of hydrated collagen with interspersed cells, acts as a barrier to hydrophobic drugs [9]. The presence of specialized efflux pumps such as P-glycoprotein (Pgp), multidrug resistance protein (MRP), and breast cancer resistance protein (BCRP) on the cell membrane also act as a barrier [10, 11]. Corneal endothelium consists of a monolayer of polygonal cells that assist in maintaining corneal hydration and transparency. The cells show high metabolic activity and can lower the absorbed dose.

### 8.4.3
### Aqueous Humor and BAB

Aqueous humor is derived through active transport, diffusion, and ultrafiltration of plasma from the ciliary capillaries. The ciliary epithelium and blood vessels together form the blood–aqueous barrier. Cells of these layers exhibit tight junctions and prevent free movement of drug molecules into the aqueous humor [12, 13]. Transport of drug molecules from the aqueous humor into ciliary circulation is less constrained. Hence, molecules present in aqueous humor can easily enter the iris and be washed away by iridial and ciliary blood vessels [14, 15]. Low molecular weight lipophilic drugs are rapidly cleared by BAB compared to high molecular weight hydrophilic drugs.

### 8.4.4
### Conjunctiva

It is a slender clear membrane that lines the inside of eyelids and spreads from the anterior surface of sclera to the limbus. The membrane is highly vascularized and forms a tight junctional barrier on the surface (TEER values more than

$1500/cm^2$) [16]. Hence, this layer controls the permeation and clearance of hydrophobic, hydrophilic, and macromolecular compounds [17, 18]. The fraction that is not picked up by the conjunctival circulation permeates across the sclera.

Sclera mainly consists of collagen and mucopolysaccharides that extend from the corneal perimeter. Like the stroma, sclera contains abundant aqueous channels [19, 20]. It is a poorly vascularized and is more permeable tissue than cornea. Drug loss through conjunctival blood and lymphatic vessels can significantly lower absorption through the conjunctival/scleral pathway. Recently, this pathway has been explored for the delivery of peptides and oligonucleotides [19].

### 8.4.5 Blood–Retinal Barrier

Blood–retinal barrier (BRB) is similar in function to blood–brain barrier (BBB), which is composed of endothelial cells. BRB can be divided into two parts: (i) outer retinal barrier and (ii) inner retinal barrier. Endothelial cells (inner retinal barrier) are sealed with zonulas occludens that act as a barrier to hydrophilic molecules, such as trypan [21]. BRB also acts as a barrier to small and large proteins [22]. BRB primarily prevents the entry of drug molecules into the posterior segment. RPE forms the outer BRB between choroid and neural retina. It regulates the transport of molecules from choroidal capillaries into retina.

## 8.5 Influx and Efflux Transporters on the Eye

Both influx (transporters that aid entry into the cell) and efflux (transporters that remove drug from the cell) transport proteins have been reported to be functionally expressed various parts of the eye. All the barriers including cornea, conjunctiva, iris–ciliary body, and retina have been reported to express both influx and efflux transporters [14]. Some of the major influx transporters that are constitutively expressed are amino acid transporters (LAT1 and LAT2), glucose transporter (Glut1), monocarboxylate transporter (MCT), and peptide transporters (PEPT1 and PEPT2). The primary role of these influx transporters is selectively transport essential nutrient molecules across cellular barriers [23]. Corneal epithelium is a major barrier to drug delivery by the topical route. Transporters and receptors expressed on cornea have been mostly utilized for targeted drug delivery to the eye.

Efflux pumps play a critical role in lowering ocular bioavailability of various therapeutic agents. These efflux pumps belong to the ATP-binding cassette (ABC) superfamily of transporters. Major transporters in this family are Pgp, MRP, and BCRP. Human and rabbit corneal epithelia express high levels of Pgp [24], MRP [25], and BCRP [26]. Expression of these proteins have also been reported on other ocular tissues such as the RPE [27], retinal capillary endothelial cells [28], the ciliary nonpigmented epithelium [29], epithelial cells of conjunctiva [30], and the endothelial cells of iris and ciliary body [30]. Many steroidal, anticancer, and antiviral agents are substrates for these transporters, which can lower their ocular absorption. Prodrug modification has been utilized to evade these efflux pumps.

## 8.6 Transporter-Targeted Prodrug Approach

Prodrugs can be designed to target transporters or receptors expressed on cell membrane such as peptide, amino acid, nucleoside and nucleobases, and monocarboxylic acid transporters. Commonly expressed receptors on various ocular tissues are folate, transferrin, and insulin receptors. In prodrug approach, promoiety such an amino acid, peptide or vitamin, which is a substrate of a transporter, is conjugated to the parent molecule. The distinct feature of this approach is that the prodrug is recognized by particular transporters or receptors expressed on the cell surface. Prodrug derivatization has significantly improved ocular bioavailability of various antiviral drugs such as acyclovir (ACV) and ganciclovir (GCV) that are discussed in the next section.

### 8.6.1 Acyclovir

Current therapy available for the treatment of herpes simplex virus (HSV) keratitis is topical formulations of trifluorothymidine (TFT), idoxuridine (IDU), and vidarabine. All these therapies are associated with cytotoxicity and poor ocular absorption, which limit their use in long-term treatment. Ophthalmic ointment of acyclovir (3% ACV) is associated with various constraints such as variable absorption and blurred vision. As a result, it is not clinically approved for use in the treatment of HSV keratitis [31]. The major constraints for topical administration of ACV are precorneal elimination, nasolacrimal drainage, conjunctival absorption, tear turnover, and poor permeability across the cornea because of its hydrophilic nature. As mentioned above, the cornea is composed of five to six layers of columnar epithelium, which act as potential barriers to hydrophilic drugs. In addition, ACV ointment is not effective against deeper ocular tissue infections such as stromal keratitis [32]. In order to overcome the problem of poor penetration of acyclovir through the cornea, various strategies have been explored. At present, ACV amino acid ester prodrug, valacyclovir (VACV) is available in the market in the form of tablets, capsules, and parenteral formulations. The formulation resulted in three- to fivefold increase in oral bioavailability of ACV [33]. Such an increase in oral bioavailability is due to the recognition and translocation of the prodrug by peptide transporter (PEPT), which is expressed on the intestinal epithelial cells [34]. Although oral bioavailability of VACV was higher than that of ACV it was only bioavailable to the extent of 55%. This could be due to premature hydrolysis of the prodrug in the intestinal lumen [35]. Such premature hydrolysis will limit the amount of the prodrug available for the transporter to bind and translocate across the intestinal epithelial cells. Hence, enzymatically stable prodrugs are essential for ocular as well as oral delivery of ACV.

Among the nutrient carriers, amino acid transporters are preferred for ocular drug delivery because of their high expression and overlapping substrate specificity. Rational for amino acid prodrug development was to improve ocular bioavailability of ACV by designing prodrugs targeted to these transporters present on the cornea. Amino acid prodrugs, such as L-alanine-ACV (AACV), L-serine-ACV (SACV), L-isoleucine-ACV (IACV), gamma-glutamate-ACV (EACV), and L-valine-ACV (VACV), were synthesized by Katragadda *et al.* [36] who examined their *in vivo* corneal absorption (Figure 8.2). Among these prodrugs, IACV was most stable whereas AACV was least stable in aqueous solution at pH 7.4. Cell cytotoxicity data revealed that all the prodrugs were safer when compared to 5 mM concentration of trifluorothymidine (TFT), a U.S. FDA-approved drug for ocular herpes. Area under curve (AUC) of the total drug (prodrug + drug) for SACV and VACV were two- to threefold compared to that of ACV in aqueous humor. Concentration at last time point was also 2-fold and 2.5-fold higher for SACV compared to VACV and ACV, respectively [36].

Later on, a series of various dipeptide prodrugs of ACV were synthesized and targeted to PEPT on corneal epithelium thereby generating enhanced ocular bioavailability. These prodrugs exhibited higher stability, solubility, and antiviral activity than the amino acid prodrugs [37]. The dipeptide prodrugs such as L-val-L-val-ACV (VVACV) and gly-L-val-ACV displayed higher affinity for PEPT and demonstrated better permeability than marketed prodrug VACV. These peptide prodrugs exhibited higher therapeutic efficacy in corneal keratitis possibly due to their enhanced solubility and permeability as compared to the parent drug. These compounds are also less cytotoxic and exhibit excellent solution stability and antiviral efficacy compared to ACV and VACV [37].

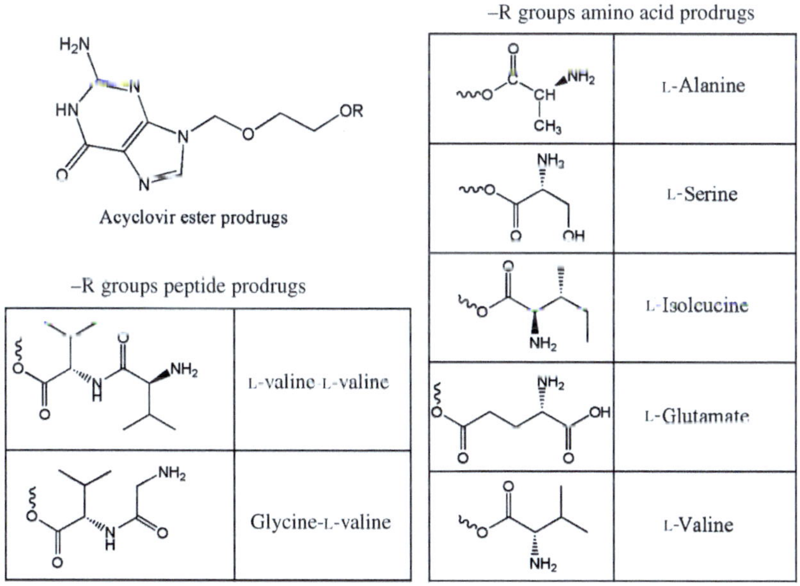


**Figure 8.2** Structure of acyclovir prodrugs.

Dipeptide ester prodrug VVACV has been further stereoisomerically modified to enhance its enzymatic stability [38]. Four diastereomeric prodrugs of ACV (L-val-L-val-ACV, L-val-D-val-ACV, D-val-L-val-ACV, and D-val-D-val-ACV) have shown different affinity toward PEPT and permeability across Caco-2 cell lines. The order of permeability was LDACV > LLACV > DDACV > DLACV [38]. Pharmacokinetics, metabolism, and corneal uptake of these stereoisomeric dipeptide prodrugs were determined and compared with VACV and ACV in rats. LLACV was found to be metabolized at a faster rate and to larger extent as compared to LDACV and DLACV following IV administration. Following oral administration of these stereoisomeric prodrugs, a higher amount of ACV (twofold) was observed at its targeted site (cornea) compared to VACV. [38] This enhanced bioavailability may be due to interaction of prodrugs with peptide transporters present on BAB and intestine [38]. It appears that due to higher stability of prodrug, a larger fraction of intact prodrug circulated in blood over a longer period.

### 8.6.2 Ganciclovir

GCV is a drug of choice for human cytomegalovirus (HCMV) retinitis. Like ACV, it has poor transcellular permeability and bioavailability (less than 10%) [39]. Low ocular bioavailability of GCV was attributed to its low lipophilicity.

Several monoester and diester prodrugs of GCV were synthesized such as L-val-GCV, L-val-L-val-GCV, gly-L-val-GCV, and L-val-gly-GCV. All these peptide prodrugs were well recognized by PEPT1. Among them, L-val-L-val-GCV and L-val-GCV showed higher aqueous solubility and lipophilicity compared to GCV. All the prodrugs were found to be less cytotoxic than the parent drug [40]. Later on, Majumdar *et al.* further synthesized and compared L-tyr-L-val-GCV, L-val-L-tyr-GCV along with L-val-L-val-GCV, L-val-gly-GCV, and gly-L-val-GCV (Figure 8.3) for stability and improvement in ocular bioavailability. These compounds did not show any measurable degradation at low pH values even after a period of 7 days at 37 °C (pH 1–5 in DPBS). L-tyr-L-val-GCV and L-val-L-tyr-GCV were found to be most lipophilic among the prodrugs and were predicted to have a log $P$ ($n$-octanol/DPBS pH 7.4) 33 times greater than that of GCV. All prodrugs generated higher aqueous solubility and greater transcorneal permeability due to better interaction with PEPT1 with L-val-L-val-GCV having eightfold higher permeability than GCV [41]. Along with the improvements in stability, solubility, affinity toward peptide transporters, these prodrugs also displayed better antiviral activity than TFT [40].

### 8.6.3 Quinidine

The chemical modification of a drug in order to reduce its affinity toward Pgp can lead to increased bioavailability. Pgp is expressed on the cornea and may limit ocular absorption of various topically administered drugs. Quinidine is a known substrate of Pgp and it was selected as a model drug to examine efflux pump evasion strategy

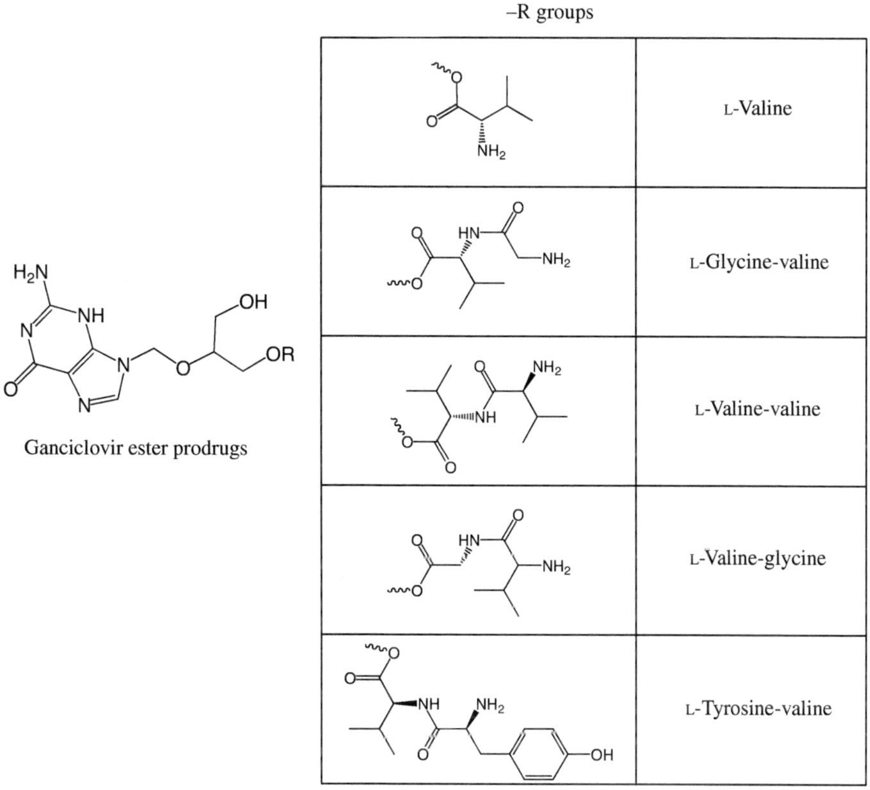


**Figure 8.3** Structure of gancyclovir prodrugs.

using prodrugs [42]. L-val-quinidine (VQ) and L-val-L-val-quinidine (VVQ) were synthesized and examined for their affinity toward Pgp and PEPT. Once recognized by PEPT, the prodrugs were no longer effluxed by Pgp [43], which might be the most probable reason for the enhanced permeability (1.5-fold for VQ and 3-fold for VVQ) across rabbit cornea [42, 43]. This concludes that by prodrug modification, ocular bioavailability of drugs can be enhanced through evasion of efflux pumps.

## 8.7 Drug Disposition in Ocular Delivery

The topical route is preferred due to several advantages such as less systemic side effects and excellent patient compliance. Still, poor permeability through the cornea, insufficient lipophilicity of drug, ionization of drug at tear pH, and precorneal factors are major reasons for the poor topical absorption. As mentioned above, nasolachrymal drainage, loss in the conjunctival blood circulation, tear dilution, loss due to normal tear drainage, reflux blinking, and enhanced tear production are the major

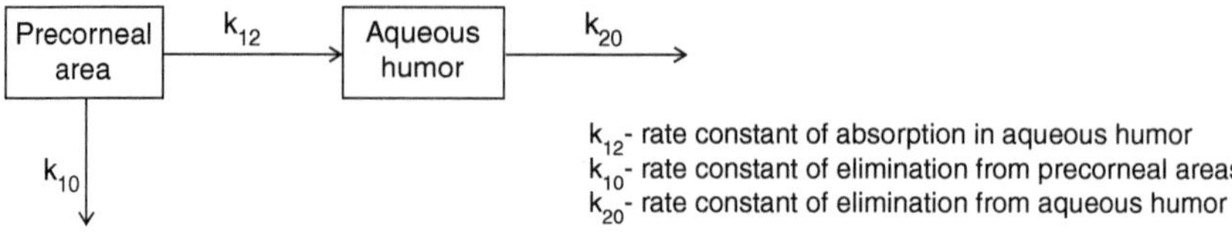


**Figure 8.4** Two-compartment model after topical administration.

precorneal factors that limit topical absorption. It is often difficult to achieve therapeutic drug levels when dosed systemically due to BAB, BRB, extensive metabolism, and large volume of distribution. In addition, systemically given drugs might show undesirable side effects. Subtherapeutic drug levels in the ocular tissue and shorter duration of action demands an increase in the dosing frequency. The two concurrent processes of precorneal loss and corneal absorption can be explained by a simple two-compartment model shown in Figure 8.4.

$k_{10}$ represents elimination rate constant and its magnitude is determined by the precorneal factors. $k_{12}$ represents the extent to which drug is able to cross the cornea and reach the aqueous humor. The magnitude of the $k_{12}$ depends on the physicochemical properties such as lipophilicity, solubility, p$K_a$ of drug, molecular radius, and charge on molecule. It is known that for any molecule to cross a biological membrane, it should have certain lipophilicity and aqueous solubility. The requirement of physicochemical properties is even stringent when molecule has to cross barriers such as cornea. The magnitude of the $k_{10}$ is much higher than $k_{12}$, which significantly decreases the bioavailability of drug upon topical instillation. Thus, in order to increase the bioavailability, it is necessary to lower the magnitude of $k_{10}$ and increase $k_{12}$.

Various formulation approaches such as particulate approach, mucoadhesives, and viscosity modifying agents may minimize drug loss by precorneal factors and thus lower the magnitude of $k_{10}$. Chemical modification of a drug to prodrug, analogue, and soft drug can be helpful by changing the physicochemical properties of drug molecules that are major determinants of the magnitude of $k_{12}$. While making the analogues, we must ensure that the newly formed compound retains its therapeutic activity. The prodrug approach is based on regeneration of active drug after metabolism in the tissue. On the other hand, the soft drug is converted to nontoxic metabolite after metabolism. Prodrug approach has been widely explored to overcome limitations of ocular drugs since the idea was introduced in the field of ophthalmology by Hussain and Truelove in 1976 [44]. In Section 8.8, we have briefly discussed importance of physicochemical properties of drug and its impact on ocular bioavailability.

## 8.8
## Effect of Physiochemical Factors on Drug Disposition in Eye

The physicochemical properties of a drug can influence its pharmacokinetic and pharmacodynamic properties. Change in the structure of molecule can lead to a change in physicochemical properties such as aqueous solubility, lipophilicity, crystal structure, and melting point. For example, in the treatment of glaucoma, a relatively higher concentrated solution of epinephrine is indicated. Due to its high polarity, a large percentage of the drug is absorbed in the systemic circulation via the nasolachrimal drainage and conjunctival absorption. Systemic absorption can result in cardiac side effects. The same is true with a beta-blockers such as timolol that exhibited cardiovascular and respiratory system-related side effects [45].

Generally, drugs cross the biological membranes via passive diffusion. Lipophilic drugs cross the membrane via transcellular pathway and the hydrophilic drugs prefer the paracellular pathway through the aqueous pore present between cell junctions. However, in cornea due to absence of aqueous pore, the drug molecules are forced to take the transcellular pathway. Therefore, drug molecules must have optimum lipophilicity to cross various ocular tissues. Partition or distribution coefficients are the terms that are used to give a measure of the lipophilicity of molecules. The relation between lipophilicity of a molecule and permeability has been well studied. Schoenwald and Ward showed the parabolic relation between the log *P* (octanol/water) and the permeability across the excised rabbit cornea (Figure 8.5) [46]. A log *P* value of 2–3 may be considered optimum for maximum corneal absorption. Therefore, by utilizing prodrug approach, one can increase the corneal permeation by increasing the lipophilicity of a molecule.

Aqueous solubility is another important factor that governs passive diffusion. Precorneal area is small and can accommodate limited volume (approximately 30 μl). So compounds must possess sufficient aqueous solubility to produce higher concentration gradient within small volume of instillation. While designing prodrug for a drug with poor log *P*, one must take into account the simultaneous decrease in

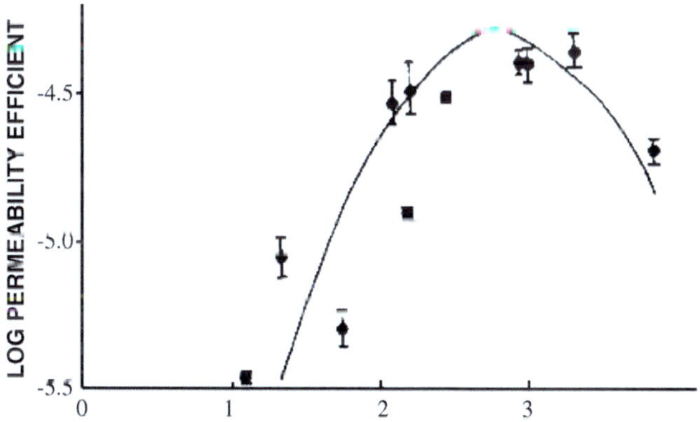


**Figure 8.5** Computer-generated curvilinear relationship between the log permeability coefficient of 11 labeled steroids and their respective log octanol–water partition coefficients. From left to right, the steroids are prednisolone, hydrocortisone, dexamithasone, fluorometholone, triamcinolone, acetonide, prednisolone acetate, cortexolone, deoxyxorticosterone, dexamethasone acetate, testosterone, and progesterone.

aqueous solubility of prodrug. Other important properties are molecular size, charge and degree of ionization. We have briefly discussed the development of prodrug approach to address the above-mentioned problems in Section 8.9.

## 8.9
## Prodrug Strategy to Improve Ocular Bioavailability (Nontransporter-Targeted Approach)

### 8.9.1
### Epinephrine

Epinephrine was a drug of choice for the treatment of glaucoma because of its ability to block the beta-adrenergic receptors. This drug exhibited poor permeation across the cornea after topical administration primarily due to its polar nature attributed to a catechol group. The poor permeation across cornea and noncorneal absorption were the major reasons for its poor bioavailability, high frequency of administration, and systemic side effects. Since epinephrine has a good aqueous solubility, a high dose of the drug was used to achieve therapeutic drug concentration. Higher dose and frequency of administration often resulted in systemic cardiovascular side effects.

Hussain and Truelove were the first who attempted to solve these problems by making dipivaloyl ester prodrug of epinephrine with suitable salt (U.S. Patent 3,809,714). The prodrug dipivaloyl epinephrine (DPE) was nontoxic and 100-fold more potent in management of glaucoma than parent drug itself [44] (U.S. Patent 3,809,714). The salt form of the prodrug compensated decrease in solubility due to esterification of two phenol groups responsible for solubility in parent drug. So the prodrug showed acceptable solubility and its partition coefficient was 600 times higher than that of the parent drug at pH 7.2 [47] that resulted in 8–10-fold better absorption via topical route across cornea. Prodrug exhibited excellent stability in solution state and therefore did not show bioreversion in precorneal area. Major site of metabolism of DPE was the cornea due to presence of esterases that converted DPE into active epinephrine (Figure 8.6). This approach has also led to decrease in drug loss to the general circulation. DPE generated 100–400 times lower systemic levels resulting in much lower incidents of cardiovascular side effects.

### 8.9.2
### Phenylephrine

Phenylephrine is a mydriatic agent used to assist surgery and eye examination. Topical solution was less bioavailable due to poor permeation across cornea, which was attributed to its low lipophilicity (log $P = -1.89$; pH 7.4). Because of this, a high dose (10%) is needed to produce the desired pharmacological response. Drainage of drug into systemic circulation also resulted in cardiovascular system-related side effects due to its $\alpha 1$ agonist activity.

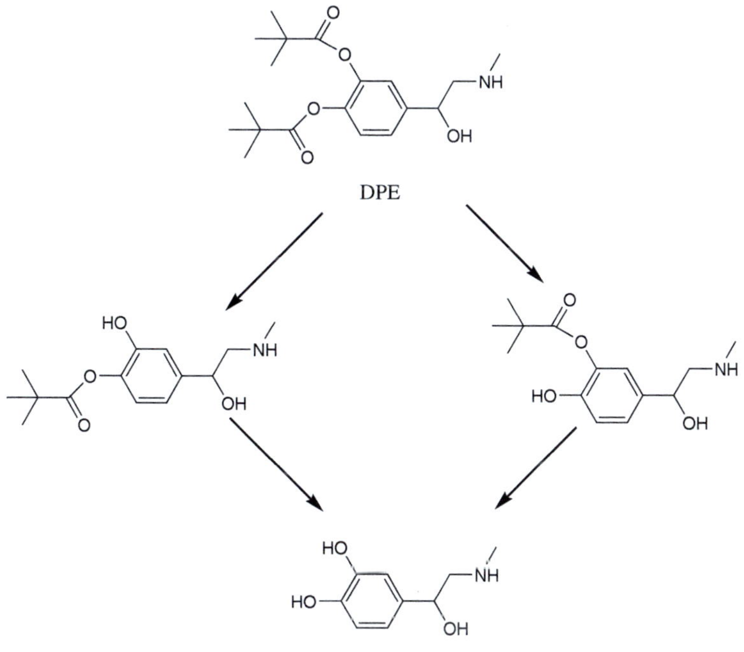


**Figure 8.6** Metabolism of dipivaloyl epinephrine prodrug (DPE) in cornea.

Lipophilic oxazolidine prodrug of phenylephrine (log $P = 1.38$; pH 7.4) with an aim to enhance corneal absorption and lower the systemic toxicities was designed (Figure 8.7) [48]. Unlike epinephrine prodrugs, oxazolidine prodrug was not obtained in salt form. Hence, its aqueous solubility was compromised and it was formulated as a suspension. Another reason for formulating an oil-based suspension was the poor aqueous stability (half-life of not more than 13 min in the pH range 1–7.4). Suspension of prodrug in 10% sesame oil raised the corneal phenylephrine level by sixfold and aqueous humor level upto eightfold higher than 10% aqueous solution of the parent drug [49]. In a study done in monkeys, investigators compared 1% phenylephrine and 10% phenylephrine oxazolidine for the ocular and systemic of drug levels. Although the strength of prodrug solution was less than parent drug, they found that 1% prodrug produces significant higher aqueous humor levels of parent drug and lower systemic drug levels. This approach lowered systemic exposure of drug and thus lowered systemic side effects.

### 8.9.3
### Pilocarpine

Pilocarpine is given topically to lower intraocular pressure associated with glaucoma. It is a polar molecule (log $P \approx 0.15$) that may be responsible for its poor corneal permeation. The drug is also a vasodilator, so it causes vasodilation of the conjunctival

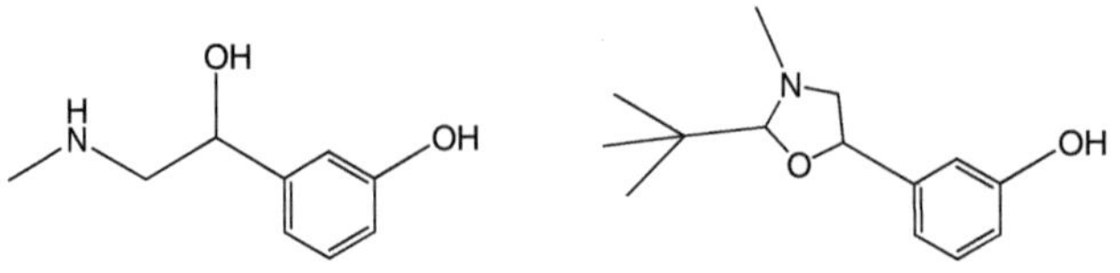


**Figure 8.7** (a) Phenylephrine and (b) Oxazolidine prodrug of phenylephrine.

circulation leading to accelerated drug loss through noncorneal pathway. The duration of action is also low (3 h), requiring repeated administration (three to six times a day).

Therefore, to improve its corneal absorption, various lipophilic alkyl and arylalkyl ester prodrugs of pilocarpine were synthesized. The prodrugs enhanced corneal permeation of pilocarpine. Unlike other ester prodrugs, regeneration of pilocarpine from its monoester prodrugs was not dependent on the activity of esterase present in tissues. Instead, cyclization to form pilocarpine lactone ring played a major role in regeneration of parent drug. General mechanism for this reaction is shown in Figure 8.8.

Cyclization was governed by activity of alcohol, which was dependent on the pH and the steric hindrance inflicted by the −R group. Nucleophilic attack by the alkoxide ion on the partially positive carbon of ester bond causes the cyclization. Since this reaction depends on the activity of alcohol group, the rate of cyclization or regeneration increases with an increment in pH from 3.5 to 10. The monoesters were not stable in solutions. However, steric hindrance by −R group enhanced the half-life ($t_{1/2}$) of prodrugs in aqueous solution. For *p*-chlorobenzyl ester, $t_{1/2}$ was 30 min and for *n*-hexyl ester it was 1105 min at 37 °C in pH 7.4 buffer. Overall, monoesters of pilocarpine exhibited higher lipophilicity resulting in enhanced corneal permeation. But even in this case, solution stability was poor. Diester derivatives of pilocarpine

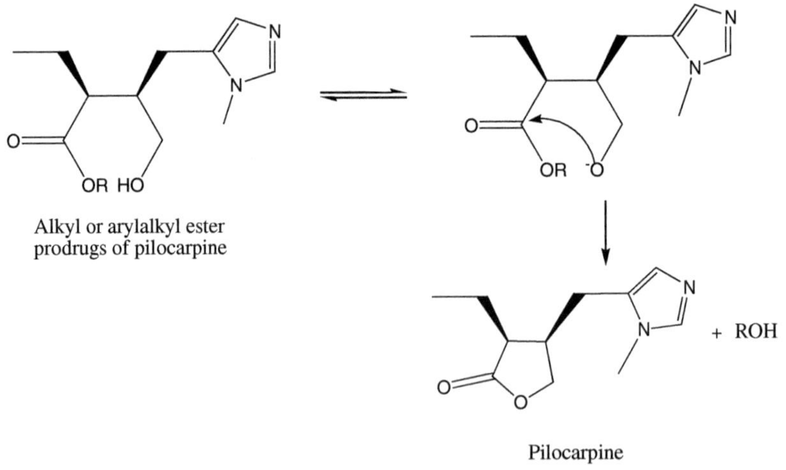


**Figure 8.8** Mechanism of lactonization and regeneration to active drug.

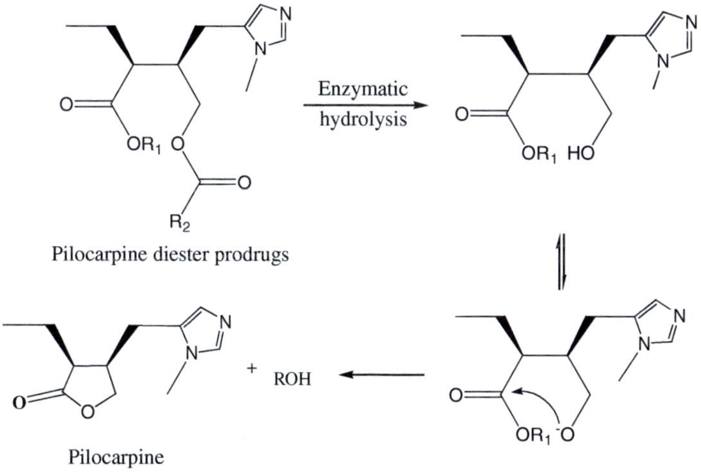


**Figure 8.9** Regeneration of pilocarpine from pilocarpic diesters.

were synthesized to address these issues [50]. These compounds exhibited higher lipophilicity than parent drug and their corresponding monoesters. In this approach, −OH group was also esterified, which blocked this functional group from being a nucleophile. Hence, the process of lactonization in the solution was avoided. As a result, diester prodrugs displayed higher stability in aqueous solution compared to monoesters. *O*-Acyl bond can be cleaved by the esterases present in the cornea and other ocular tissues to generate the monoester, which can spontaneously undergo lactonization to produce the active parent drug (Figure 8.9).

Both the pilocarpine monoester and diesters showed higher lipophilicity than pilocarpine and thus increased the corneal permeation. Moreover, monoester and diester prodrugs generated longer duration of action by 1.5-fold and by 2.25-fold, respectively, at half of the dose of parent drug [51]. So, the diester prodrugs improved bioavailability and duration of action of pilocarpine. This approach, however, reduced aqueous solubility of the prodrug.

Järvinen *et al.* synthesized bispilocarpic acid diester prodrugs of pilocarpine (Figure 8.10) [52, 53]. These prodrugs were more lipophilic than diesters of pilocarpine and showed similar permeability across excised cornea [54]. Like diesters, bispilocarpic acid diesters also permeated across corneal epithelium rapidly due to high lipophilicity and converted to pilocarpine in the cornea by the esterases. Due to the high esterases activity in the cornea, all the prodrugs were converted into parent drug during their passage to corneal endothelium.

### 8.9.4
### Timolol

Timolol is a nonselective beta-adrenergic receptor antagonist used for a long time for the treatment of open angle glaucoma. Ever since it was introduced in the market, the

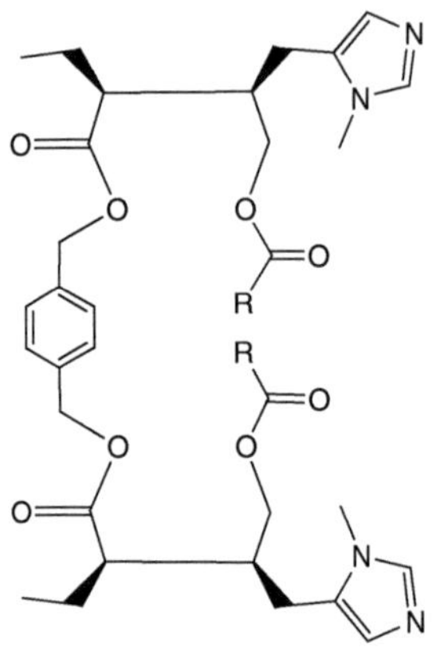

**Figure 8.10** General structure of bispilocarpic acid prodrug, where –R can be alkyl or cycloalkyl group.

major problem was the systemic side effects associated with its topical use. The drug is basic having a p$K_a$ of 9.2. Therefore, at pH 7.4, 98% of the drug is in ionized form. Log *P* for this drug is very low (-0.04; pH 7.4) and thus the drug exhibited very poor permeability across lipoidal corneal membrane. Prodrugs of timolol were developed to facilitate corneal absorption and lower systemic exposure to avoid its cardiovascular and respiratory-related side effects.

Bundgaard *et al.* synthesized lipophilic ester prodrugs of timolol and studied lipophilicity and stability of these prodrugs. All these prodrugs were more lipophilic than parent drug and they regenerated timolol in the corneal tissue. Among all, corneal absorption for *O*-butyryl timolol was highest. But none of the compounds reduced systemic absorption of timolol. Systemic absorption was lowered due to lowering the dose of the *O*-butyryl timolol from 15 to 3.75 mM. Dose reduction resulted in optimal aqueous humor drug level along with decrease in plasma drug levels. *O*-Butyryl timolol also prolonged duration of action. However, these prodrugs exhibited poor stability in phosphate buffer. So, it was difficult to design a stable formulation. Therefore, a series of amphiphilic esters of timolol malonate were developed and studied for antagonistic effect against isoproterenol-induced ocular hypotension [55]. Palmitoyl timolol malonate (PTM) was found to be the most active. Permeability of PTM and timolol malonate was found to be $0.42 \times 10^{-6}$ and $2.2 \times 10^{-6}$ cm/s, respectively. Despite of the poor permeability, PTM showed much better efficacy in lowering ocular hypertension with longer duration of action. It was speculated that longer duration of effect was due to sustained release of drug from the corneal epithelium and intense IOP reduction at early time points was due to its transscleral drug absorption. Hydrolytic kinetics of PTM in aqueous solution showed that it is more stable than previously synthesized acylester prodrugs due to increase in carbon chain length [56]. Structures of various prodrugs of timolol have been summarized in Figure 8.11.

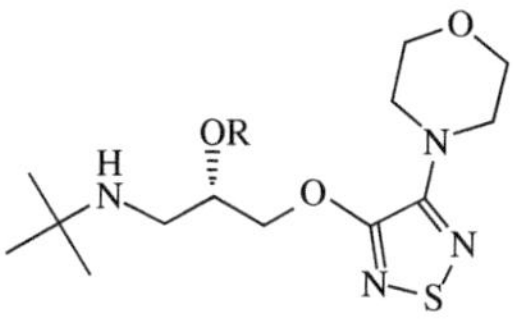

R group

| | |
|---|---|
| octanoyl | 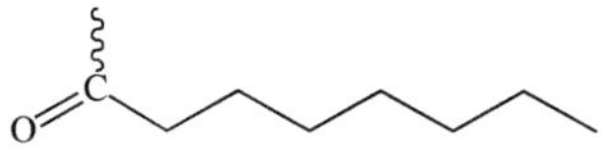 |
| decanoyl | 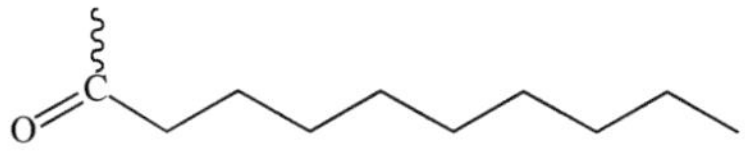 |
| dodecanoyl | 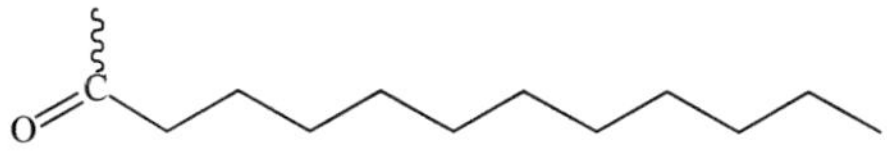 |
| myristoyl | 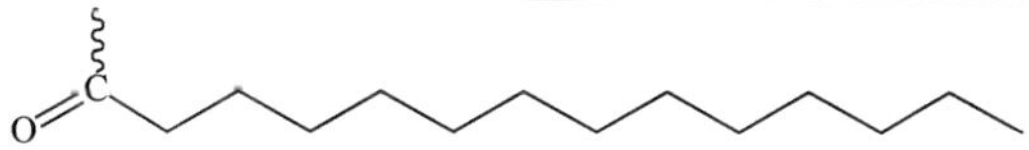 |
| palmitoyl | 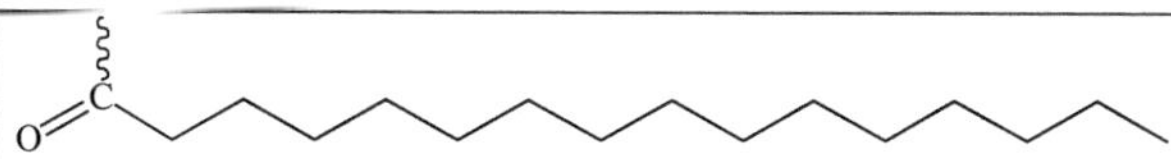 |

**Figure 8.11** Amphiphilic ester prodrug of timolol malonate, where –R can be octanoyl, decanoyl, dodecanoyl, myristoyl, and palmitoyl groups.

### 8.9.5
### Prostaglandin $F_{2\alpha}$

Various prostaglandin analogues and prodrugs have been developed to treat open angle glaucoma. [57]. Unlike timolol, prostaglandin F analogues did not cause systemic side effects. However, several ocular side effects such as conjunctival hyperemia, color changes in eyelashes, periocular skin pigmentation, and darkening of iris were observed [58]. So it was necessary to overcome ocular side effects related to prostaglandin (PG) analogues to enhance patient compliance.

Initially, prodrug approach was adopted by investigators to increase lipophilicity and thereby corneal permeability. Esterification of acid and/or alcohol at position 1 and 15 resulted in monoester and diesters of $PGF_{2\alpha}$. Prodrugs were highly lipophilic and showed higher corneal permeability and IOP lowering capacity than parent drug [59]. However, none of the prodrugs reduced conjunctival hyperemia [60].

A series of acyl ester prodrugs were synthesized by making chemical modifications at positions 9, 11, and 15 of $PGF_{2\alpha}$. They also studied their bioreversion in ocular tissues, efficacy to lower the IOP and conjunctival hyperemia produced by each prodrug and compared with $PGF_{2\alpha}$-1-isopropyl ester [61]. They observed that all the compounds modified at position 9 could not be hydrolyzed to parent drug and so cannot be considered as a prodrug. Monoester and diester produced by modifications at positions 11 and 15 were considered as prodrugs. All prodrugs were more lipophilic than the parent drug and were found to be cleared by carboxylesterase and not by acetyl choline esterase or butyryl choline esterase. A prodrug modified at position 11 and/or position 15 exhibited much slower hydrolysis rate than $PGF_{2\alpha}$-1-isopropyl ester. They observed a delay in the conjunctival hyperemia with these prodrugs. Although these prodrugs were hydrolyzed at a slower rate than $PGF_{2\alpha}$-1-isopropyl ester, these compounds were as effective as $PGF_{2\alpha}$-1-isopropyl ester in producing ocular hypotension. So it was concluded that adverse effects of parent drug can be overcome by slowing down the conversion rate of prodrug to drug [62].

Later on, analogues of $PGF_{2\alpha}$ were synthesized for increasing selectivity toward $PGF_{2\alpha}$ receptors. Latanoprost was synthesized which is an isopropyl ester of $PGF_{2\alpha}$ analogue. Latanoprost was able to reduce conjunctival hyperemia due to the modification done on one of the side chain by attaching phenyl ring. This modification enhanced the affinity of latanoprost to the prostaglandin F (FP) receptors and lowered its affinity toward nonspecific receptors [58]. Travoprost is also ester prodrug of $PGF_{2\alpha}$ analogue with higher selectivity for FP receptors. Bimatoprost is more efficacious as ocular hypotensive agent than latanoprost and travoprost [63]. However, it is a structural analogue of prostamide $F_{2\alpha}$ (Figure 8.12).

Various other prodrugs utilizing targeted and nontargeted approaches have been synthesized and studied. To discuss all of them is beyond the scope of this chapter. Some of the prodrugs that are not discussed in this chapter have been listed in Table 8.1.

## 8.10
## Recent Patents and Marketed Ocular Prodrugs

In a recent patent from Allergan, inventors have prepared prodrugs of various therapeutic molecules coupled with amino acid, peptide, monocarboxylic acid, organic anion, and cation nucleoside to target transporters. D-Glucopyranosyl ester of dexamethasone and gly-sar ester of bimatoprost (Figure 8.13) have been developed to overcome the limitations of parent molecules [64].

Recently, inventors from Allergan have also developed a prodrug molecule by conjugating a therapeutic molecule used in glaucoma with acetylcholinesterase or acetylcholine. Due to this prodrug modification, they presumed a higher and selective uptake of prodrug by acetylcholine or acetylcholinesterase receptors present on the cell surface. Upon entry into the cell, this prodrug will regenerate its parent drug due to enzymatic hydrolysis [65].

In another approach to treat posterior segment diseases, researchers have developed prodrug by conjugating carotenoid to the drug molecule. Carotenoid is a naturally occurring xanthophyll, which has a tendency to accumulate in the macula from the diet. This property of xanthophyll was exploited by attaching it to a

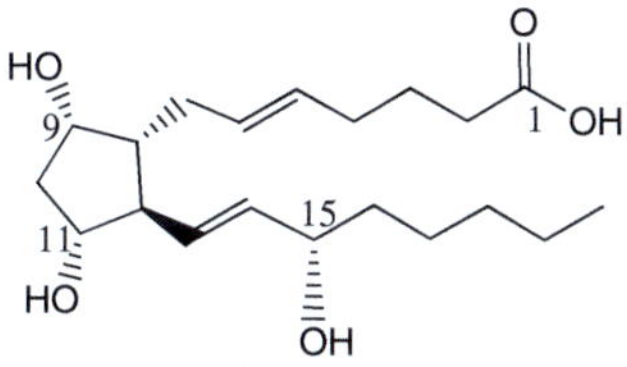


Prostaglandin $F_{2\alpha}$

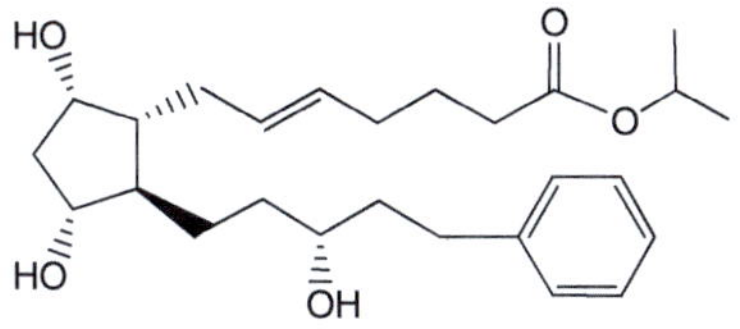


Latanoprost

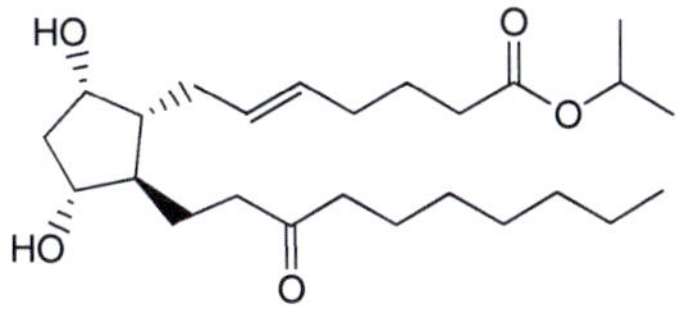


Prostaglandin $F_{2\alpha}$-1-isopropyl

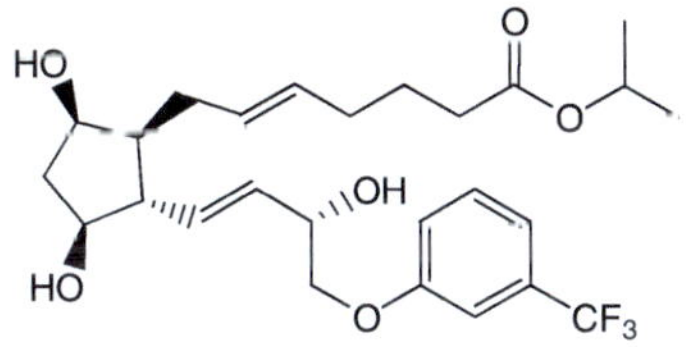


Travoprost

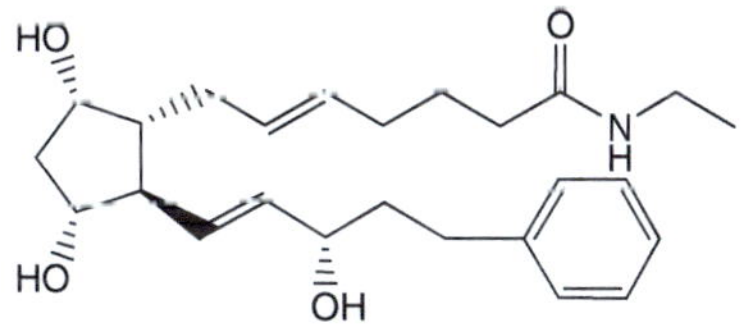


Bimatoprost

**Figure 8.12** Clinically used prostaglandins.

therapeutic molecule. Investigators have used this strategy to make prodrugs of etoposide, vincristine, fluocinolone, and other steroids [66].

Steroidal molecules upon long-term administration cause IOP elevation and cataract formation. In a novel approach to deliver steroidal molecule over a long period without causing side effects, some inventors have hypothesized a lipophilic ester prodrug of steroidal molecule. A lipophilic ester prodrug of dexamethasone was developed. This conjugate could be selectively taken up by macrophages. Once administered via intravitreal injection, prodrug may not allow partition into the aqueous humor and lens, which may lower side effects such as elevation in IOP and cataract formation. These researchers have also reported a sustained release of dexamethasone from its prodrug (dexamethasone palmitate) for more than 2 months following a single administration [67].

A sustained release microsphere formulation of tazarotene has also been developed. Esterification of tazarotenic acid forms tazarotene. This compound shows significantly lower side effects relative to the active drug, tazarotenic acid. Following sustained release of tazarotene from PLGA microparticles the prodrug is converted into the active moiety tazarotenic acid by enzymes present in choroid and retina. The prodrug can be administered by periocular route to obtain a sustained release for over 2 weeks [68].

**Table 8.1** Summary of recent developments of formulating prodrugs of drug molecules.

| Drug | Prodrug | Characteristic/major advantage of prodrug | Reference |
|---|---|---|---|
| Ethacrynic acid (ECA) | SA9000, an ECA analogue and SA9000-cysteine adduct | Higher corneal penetration, less irritation, and significant decrease in intraocular pressure | [72] |
| L-Carnosine | *N*-acetylcarnosine (NAC) | Codrug and prodrug approach has enhanced transcorneal permeation resulting in higher drug levels in aqueous humor and lens for treatment of senile cataract | [73] |
| TG100 801 | Generates TG100 572 after de-esterification. | After topical administration, less systemic drug bioavailability, less side effects, and higher intraocular penetration for retinal diseases | [74] |
| Cyclosporine A | UNIL088 | Water-soluble prodrug formed by esterification of cyclosporine A | [75] |
| Tafluprost | An ester prodrug of 15,15-difluoro-$PGF_{2\alpha}$ | Enhanced transcorneal permeation | [76] |
| Penciclovir | Famciclovir | Oral administration achieved therapeutic levels in vitreous humor to treat herpes simplex 1, herpes simplex 2, and varicella zoster virus | [77] |

In 2005, U.S. FDA approved a topical prodrug-based formulation of nepafenac, which is a nonsteroidal anti-inflammatory drug. This formulation is applied topically to treat postoperative inflammation and pain occurring after cataract surgery. Nepafenac permeates more efficiently into the corneal tissue. This prodrug then metabolizes into amfenac by enzymatic hydrolysis (Figure 8.14) [69].

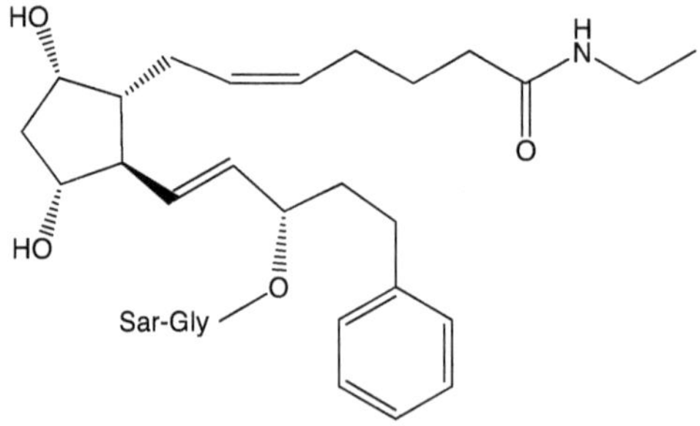


**Figure 8.13** Gly-Sar ester of Bimatoprost.

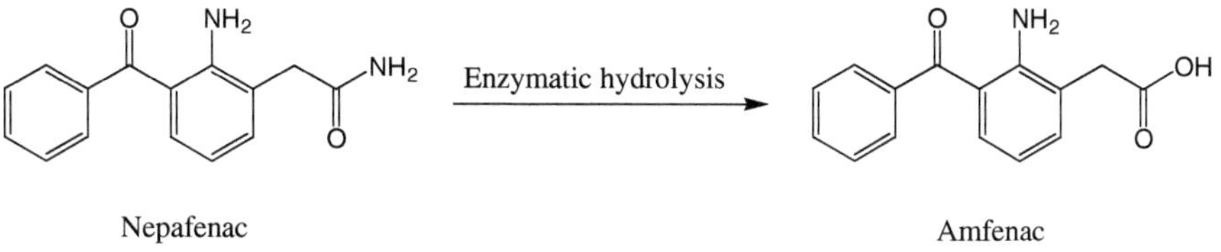


**Figure 8.14** Bioconversion of nepafenac to amfenac.

## 8.11 Novel Formulation Approaches for Sustained Delivery of Prodrugs

Sustaining drug levels at targeted site after administration is an important aspect of ocular delivery. Various colloidal carriers such as microparticles, nanoparticles, and liposomes have been developed. These delivery systems can be administered alone or by suspending into a gel-based formulation to tailor the drug release following ocular administration [70]. To prevent drug loss from precorneal area, sustained release formulations can also be developed. After subconjunctival administration, drug loss via conjunctival capillaries and lymphatic circulation can be partially or completely avoided by making a hydrophilic prodrug of a lipophilic molecule such as steroidal molecules. Lymphatic circulation and conjunctival circulation preferentially pick up hydrophobic molecules, which can also be avoided by suspending prodrug-based formulation into a thermosensitive gel. Drug levels in vitreous humor and retina can be sustained by developing controlled release intraocular formulation such as microsphere, nanoparticles, and liposomes that can be administered via intravitreal injection. Development of various biodegradable and biocompatible polymers has gained considerable attention in last decade. Drug release from various block copolymers can be tailored depending upon requirement of disease state. Our laboratory has developed pentablock polymers to sustain drug release from nanoparticles. We are also developing pentablock-based gel formulation to sustain even longer release without any burst effect. Each polymer block used in the preparation of the polymer is biocompatible, biodegradable, and approved by U.S. FDA for human use. This approach can be widely exploited because of its tremendous potential to sustain drug release for longer duration (6–12 months), which has particular importance for the treatment of posterior segment disease such as wet age-related macular degeneration (AMD), diabetic retinopathy, and macular edema development of nanocarriers can also overcome drug efflux from targeted macular cells. Various excipients such as surfactants and polymers inhibit various efflux pumps [71].

## 8.12 Conclusion

The prodrug approach must be applied at a much earlier stage in drug development process. A multidisciplinary approach toward prodrug design as well as a combination of novel formulation strategies along with prodrug strategy may eventually generate ideal therapy for ocular disease.

## Acknowledgments

Supported by National Eye Institute Grants RO1EY09 171 and RO1EY10 659.

## References


1 Dingeldein, S.A. and Klyce, S.D. (1988) Imaging of the cornea. *Cornea*, **7** (3), 170–182.
2 Lacouture, A. (2006) Anatomy–physiology of the eye. *Revue de l'Infirmiere* (120), 16–17.
3 Edelhauser, H. and Ubels, J. (2003) Cornea and sclera, in *Physiology of the Eye* (eds P. Kaufman and A. Alm), Mosby, St. Louis, pp. 47–116.
4 Sharma, R. and Ehinger, B. (2003) Development and structure of retina, in *Physiology of the Eye* (eds P. Kaufman and A. Alm), Mosby, St. Louis, pp. 319–347.
5 Lund-Andersen, H. and Sander, B. (2003) The vitreous, in *Physiology of the Eye* (eds P. Kaufman, A. Aam, and R.A. Moses,) Mosby, CV, St. Louis, pp. 293–216.
6 Dartt, D.A., Hodges, R.R., and Zoukhri, D. (2006) Tear and their secretion, in *The Biology of Eye* (ed. J. Fischbarg), Academic Press, New York, pp. 21–82.
7 Cai, X., Conley, S., and Naash, M. (2008) Nanoparticle applications in ocular gene therapy. *Vision Research*, **48** (3), 319–324.
8 Sunkara, G. and Kompella, U. (2003) Membrane transport processes in the eye, in *Ophthalmic Drug Delivery Systems* (ed. A. Mitra), Marcel Dekker, New York, pp. 13–58.
9 Huang, H.S., Schoenwald, R.D., and Lach, J.L. (1983) Corneal penetration behavior of beta-blocking agents. II. Assessment of barrier contributions. *Journal of Pharmaceutical Sciences*, **72** (11), 1272–1279.
10 Jorge, F. (2003) On the mechanism of fluid transport across corneal endothelium and epithelia in general. *Journal of Experimental Zoology. Part A. Comparative Experimental Biology*, **300A** (1), 30–40.
11 Kuang, K. *et al.* (2004) Intracellular [$Na^+$], $Na^+$ pathways, and fluid transport in cultured bovine corneal endothelial cells. *Experimental Eye Research*, **79** (1), 93–103.
12 Cunha-Vaz, J.G. (1997) The blood–ocular barriers: past, present, and future. *Documenta Ophthalmologica*, **93** (1–2), 149–157.
13 Freddo, T.F. (2001) Shifting the paradigm of the blood–aqueous barrier. *Experimental Eye Research*, **73** (5), 581–592.
14 Mannermaa, E., Vellonen, K.S., and Urtti, A. (2006) Drug transport in corneal epithelium and blood–retina barrier: emerging role of transporters in ocular pharmacokinetics. *Advanced Drug Delivery Reviews*, **58** (11), 1136–1163.
15 Urtti, A. (2006) Challenges and obstacles of ocular pharmacokinetics and drug delivery. *Advanced Drug Delivery Reviews*, **58** (11), 1131–1135.
16 Saha, P., Kim, K.J., and Lee, V.H. (1996) A primary culture model of rabbit conjunctival epithelial cells exhibiting tight barrier properties. *Current Eye Research*, **15** (12), 1163–1169.
17 Einmahl, S. *et al.* (2001) Therapeutic applications of viscous and injectable poly(ortho esters). *Advanced Drug Delivery Reviews*, **53** (1), 45–73.
18 Liaw, J., Chang, S.F., and Hsiao, F.C. (2001) *In vivo* gene delivery into ocular tissues by eye drops of poly(ethylene oxide)-poly (propylene oxide)-poly(ethylene oxide) (PEO-PPO-PEO) polymeric micelles. *Gene Therapy*, **8** (13), 999–1004.
19 Hamalainen, K.M. *et al.* (1997) Characterization of paracellular and

aqueous penetration routes in cornea, conjunctiva, and sclera. *Investigative Ophthalmology & Visual Science*, **38** (3), 627–634.

**20** Kim, S.H. *et al.* (2007) Transport barriers in transscleral drug delivery for retinal diseases. *Ophthalmic Research*, **39** (5), 244–254.

**21** Cunha-Vaz, J. (1979) The blood–ocular barriers. *Survey of Ophthalmology*, **23** (5), 279–296.

**22** Smith, R.S. and Rudt, L.A. (1975) Ocular vascular and epithelial barriers to microperoxidase. *Investigative Ophthalmology*, **14** (7), 556–560.

**23** Omidi, Y. and Gumbleton, M. (2005) Biological membranes and barriers, in *Biomaterials for delivery and targeting of proteins nucleic acids* (ed. R. Mahato), CRC Press, New York, pp. 232–274.

**24** Dey, S. *et al.* (2003) Molecular evidence and functional expression of P-glycoprotein (MDR1) in human and rabbit cornea and corneal epithelial cell lines. *Investigative Ophthalmology & Visual Science*, **44** (7), 2909–2918.

**25** Karla, P.K. *et al.* (2007) Molecular evidence and functional expression of a novel drug efflux pump (ABCC2) in human corneal epithelium and rabbit cornea and its role in ocular drug efflux. *International Journal of Pharmaceutics*, **336** (1), 12–21.

**26** Karla, P.K. *et al.* (2009) Molecular expression and functional evidence of a drug efflux pump (BCRP) in human corneal epithelial cells. *Current Eye Research*, **34** (1), 1–9.

**27** Duvvuri, S., Gandhi, M.D., and Mitra, A.K. (2003) Effect of P-glycoprotein on the ocular disposition of a model substrate, quinidine. *Current Eye Research*, **27** (6), 345–353.

**28** Holash, J.A. and Stewart, P.A. (1993) The relationship of astrocyte-like cells to the vessels that contribute to the blood–ocular barriers. *Brain Research*, **629** (2), 218–224.

**29** Wu, J. *et al.* (1996) P-glycoprotein regulates a volume-activated chloride current in bovine non-pigmented ciliary epithelial cells. *The Journal of Physiology*, **491**Pt (3), 743–755.

**30** Saha, P., Yang, J.J., and Lee, V.H. (1998) Existence of a p-glycoprotein drug efflux pump in cultured rabbit conjunctival epithelial cells. *Investigative Ophthalmology & Visual Science*, **39** (7), 1221–1226.

**31** Richards, D.M. *et al.* (1983) Acyclovir. A review of its pharmacodynamic properties and therapeutic efficacy. *Drugs*, **26** (5), 378–438.

**32** Sanitato, J.J. *et al.* (1984) Acyclovir in the treatment of herpetic stromal disease. *American Journal of Ophthalmology*, **98** (5), 537–547.

**33** Perry, C.M. and Faulds, D. (1996) Valaciclovir. A review of its antiviral activity, pharmacokinetic properties and therapeutic efficacy in herpesvirus infections. *Drugs*, **52** (5), 754–772.

**34** Anand, B.S., Patel, J., and Mitra, A.K. (2003) Interactions of the dipeptide ester prodrugs of acyclovir with the intestinal oligopeptide transporter: competitive inhibition of glycylsarcosine transport in human intestinal cell line-Caco-2. *The Journal of Pharmacology and Experimental Therapeutics*, **304** (2), 781–791.

**35** Han, H. *et al.* (1998) 5′-Amino acid esters of antiviral nucleosides, acyclovir, and AZT are absorbed by the intestinal PEPT1 peptide transporter. *Pharmaceutical Research*, **15** (8), 1154–1159.

**36** Katragadda, S. *et al.* (2008) Ocular pharmacokinetics of acyclovir amino acid ester prodrugs in the anterior chamber: evaluation of their utility in treating ocular HSV infections. *International Journal of Pharmaceutics*, **359** (1–2), 15–24.

**37** Anand, B., Nashed, Y., and Mitra, A. (2003) Novel dipeptide prodrugs of acyclovir for ocular herpes infections: Bioreversion, antiviral activity and transport across rabbit cornea. *Current Eye Research*, **26** (3–4), 151–163.

**38** Talluri, R.S. *et al.* (2008) Synthesis, metabolism and cellular permeability of enzymatically stable dipeptide prodrugs of acyclovir. *International Journal of Pharmaceutics*, **361** (1–2), 118–124.

**39** Dunn, D.L. *et al.* (1994) A prospective randomized study of acyclovir versus ganciclovir plus human immune globulin prophylaxis of cytomegalovirus infection after solid organ transplantation. *Transplantation*, **57** (6), 876–884.

40 Patel, K. *et al.* (2005) Synthesis, physicochemical properties and antiviral activities of ester prodrugs of ganciclovir. *International Journal of Pharmaceutics*, **305** (1–2), 75–89.

41 Majumdar, S. *et al.* (2005) Dipeptide monoester ganciclovir prodrugs for treating HSV-1-induced corneal epithelial and stromal keratitis: *in vitro* and *in vivo* evaluations. *Journal of Ocular Pharmacology and Therapeutics*, **21** (6), 463–474.

42 Katragadda, S., Talluri, R.S., and Mitra, A.K. (2006) Modulation of P-glycoprotein-mediated efflux by prodrug derivatization: an approach involving peptide transporter-mediated influx across rabbit cornea. *Journal of Ocular Pharmacology and Therapeutics*, **22** (2), 110–120.

43 Jain, R. *et al.* (2004) Circumventing P-glycoprotein-mediated cellular efflux of quinidine by prodrug derivatization. *Molecular Pharmacology*, **1** (4), 290–299.

44 Hussain, A. and Truelove, J.E. (1976) Prodrug approaches to enhancement of physicochemical properties of drugs. IV. novel epinephrine prodrug. *Journal of Pharmaceutical Sciences*, **65** (10), 1510–1512.

45 Chang, S.C. *et al.* (1987) Improved corneal penetration of timolol by prodrugs as a means to reduce systemic drug load. *Investigative Ophthalmology & Visual Science*, **28** (3), 487–491.

46 Schoenwald, R.D. and Ward, R.L. (1978) Relationship between steroid permeability across excised rabbit cornea and octanol–water partition coefficients. *Journal of Pharmaceutical Sciences*, **67** (6), 786–788.

47 Wei, C.P., Anderson, J.A., and Leopold, I. (1978) Ocular absorption and metabolism of topically applied epinephrine and a dipivalyl ester of epinephrine. *Investigative Ophthalmology & Visual Science*, **17** (4), 315–321.

48 Chien, D.S. and Schoenwald, R.D. (1986) Improving the ocular absorption of phenylephrine. *Biopharmaceutics & Drug Disposition*, **7** (5), 453–462.

49 Schoenwald, R.D. and Chien, D.S. (1988) Ocular absorption and disposition of phenylephrine and phenylephrine oxazolidine. *Biopharmaceutics & Drug Disposition*, **9** (6), 527–538.

50 Bundgaard, H. *et al.* (1986) Pilocarpine prodrugs. II. Synthesis, stability, bioconversion, and physicochemical properties of sequentially labile pilocarpine acid diesters. *Journal of Pharmaceutical Sciences*, **75** (8), 775–783.

51 Mosher, G.L. *et al.* (1987) Ocular bioavailability of pilocarpic acid mono- and diester prodrugs as assessed by miotic activity in the rabbit. *International Journal of Pharmaceutics*, **39** (1–2), 113–120.

52 Järvinen, T. *et al.* (1991) O,O′-(1,4-Xylylene) bispilocarpic acid esters as new potential double prodrugs of pilocarpine for improved ocular delivery. I. Synthesis and analysis. *International Journal of Pharmaceutics*, **75** (2–3), 249–258.

53 Järvinen, T. *et al.* (1991) O,O′-(1,4-Xylylene) bispilocarpic acid esters as new potential double prodrugs of pilocarpine for improved ocular delivery. II. Physicochemical properties, stability, solubility and enzymatic hydrolysis. *International Journal of Pharmaceutics*, **75** (2–3), 259–269.

54 Suhonen, P. *et al.* (1991) Improved corneal pilocarpine permeability with O,O′-(1,4-xylylene) bispilocarpic acid ester double prodrugs. *Pharmaceutical Research*, **8** (12), 1539–1542.

55 Pech, B. *et al.* (1993) Preliminary evaluation of a series of amphiphilic timolol prodrugs: possible evidence for transscleral absorption. *Journal of Ocular Pharmacology*, **9** (2), 141–150.

56 Pech, B. *et al.* (1996) A timolol prodrug for improved ocular delivery: synthesis, conformational study and hydrolysis of palmitoyl timolol malonate. *International Journal of Pharmaceutics*, **128** (1–2), 179–188.

57 Bito, L.Z. *et al.* (1983) Long-term maintenance of reduced intraocular pressure by daily or twice daily topical application of prostaglandins to cat or rhesus monkey eyes. *Investigative Ophthalmology & Visual Science*, **24** (3), 312–319.

58 Alm, A., Grierson, I., and Shields, M.B. (2008) Side effects associated with prostaglandin analog therapy. *Survey of Ophthalmology*, **53** (6 Supp. 1), S93–S105.

59 Camras, C.B. *et al.* (1989) Maintained reduction of intraocular pressure by prostaglandin $F_{2\alpha}$-1-isopropyl ester applied in multiple doses in ocular hypertensive and glaucoma patients. *Ophthalmology*, **96** (9), 1329–1336; discussion 1336–1337.

60 Villumsen, J. and Alm, A. (1990) Ocular effects of two different prostaglandin $F_{2\alpha}$ esters. A doublemasked cross-over study on normotensive eyes. *Acta Ophthalmologica*, **68** (3), 341–343.

61 Cheng-Bennett, A. *et al.* (1994) Studies on a novel series of acyl ester prodrugs of prostaglandin $F_{2\alpha}$. *The British Journal of Ophthalmology*, **78** (7), 560–567.

62 Woodward, D.F. *et al.* (1996) *In-vivo* activity and enzymatic hydrolysis of novel prostaglandin $F_{2\alpha}$ prodrugs in ocular tissues. *Experimental Eye Research*, **63** (4), 411–423.

63 Woodward, D.F. *et al.* (2004) Bimatoprost: a novel antiglaucoma agent. *Cardiovascular Drug Reviews*, **22** (2), 103–120.

64 Hughes, P.M., Olejnik, O., and Chang-lin, J.-E. (2007) Compositions and methods for the intraocular transport of therapeutic agents. Allergan, Inc., Irvine, CA.

65 Garst, M.E. and Adorante, J.S. (2002) Methods and compositions for drug delivery. Allergan Sales, Inc., Irvine, CA.

66 Marcus, D.M. and Chu, C.K. (2007) Methods and compositions for treatment of macular and retinal disease. University of Georgia Research Foundation, Inc., Athens, GA; Medical College of Georgia Research Institute, Inc., Augusta, GA.

67 Rabinovich-guilatt, L.P. and Lambert, G. (2007) Use of a steroid prodrug for the treatment of disease of the posterior segment of the eye. U.S. Patent Application 20070281914.

68 Hughes, P.M. and Olejnik, O. (2005) Delivery of an active drug to the posterior part of the eye via subconjunctival or periocular delivery of a prodrug. Allergan, Inc., Irvine, CA.

69 Lindstrom, R. and Kim, T. (2006) Ocular permeation and inhibition of retinal inflammation: an examination of data and expert opinion on the clinical utility of nepafenac. *Current Medical Research and Opinion*, **22** (2), 397–404.

70 Gaudana, R. *et al.* (2009) Recent perspectives in ocular drug delivery. *Pharmaceutical Research*, **26** (5), 1197–1216.

71 Werle, M. (2008) Natural and synthetic polymers as inhibitors of drug efflux pumps. *Pharmaceutical Research*, **25** (3), 500–511.

72 Arnold, J.J. *et al.* (2009) Eyedrops containing SA9000 prodrugs result in sustained reductions in intraocular pressure in rabbits. *Journal of Ocular Pharmacology and Therapeutics*, **25** (3), 179–186.

73 Babizhayev, M.A. (2008) Ocular drug metabolism of the bioactivating antioxidant *N*-acetylcarnosine for vision in ophthalmic prodrug and codrug design and delivery. *Drug Development and Industrial Pharmacy*, **34** (10), 1071–1089.

74 Doukas, J. *et al.* (2008) Topical administration of a multi-targeted kinase inhibitor suppresses choroidal neovascularization and retinal edema. *Journal of Cellular Physiology*, **216** (1), 29–37.

75 Lallemand, F. *et al.* (2005) A water-soluble prodrug of cyclosporine A for ocular application: a stability study. *European Journal of Pharmaceutical Sciences*, **26** (1), 124–129.

76 Fukano, Y. and Kawazu, K. (2009) Disposition and metabolism of a novel prostanoid antiglaucoma medication, tafluprost, following ocular administration to rats. *Drug Metabolism and Disposition: The Biological Fate of Chemicals*, **37** (8), 1622–1634.

77 Chong, D.Y. *et al.* (2009) Vitreous penetration of orally administered famciclovir. *American Journal of Ophthalmology*, **148** (1), 38–42 e1.

# 9
# Reducing Presystemic Drug Metabolism

*Majid Y. Moridani*

## 9.1
## Introduction

Oral administration is a convenient route of drug delivery for systemic drug therapy as well as local treatment of gastrointestinal tract-related diseases such as gastrointestinal inflammation, cancer, and infection. However, this route of drug delivery is a major contributing source of interindividual variations in drug response due to variations in drug bioavailability. Drugs that have high absorption rates generally demonstrate lower rates of interindividual variations in drug bioavailability whereas drugs with lower oral absorption demonstrate greater interindividual variability in bioavailability. Factors that result in a lower drug bioavailability include (1) incomplete drug absorption due to poor drug solubility in water or low membrane and lipid permeability; (2) the chemical instability in gastrointestinal tract; and (3) pre-systemic drug metabolism in gastrointestinal tract and liver. Hence, enhancing the oral bioavailability of drugs can in principle minimize the variations in drug response. Such strategy in enhancing of the oral bioavailability of drugs can also minimize unnecessary exposure of the body to potential inactive, active, and toxic metabolites that may be formed as a result of presystemic drug metabolism in gastrointestinal tract and/or liver. In addition, enhancing the drug's bioavailability minimizes the need for a larger dose, which in turn reduces costs associated with production of highly expensive drugs.

It is possible to employ strategies such as prodrug design and drug formulation optimizations to overcome problems associated with incomplete drug absorption due to chemical instability, poor water solubility, and/or poor lipid/membrane permeability. The prodrug approaches that deal with physicochemical properties, which enhance drug lipid solubility, are discussed in Chapter 3. In this chapter, we will discuss only those prodrug approaches that overcome problems related to presystemic drug metabolism by gastrointestinal tract and liver. In addition, we will briefly discuss prodrug approaches that are useful in targeting colon and lymphatic system as routes of drug delivery void of presystemic drug metabolism.

Figure 9.1 illustrates a summary scheme using prodrug approaches to overcome presystemic metabolic barriers mediated by esterases, proteases, peptidases, and

*Prodrugs and Targeted Delivery: Towards Better ADME Properties.* Edited by Jarkko Rautio

ISBN: 978-3-527-32603-7

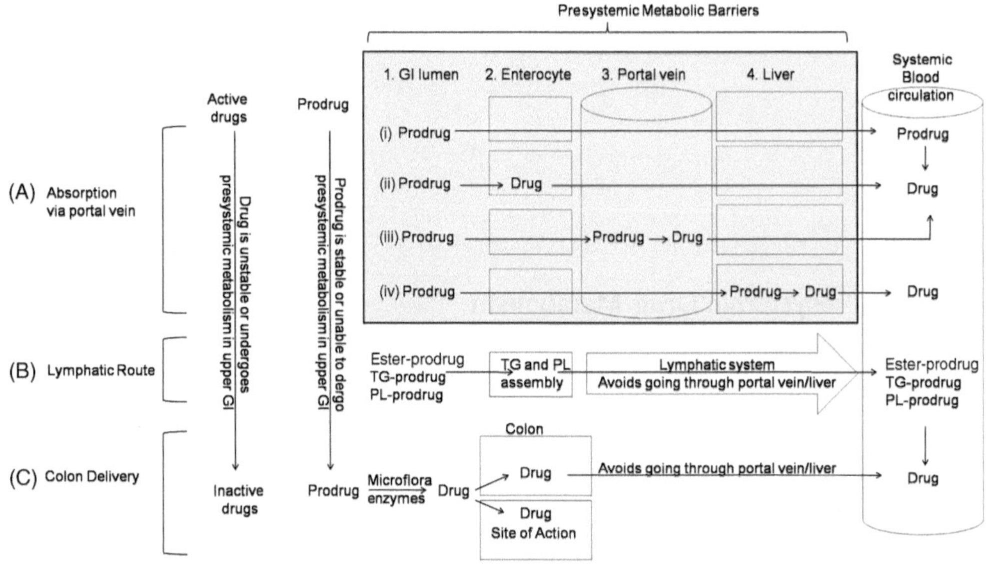


**Figure 9.1** Prodrug approaches to minimize presystemic metabolism in intestine, hepatic portal vein and liver. TG-prodrug (triglyceride ester drug), PL-prodrug (phospholipid ester drug), TG (triglyceride), and PL (phospholipid). In the hepatic portal system, venous blood carries nutrients and drugs from small intestine, portions of large intestine, stomach, and pancreas. In this case, the blood from hepatic portal vein drains to liver, a major site for drug metabolism, before reaching inferior vena cava (systemic blood circulation). However, other veins that collect blood from pelvic area, abdominal cavity, and portions of large intestine flow directly to inferior vena cave without passing through hepatic portal vein system.

cytochrome P450 enzymes that are found in gastrointestinal lumen, enterocytes, portal vein and hepatocytes. These metabolic barriers can substantially reduce the bioavailability of drugs via oral route. However, prodrugs are designed to have significantly diminished presystemic metabolisms so that a larger portion of the drugs can reach systemic blood circulation where it can undergo spontaneous hydrolysis/decomposition or enzyme-mediated hydrolysis in liver and/or plasma to release active drugs.

A drug may be unstable in a portion of gastrointestinal tract such as in stomach where the acid content is high. Formulation and prodrug approaches can increase the chemical stability of the drug enabling it to pass through stomach and reach gastrointestinal tract. Then the prodrug can be metabolized by esterases and lipases present in gastrointestinal lumen and enterocyte brush border releasing the active drug. Subsequently, the released drug can be absorbed and transported by portal vein to liver. Alternatively, the designed prodrug may be stable throughout the gastrointestinal lumen where it can be absorbed into hepatic portal vein to reach liver in its intact form where subsequently it can undergo hydrolyses by liver esterases to active drug component.

Figure 9.1 also depicts lymphatic route and colon-targeted drug delivery void of presystemic metabolism. For example, ester prodrugs with high lipid solubility can be designed to be absorbed via lymphatic route only (Figure 9.1B). In this route, prodrug will be incorporated in chylomicrons and VLDL particles biosynthesized in enterocytes, transported into lymphatic system, subsequently draining into systemic blood circulation bypassing hepatic portal vein and liver; hence, enhancing the oral bioavailability of the drugs by minimizing their presystemic metabolism by liver and gastrointestinal enzymes. As shown in Figure 9.1C, prodrugs can also be designed for targeted drug delivery to colon as the site of drug action or drug absorption in the treatment of colon-specific diseases such as Crohn's disease.

In the following, we briefly discuss a number of prodrug approaches that are employed to enhance the oral bioavailability of drugs. Such approaches generally can either reduce presystemic drug metabolism or enhance drug absorption into hepatic portal vein and lymphatic systems, or target colon as the site of drug delivery/absorption/action (Figure 9.1).

## 9.2 Presystemic Metabolic Barriers

A number of enzymatic barriers exist in gastrointestinal tract lumen, enterocytes, plasma, and liver that significantly contribute in the presystemic drug metabolism. Examples of the enzymes, which are the major contributors in reducing the oral bioavailability, include esterases, lipases, cytochrome P450 enzymes, Phase II drug metabolizing enzymes, proteases and peptidases, which will be discussed briefly in this chapter.

### 9.2.1 Esterases

Often, esterification is one of the most widely used chemical modifications in prodrug design. In principle, the goal of esterification is to enhance the membrane permeability of a drug by increasing its lipid solubility properties. However, ester-based prodrugs are extensively hydrolyzed by intestinal and hepatic esterases (Figure 9.2). In addition, the hydrolyzed product may subsequently undergo Phase

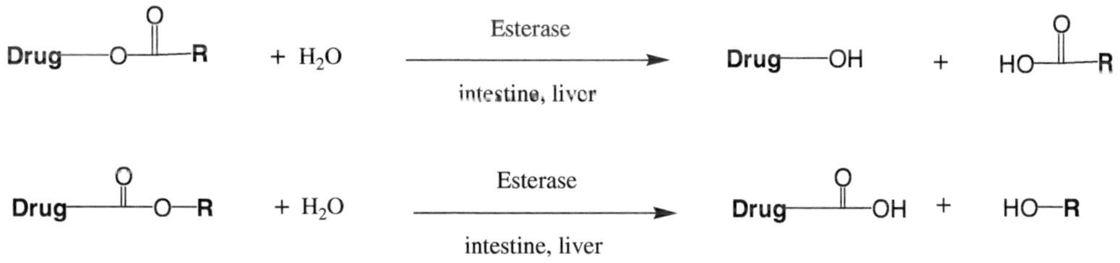


**Figure 9.2** Presystemic metabolism of ester-based drug and prodrugs by intestinal and liver esterases. The carboxylic, alcoholic, or phenolic functional groups are masked by an alkyl or acyl group, which can undergo hydrolysis by intestinal and hepatic esterases.

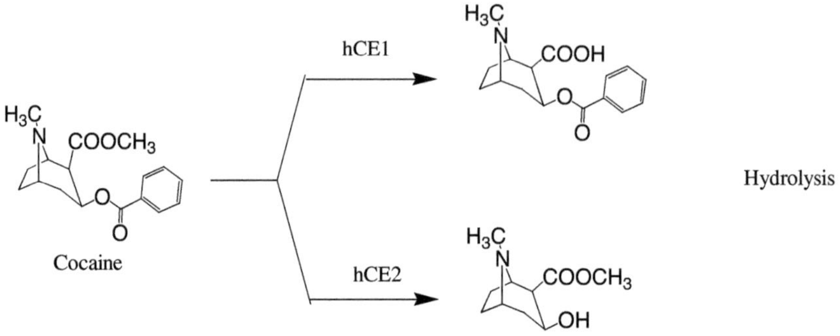


**Figure 9.3** Cocaine hydrolysis by human carboxylesterase 1 (hCE1) and carboxylesterase 2 (hCE2).

I and Phase II drug metabolism. Therefore, to enhance the oral bioavailability, the ester prodrugs should be resistant to hydrolysis by esterases found in gastrointestinal tract.

Esterases belong to the class of hydrolases and are generally responsible for the hydrolysis of ester- and amide-based drugs and prodrugs. Examples of gastrointestinal tract esterases that can hydrolyze ester-based prodrugs include carboxylesterase, acetylesterase, arylesterase, lipase, and phospholipase. Human carboxylesterase 1 (hCE1) and carboxylesterase 2 (hCE2) are involved in drug metabolism/inactivation or drug activation as well as food digestion [1]. For example, Figure 9.3 depicts hydrolysis of cocaine by esterases hCE1 and hCE2, which significantly reduces the oral bioavailability of cocaine. Although both carboxylesterases are expressed in many organs but their hydrolase activities are high in liver and intestine, which mainly attributed to hCE1 and hCE2, respectively [2]. Mammalian intestine possesses several hCE2 isozymes. Ester prodrugs can be taken into enterocyte and then hydrolyzed by enterocyte esterases. After hydrolysis the drugs either reach hepatic portal vein or efflux back to intestinal lumen. One such example includes *O*-isovaleryl-propranolol prodrug that is first absorbed via passive diffusion to enterocyte where it is hydrolyzed by enterocyte carboxylesterases to propranolol and isovaleryl moiety [3]. However, propranolol is effluxed back to intestinal lumen whereas isovaleryl moiety is found more in vascular side (Figure 9.4). Therefore, *O*-isovaleryl-propranolol prodrug is not a successful strategy in increasing the oral bioavailability of propranolol. Considering the metabolic pathway of propranolol (Figure 9.5), for a prodrug approach to be successful, the propranolol ester prodrug needs to be relatively more stable than *O*-isovaleryl-propranolol in gastrointestinal lumen and enterocytes so that it can reach liver and/or perhaps bypass the liver avoiding drug metabolism by liver enzymes.

Other esterase enzymes that are involved in hydrolyses of prodrugs include pancreatic phospholipase A2 [4, 5] and pancreatic, hepatic, and lipoprotein lipases [1]. Pancreatic phospholipase A2 and pancreatic lipase, its protein cofactor, colipase, and bile acids are required for efficient digestion of dietary triglycerides and phospholipids. Both phospholipase A2 and pancreatic lipase enzymes have important roles in the hydrolysis of triglycerides and phospholipids ester-based prodrugs for delivery through lymphatic system.

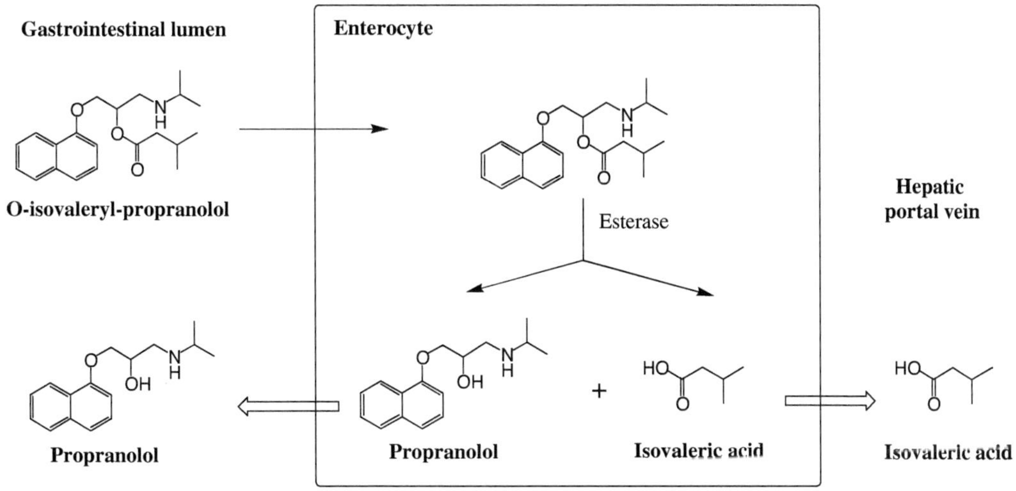


**Figure 9.4** Presystemic metabolism of O-isovaleryl-propranolol prodrug by enterocyte esterases.

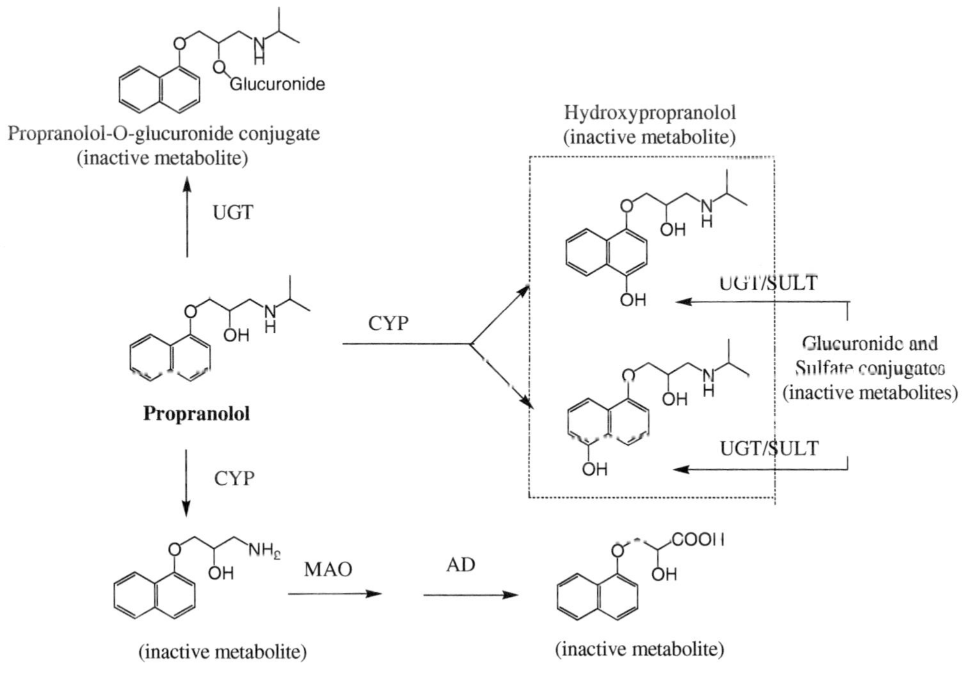


**Figure 9.5** Presystemic metabolism of propranolol by liver enzymes [6–9]. UGTs, SULTs, MAO, AD, and cytochrome P450 (CYP).

In addition to esterases, other hydrolases such as glycosidases, phosphatases, thioesterases, phosphodiesterases, sulfatase, deoxyribonuclease, and ribonuclease may also find important roles in prodrug designs.

### 9.2.2 Cytochrome P450 Enzymes

Cytochrome P450, also known as CYP, is a large group of enzymes found in various organs including gastrointestinal tract, liver, lung, and kidneys; however, liver and intestine CYPs are widely studied. CYPs are membrane-associated proteins and located on mitochondria or cellular endoplasmic reticulum. They are heme containing enzymes that can metabolize a large number of endogenous and exogenous compounds including drug molecules. CYP-mediated metabolism often produces both active (Figure 9.6) and inactive (Figures 9.7–9.9) metabolites, accounting for 75% of the total drug metabolism [10]. The most common reaction mediated by CYPs includes monooxygenase reactions where oxygen atoms are involved in the oxidation of exogenous and endogenous molecules. Examples of such reactions include hydroxylation, oxidation, expoxidation, and dealkylation.

Humans have 57 genes and more than 59 pseudogenes grouped in 18 and 43 families and subfamilies, respectively. Cytochrome enzymes are designated with the abbreviation CYP, followed by a number, a letter, and a number. For example, CYP2D6 enzyme belongs to "CYP2" family of cytochrome P450, subfamily "D", and the individual isoform "6". In addition, polymorphisms can influence the extent and degree by which a specific isoform can metabolize endogenous and exogenous compounds. In general, polymorphisms affect all Phase I and Phase II drug metabolizing enzymes, transporters, and esterases in the body. The effect of polymorphisms on drug bioavailability, metabolism, efficacy, and toxicity are discussed in chapter 16 in this book. For nomenclature of CYPs and their alleles see Ref. [11, 12]. Examples of the CYPs that are expressed in intestine and liver include CYP1A1, CYP1A2, CYP2C9, CYP2C19, CYP2D6, CYP2E1, and CYP3A4/5. CYPP450s are also extensively investigated in mice, rats, rabbits, dogs, and monkeys to facilitate their use as models in drug discovery, metabolism, and toxicology.

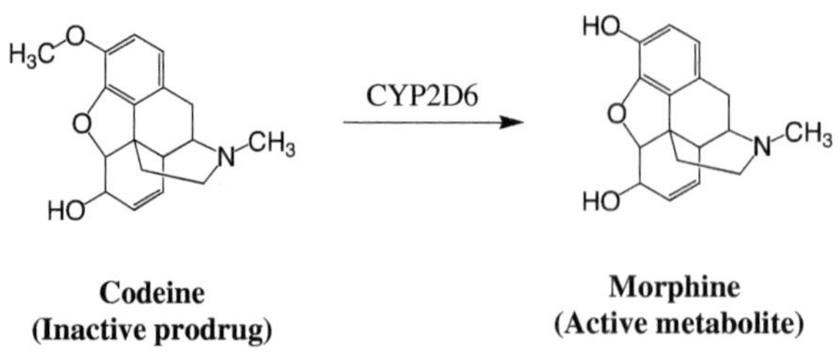


**Figure 9.6** Bioactivation of codeine to morphine by CYP2D6.

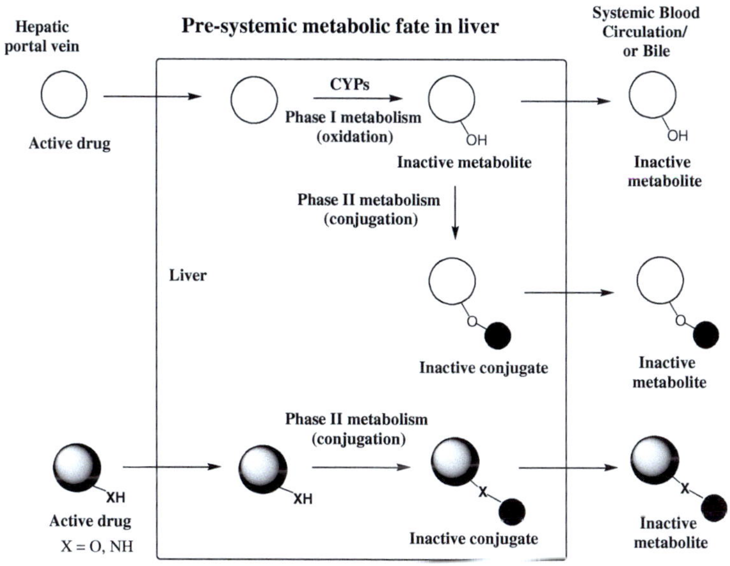


**Figure 9.7** Presystemic drug metabolism mediated by liver. Phase I CYP drug metabolizing enzymes and Phase II drug metabolizing enzymes such as UGTs, COMT, NAT, GST, and SULTs can inactivate drugs by chemical modifications.

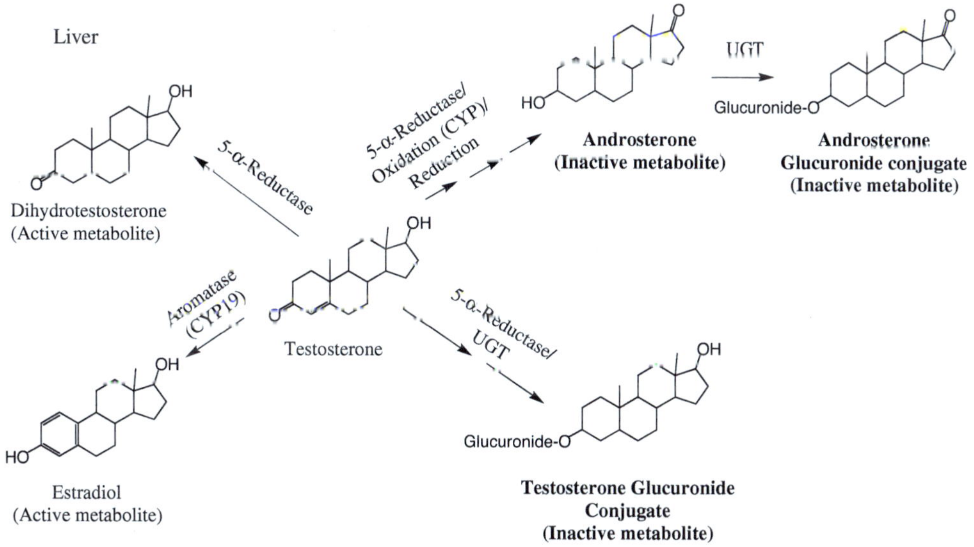


**Figure 9.8** Testosterone inactivation by liver enzymes limits its bioavailability when administered orally [13–16].

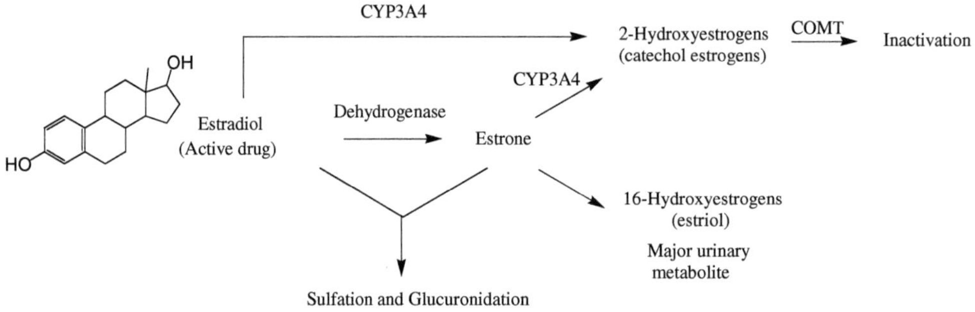


**Figure 9.9** Extensive metabolic first-pass effects by liver limiting the oral bioavailability of estradiol [16, 17].

### 9.2.3
### Phase II Drug Metabolizing Enzymes

Many exogenous and endogenous compounds are lipid soluble, which are readily absorbed via gastrointestinal tract. Phase I and Phase II drug metabolizing enzymes are evolved to alter the lipid-soluble drugs to more water-soluble agents to facilitate the termination of their pharmacological effects. These objectives are achieved by (1) changing the three-dimensional shape of the molecule so that drug cannot fit to its receptor; (2) making the molecule more water soluble so that it can be excreted via urine, and (3) making the molecule larger by conjugating it with glucuronide or glutathione so that the metabolites can be readily excreted in bile and/or urine.

CYP metabolizing enzymes make sure to create water-soluble moieties in the molecule by introducing a hydroxyl group or unmaking a moiety such as alcoholic, phenolic, amine, and carboxylic group by dealkylation reactions. These functional groups can then undergo a Phase II conjugation reactions by enzymes such as UDP-glucuronosyltransferases (UGTs), catechol-*O*-methyltransferases (COMTs), *N*-acetyltransferases (NATs), glutathione *S*-transferases (GSTs), and sulfotransferases (SULTs) (Figure 9.7). When a drug already possesses a suitable functional group such as a phenol or an alcohol group, it may directly undergo conjugation reactions. Because many of these Phase II conjugation enzymes are present in liver and intestine, they can act as presystemic metabolic barriers leading to a reduced oral bioavailability. In the following, we briefly discuss UGT, SULT, GST, NAT, and COMT as examples of Phase II drug metabolizing enzymes.

Glucuronidation is a Phase II drug metabolic pathway with a large metabolic capacity in humans. UDP-glucuronosyltransferase (UGT) has many isoforms that are widely expressed in intestine (UGT1A7, UGT1A8, and UGT1A10) and liver (UGT1A1, UGT1A3, UGT1A4, UGT1A6, UGT1A9, UGT2B4, UGT2B7, UGT2B15, and UGT2B17) with ability to metabolize a wide variety of substrates. These enzymes are located at inner portion of endoplasmic reticulum in proximity to CYP enzymes, which are also located in endoplasmic reticulum to ensure maximum efficiency in conjugation of newly formed metabolites by CYP enzymes. Moreover, it is possible that highly lipid-soluble drugs can readily partition to endoplasmic reticulum, then undergo glucuronide conjugation without undergoing Phase I drug metabolism. In brief, UGT enzymes are generally able to form *O*-ether, *O*-ester, and *N*-glucuronide drug conjugates leading to reduced drug bioavailability via oral route.

SULTs are another group of enzymes that are found in most organs. Their major sites of activities include liver, small intestine, and large intestine. SULTs are cytosolic enzymes. The main goal of sulfation is to make the drug more water soluble; hence, pharmacologically less active. The metabolites are readily eliminated via urine and bile. There are nearly 50 SULT isoforms among which SULT1 (A, B, C, and E) and SULT2 (A and B) isoforms are more important in humans. SULTs are involved in conjugation of phenols, aryl amines, steroids, sex hormones, and their hydroxysteroids.

GSTs are enzymes that facilitate a reaction between glutathione (GSH) and electrophilic drugs and reactive metabolites (e.g., quinones and epoxides), which are generated during drug metabolism by CYP enzymes. The majorities of GSTs are found in the cytosolic portion of the cells but some are also found in endoplasmic reticulum that are involved in GSH conjugation of more lipophilic compounds such as leukotrienes and prostaglandins. The major GST classes include alpha (e.g., GSTA2, 3, and 4), mu (e.g., GSTM1-1), pi (GSTP), theta (GST-T), and omega (GSTO), which are widely expressed in various organs including liver and intestine. The GSH-conjugated metabolites are water soluble, larger, and heavier than the parent drug; hence, they can be eliminated via urine and bile.

In contrast to Phase II drug metabolizing enzymes that are discussed above, conjugation mediated by COMT and NAT make the molecules actually less water soluble. Moreover, the COMT and NAT conjugation processes do not change the molecular weight of the metabolite significantly, a requirement to make the metabolite more suitable for elimination via bile. Despite these, their functions mostly make the molecules pharmacologically less active. The acetyl transferases that are mostly relevant to human drug metabolism include NAT-1 and NAT-2, which are expressed in intestine and liver, respectively. COMT is responsible for the methylation of a number of endogenous compounds such as norepinephrine, epinephrine, and dopamine (Figure 9.10). Additional examples of metabolic reactions mediated by a number of conjugating enzymes are shown in Figure 9.11.

### 9.2.4
### Peptidases

Human body has numerous enzymes capable of breaking amide bonds present in various drugs, proteins, and peptides. In general, amides are chemically more stable toward hydrolysis than ester analogues. Similarly, they are also more resistant to enzymatic hydrolyses by peptidases and esterases present in gastrointestinal tract. Gastrointestinal tract contains a number of proteolytic enzymes that are secreted into gastrointestinal lumen, which catalyze the hydrolysis and break down of food proteins to respective amino acids. These peptidases are categorized as

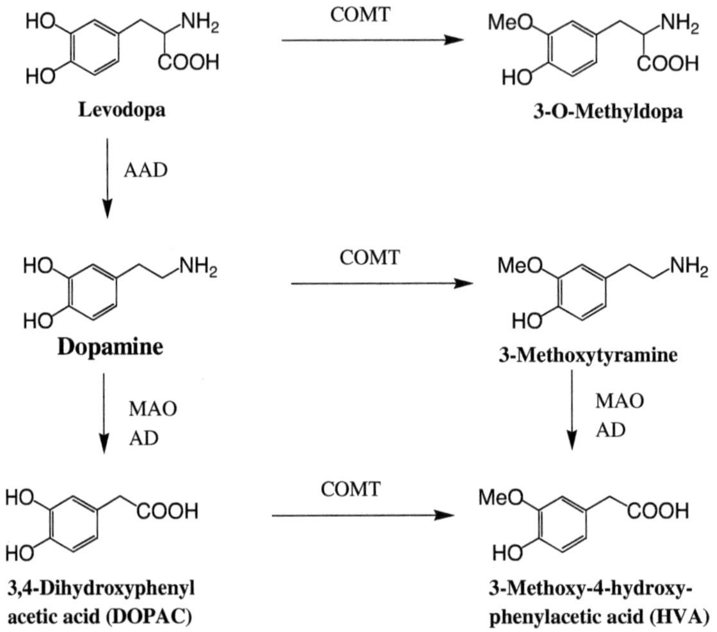


**Figure 9.10** Presystemic metabolism of levodopa and dopamine by liver enzymes. Cytosolic COMT and membrane-bound MAO-A and MAO-B are expressed widely in the body; however, the highest concentrations of each are found in liver and kidneys [18–21]. Aromatic L-amino acid decarboxylase (AAD) [22–28] and AD [24–28] are expressed in liver. Norepinephrine and epinephrine can also undergo similar metabolic pathways as mentioned above [16].

endopeptidases and exopeptidases. Examples of endopeptidases include trypsin, chymotrypsin, and elastases. Examples of exopeptidases include carboxypeptidase A and carboxypeptidase B. In general, peptidases along with esterases are able to metabolize amide-based drugs, which limit the use of oral administration of polypeptides and protein-based drugs and prodrugs, in which case other routes of drug delivery such as injection and transmucosal drug delivery become more appropriate.

### 9.2.5 Other Oxidative Metabolizing Enzymes

In addition to CYP enzymes, many other oxidative enzymes are involved in metabolism and elimination of lipophilic and hydrophilic xenobiotics, contributing significantly into presystemic drug metabolism. The examples of these oxidative enzymes that are expressed in liver include peroxidases, flavin monooxygenase (FMOs), alcohol dehydrogenases (ALDs), aldehyde dehydrogenases (ADs), monoamine oxidases (MAO-A and MAO-B), xanthine oxidase (XOR), and aldehyde oxidase (AO). For additional information on the drug metabolizing enzymes, see Refs [29, 30].

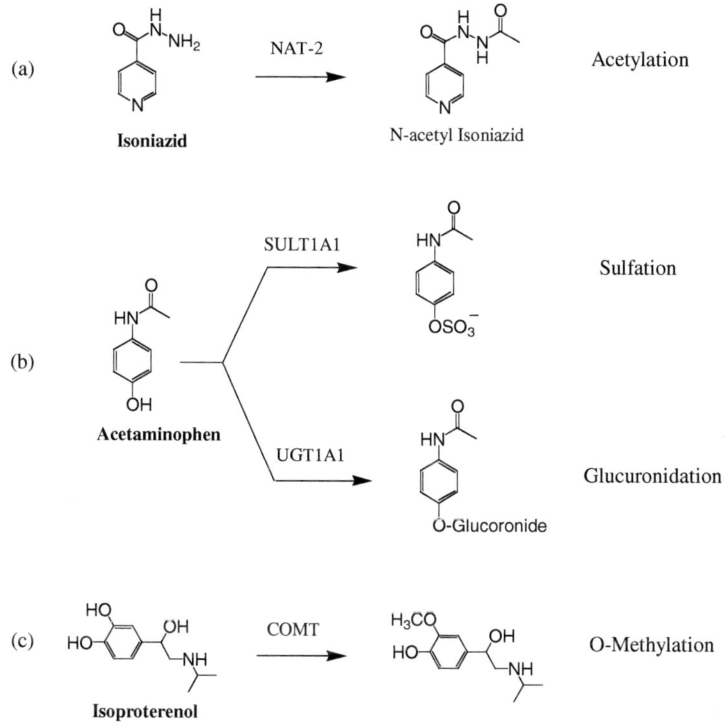


**Figure 9.11** Examples of drugs undergoing Phase II conjugations.

## 9.3 Prodrug Approaches to Reduce Presystemic Drug Metabolism

This section discusses the application of prodrug approaches aiming to improve oral bioavailability by diminishing presystemic drug metabolism at gastrointestinal tract and liver. Examples of the chemical approaches used to reduce presystemic drug metabolism include (i) direct chemical modification of the functional group undergoing extensive metabolism; for example, with an ester bond preventing it from undergoing extensive metabolism; (ii) chemical modifications of a site at nearby or distant to the functional group undergoing extensive metabolism, and (iii) chemical alteration of bioactive peptide-based drugs. Some of these prodrug chemical modifications may require enzymatic bioactivation to release the drug whereas others may release the drug as the result of the spontaneous decomposition of the prodrugs.

Masking groups can be introduced to the drug chemical structure to protect the functional groups undergoing extensive metabolism. In general, these prodrugs require enzymatic bioactivation to release the active parent drug. Examples of substitutes that are used as masking groups include sulfamate, linear and branched alkyl, acyloxyalkyl, cycloalkyl, and anthranilate ester and amide bonds to mask functional groups such as phenol, alcohol, carboxylic, amine groups that undergo extensive presystemic drug metabolism such as sulfation, glucuronidation, *O*-methylation, oxidation, decarboxylation, and amine oxidation (Figure 9.12). Prodrugs can also be designed that do not require enzymatic bioactivation to release the active

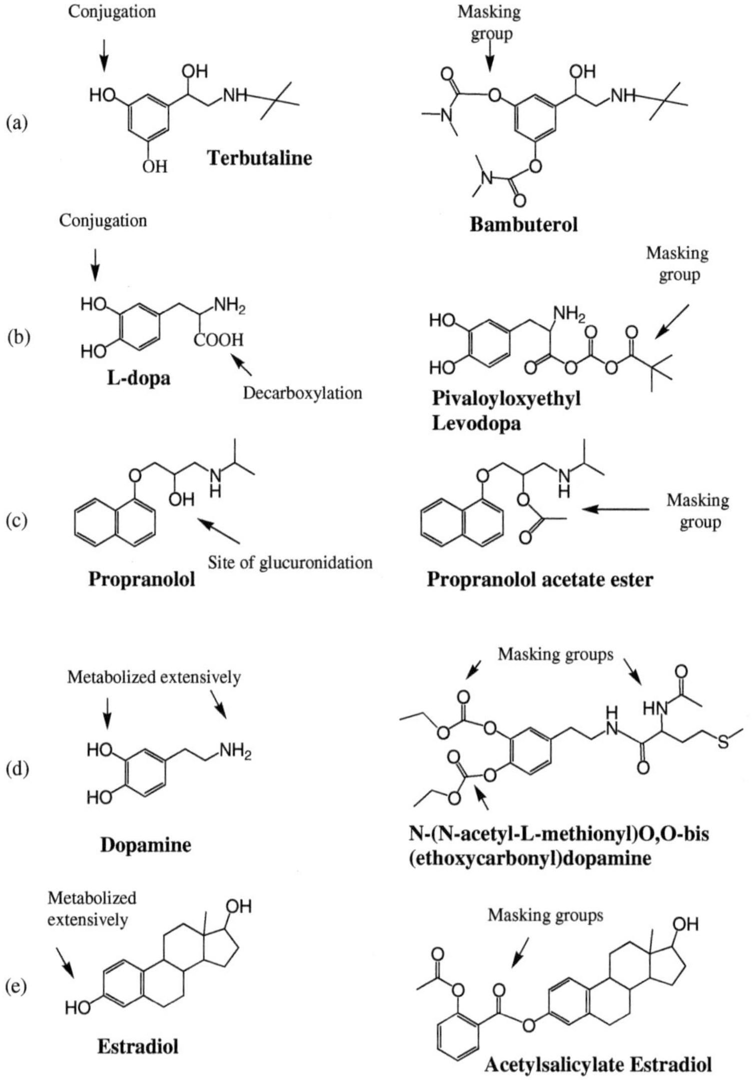


**Figure 9.12** Examples of masking groups that require enzymatic bioactivation. The chemical structures on the left show parent drugs that undergo extensive Phase I drug metabolism, Phase II drug metabolism, or decarboxylation. Masking group prevents extensive presystemic drug metabolism. For metabolic pathways of propranolol, estradiol, and dopamine, see Figures – 9.4, 9.5, 9.9, and 9.10, respectively. Bambuterol [32], pivaloyloxyethyl levodopa [32, 33], propranolol acetate ester [34], *N*-(*N*-acetyl-L-methionyl)*O*,*O*-bis(ethoxycarbonyl) dopamine [35], and acetylsalicylate estradiol [36].

drug. This is especially important in situations that interindividual variations in drug metabolism and release can impact oral bioavailability of the drug. Another advantage of designing a prodrug that does not require nonenzymatic hydrolysis is that it usually provides a predictable kinetic profile for releasing the active drug. Such chemical modifications can be achieved by carbamate derivatization of the amines such as dopamine derivatives [31]. The prodrug can then undergo spontaneous hydrolysis once absorbed (Figure 9.13).

In addition to the above examples, chemical modifications are used to enhance metabolic stability of bioactive peptides in gastrointestinal tract for oral drug delivery and transmucosal delivery (buccal, nasal, rectum, and lung). In principle, a major problem associated with using peptides as drugs is their susceptibility to various enzymatic barriers present in gastrointestinal tract. Peptides are good substrates for peptidases found in gastrointestinal lumen and enterocytes brush borders. In addition, peptides are hydrophilic compounds that show poor membrane permeability. Therefore, a possible approach to increase the stability of peptide is to use chemical approaches to enhance their physicochemical properties to have increased chemical and metabolic stabilities in gastrointestinal environment or to be administered from an alternative route of delivery. Such chemical modifications increase the lipid solubility of the drugs and hinder their degradations by enzymes present in gastrointestinal lumen and at mucosal barriers [37–48]. However, the modified derivatives should be capable of releasing the parent bioactive peptide either spontaneously or as the result of enzymatic hydrolysis after their absorption into systemic blood circulation [49]. Examples of chemical modifications, that are employed to enhance the chemical stability of peptides include (i) esterification of C-terminal amide groups with aliphatic and carbonate ester prodrugs; (ii) esterification of phenolic group of tyrosine amino acid; (iii) addition of α-hydroxyglycine to C-terminal; (iv) N-α-hydroxylakylation that can spontaneously release the parent

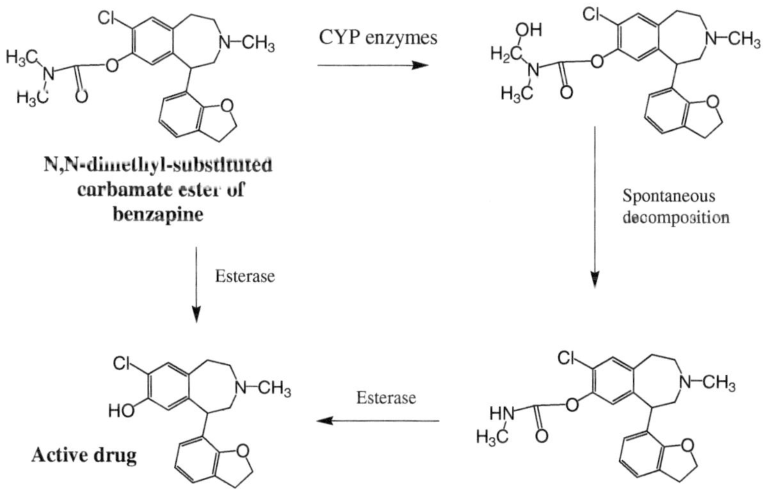


**Figure 9.13** Example of carbamate-based prodrug [31].

drug; (v) cyclization of the peptides by joining the N- and C-terminals of the peptides using coumarinic or phenylpropionic acids as linker groups; (vi) PEGylation of the peptides; (vii) acylation of the peptide N-terminal; and (viii) derivatization of peptides with fatty acid to enhance their lipid solubility properties and absorption from gastrointestinal tract. Examples of the bioactive peptides that are suitable candidates for chemical modifications include desmopressin, enkephalins, cholecystokinin tetrapeptide, and thyrotropin-releasing hormone (Figure 9.14).

## 9.4 Targeting Colon

Prodrug approaches for colon-targeted drug delivery have obtained increasing importance in the treatment of colon-specific diseases and for bioactive peptide delivery to systemic circulation [50–60]. In addition to chemical modification that relies upon microflora enzyme prodrug bioactivation and drug release, other methods that are widely used for colon-targeted drug delivery include pH, pressure sensitive, osmolal pump, time-dependent activated systems.

For successful colon-targeted prodrug delivery, the prodrug needs to be chemically stable in acidic environment of stomach, protected from various enzymes present in small intestine, and has minimal absorption into the blood circulation before

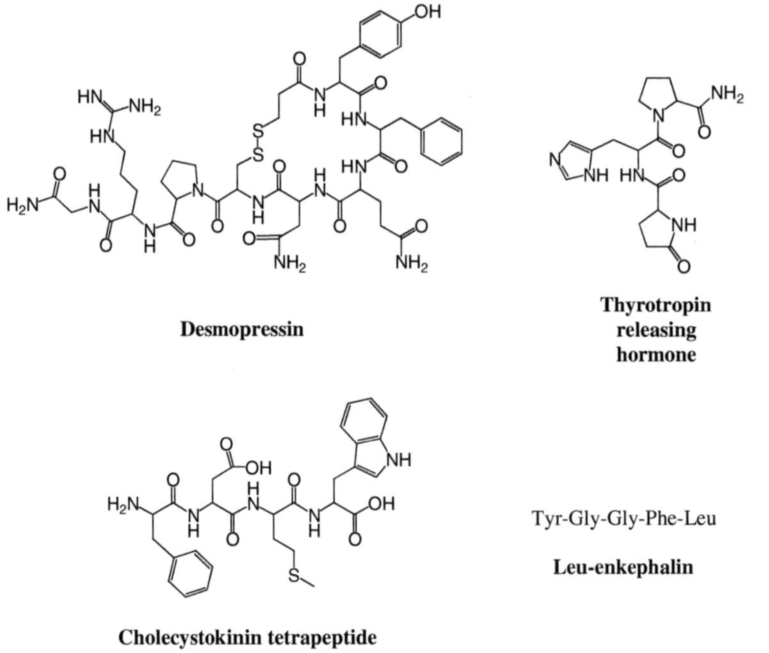


**Figure 9.14** The chemical structures of a number of bioactive peptides as suitable candidates for prodrug designs.

reaching colon. Such prodrug strategies can minimize drug-induced side effects associated with upper gastrointestinal tract. Moreover, the minimization of drug absorption from upper gastrointestinal tract also prevents presystemic drug metabolism by liver. Therefore, after its journey through small intestine and arrival at colon, untouched and unabsorbed prodrug can undergo bioactivation by microbial enzymes that are present in colon to release its active drug. Examples of prodrug chemical modifications that are widely investigated in colon drug delivery include azo-based compounds [53, 54, 60], amino acid as linkers [61–64], glucoside [65–69] and glucuronide conjugations [70–74], and cyclodextrin and polymers as linkers. The bacterial enzymes such as reductase, β-D-glucosidase, and β-D-glucoronidase, which are found relatively in large amount in colon than in small intestine, can then bioactivate azo, glucoside, and glucuronide prodrugs, respectively, to their active components. The locally released drug can then exert its pharmacological effects in colon as the site of drug action or can be absorbed from colon into systemic blood circulation without passing through liver; hence, void of presystemic drug metabolism by liver, which can in turn enhance the oral bioavailability. For a drug to be absorbed from colon, it should have optimum physicochemical properties to cross biological membranes. For a successful colon-target delivery where colon is the site of drug action, the drug should have lower lipid solubility so that they cannot extensively cross biological membrane or it should be administered in quantity sufficient for the treatment of colon-specific diseases such as inflammation, infection, and cancer without significant systemic absorption. As examples, Figure 9.15 illustrates sulfasalazine and olsalazine, azo-based prodrugs, that undergo metabolic bioactivation by colon's microbial reductase enzymes. The development of these two prodrugs was based on prontosil, an azo-based antibiotic prodrug, that undergoes bioactivation by colon's microbial reductase enzymes to release sulfanilamide (Figure 9.16). Prontosil was the first commercially available antibacterial antibiotic, which is no longer in use now. The discovery and development of this first sulfonamide drug opened a new era in medicine. All the azo-based prodrugs are modeled after prontosil.

Figure 9.17 shows prodrugs using glucose, glucuronic acid, amino acids, and cyclodextrin as the linker/carrier for colon-targeted prodrug delivery. Examples of cyclodextrin prodrugs include nonsteroidal anti-inflammatory agents, corticosteroids, and 5-fluoruracil [75–81]. Figure 9.18 depicts corticosteroid drugs, dexamethasone, and budesonide that are suitable candidates as glucoside and glucuronide prodrugs. Because they are released locally and absorbed minimally into systemic circulation, corticosteroid glucoside and glucuronide prodrugs have minimal adrenal gland suppression as side effects.

## 9.5 Targeting Lymphatic Route

Drugs that are administered orally are absorbed into portal vein or lymphatic system or via colon directly to systemic circulation. One should also note that the drug absorption through lymphatic system and colon site minimizes presystemic drug

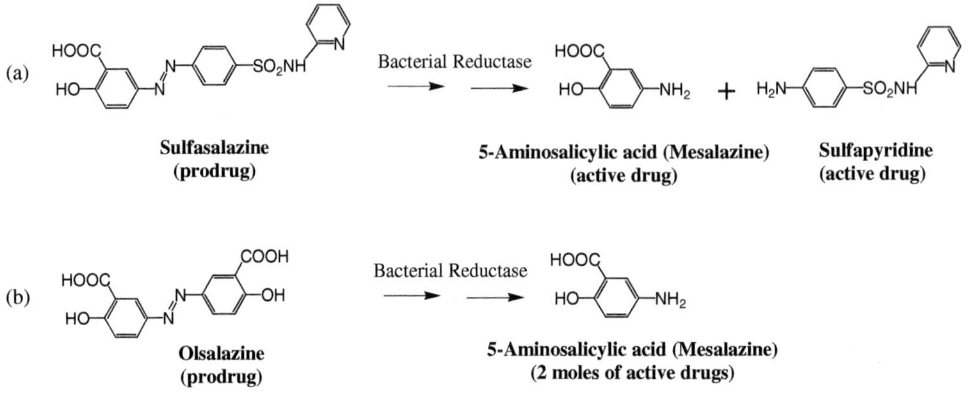


**Figure 9.15** Azo-based prodrugs targeting colon-related disorders. These prodrugs undergo reductions by bacterial reductase to release the active drug 5-aminosalicylic acid in colon. Both sulfasalazine and olsalazine are used in targeting colon-related disorders. The use of sufasalazine is declined due to the fact that it yields the metabolite sulfapyrindine. Although sulfapyridine is a good antibacterial agent it is prescribed no longer. Because sulfapyridine's water solubility is pH dependent there is a risk of crystallization within bladder or urethra, which could lead to pain or blockage. In addition, although rare, sulfasalazine can cause serious, even fatal, side effects such as a severe skin rash known as Stevens–Johnson syndrome, agranulocytosis, aplastic anemia, or liver damage, limiting its use in the treatment of colon-related disorders. 5-Aminosalicylic acid is the active component of sulfasalazine used in the treatment of colon-related disorder. Olsalazine was designed by attaching two moles of 5-aminoslaicylic acid via an azo linking group. Note that two moles of 5-aminosalicylic acid are released from one mole of olsalazine.

metabolism by liver. In order to be absorbed via lymphatic route, a drug should have a high log *P* value of greater than 5 and reasonable lipid solubility in a long-chain triglyceride [82]. Often this goal is achieved by esterification of the drug with long-chain alkyl ester, triglyceride, and phospholipid ester prodrugs (Figure 9.19). Therefore, understanding how triglycerides and phospholipids are digested and absorbed from gastrointestinal tracts and how they are metabolized and reassembled in enterocytes is important in targeting lymphatic route in order to minimize chemical instability in gastrointestinal tract and presystemic drug metabolism by gastrointestinal and hepatic enzymes. Figure 9.20 illustrates the absorption and metabolism of triacylglycerides (triglyceride) and phospholipids in gastrointestinal tract and enterocytes. Triglycerides present in the meal are partially hydrolyzed by lipases present in saliva and stomach to 1,2-diacylglyceride. During this step, fatty acids at

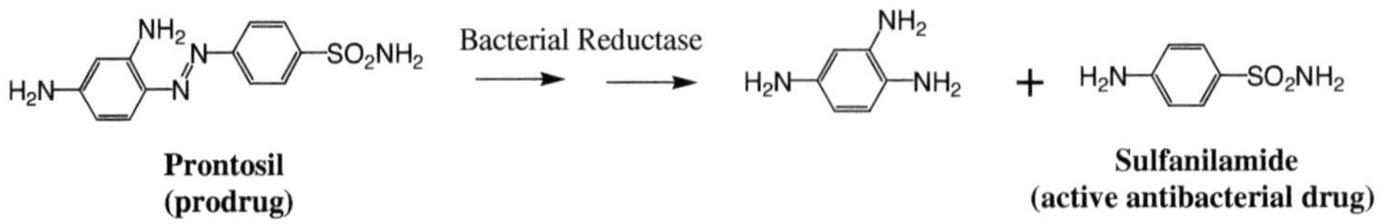


**Figure 9.16** Prontosil is an azo-based prodrug, which after reductions by bacterial reductase releases sulfanilamide as an active antibacterial drug.

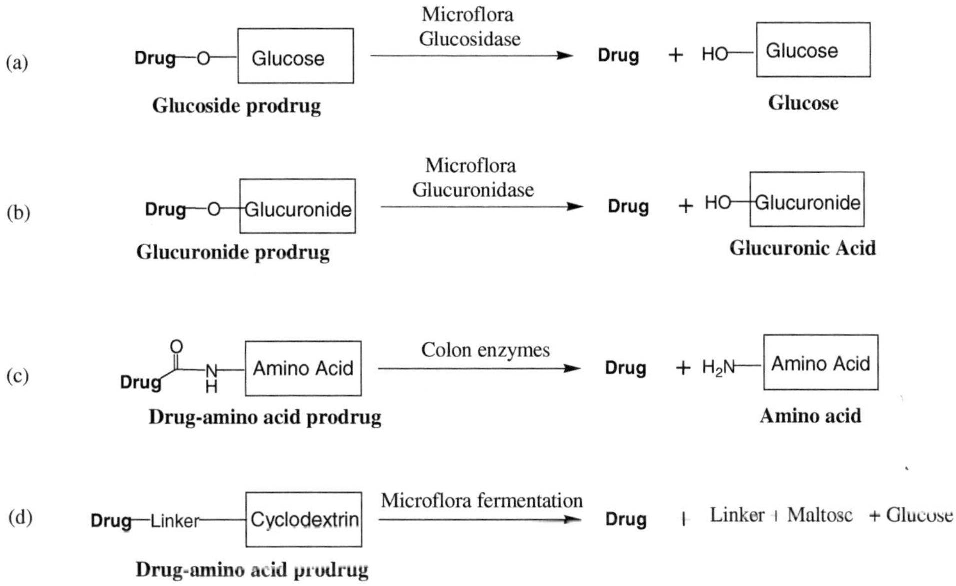


**Figure 9.17** Prodrug examples for colon drug delivery. Colon as the site of drug delivery, drug action, drug release, and/or as the site of drug absorption into systemic blood circulation void of presystemic drug metabolism by liver.

position 2 are selectively removed by lipases. Subsequently, 1,2-diacylglycerides undergo hydrolyses by pancreatic lipases that selectively removes the first acyl group to form 2-monoacylglyceride. Therefore, the acyl group at position 2 seems to be more stable and less likely undergo further hydrolyses in gastrointestinal tract. Because of this, most of the triglyceride-based prodrugs have the drug attached to position 2 on the triglycerides. Monoglycerides and phospholipids present in the meal or secreted as part of the bile along with the partially hydrolyzed prodrug are then incorporated in micelles that can be absorbed via intestine into enterocytes. In

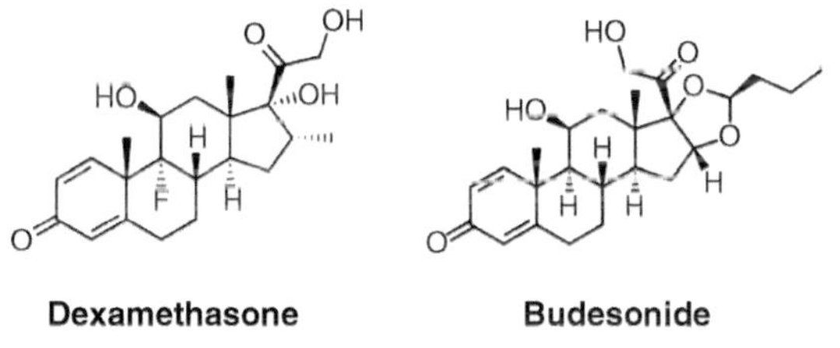


**Figure 9.18** Corticosteroid glucoside and glucuronide prodrugs. Corticosteroids such as dexamethosone are highly lipid soluble and are effectively absorbed from gastrointestinal tract. They have serious systemic side effects such as suppression of hypothalamus–pituitary–adrenal axis and immune system. However, their glucoside and glucuronide prodrugs are water soluble and are not absorbed from small intestine. Once reaching colon, the glucoside and glucuronide prodrugs undergo hydrolysis mediated by microbial enzyme at colon releasing the active drug locally minimizing systemic drug adverse reactions.

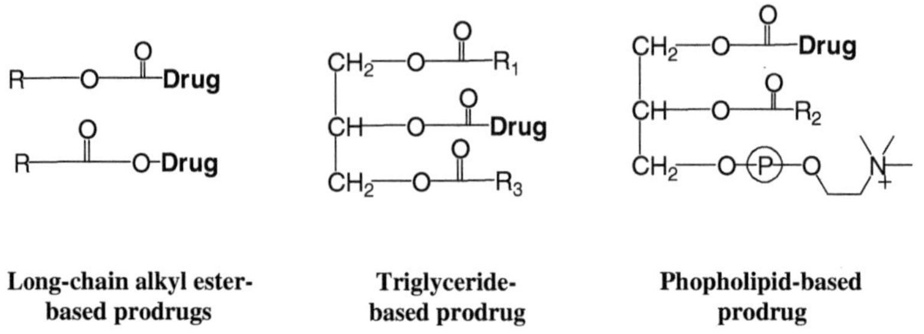


**Figure 9.19** Examples of prodrug approaches to divert drug absorption via portal vein and/or to target lymphatic route minimizing presystemic drug metabolism.

the enterocytes, 2-monoacylglycerides and the glyceride prodrug ester undergo re-esterification with long-chain fatty acids via monoacylglycerol pathways to form triacylglycerides. These triacylglycerol along with the prodrug will be incorporated at the core of chylomicron particles at fed state and in VLDL particles at fasting state [83]. Chylomicron and VLDL are then transferred to lymphatic system, which will be drained into the systemic circulation via thoracic duct; hence, bypassing presystemic metabolism by liver.

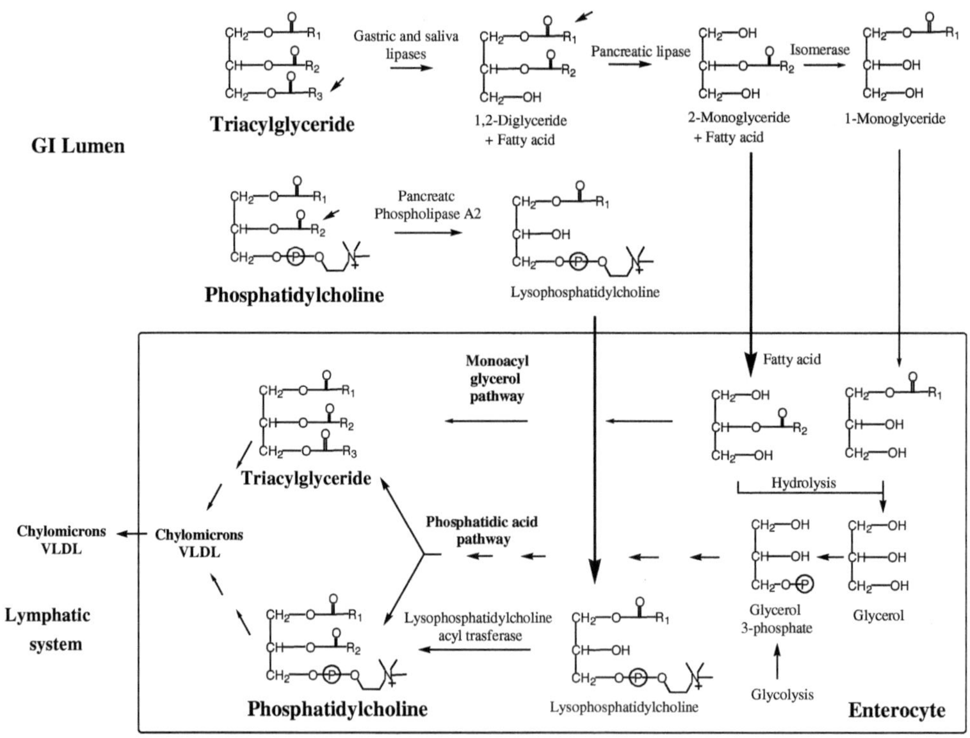


**Figure 9.20** Digestion, absorption, and metabolism of triacylglyceride and phospholipids in gastrointestinal tract and enterocytes.

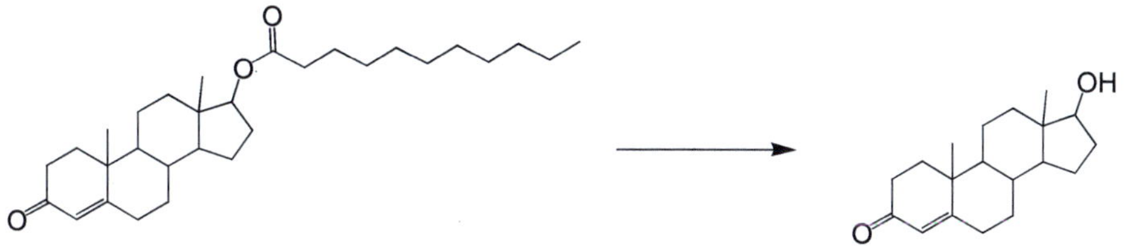


**Figure 9.21** Testosterone undecanoate.

As shown in Figure 9.20, the 2-monoglyceride can also partially undergo isomerization to form 1-monoacylglyceride that can be absorbed along with 2-monoglyceride as described above. 1-Monoacylglycerides are hydrolyzed in enterocytes to produce glycerol and free fatty acids. Glycerol can either be absorbed directly into the portal vein or converted into glycerol 3-phosphate that can subsequently form triacylglycerides and phospholipids through phosphatidic acid pathway. Glycolysis is therefore another source for glycerol 3-phosphate formation, which can be incorporated in lipid synthesis.

Phospholipids present in the food undergo hydrolyses by pancreatic phopholipase A2, which selectively removes the second acyl group to form lysophospholipids that can be then incorporated in the micelles [83]. Absorbed lysophospholipids undergo reacylation by lysophospholipid acyl transferase present in enterocyte to form phospholipids, which are then incorporated on the surface of chylomicron and VLDL particles.

Using above strategies, a number of lipid-based prodrugs were investigated for antiviral drugs, anticancer agents, aspirin, indomethacin, phenytoin, and L-dopa, to name a few. Lipid-based prodrugs are generally used to enhance the lipid solubility and oral bioavailability of drugs. In such design, the lipids moieties are linked to the drug through ester or ether bonds. For example, free testosterone is highly lipid soluble but it is effectively absorbed from small intestine to portal vein, subsequently passing through liver (Figures 9.1 and 9.21). However, testosterone undergoes extensive presystemic metabolism by liver enzymes, which limits its oral bioavailability as shown in Figure 9.8. In contrast, because testosterone undecanoate is highly lipid soluble, it is incorporated into micelles formed in gastrointestinal lumen. It can then be absorbed through lymphatic route bypassing hepatic portal vein and liver metabolism [84–86]. In addition to minimizing presystemic drug metabolism by liver, lipid-based prodrug approaches have potential to reduce drug-induced irritation to gastrointestinal lining and targeting the lymphatic system as the site of drug action.

## 9.6 Conclusion

Physicochemical properties, presystemic drug metabolism by gastrointestinal and liver enzymes and chemical instability in gastrointestinal tract are the major barriers that limit oral bioavailability. Chemical modifications can be used to enhance the oral bioavailability of drugs by reducing presystemic drug metabolism. Such approaches generally (1) prevent the molecules undergoing drug metabolic pathways such as methylation, glucuronidation, and sulfation in liver; (2) deliver the drug to colon as the site of drug release/drug action/drug absorption; or (3) target the lymphatic route as the site of drug delivery. In addition to toxicological and pharmacokinetics studies, learning about drug's metabolic pathways can also generate ideas for prodrug opportunities to diminish presystemic drug metabolism and enhance its oral bioavailability; hence, making it necessary to implement drug metabolic studies as early as possible in a drug discovery program.

## References


1 Lowe, M.E. (2002) The triglyceride lipases of the pancreas. *Journal of Lipid Research*, **43** (12), 2007–2016.

2 Imai, T. (2006) Human carboxylesterase isozymes: catalytic properties and rational drug design. *Drug Metabolism and Pharmacokinetics*, **21** (3), 173–185.

3 Masaki, K., Taketani, M., and Imai, T. (2006) First-pass hydrolysis of a propranolol ester derivative in rat small intestine. *Drug Metabolism and Disposition: The Biological Fate of Chemicals*, **34** (3), 398–404.

4 Watkins, J.B. (1985) Lipid digestion and absorption. *Pediatrics*, **75** (1 Pt2), 151–156.

5 Müller, J., Petković, M., Schiller, J., and Arnhold, J. (2001) Pancreatic phospholipase A2-mediated enhancement of the respiratory burst response of human neutrophils. *Zeitschrift Fur Naturforschung C Journal of Biosciences*, **56** (11–12), 1150–1156.

6 Gibaldi, M. (1971) Pharmacokinetic aspects of drug metabolism. *Annals of the New York Academy of Sciences*, **179**, 19–31.

7 Routledge, P.A. and Shand, D.G. (1979) Clinical pharmacokinetics of propranolol. *Clinical Pharmacokinetics*, **4** (2), 73–90.

8 Drieman, J.C., Thijssen, H.H., and Struyker-Boudier, H.A. (1993) Renal selective *N*-acetyl-L-gamma-glutamyl prodrugs: studies on the selectivity of some model prodrugs. *British Journal of Pharmacology*, **108** (1), 204–208.

9 Walle, T., Walle, U.K., Olanoff, L.S., and Conradi, E.C. (1986) Partial metabolic clearances as determinants of the oral bioavailability of propranolol. *British Journal of Clinical Pharmacology*, **22** (3), 317–323.

10 Guengerich, F.P. (2008) Cytochrome p450 and chemical toxicology. *Chemical Research in Toxicology*, **21** (1), 70–83.

11 Nelson, D., *Cytochrome P450 Homepage*, University of Tennessee, http://drnelson.utmem.edu/cytochromeP450.html (accessed 19 Jan 2010).

12 Human Cytochrome P450 Allele Nomenclature Committee http://www.cypalleles.ki.se/ (accessed 19 Jan 2010).

13 Daggett, P.R., Wheeler, M.J., and Nabarro, J.D. (1978) Oral testosterone, a reappraisal. *Hormone Research*, **9** (3), 121–129.

14 Nieschlag, E., Cüppers, H.J., and Wickings, E.J. (1977) Influence of sex, testicular development and liver function on the bioavailability of oral testosterone. *European Journal of Clinical Investigation*, **7** (2), 145–147.

15 Frey, H., Aakvaag, A., Saanum, D., and Falch, J. (1979) Bioavailability of oral testosterone in males. *European Journal of Clinical Pharmacology*, **16** (5), 345–349.

16 Brunton, L.L., Lazo, J.S., and Parker, K.L. (eds.) (2006) *Goodman & Gilman's the Pharmacological Basis of Therapeutics*, 11th edn, McGraw-Hill, New York.

17 Fotherby, K. (1996) Bioavailability of orally administered sex steroids used in oral contraception and hormone replacement therapy. *Contraception*, **54** (2), 59–69.

18 Männistö, P.T. and Kaakkola, S. (1999) Catechol-*O*-methyltransferase (COMT): biochemistry, molecular biology, pharmacology, and clinical efficacy of the new selective COMT inhibitors. *Pharmacological Reviews*, **51** (4), 593–628.

19 Axelrod, J. (1966) Methylation reactions in the formation and metabolism of catecholamines and other biogenic amines. *Pharmacological Reviews*, **18** (1), 95–113.

20 Edmondson, D.E., Binda, C., and Mattevi, A. (2007) Structural insights into the mechanism of amine oxidation by monoamine oxidases A and B. *Archives of Biochemistry and Biophysics*, **464** (2), 269–276.

21 Coper, J.R., Bloom, F.E., and Roth, H.R. (eds.) (1996) *The Biochemical Basis of Neuropharmacology*, 7th edn, Oxford University Press, New York.

22 Rooke, N., Li, D.J., Li, J., and Keung, W.M. (2000) The mitochondrial monoamine oxidase aldehyde dehydrogenase pathway: a potential site of action of daidzin. *Journal of Medicinal Chemistry*, **43** (22), 4169–4179.

23 Tank, A.W., Deitrich, R.A., and Weiner, H. (1986) Effects of induction of rat liver cytosolic aldehyde dehydrogenase on the oxidation of biogenic aldehydes. *Biochemical Pharmacology*, **35** (24), 4563–4569.

24 MacKerell, A.D. Jr., Blatter, E.E., and Pietruszko, R. (1986) Human aldehyde dehydrogenase: kinetic identification of the isozyme for which biogenic aldehydes and acetaldehyde compete. *Alcoholism, Clinical and Experimental Research*, **10** (3), 266–270.

25 Tank, A.W., Weiner, H., and Thurman, J.A. (1981) Enzymology and subcellular localization of aldehyde oxidation in rat liver. Oxidation of 3,4-dihydroxyphenylacetaldehyde derived from dopamine to 3,4-dihydroxyphenylacetic acid. *Biochemical Pharmacology*, **30** (24), 3265–3275.

26 Ehrig, T., Bosron, W.F., and Li, T.K. (1990) Alcohol and aldehyde dehydrogenase. *Alcohol*, **25** (2–3), 105–116.

27 Zhu, M.Y. and Juorio, A.V. (1995) Aromatic L-amino acid decarboxylase: biological characterization and functional role. *General Pharmacology*, **26** (4), 681–696.

28 Hayashi, H., Mizuguchi, H., and Kagamiyama, H. (1993) Rat liver aromatic L-amino acid decarboxylase: spectroscopic and kinetic analysis of the coenzyme and reaction intermediates. *Biochemistry*, **32** (3), 812–818.

29 Uetrecht, J.P. and Trager, W. (eds.) (2007) *Drug Metabolism: Chemical and Enzymatic Aspects*, Informa Healthcare USA, Inc., New York.

30 Coleman, M.D. (ed.) (2005) *Human Drug Metabolism: An Introduction*, John Wiley & Sons, Ltd., UK.

31 Hansen, K.T., Faarup, P., and Bundgaard, H. (1991) Carbamate ester prodrugs of dopaminergic compounds: synthesis, stability, and bioconversion. *Journal of Pharmaceutical Sciences*, **80** (8), 793–798.

32 Holstein-Rathlou, N.H., Laursen, L.C., Madsen, F., Svendsen, U.G., Gnosspelius, Y., and Weeke, B. (1986) Bambuterol: dose response study of a new terbutaline prodrug in asthma. *European Journal of Clinical Pharmacology*, **30** (1), 7–11.

33 Vickers, S., Duncan, C.A., Ramjit, H.G., Dobrinska, M.R., Dollery, C.T., Gomez, H.J., Leidy, H.L., and Vincek, W.C. (1984) Metabolism of methyldopa in man after oral administration of the pivaloyloxyethyl ester. *Drug Metabolism and Disposition: The Biological Fate of Chemicals*, **12** (2), 242–246.

34 Anderson, B.D., Chu, W.W., and Glinksy, R.E. (1988) Reduction of first pass metabolism of propranolol after oral administration of ester prodrugs. *International Journal of Pharmaceutics*, **43**, 261–265.

35 Murata, K., Noda, K., Kohno, K., and Samejima, M. (1989) Bioavailability and pharmacokinetics of an oral dopamine prodrug in dogs. *Journal of Pharmaceutical Sciences*, **78** (10), 812–814.

36 Hussain, M.A., Aungst, B.J., and Shefter, E. (1988) Prodrugs for improved oral beta-estradiol bioavailability. *Pharmaceutical Research*, **5**, 44–47.

37 Gomes, P., Vale, N., and Moreira, R. (2007) Cyclization-activated prodrugs. *Molecules*, **12** (11), 2484–2506.

38 Filpula, D. and Zhao, H. (2008) Releasable PEGylation of proteins with customized linkers. *Advanced Drug Delivery Reviews*, **60** (1), 29–49.

39 Hamman, J.H., Enslin, G.M., and Kotzé, A.F. (2005) Oral delivery of peptide drugs: barriers and developments. *BioDrugs: Clinical Immunotherapeutics, Biopharmaceuticals and Gene Therapy*, **19** (3), 165–177.

40 Tirucherai, G.S., Yang, C., and Mitra, A.K. (2001) Prodrugs in nasal drug delivery. *Expert Opinion on Biological Therapy*, **1** (1), 49–66.

41 Wang, W., Jiang, J., Ballard, C.E., and Wang, B. (1999) Prodrug approaches to the improved delivery of peptide drugs. *Current Pharmaceutical Design*, **5** (4), 265–287.

42 Yamamoto, A. (1998) Improvement of intestinal absorption of peptide and protein drugs by chemical modification with fatty acids. *Nippon Rinsho*, **56** (3), 601–607.

43 Fujita, T. and Muranishi, S. (1998) Methodologies for regulation of intestinal absorption of biologically active peptides. *Nippon Rinsho*, **56** (3), 589–594.

44 Shan, D., Nicolaou, M.G., Borchardt, R.T., and Wang, B. (1997) Prodrug strategies based on intramolecular cyclization reactions. *Journal of Pharmaceutical Sciences*, **86** (7), 765–767.

45 Bai, J.P., Chang, L.L., and Guo, J.H. (1995) Targeting of peptide and protein drugs to specific sites in the oral route. *Critical Reviews in Therapeutic Drug Carrier Systems*, **12** (4), 339–371.

46 Catnach, S.M., Fairclough, P.D., and Hammond, S.M. (1994) Intestinal absorption of peptide drugs: advances in our understanding and clinical implications. *Gut*, **35** (4), 441–444.

47 Amidon, G.L. and Lee, H.J. (1994) Absorption of peptide and peptidomimetic drugs. *Annual Review of Pharmacology and Toxicology*, **34**, 321–341.

48 Oliyai, R. and Stella, V.J. (1993) Prodrugs of peptides and proteins for improved formulation and delivery. *Annual Review of Pharmacology and Toxicology*, **33**, 521–544.

49 Bundgaard, H. and Rasmussen, G.J. (1991) Prodrugs of peptides. 9. Bioreversible *N*-alpha-hydroxyalkylation of the peptide bond to effect protection against carboxypeptidase or other proteolytic enzymes. *Pharmaceutical Research*, **8** (3), 313–322.

50 Kumar, P. and Mishra, B. (2008) Colon targeted drug delivery systems–an overview. *Current Drug Delivery*, **5** (3), 186–198.

51 Jain, A., Gupta, Y., and Jain, S.K. (2007) Perspectives of biodegradable natural polysaccharides for site-specific drug delivery to the colon. *Journal of Pharmacy & Pharmaceutical Sciences*, **10** (1), 86–128.

52 Lichtenstein, G.R. and Kamm, M.A. (2008) Review article: 5-aminosalicylate formulations for the treatment of ulcerative colitis: methods of comparing release rates and delivery of 5-aminosalicylate to the colonic mucosa. *Alimentary Pharmacology & Therapeutics*, **28** (6), 663–673.

53 Roldo, M., Barbu, E., Brown, J.F., Laight, D.W., Smart, J.D., and Tsibouklis, J. (2007) Azo compounds in colon-specific drug delivery. *Expert Opinion Drug Delivery*, **4** (5), 547–560.

54 Jain, A., Gupta, Y., and Jain, S.K. (2006) Azo chemistry and its potential for colonic delivery. *Critical Reviews in Therapeutic Drug Carrier Systems*, **23** (5), 349–400.

55 Klotz, U. (2005) Colonic targeting of aminosalicylates for the treatment of ulcerative colitis. *Digestive and Liver Disease*, **37** (6), 381–388.

56 Friend, D.R. (2005) New oral delivery systems for treatment of inflammatory bowel disease. *Advanced Drug Delivery Reviews*, **57** (2), 247–265.

57 Chourasia, M.K. and Jain, S.K. (2003) Pharmaceutical approaches to colon targeted drug delivery systems. *Journal of Pharmacy & Pharmaceutical Sciences*, **6** (1), 33–66.

58 Van den Mooter, G., Maris, B., Samyn, C., Augustijns, P., and Kinget, R. (1997) Use of azo polymers for colon-specific drug delivery. *Journal of Pharmaceutical Sciences*, **86** (12), 1321–1327.

59 Travis, S.P. and Jewell, D.P. (1994) Salicylates for ulcerative colitis: their mode of action. *Pharmacology & Therapeutics*, **63** (2), 135–161.

60 Klotz, U. (1985) Clinical pharmacokinetics of sulphasalazine, its metabolites and other prodrugs of 5-aminosalicylic acid. *Clinical Pharmacokinetics*, **10** (4), 285–302.

61 Oz, H.S., Chen, T.S., and Nagasawa, H. (2007) Comparative efficacies of 2 cysteine prodrugs and a glutathione delivery agent in a colitis model. *Translation of Resolution*, **150** (2), 122–129.

62 Kim, H., Huh, J., Jeon, H., Choi, D., Han, J., Kim, Y., and Jung, Y. (2009) *N,N'*-Bis(5-aminosalicyl)-L-cystine is a potential colon-specific 5-aminosalicylic acid prodrug with dual therapeutic effects in experimental colitis. *Journal of Pharmaceutical Sciences*, **98** (1), 159–168.

63 Kim, D., Hong, S., Jung, S., Jung, Y., and Kim, Y.M. (2009) Synthesis and evaluation of *N*-nicotinoyl-2-{2-(2-methyl-5-nitroimidazol-1-yl)ethyloxy}-D,L-glycine as a colon-specific prodrug of metronidazole. *Journal of Pharmaceutical Sciences*, **98** (11), 4161–4169.

64 Cassano, R., Trombino, S., Cilea, A., Ferrarelli, T., Muzzalupo, R., and Picci, N. (2010) l-Lysine pro-prodrug containing *trans*-ferulic acid for 5-amino salicylic acid colon delivery: synthesis, characterization and *in vitro* antioxidant activity evaluation. *Chemical & Pharmaceutical Bulletin*, **58** (1), 103–105.

65 Albrecht, C.F., Theron, E.J., and Kruger, P.B. (1995) Morphological characterisation of the cell growth inhibitory activity of rooperol and pharmacokinetic aspects of hypoxoside as an oral prodrug for cancer therapy. *South African Medical Journal*, **85** (9), 853–860.

66 Tozer, T.N., Rigod, J., McLeod, A.D., Gungon, R., Hoag, M.K., and Friend, D.R. (1991) Colon-specific delivery of dexamethasone from a glucoside prodrug in the guinea pig. *Pharmaceutical Research*, **8** (4), 445–454.

67 Friend, D.R., Chow, J.J., and Chang, G.W. (1990) Effect of antibiotic pretreatment on glycoside/glycosidase-based colonic drug delivery. *Drug design and Delivery*, **6** (4), 311–318.

68 Friend, D.R. and Chang, G.W. (1985) Drug glycosides: potential prodrugs for colon-specific drug delivery. *Journal of Medicinal Chemistry*, **28** (1), 51–57.

69 Friend, D.R. and Chang, G.W. (1984) A colon-specific drug-delivery system based on drug glycosides and the glycosidases of colonic bacteria. *Journal of Medicinal Chemistry*, **27** (3), 261–266.

70 Haeberlin, B., Rubas, W., Nolen, H.W. 3rd, and Friend, D.R. (1993) *In vitro* evaluation of dexamethasone-beta-D-glucuronide for colon-specific drug delivery. *Pharmaceutical Research*, **10** (11), 1553–1562.

71 Nolen, H.W. 3rd, Fedorak, R.N., and Friend, D.R. (1997) Steady-state pharmacokinetics of corticosteroid delivery from glucuronide prodrugs in normal and colitic rats. *Biopharmaceutics & Drug Disposition*, **18** (8), 681–695.

72 Fedorak, R.N., Haeberlin, B., Empey, L.R., Cui, N., Nolen, H. 3rd, Jewell, L.D., and Friend, D.R. (1995) Colonic delivery of dexamethasone from a prodrug accelerates healing of colitis in rats without adrenal suppression. *Gastroenterology*, **108** (6), 1688–1699.

73 Nolen, H.W. 3rd and Friend, D.R. (1994) Menthol-beta-D-glucuronide: a potential prodrug for treatment of the irritable bowel syndrome. *Pharmaceutical Research*, **11** (12), 1707–1711.

74 Cui, N., Friend, D.R., and Fedorak, R.N. (1994) A budesonide prodrug accelerates treatment of colitis in rats. *Gut*, **35** (10), 1439–1446.

75 Zou, M.J., Cheng, G., Okamoto, H., Hao, X.H., An, F., Cui, F.D., and Danjo, K. (2005) Colon-specific drug delivery systems based on cyclodextrin prodrugs: *in vivo* evaluation of 5-aminosalicylic acid from its cyclodextrin conjugates. *World Journal of Gastroenterology*, **11** (47), 7457–7460.

76 Yano, H., Hirayama, F., Kamada, M., Arima, H., and Uekama, K. (2002) Colon-specific delivery of prednisolone-appended alpha-cyclodextrin conjugate: alleviation of systemic side effect after oral administration. *Journal of Controlled Release*, **79** (1–3), 103–112.

77 Sinha, V.R. and Kumria, R. (2001) Polysaccharides in colon-specific drug delivery. *International Journal of Pharmaceutics*, **224** (1–2), 19–38.

78 Yano, H., Hirayama, F., Arima, H., and Uekama, K. (2001) Preparation of prednisolone-appended alpha-, beta- and gamma-cyclodextrins: substitution at secondary hydroxyl groups and *in vitro* hydrolysis behavior. *Journal of Pharmaceutical Sciences*, **90** (4), 493–503.

79 Hirayama, F. and Uekama, K. (1999) Cyclodextrin-based controlled drug release system. *Advanced Drug Delivery Reviews*, **36** (1), 125–141.

80 Minami, K., Hirayama, F., and Uekama, K. (1998) Colon-specific drug delivery based on a cyclodextrin prodrug: release behavior of biphenylylacetic acid from its cyclodextrin conjugates in rat intestinal tracts after oral administration. *Journal of Pharmaceutical Sciences*, **87** (6), 715–720.

81 Uekama, K., Minami, K., and Hirayama, F. (1997) 6*A*-*O*-[(4-biphenylyl)acetyl]-alpha-, -beta-, and -gamma-cyclodextrins and 6*A*-deoxy-6*A*-[[(4-biphenylyl)acetyl] amino]-alpha-, -beta-, and -gamma-cyclodextrins: potential prodrugs for colon-specific delivery. *Journal of Medicinal Chemistry*, **40** (17), 2755–2761.

82 Charman, W.N. (2000) Lipids, lipophilic drugs, and oral drug delivery: some emerging concepts. *Journal of Pharmaceutical Sciences*, **89** (8), 967–978.

83 Murray, R.K., Granner, D.K., Mayes, P.A. and Rodwell, V.M. (eds.) (2003) *Harper's Illustrated Biochemistry*, 26th edn, Lange Medical Books/McGraw-Hill.

84 Shackleford, D.M., Faassen, W.A., Houwing, N., Lass, H., Edwards, G.A., Porter, C.J., and Charman, W.N. (2003) Contribution of lymphatically transported testosterone undecanoate to the systemic exposure of testosterone after oral administration of two andriol formulations in conscious lymph duct-cannulated dogs. *The Journal of Pharmacology and Experimental Therapeutics*, **306** (3), 925–933.

85 Horst, H.J., Höltje, W.J., Dennis, M., Coert, A., Geelen, J., and Voigt, K.D. (1976) Lymphatic absorption and metabolism of orally administered testosterone undecanoate in man. *Klinische Wochenschrift*, **54** (18), 875–879.

86 Coert, A., Geelen, J., de Visser, J., and van der Vies, J. (1975) The pharmacology and metabolism of testosterone undecanoate (TU), a new orally active androgen. *Acta Endocrinologica*, **79** (4), 789–800.

# 10
# Enzyme-Activated Prodrug Strategies for Site-Selective Drug Delivery

*Krista Laine and Kristiina Huttunen*

## 10.1
## Introduction

The concept of site-selective drug delivery or drug targeting has evolved since Nobelist Dr. Paul Erlich launched his "magic bullet," a drug that acted precisely at disease site in the body and left the healthy tissues unharmed, over a century ago. Since then, the ultimate goal to develop safer therapeuticals ("magic bullets") that are efficiently and selectively delivered to the desired site of action without affecting nontarget cells has begun an attractive and actively pursued objective in both pharmaceutical research and industry.

In prodrug approach, targeted drug delivery can in general be achieved either by site-specific drug bioactivation or site-directed drug delivery. With site-directed drug delivery, the intact prodrug is selectively or primarily transported to the site of drug action; for example, when prodrug is applied directly to the target organ as in the case of ocular and dermal drug delivery. Site-directed drug delivery after systemic administration constitutes very challenging task due to various complex and unpredictable barriers in the body but has demonstrated some success, for example, in brain delivery [1–3]. With site-specific bioactivation, the prodrug can be widely distributed through the body, but undergoes bioactivation and exerts pharmacological activity only at the desired site. In site-specific bioactivation, the active therapeutic agent is typically detached from a carefully designed promoiety, which can act as tissue/organ-selective carrier, or results from a prodrug itself after series of biotransformations *in situ* [4].

In prodrug strategy, the site-specific drug activation can be accomplished by either (a) exploiting endogenous enzymes or physiological conditions, such as hypoxia or pH, of target tissue, (b) delivering of genes that encode prodrug-activating (exogenous) enzyme into target tissue (e.g., GDEPT and VDEPT), or (c) delivering of active (exogenous) enzymes into target tissue via monoclonal antibodies (ADEPT). In this chapter, only the site-specific prodrug strategies where activation of prodrug candidate occurs via endogenous tissue-specific enzymes are discussed. ADEPT, GDEPT, and VDEPT strategies are discussed in Chapter 15.

*Prodrugs and Targeted Delivery: Towards Better ADME Properties.* Edited by Jarkko Rautio

ISBN: 978-3-527-32603-7

## 10.2
## General Requirements for Enzyme-Activated Targeted Prodrug Strategy

For successful site-selective drug delivery via enzyme-activated prodrug strategy, several important properties of prodrug, parent drug, and target enzyme should be taken into consideration [5–8]. First, the potential prodrug activating target enzyme should belong in well-characterized enzyme or enzyme family that has a known role in the target tissue phenotype or in the development and progression of the disease. The enzyme should be preferably unique for the target tissue or be present at a significantly higher concentrations compared with healthy tissues. The enzyme should possess a high catalytic activity for the prodrug candidate to rapidly and selectively liberate the active parent drug, and the levels of enzyme should be adequate to generate pharmacologically relevant concentrations of active drug in target tissue. Finally, the expression of target enzyme should be minimal or even absent in patient serum and other healthy tissues [5].

Correspondingly, the enzyme-activated targeted prodrug candidate should be readily transported to the target site and its uptake to target tissue should be reasonable fast [5, 6, 8]. The prodrug should be an excellent substrate for tissue-specific target enzyme. The conversion of prodrug to the active parent drug should be selective at the target site and its conversion at other sites of the body should be minimal. The toxicity of prodrug candidate should be significantly lesser than toxicity of parent drug. Additionally, once selectively released at the target site, the active drug should maintain in target tissue for a period of time sufficient to produce pharmacological action.

## 10.3
## Examples of Targeted Prodrug Strategies

### 10.3.1
### Tumor-Selective Prodrugs

Site-selective drug delivery has originated from the field of cancer chemotherapy where therapeutic drugs are highly reactive and poorly separate their cell-destroying action between healthy cells and tumor cells [9]. Many antitumor drugs possess narrow therapeutic index, indicating that there is only minor difference between the dose needed for therapeutical response and the dose causing potentially life-threatening hazardous adverse effects to the patient [10].

Increased knowledge in the molecular biology of tumors has enabled the development of more tumor-selective anticancer drugs. Numerous tumor-associated enzymes have been utilized to cleave prodrugs of antitumor agents to active form. Those enzymes include either unique tumor-specific enzymes or endogenous enzymes with significant overexpression between tumor cells and healthy cells.

#### 10.3.1.1 Prodrugs Activated by Hypoxia-Associated Reductive Enzymes

Many solid tumors are characterized with abnormal vasculature, which lead to hypoxia and reduced nutrient delivery to the tissue. The low oxygen content increases tumor resistance to drug or radiation therapy and favors tumor progression [11, 12]. This hypoxic state of solid tumors can be, however, turned to the therapeutic advance by designing cytotoxic prodrugs that are converted to the active drug in hypoxic environment of tumor tissue leaving the healthy well-vascularized tissues unaffected. In hypoxia-selective cytotoxic prodrugs, functionalities, such as quinones, *N*-oxides, and aromatic nitro groups that are readily reducible by endogenous reductive enzymes, are usually incorporated in the active cytotoxic drug [13, 14]. Even though the bioreductive enzymes are often expressed in a variety of tissues, the hypoxia-specific activation of antitumor drug can still be obtained, since the initial reduction intermediate is rapidly reoxidized back to the inactive prodrug in the oxygen-rich healthy tissues [9]. In hypoxic solid tumors, this oxidation is significantly slower and results in higher concentrations of active anticancer agent. Examples of reductive enzymes that have been successfully exploited in bioreversible activation of antitumor prodrugs include cytochrome P450 reductase and cytochrome P450s.

**Tirapazamine** Cytochrome P450 reductase activates efficiently tirapazamine (SR 4233) [15, 16], a heteroaromatic *N*-oxide, which has undergone extensive clinical trial. In the hypoxic environment, the proposed activation mechanism for tirapazamine involves an enzymatic one-electron reduction to yield a highly reactive benzotriazinyl radical that can attack tumor DNA (Figure 10.1) prior to its subsequent reduction to the nontoxic metabolite [17, 18]. In the presence of oxygen, the unstable radical intermediate can be rapidly oxidized back to inactive parent prodrug with concomitant generation of moderately cytotoxic superoxide radical and other reactive oxygen species that mediate the anticancer effects of tirapazamine under aerobic conditions [17, 19]. Tirapazamine has shown 15–200-fold activity against hypoxic

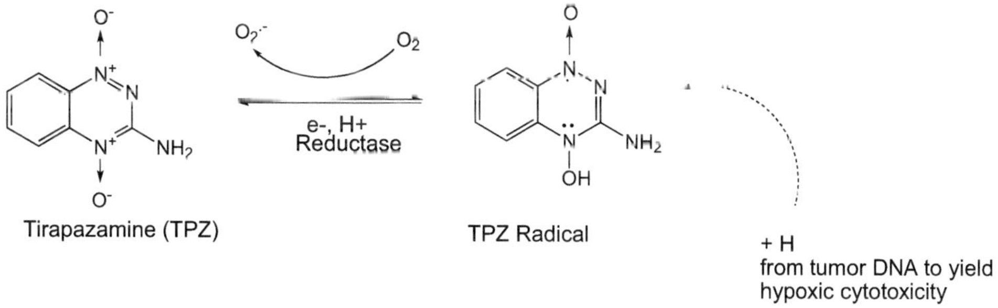


**Figure 10.1** Suggested activation pathway for tirapazamine (TPZ) [18].

cells versus oxic cells in mammalian cells [20], whereas in tumor-bearing mice this ratio has been only threefold, suggesting that the effect of tirapazamine is strongly dependent on oxidation level of tissue [21]. In fact, it is reported that after tirapazamine administration, cells close to blood vessels survive with less DNA damage than cells distant from blood vessels [22].

**PR-104** The first hypoxia-activated alkylating nitrogen mustard prodrug PR-104 is currently undergoing Phase II clinical trials by Proacta, Inc. Activation of this dinitrobenzamide mustard is preceded by a systemic cleavage of water-soluble phosphate ester by phosphatases to yield the corresponding more lipophilic alcohol metabolite PR-104A [23]. In hypoxic regions of tumor, the 5-nitro group of PR-104A is reduced selectively by cytochrome P450 reductase to the corresponding hydroxylamine (PR-104H) that exerts the cytotoxic effects through activation of the mustard to form DNA interstrand cross-links. Subsequently, PR-104H is reduced to its 5-amine metabolite (PR-104M) [23, 24] (Figure 10.2). Albeit the cytochrome P450 reductase has been reported to have the predominant role in bioreductive activation of PR-104A, other intratumoral flavoenzymes may also contribute to its activation [23]. In human cervical tumor cells, PR-104 has shown selective cytotoxicity toward hypoxia with 22-fold increased activity against hypoxic cells versus aerobic cells [25].

**Apaziquone** An indoloquinone compound apaziquone (EO-9) (Figure 10.3) is a bioreductive anticancer prodrug that generates a highly oxygen-sensitive drug radical and other reactive oxygen species after activation by intracellular reductases [26–29]. The mechanism of activation of apaziquone is not yet completely clear. Apaziquone is

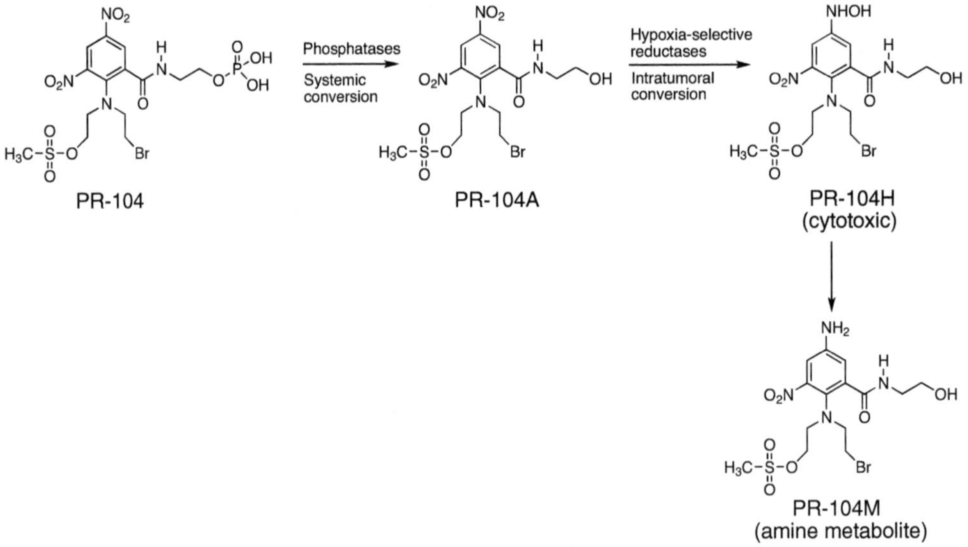


**Figure 10.2** Two-step enzymatic activation pathway for PR-104 to form an active cytotoxic drug PR-104H and its subsequent metabolite PR-104M [24].

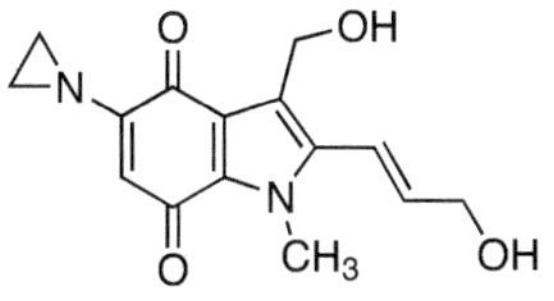


**Figure 10.3** Chemical structure of apaziquone (EO-9).

a good substrate for DT-diaphorase (NQO1), which has been proposed to be the main enzyme involved in activation of apaziquone under aerobic conditions [27]. However, the cytochrome P450 reductase may also contribute to its antitumor cytotoxity in hypoxic cells [28]. Earlier, apaziquone has been failed to demonstrate clinical efficacy in Phase II studies after intravenous administration, but recently its intravesical formulation has been entered to Phase III clinical evaluation against noninvasive bladder cancer (EOquin®) (Spectrum Pharmaceuticals, Inc.).

*CB1954* is an anticancer prodrug that requires nitroreduction of its 2- or 4-nitro group prior to cytotoxic action (Figure 10.4). Additionally, both nitro groups of CB1954 can be metabolized to the corresponding hydroxylamine derivatives, which can further be transformed to amines by two-electron reduction. The most cytotoxic metabolite of CB1954 is the 5-(aziridin-1-yl)-4-hydroxyamino-2-nitrobenzamide that can react with acetyl coenzyme A and produce a highly reactive nitrenium intermediate [30]. Other metabolites may also contribute to the cytotoxic DNA cross-linking action of CB1954 [31]. The bioactivation of CB1954 has been reported to occur by the reductive DT-diaphorase enzyme NQO2, which activity is related to expression of NQO1 [32]. Other reductive enzymes such as rat NQO1, nitric oxide synthases (NOS) and nitroreductase has also been shown to metabolize CB1954 [33–35]. In mice, the tumor tissue penetration of CB1954 has proven slow but generally good with tumor to plasma rations ranging from 50 to 90% [36].

**Banoxantrone** AQ4N (banoxantrone) (Figure 10.5) is a novel *N*-oxide prodrug of active topoisomerase II inhibitor AQ4. Activation of AQ4N is not targeted to a specific CYP enzyme, but a local CYP expression is required for its activation. AQN4 is reduced to its active basic amine AQ4 in the hypoxic tumor environment by CYP3A4, CYP1A, and CYP1B1 enzyme isoforms [37]. Recent Phase I study has indicated a

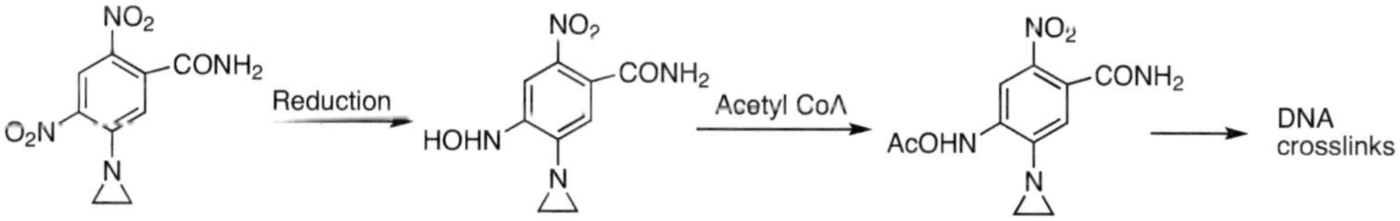


**Figure 10.4** Activation of CB1954 to cytotoxic intermediate by enzyme-catalyzed reduction of 4-nitro group [31].

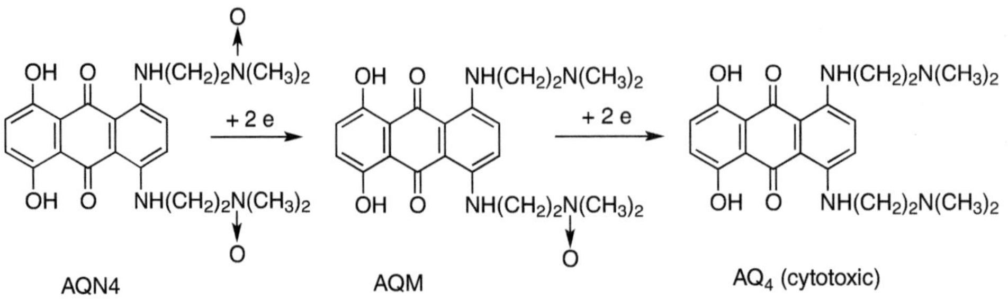


**Figure 10.5** CYP450-catalyzed reduction of AQN4 to active antitumor drug AQ4 through a formation of mono-*N*-oxide intermediate (AQM) [37].

tumor-targeted and hypoxia-selective action of AQN4 in patients with advanced solid tumors [38]. Additionally, AQ4N has been shown to rapidly penetrate throughout multilayered cultured cells and tumor tissue in mice [39]. AQ4N or its active reduced form AQ4 has been found with high concentrations in hypoxic regions far from blood vessels *in vivo* whereas the concentrations of drug have been low in oxic regions around blood vessel [39]. AQ4N is currently under clinical development by Novacea, Inc.

#### 10.3.1.2 **Prodrugs Activated by Glutathione S-Transferase**

**Canfosfamide** A novel glutathione analog prodrug, canfosfamide (TLK286, formerly TER286), exploits the tumor tissue overexpression of glutathione *S*-transferase P1-1 in its cleavage to cytotoxic DNA alkylating phosphoroamidate mustard and vinyl sulfate derivative (Figure 10.6) [40, 41]. Cytotoxicity of canfosfamide correlates well with glutathione *S*-transferase P1-1 expression, that is, the cells that have increased levels of glutathione *S*-transferase P1-1 expression are more sensitive to the therapeutic effects of prodrug [42]. Furthermore, downregulation of the glutathione *S*-transferase P1-1 by long-term chronic exposure to canfosfamide may also increase the therapeutic efficacy of other antitumor agents that have developed glutathione *S*-transferase-mediated drug resistance to the tumor [43]. Canfosfamide has been recently shown to have clinical benefit in the advanced non-small cell lung cancer and in platinum-resistant ovarian cancer [43].

**JS-K** Another interesting example of glutathione *S*-transferase-activated prodrug candidates is $O^2$-aryl diazeniumdiolate compound JS-K (Figure 10.7). JS-K is cleaved by glutathione *S*-transferase to selectively release nitric oxide (NO), which ability to inhibit tumor growth has made it an interesting molecule for tumor therapy [44, 45]. Activation of JS-K occurs via two-step reaction. First, the glutathione or other strong nucleophilic biomolecule is arylated with JS-K by glutathione *S*-transferase to form 4-ethoxycarbonylpiperazine/NO, which subsequently releases NO spontaneously at physiological pH [45]. The antitumor activity of JS-K is currently under investigation. Previously, it has been shown to be both effective against human leukemia, hepatoma, and prostate cancer *in vivo* [45, 46] and selectively toxic toward cultured

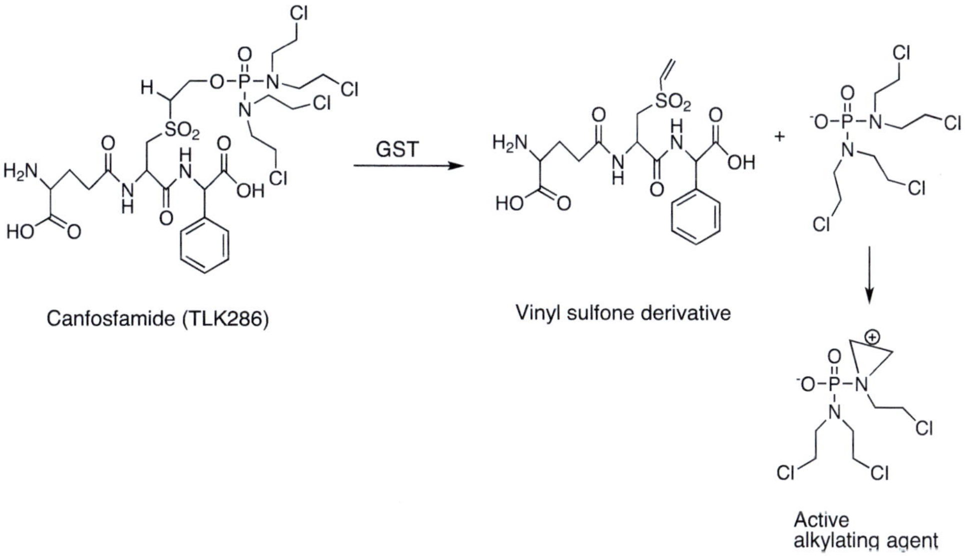


**Figure 10.6** Chemical structure and metabolites of antitumor prodrug, canfosfamide (TLK286), which requires glutathione *S*-transferase P1-1 for its activation [42].

renal cancer cells at concentrations that did not significantly affect the proliferation of normal renal epithelial cells [47].

### 10.3.1.3 **Prodrugs Activated by Thymidine Phosphorylase**

**Doxifluridine** 5′-Deoxy-5-fluorouridine (5′-DFUR) (Doxifluridine) (Figure 10.8) is an orally administrated anticancer prodrug that was developed to improve the tumor selectivity of an active antimetabolite drug 5-fluorouracil (5-FU). Conversion of 5′-DFUR to active 5-FU occurs by thymidine phosphorylase, which is present at least 10% elevated levels in many types of tumors compared to healthy normal tissue [48]. However, since tymidine phosphorylase also exists in intestinal tissue, the conversion of 5′-DFUR to 5-FU in gastrointestinal tract caused dose-related diarrhea in clinical trials. This unwanted gastrointestinal toxicity limits its oral administration [49, 50].

**Capecitabine** Highly innovative fluoropyrimidine prodrug capecitabine (Figure 10.8) [49] was rationally developed to be more effective and overcome the

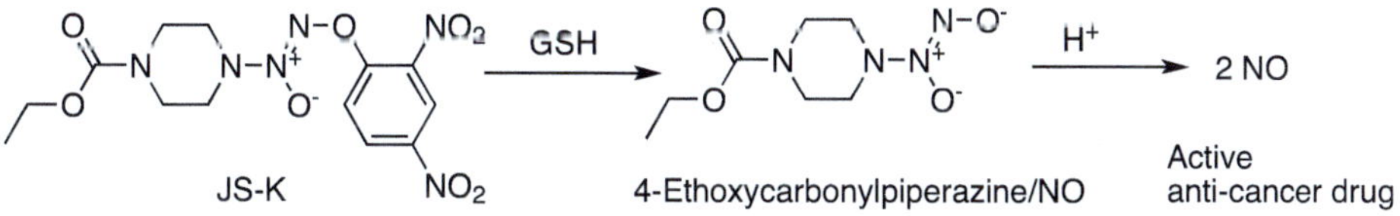


**Figure 10.7** Glutathione *S*-transferase-dependent mechanism of NO release from antitumor prodrug JS-K [44].

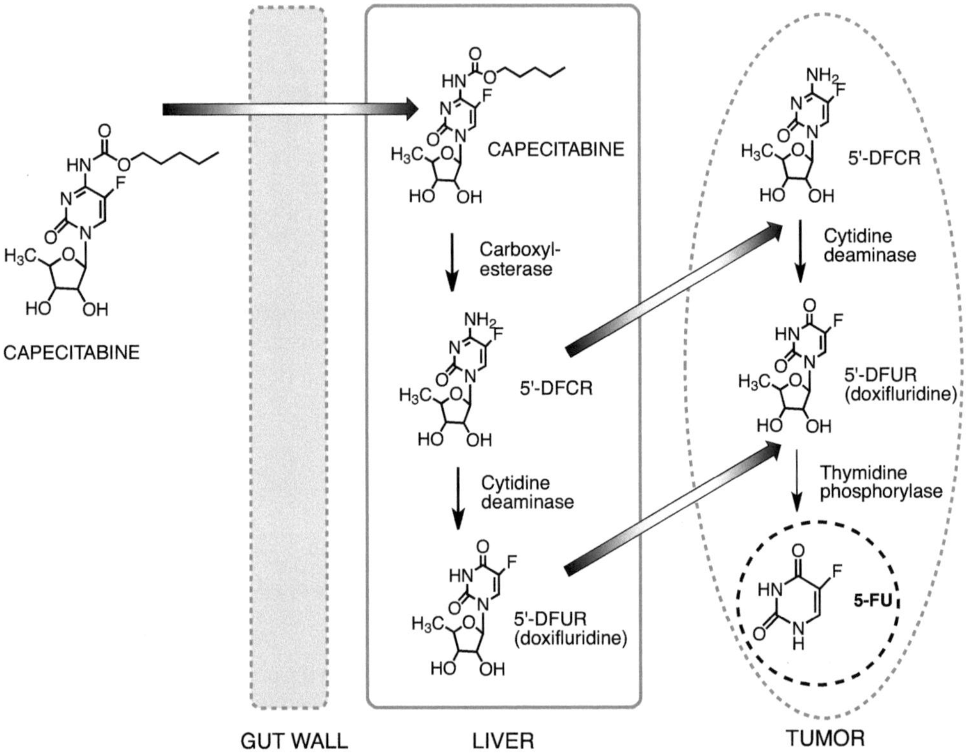


**Figure 10.8** Three-step enzymatic activation pathway of capecitabine to cytotoxic 5-FU.

unwanted gastrointestinal adverse effects of 5′-DFUR. Capecitabine is activated to 5-FU through three reaction steps, which all are enzymatic. After rapid and extensive absorption from gastrointestinal tract, capecitabine is first effectively hydrolyzed to 5′-deoxy-5-fluorocytidine (5′-DFCR) in liver by hepatic carboxylesterase activity. Consequently, 5′-DFCR is converted into 5′-DFUR by cytidine deaminase either in liver or in tumor tissue. Finally, the release of cytotoxic 5-FU occurs selectively through thymidine phosphorylase activity at the tumor site [48]. Orally administered capecitabine has resulted in 114- to 209-fold higher 5-FU levels in the tumor tissue compared to the plasma in mice bearing human cancer xenografts [51]. Additionally, the tumor concentrations of 5-FU produced by an orally administered capecitabine compared to the intraperitoneally administered 5-FU has resulted an area under curve (AUC) over 20-fold greater *in vivo* [51]. The tumor selectivity of capecitabine has confirmed also in patients with advanced breast cancer [52]. After capecitabine administration to patients, the 5-FU levels in tumor tissue were 2.5-fold greater compared to healthy tissue and 14-fold greater compared to plasma. Capecitabine has shown thymidine phosphorylase-dependent antitumor activity, and it is currently approved for the treatment of metastatic colorectal and breast cancer in more than 70 countries worldwide. An interesting curiosity with this prodrug is an observation that the long-term treatment with capecitabine can induce loss of fingerprints and cause problems for patients traveling to countries that require fingerprint identification when entering to custom officers [53].

## 10.3.2 Organ-Selective Prodrugs

### 10.3.2.1 Liver-Targeted Prodrugs

The liver is the first organ to encounter nutrients, drugs, and toxins after their absorption from the stomach and intestine, and it plays a primary role in the synthesis and/or metabolism of biomolecules and xenobiotics [54, 55]. Therefore, the liver possesses a battery of cell surface carriers, transport proteins, and metabolizing enzymes that may be used as targets for the liver-specific drug delivery to improve efficacy and safety of drug molecules. The major cells of the liver are the hepatocytes, which are responsible for the main metabolic properties of the organ. The metabolism in the hepatocytes usually leads to detoxification of xenobiotics and the formed more hydrophilic metabolites are then eliminated via the bile or kidneys from the body. Various acute and chronic liver diseases (e.g., several viral infections, overdose of particular drugs, toxins, or alcohol), several metabolic disorders (e.g., diabetes and hyperlipidemia), and chronic congenital disorders (e.g., hemochromatosis, Wilson disease, Gilbert syndrome, and α1-antitrypsin deficiency) can affect the normal functions of the liver. If untreated, these diseases can progress to cirrhosis and eventually kill the patient due to the liver failure or liver cancer. Although many drugs used in the treatment of liver diseases do reach the liver in sufficient amounts, they may cause unwanted extrahepatic adverse effects.

Attempts have been made to exploit liver-specific receptors and transporters to achieve the liver-specific drug delivery, but the most successful strategy today targets liver-specific enzymes, such as cytochrome P450 enzymes, which biotransform the prodrugs to the active drug molecules in the hepatocytes. CYP enzymes are a large class of heme-containing microsomal proteins that catalyze more than 40 different types of oxidation and reduction reactions of a great number of endogenous and exogenous substrates [56]. The liver is the predominant site for CYP-mediated reactions, although CYP enzymes are also expressed to the lesser extent in the intestine, kidney, brain, lung, testis, skin, and spleen (Table 10.1). Xenobiotic

**Table 10.1** Total cytochrome P450 enzyme content in selected human tissues [62].

| Tissue | CYP content (nmol/mg microsomal protein) |
|---|---|
| Liver | 0.30–0.60 |
| Adrenal gland | 0.23–0.54 |
| Small intestine | 0.03–0.21 |
| Brain | 0.10 |
| Kidney | 0.03 |
| Lung | 0.01 |
| Testis | 0.01 |

metabolizing CYPs (CYP forms in families 1, 2, and 3) have a wide substrate specificity, whereas CYP enzymes metabolizing endogenous compounds, such as steroid hormones and fatty acids (CYP forms in families 4, 5, 7, 8, 11, 17, 19, 21, 24, 27, and 51) have a very strict substrate specificity, although in general, a typical CYP substrate is highly lipophilic [56–59]. However, when targeting CYP enzymes, special attention needs to be paid to potential species-related and patients-related specificities, genetic polymorphisms, and drug–drug interactions during the development phases [60]. There are also several challenges in designing CYP-activated prodrugs, because the crystal structures for most of the CYP enzymes are yet to be determined. Presently, drug design strategies are based on the knowledge of the substrate structure and the enzyme's mechanism of action [61].

Knowledge of CYP-catalyzed bioconversion mechanisms of anticancer prodrugs cyclophosphamide (CPA), ifosfamide (IFA), and trofosfamide has led to the development of liver-specific cyclic phosphate and phosphonate prodrugs called HepDirect® prodrugs [62–68]. Originally, HepDirect prodrugs were designed and applied to nucleosides, which were widely used for the treatment of viral infections and leukemia, in attempts to improve the poor intracellular bioconversion of nucleosides to nucleoside monophosphates (NMPs) inside the cells. Before these compounds can inhibit viral replication and cell proliferation, the nucleosides need to be bioconverted to nucleoside triphosphates (NTPs). The C4 aryl substituent of cyclic 1,3-propanyl esters of phosphates and phosphonates renders prodrugs sensitive to the hydroxylation of the C4 methine, the benzylic carbon atom adjacent to a phosph(on)ate oxygen, which is catalyzed specifically by CYP3A4 (Figure 10.9). Hydroxylation results in irreversible ring opening and the formation of a transient intermediate, which is a negatively charged form. A subsequent β-elimination reaction releases the phosphate or phosphonate, and an aryl vinyl ketone as a by-product. Different electron-withdrawing aryl substituents, such as chlorine in the

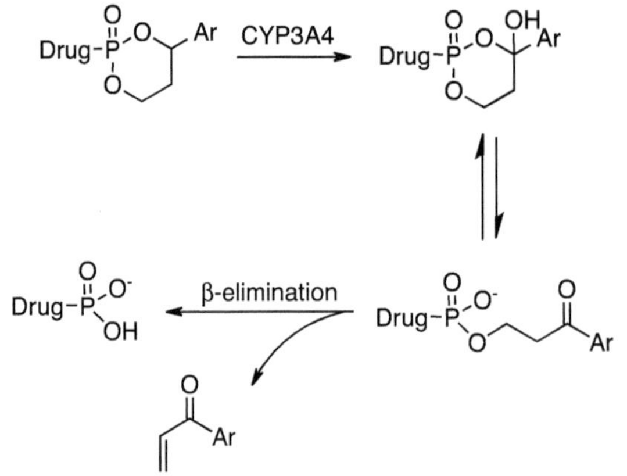


**Figure 10.9** Bioconversion of HepDirect prodrugs to the corresponding phosphates or phosphonates and aryl vinyl ketone after a CYP3A4-catalyzed hepatic oxidation and consequent ring opening and β-elimination.

*meta*-position of C4 aryl ring or pyridine, enhance the cleavage of the highly electrophilic aryl vinyl ketone, which, along with other vinyl ketones, is associated with significant toxicity. However, it is rapidly detoxified by intracellular glutathione, as long as the glutathione levels remain at 20% of normal liver levels (0.5–1 mM). The anionic intermediate and the product after prodrug cleavage have poor diffusion across the cell membranes. They are, therefore, retained in the hepatocytes, which augment the liver specificity.

Presently, two aryl substituted cyclic phosphonate prodrugs have advanced to the clinical trials. These are pradefovir (MB06866, remofovir) and MB07133, which are prodrugs of adefovir (PMEA) and cytarabine (araC), respectively (Figure 10.10) [63, 65, 66, 68]. Pradefovir was developed to improve the therapeutic potential of the hepatitis B (HBV) prodrug, adefovir dipivoxil (Hepsera®). Adefovir dipivoxil is a bispivaloyloxymethyl (POM) ester of PMEA and cleaved nonspecifically by esterases in the body. However, the Phase III clinical studies have revealed that the exposure of PMEA to the kidneys and the subsequent kidney toxicity limits the use of adefovir dipivoxil [69]. In contrast, the HepDirect prodrug of PMEA, pradefovir, has higher liver/kidney (12-fold) and liver/intestine (84-fold) targeting ratio relative to adefovir dipivoxil *in vivo*. Furthermore, the systemic adefovir levels are low and the prodrug has good therapeutic efficacy in patients with hepatitis B [70, 71]. The antileukemic agent, araC, is converted to araC triphosphate via araC monophosphate, mainly in the leukemic cells, but to a lesser extent also in the bone marrow cells, which results in the bone marrow toxicity. On the contrary, the HepDirect prodrug MB07133 is bioactivated to araC triphosphate in the hepatocytes, effluxed into the circulation, and transported directly to the leukemic cells. *In vivo* studies have shown that MB07133 has much higher liver/bone marrow targeting ratio (45-fold) for araC triphosphate, since there is no CYP3A4 activity present in bone marrow.

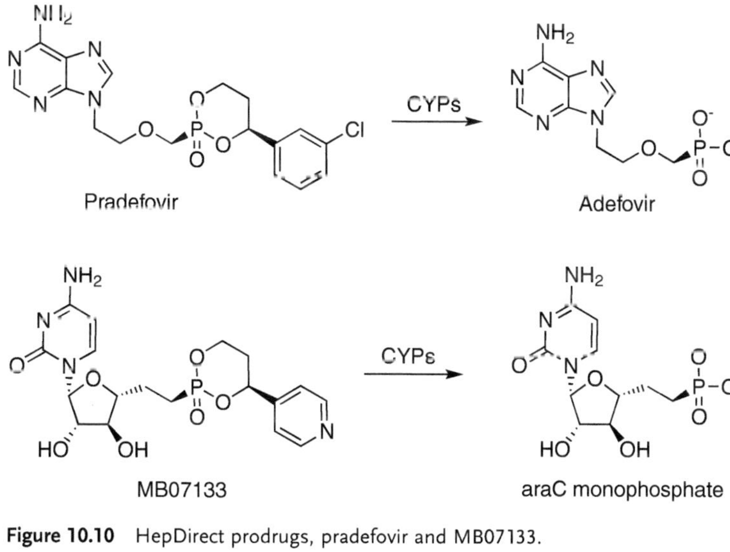


**Figure 10.10** HepDirect prodrugs, pradefovir and MB07133.

The cyclic phosphate prodrug approach may as well be used for other drug compounds than nucleoside phosphates and phosphonates, since hepatocytes possess phosphatases that can hydrolyze the phosphate group from the parent drug molecule after CYP-catalyzed oxidation and subsequent β-elimination of aryl vinyl ketone [72]. However, more research is still needed to evaluate completely the nature of this novel liver targeting approach.

#### 10.3.2.2 **Kidney-Targeted Prodrugs**

While the liver is the most important metabolizing organ in the body, renal excretion is a major route of elimination. In addition, the kidneys also control the blood pressure and the manufacture of red blood cells in the bone marrow, as well as maintain the balance of calcium and phosphate [73, 74]. The renal clearance of a drug consists of four different processes: (1) glomerular filtration (in the glomerulus), (2) active secretion (mainly in the proximal tubule), (3) passive reabsorption (mainly in the distal tubule), and (4) renal metabolism, which occur in the functional kidney unit called the nephron. Several diseases, such as nephritis, inherited polycystic kidney disease, pyelonephritis, renovascular disease, *diabetes mellitus*, and obstructive nephropathy, can cause chronic kidney failure, which often progress to a condition called end-stage renal failure where the kidneys stop working almost completely. Today, the only treatments for renal failure are dialysis or kidney transplantation. Although most of drugs are eventually excreted by the kidneys, some of them are inactivated before they reach the kidneys. However, those drugs that reach the kidneys in active form may cause unwanted extrarenal adverse effects. In spite of years of research, no renal-specific prodrug has reached the clinic, and therefore, the recent research results in the field of the kidney-specific prodrug delivery will be briefly described.

The mesangial cells of the glomerulus and the proximal tubular cells are the primary choice of targets for the renal-specific drug delivery, since they play a pivotal role in many kidney diseases [75]. To date, only a limited number of studies have focused on the drug delivery to the mesangial cells and have revealed only a modest degree of selectivity. More extensive research has been performed on targeting drugs to the proximal tubular cells, which are the most active cells in the kidneys, since they are involved in both active transport and metabolism of drugs. Certain amino acid prodrugs can be delivered selectively into the proximal tubular cells, where they are activated by specific enzymes, for example, γ-glutamyl transpeptidase at the brush border or basolateral side of the proximal tubular cells, or β-lyase, *N*-acetyl transferase, or L-amino acid decarboxylase in the cytosolic side of the proximal tubular cells. L-γ-Glutamyl-L-dopa (gludopa) (Figure 10.11) is a double prodrug of dopamine

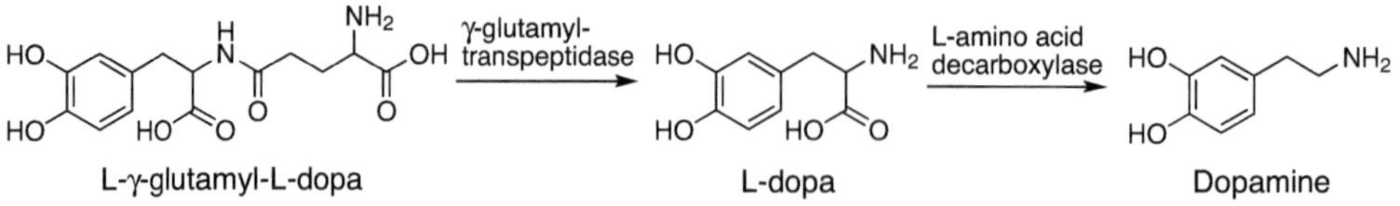


**Figure 10.11** Investigational renal-specific prodrug of dopamine.

that is activated selectively in the proximal tubular cells by γ-glutamyl transpeptidase to L-dopa, and subsequently by L-amino acid decarboxylase to the active dopamine. It may be used as a renal vasodilator [76–78], although the oral bioavailability of gludopa appears to be poor [79]. Similarly, *N*-acyl-L-γ-glutamyl derivatives of bacteriostatic sulfamethoxazole and the vasodilative drug CGP 18137 (2-hydrazine-5-*n*-butyl pyridine) are selectively activated in the proximal tubular cells by the sequential action of kidney-specific acylase and γ-glutamyl transpeptidase [80–82]. However, not every (*N*-acyl)-L-γ-glutamyl prodrug is transported into the proximal tubular cells. For example, *N*-acyl-L-γ-glutamyl-4′-aminowarfarin is not renally selective. This may be due to the lack of carrier-mediated transport and its high plasma protein binding [83, 84]. In addition, the chemotherapeutic prodrugs, *S*-(purin-6-yl)-L-cysteine and selenocysteine Se-conjugates have been studied as kidney-selective prodrugs of 6-mercaptopurine [83–88] and selenol compounds [89–91], respectively. These prodrugs are activated by renal cysteine conjugate β-lyases.

#### 10.3.2.3 **Colon-Targeted Prodrugs**

The colon is a highly efficient part of the lower GI tract. The main functions of the colon are to reabsorb water from the waste material, store the solid waste, and finally to eliminate the fecal waste [92, 93]. A number of colonic diseases, such as ulcerative colitis, Crohn's disease, and colorectal cancer, are still lacking appropriate medical treatments. Therefore, these diseases would benefit from colon-specific drug delivery, which could permit lower dosing, resulting in increased therapeutic efficacy and fewer adverse effects. The objective of the colon-targeted drug delivery is to avoid absorption and degradation of drugs in the upper GI tract allowing them act site specifically in the colon. Various approaches, such as pH-, time-, and pressure-sensitive polymers, and enzyme-activated drug delivery systems (e.g., prodrugs, coatings, and matrices), have been studied over the last decades [94, 95]. In colon-targeted prodrug approaches, the active drug molecule is liberated by colonic bacterial enzymes, for example, azoreductases, β-glucosidases, or β-glucuronidases [96].

A classic example of a colon-specific prodrug is an azo-prodrug of the anti inflammatory agent 5-aminosalicylic acid (5-ASA), salicylazosulfapyridine (SASP; Sulfasalazine®, Azulfidine®). The highly polar SASP is poorly absorbed from the upper GI tract and considerable amounts (>80%) of SASP reach the colon, where it is bioactivated to 5-ASA and sulfapyridine by azoreductases [97, 98]. However, sulfapyridine poses toxic adverse effects, and therefore, various similar azo-prodrugs, such as olsalazine (Dipentum®) [99, 100], balsalazide (Colazal®) [101], and ipsalazine [94] with less toxic promoieties (benzoyl-β-alanine, 5-ASA, and 4-amino benzoyl glycine, respectively) have been developed (Figure 10.12).

Another colon-targeted prodrug example is the glucoside prodrug of the glucocorticoid, dexamethasone 21-β-D-glucoside, which is bioactivated to the active parent drug molecule, dexamethasone, by bacterial glucosidases when it reaches the colon (Figure 10.13). Dexamethasone 21-β-D-glucoside is highly hydrophilic, and thus, poorly absorbed in the upper GI tract, and therefore, nearly 60% of the oral dose of dexamethasone 21-β-D-glucoside reaches the cecum [102]. Similarly, β-D-glucuronide

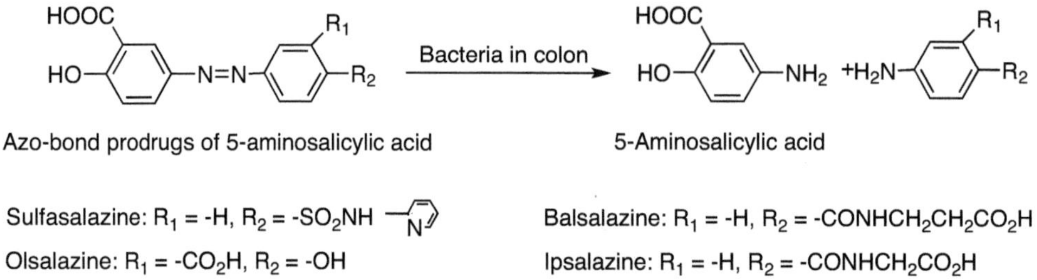


**Figure 10.12** Azo prodrugs of 5-aminosalicylic acid (5-ASA).

prodrug of dexamethasone has shown improved colon delivery [103], although neither of these prodrugs has advanced into the clinic yet. In the most recent study, 5-ASA and prednisolone has been linked together as a mutual prodrug via 1,4-self-immolative spacer by azo and ester bonds [104]. This codrug is bioactivated initially by azoreductases and subsequently by spontaneous intramolecular lactamization of the of the 1,4-elimination spacer. In addition to azo and glucoside/glucuronide prodrugs, attempts have been made to develop various other colon-specific prodrugs, such as amino acid esters and cyclodextrin prodrugs, in efforts to improve the colon targeting of anti-inflammatory drugs [105, 106].

### 10.3.3
### Virus-Selective Prodrugs

Viruses are ubiquitous microscopic infectious agents that can only reproduce inside host cells and can therefore cause harm to the infected organism [107]. As discussed in Section 10.3.2.1, the cyclic 1,3-propanyl esters (HepDirect prodrugs) [70] and the other similar prodrugs, such as bis-isopropyloxymethylcarbonyl (bisPOC) esters [108] and nucleotide dimers [109], have been widely used to target nucleoside triphosphates and phosphonates to viruses. Interestingly, acyclovir itself is probably the oldest example of virus-selective prodrug. Acyclovir is bioconverted to its monophosphate by virus-specific pyrimidine deoxynucleoside kinase (thymidine kinase) and subsequently phosphorylated to its di- and triphosphates by other cellular kinases (Figure 10.14). These phosphorylations occur to a very limited extent in the

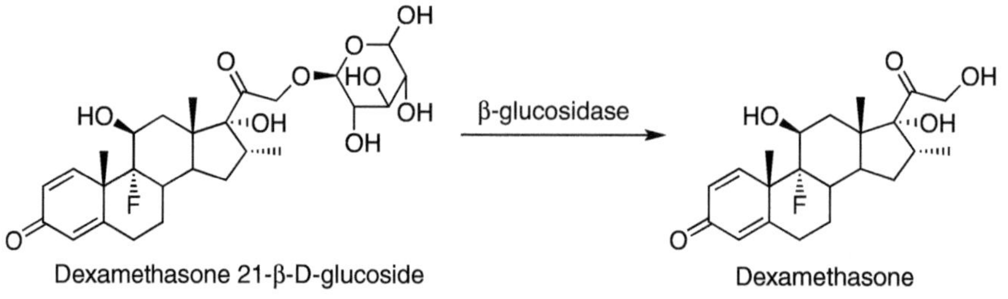


**Figure 10.13** Dexamethasone 21-β-D-glucoside.

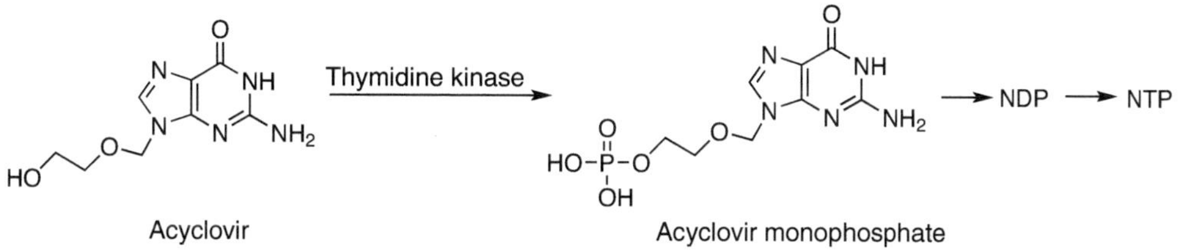


**Figure 10.14** Viral-targeted prodrug acyclovir.

uninfected host cells and a 300-fold greater concentration of acyclovir is needed to inhibit uninfected cell multiplication in comparison to the inhibition of virus-infected cell multiplication [110]. In addition to acyclovir, several other antiviral nucleoside analogues, such as ganciclovir, penciclovir didanosine, zalsitabine, tenofovir, and lamivudine, can be classified to virus-selective prodrugs since their activation require intracellular phosphorylation by virus-specific enzymes.

Sialated diazeniumdiolates is another example of an investigational virus-targeted nitric oxide releasing prodrug, which could be used to impair the replication of influenza A and B viruses [111]. Nitric oxide is an important signaling molecule in various physiological processes, but it also plays a key role in host defense against bacteria, viruses, protozoa, and tumor cells [112]. Since influenza viruses have specific sialic acid conjugates hydrolyzing proteins, such as hemagglutinin and neuramidases, on their surface, sialated diatseniumdiolates can deliver the nitric oxide selectively to the proximity of influenza viruses and obtain the targeting effect (Figure 10.15).

## 10.4 Summary

Rationally designed drug targeting is one of the most interesting and actively pursued objectives of prodrug approach. In fact, during 1993–2003, 14.9% of all prodrug patents claimed drug targeting [113]. Since drug targeting is particularly attractive for highly toxic drugs and for drugs having a narrow therapeutical window, it is not surprising that majority of patents mentioning drug targeting was directed toward cancer treatment. In addition to very innovative anticancer prodrugs with site-selective activation, such as capecitabine, the targeted delivery of therapeuticals to

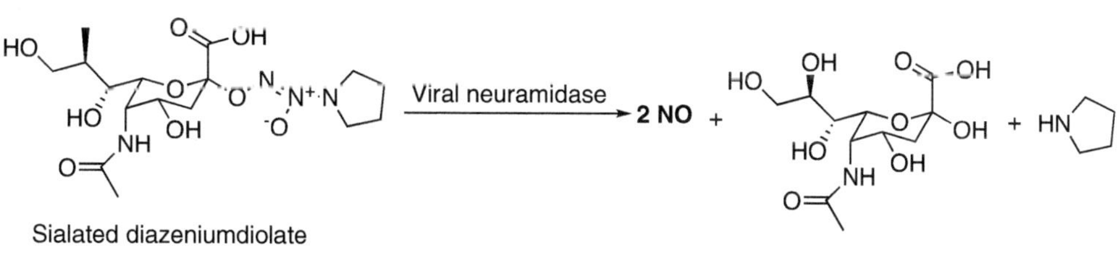


**Figure 10.15** Investigational viral-targeted sialated diazeniumdiolate.

other organs, for example, liver and colon, has been successfully provided by enzyme-activated prodrug strategies.

In prodrug design, the site-selective drug delivery is commonly achieved by unique tissue/organ-specific enzymes or by endogenous enzymes with significant over-expression in target tissue/organ. However, the ubiquitous distribution of several endogenous enzymes responsible for bioactivation of prodrug candidates hinders the possibilities of selective activation, and consequently, the targeting. Therefore, the prodrug approaches that rely on bioactivation by exogenous enzymes delivered selectively via monoclonal antibodies (ADEPT), genes (GDEPT), or viruses (VDEPT) have received considerable attention over the last decade especially in cancer therapy.

Increasing understanding in molecular biology beyond different disease processes may reveal completely new targets for site-selective enzyme-activated prodrug strategies in the future. For example, development of prodrug candidates those are bioactivated by the increased activity of tumor endoproteases, proteolytic enzymes that play important role in tumor invasion and metastasis [114, 115], may prove potential and provide promise for tumor-targeted prodrug approaches.

## Acknowledgment

Academy of Finland is acknowledged for the grants 108569 and 214334 (KL).

## References

1 Bodor, N. and Buchwald, P. (1999) Recent advances in the brain targeting of neuropharmaceuticals by chemical delivery systems. *Advanced Drug Delivery Reviews*, **36**, 229–254.

2 Bodor, N. and Buchwald, P. (2002) Barriers to remember: brain-targeting chemical delivery systems and Alzheimer's disease. *Drug Discovery Today*, **7**, 766–774.

3 Gynther, M. *et al.* (2008) Large neutral amino acid transporter enables brain drug delivery via prodrugs. *Journal of Medicinal Chemistry*, **51**, 932–936.

4 Testa, B. (2009) Prodrugs: bridging pharmacodynamic/pharmacokinetic gaps. *Current Opinion in Chemical Biology*, **13**, 338–344.

5 Atkinson, J.M., Siller, C.S., and Gill, J.H. (2008) Tumour endoproteases: the cutting edge of cancer drug delivery? *British Journal of Pharmacology*, **153**, 1344–1352.

6 de Groot, V.F.M.H. (2007) in *Prodrugs: Challenges and Rewards* (eds. V.J. Stella *et al.*.), AAPS Press, Springer, New York, pp. 447–506.

7 Stella V.J. and Himmelstein, K.J. (1985) *Design of Prodrugs* (ed. H. Bundgaard), Elsevier Science Publishers BV, Amsterdam, pp. 177–198.

8 Stella, V.J. and Himmelstein, K.J. (1985) *Directed Drug Delivery* (eds R.T. Borchardt, A.J., Repta, and V.J. Stella), Humana Press, Clifton, NJ, pp. 247–267.

9 Denny F W.A. (2004) Tumor-activated prodrugs: a new approach to cancer therapy. *Cancer Investigation*, **22**, 604–619.

10 Huang, P.S. and Oliff, A. (2001) Drug-targeting strategies in cancer therapy. *Current Opinion in Genetics & Development*, **11**, 104–110.

11 Brahimi-Horn, M.C., Chiche, J., Pouyssegur, J., and Hypoxia and, cancer.

(2007) *Journal of Molecular Medicine*, **85**, 1301–1307.

12 Brown, J.M. (1999) The hypoxic cell: a target for selective cancer therapy: eighteenth Bruce F. Cain Memorial Award lecture. *Cancer Research*, **59**, 5863–5870.

13 Denny, W.A. (2001) Prodrug strategies in cancer therapy. *European Journal of Medicinal Chemistry*, **36**, 577–595.

14 Jaffar, M., Williams, K.J., and Stratford, I.J. (2001) Bioreductive and gene therapy approaches to hypoxic diseases. *Advanced Drug Delivery Reviews*, **53**, 217–228.

15 Patterson, A.V. *et al.* (1995) Importance of P450 reductase activity in determining sensitivity of breast tumour cells to the bioreductive drug, tirapazamine (SR 4233). *British Journal of Cancer*, **72**, 1144–1150.

16 Saunders, M.P., Patterson, A.V., Chinje, E.C., Harris, A.L., and Stratford, I.J. (2000) NADPH: cytochrome c (P450) reductase activates tirapazamine (SR4233) to restore hypoxic and oxic cytotoxicity in an aerobic resistant derivative of the A549 lung cancer cell line. *British Journal of Cancer*, **82**, 651–656.

17 Lloyd, R.V., Duling, D.R., Rumyantseva, G.V., Mason, R.P., and Bridson, P.K. (1991) Microsomal reduction of 3-amino-1,2,4-benzotriazine 1,4-dioxide to a free radical. *Molecular Pharmacology*, **40**, 440–445.

18 Anderson, R.F., Shinde, S.S., Hay, M.P., Gamage, S.A., and Denny, W.A. (2003) Activation of 3-amino-1,2,4-benzotriazine 1,4-dioxide antitumor agents to oxidizing species following their one-electron reduction. *Journal of the American Chemical Society*, **125**, 748–756.

19 Elwell, J.H., Siim, B.G., Evans, J.W., and Brown, J.M. (1997) Adaptation of human tumor cells to tirapazamine under aerobic conditions: implications of increased antioxidant enzyme activity to mechanism of aerobic cytotoxicity. *Biochemical Pharmacology*, **54**, 249–257.

20 Zeman, E.M., Brown, J.M., Lemmon, M.J., Hirst, V.K., and Lee, W.W. (1986) SR-4233: a new bioreductive agent with high selective toxicity for hypoxic mammalian cells. *International Journal of Radiation Oncology, Biology, Physics*, **12**, 1239–1242.

21 Durand, R.E. and Olive, P.L. (1997) Physiologic and cytotoxic effects of tirapazamine in tumor-bearing mice. *Radiation Oncology Investigations*, **5**, 213–219.

22 Olive, P.L. (1995) Detection of hypoxia by measurement of DNA damage in individual cells from spheroids and murine tumours exposed to bioreductive drugs. I. Tirapazamine. *British Journal of Cancer*, **71**, 529–536.

23 Patterson, A.V. *et al.* (2007) Mechanism of action and preclinical antitumor activity of the novel hypoxia-activated DNA cross-linking agent PR-104. *Clinical Cancer Research*, **13**, 3922–3932.

24 Guise, C.P. *et al.* (2007) Identification of human reductases that activate the dinitrobenzamide mustard prodrug PR-104A: a role for NADPH: cytochrome P450 oxidoreductase under hypoxia. *Biochemical Pharmacology*, **74**, 810–820.

25 Singleton, R.S. *et al.* (2009) DNA cross-links in human tumor cells exposed to the prodrug PR-104A: relationships to hypoxia, bioreductive metabolism, and cytotoxicity. *Cancer Research*, **69**, 3884–3891.

26 Speckamp, W.N. and Oostveen, E.A. (1992) United States Patent 5079257.

27 Bailey, S.M. *et al.* (1998) Reduction of the indoloquinone anticancer drug EO9 by purified DT-diaphorase: a detailed kinetic study and analysis of metabolites. *Biochemical Pharmacology*, **56**, 613–621.

28 Bailey, S.M. *et al.* (2001) Involvement of NADPH: cytochrome P450 reductase in the activation of indoloquinone EO9 to free radical and DNA damaging species. *Biochemical Pharmacology*, **62**, 461–468.

29 Hendriks, H.R. *et al.* (1993) EO9: a novel bioreductive alkylating indoloquinone with preferential solid tumour activity and lack of bone marrow toxicity in preclinical models. *European Journal of Cancer*, **29A**, 897–906.

30 Knox, R.J., Friedlos, F., Marchbank, T., and Roberts, J.J. (1991) Bioactivation of CB1954: reaction of the active

4-hydroxylamino derivative with thioesters to form the ultimate DNA–DNA interstrand crosslinking species. *Biochemical Pharmacology*, **42**, 1691–1697.

**31** Helsby, N.A., Ferry, D.M., Patterson, A.V., Pullen, S.M., and Wilson, W.R. (2004) 2-Amino metabolites are key mediators of CB1954 and SN 23862 bystander effects in nitroreductase GDEPT. *British Journal of Cancer*, **90**, 1084–1092.

**32** Knox, R.J. *et al.* (2000) Bioactivation of 5-(aziridin-1-yl)-2,4-dinitrobenzamide (CB1954) by human NAD(P)H quinone oxidoreductase 2: a novel co-substrate-mediated antitumor prodrug therapy. *Cancer Research*, **60**, 4179–4186.

**33** Anlezark, G.M. *et al.* (1992) The bioactivation of 5-(aziridin-1-yl)-2,4-dinitrobenzamide (CB1954). I. Purification and properties of a nitroreductase enzyme from *Escherichia coli*: a potential enzyme for antibody-directed enzyme prodrug therapy (ADEPT). *Biochemical Pharmacology*, **44**, 2289–2295.

**34** Chandor, A. *et al.* (2008) Metabolic activation of the antitumor drug 5-(aziridin-1-yl)-2,4-dinitrobenzamide (CB1954) by NO synthases. *Chemical Research in Toxicology*, **21**, 836–843.

**35** Knox, R.J. *et al.* (1988) The nitroreductase enzyme in Walker cells that activates 5-(aziridin-1-yl)-2,4-dinitrobenzamide (CB1954) to 5-(aziridin-1-yl)-4-hydroxylamino-2-nitrobenzamide is a form of NAD(P)H dehydrogenase (quinone) (EC 1. 6. 99. 2). *Biochemical Pharmacology*, **37**, 4671–4677.

**36** Workman, P., White, R.A., and Talbot, K. (1986) CB1954 revisited. I. Disposition kinetics and metabolism. *Cancer Chemotherapy and Pharmacology*, **16**, 1–8.

**37** Patterson, L.H. and McKeown, S.R. (2000) AQ4N: a new approach to hypoxia-activated cancer chemotherapy. *British Journal of Cancer*, **83**, 1589–1593.

**38** Albertella, M.R. *et al.* (2008) Hypoxia-selective targeting by the bioreductive ProDrug AQ4N in patients with solid tumors: results of a Phase I study. *Clinical Cancer Research*, **14**, 1096–1104.

**39** Tredan, O., Garbens, A.B., Lalani, A.S., and Tannock, I.F. (2009) The hypoxia-activated ProDrug AQ4N penetrates deeply in tumor tissues and complements the limited distribution of mitoxantrone. *Cancer Research*, **69**, 940–947.

**40** Lyttle, M.H. *et al.* (1994) Glutathione-*S*-transferase activates novel alkylating agents. *Journal of Medicinal Chemistry*, **37**, 1501–1507.

**41** Satyam, A. *et al.* (1996) Design, synthesis, and evaluation of latent alkylating agents activated by glutathione *S*-transferase. *Journal of Medicinal Chemistry*, **39**, 1736–1747.

**42** Rosario, L.A., O'Brien, M.L., Henderson, C.J., Wolf, C.R., and Tew, K.D. (2000) Cellular response to a glutathione *S*-transferase P1-1 activated prodrug. *Molecular Pharmacology*, **58**, 167–174.

**43** Townsend, D.M. and Tew, K.D. (2003) The role of glutathione-*S*-transferase in anti-cancer drug resistance. *Oncogene*, **22**, 7369–7375.

**44** Chakrapani, H. *et al.* (2008) Synthesis and *in vitro* anti-leukemic activity of structural analogues of JS-K, an anti-cancer lead compound. *Bioorganic & Medicinal Chemistry Letters*, **18**, 950–953.

**45** Shami, P.J. *et al.* (2003) JS-K, a glutathione/glutathione *S*-transferase-activated nitric oxide donor of the diazeniumdiolate class with potent antineoplastic activity. *Molecular Cancer Therapeutics*, **2**, 409–417.

**46** Shami, P.J. *et al.* (2006) Antitumor activity of JS-K [$O^2$-(2,4-dinitrophenyl) 1-[(4-ethoxycarbonyl)piperazin-1-yl]diazen-1-ium-1,2-diolate] and related $O^2$-aryl diazeniumdiolates *in vitro* and *in vivo*. *Journal of Medicinal Chemistry*, **49**, 4356–4366.

**47** Chakrapani, H. *et al.* (2008) Synthesis, mechanistic studies, and anti-proliferative activity of glutathione/glutathione *S*-transferase-activated nitric oxide prodrugs. *Bioorganic and Medicinal Chemistry*, **16**, 9764–9771.

**48** Miwa, M. *et al.* (1998) Design of a novel oral fluoropyrimidine carbamate, capecitabine, which generates 5-fluorouracil selectively in tumours by enzymes concentrated in human liver and cancer tissue. *European Journal of Cancer*, **34**, 1274–1281.

**49** Budman, D.R. (2000) Capecitabine. *Investment in New Drugs*, **18**, 355–363.

**50** Ebi, H. *et al.* (2005) Pharmacokinetic and pharmacodynamic comparison of fluoropyrimidine derivatives, capecitabine and 5′-deoxy-5-fluorouridine (5′-DFUR). *Cancer Chemotherapy and Pharmacology*, **56**, 205–211.

**51** Ishikawa, T. *et al.* (1998) Tumor selective delivery of 5-fluorouracil by capecitabine, a new oral fluoropyrimidine carbamate, in human cancer xenografts. *Biochemical Pharmacology*, **55**, 1091–1097.

**52** Mader, R.M. *et al.* (2003) Penetration of capecitabine and its metabolites into malignant and healthy tissues of patients with advanced breast cancer. *British Journal of Cancer*, **88**, 782–787.

**53** Wong, M., Choo, S.P., and Tan, E.H. (2009) Travel warning with capecitabine. *Annals of Oncology*, **20**, 1281.

**54** Boyer, T.D., Wright, W.L., and Manns, M.P. (2006) *Zakim and Boyer's Hepatology: A Textbook of Liver Diseases*, Elsevier, Inc., Philadelphia, PA.

**55** Worman, H.J. (2006) *The Liver Disorders and Hepatic Sourcebook*, McGraw-Hill, Inc., New York, NY.

**56** Guengerich, F.P. (2001) Common and uncommon cytochrome P450 reactions related to metabolism and chemical toxicity. *Chemical Research in Toxicology*, **14**, 611–650.

**57** Lewis, D.F. and Dickins, M. (2002) Substrate SARs in human P450s. *Drug Discovery Today*, **7**, 918–925

**58** Nebert, D.W. and Russell, D.W. (2002) Clinical importance of the cytochromes P450. *Lancet*, **360**, 1155–1162.

**59** Smith, D.A., Ackland, M.J., and Jones, B.C. (1997) Properties of cytochrome P450 isoenzymes and their substrates. Part 1. Active site characteristics. *Drug Discovery Today*, **2**, 406–414.

**60** Ettmayer, P., Amidon, G.L., Clement, B., and Testa, B. (2004) Lessons learned from marketed and investigational prodrugs. *Journal of Medicinal Chemistry*, **47**, 2393–2404.

**61** Bruno, R.D. and Njar, V.C. (2007) Targeting cytochrome P450 enzymes: a new approach in anti-cancer drug development. *Bioorganic and Medicinal Chemistry*, **15**, 5047–5060.

**62** Pelkonen, O. *et al.* (2008) Inhibition and induction of human cytochrome P450 enzymes: current status. *Archives of Toxicology*, **82**, 667–715.

**63** Boyer, S.H. *et al.* (2006) Synthesis and characterization of a novel liver-targeted prodrug of cytosine-1-beta-D-arabinofuranoside monophosphate for the treatment of hepatocellular carcinoma. *Journal of Medicinal Chemistry*, **49**, 7711–7720.

**64** Erion, M.D. *et al.* (2007) Targeting thyroid hormone receptor-beta agonists to the liver reduces cholesterol and triglycerides and improves the therapeutic index. *Proceedings of the National Academy of Sciences of the United States of America*, **104**, 15490–15495.

**65** Erion, M.D. *et al.* (2004) Design, synthesis, and characterization of a series of cytochrome P(450) 3A-activated prodrugs (HepDirect prodrugs) useful for targeting phosph(on)ate-based drugs to the liver. *Journal of the American Chemical Society*, **126**, 5154–5163.

**66** Erion, M.D. *et al.* (2005) Liver-targeted drug delivery using HepDirect prodrugs. *The Journal of Pharmacology and Experimental Therapeutics*, **312**, 554–560.

**67** Hecker, S.J. *et al.* (2007) Liver-targeted prodrugs of 2′-*C*-methyladenosine for therapy of hepatitis C virus infection. *Journal of Medicinal Chemistry*, **50**, 3891–3896.

**68** Reddy, K.R. *et al.* (2008) Pradefovir: a prodrug that targets adefovir to the liver for the treatment of hepatitis B. *Journal of Medicinal Chemistry*, **51**, 666–676.

**69** Dando, T. and Plosker, G. (2003) Adefovir dipivoxil: a review of its use in chronic hepatitis B. *Drugs*, **63**, 2215–2234.

**70** Erion, M.D., Bullough, D.A., Lin, C.C., and Hong, Z. (2006) HepDirect prodrugs for targeting nucleotide-based antiviral drugs to the liver. *Current Opinion in Investigational Drugs*, **7**, 109–117.

**71** Tillmann, H.L. (2007) Pradefovir, a liver-targeted prodrug of adefovir against HBV infection. *Current Opinion in Investigational Drugs*, **8** 682–690.

**72** Huttunen, K.M. *et al.* (2007) Novel cyclic phosphate prodrug approach for cytochrome P450-activated drugs containing an alcohol functionality. *Pharmaceutical Research*, **24**, 679–687.

**73** Stein, A. and Wild, J. (2002) *Kidney Failure Explained*, Class Publishing, London, UK.

**74** Benner, B.M. (2004) *Benner & Rector's The Kidney*, Elsevier, Inc., Philadelphia, PA.

**75** Haas, M., Moolenaar, F., Meijer, D.K., and de Zeeuw, D. (2002) Specific drug delivery to the kidney. *Cardiovascular Drugs Therapeutics*, **16**, 489–496.

**76** Barthelmebs, M., Caillette, A., Ehrhardt, J.D., Velly, J., and Imbs, J.L. (1990) Metabolism and vascular effects of gamma-L-glutamyl-L-dopa on the isolated rat kidney. *Kidney International*, **37**, 1414–1422.

**77** Drieman, J.C. *et al.* (1994) Regional haemodynamic effects of dopamine and its prodrugs L-dopa and gludopa in the rat and in the glycerol-treated rat as a model for acute renal failure. *British Journal of Pharmacology*, **111**, 1117–1122.

**78** Wilk, S., Mizoguchi, H., and Orlowski, M. (1978) gamma-Glutamyl dopa: a kidney-specific dopamine precursor. *The Journal of Pharmacology and Experimental Therapeutics*, **206**, 227–232.

**79** Lee, M.R. (1990) Five years' experience with gamma-L-glutamyl-L-dopa: a relatively renally specific dopaminergic prodrug in man. *Journal of Autonomic Pharmacology*, **10** (Suppl. 1), S103–S108.

**80** Drieman, J.C., Thijssen, H.H., and Struyker-Boudier, H.A. (1990a) Renal selective *N*-acetyl-gamma-glutamyl prodrugs. II. Carrier-mediated transport and intracellular conversion as determinants in the renal selectivity of *N*-acetyl-gamma-glutamyl sulfamethoxazole. *The Journal of Pharmacology and Experimental Therapeutics*, **252**, 1255–1260.

**81** Drieman, J.C., Thijssen, H.H., Zeegers, H.H., Smits, J.F., and Struyker Boudier, H.A. (1990b) Renal selective *N*-acetyl-gamma-glutamyl prodrugs: a study on the mechanism of activation of the renal vasodilator prodrug CGP 22979. *British Journal of Pharmacology*, **99**, 15–20.

**82** Orlowski, M., Mizoguchi, H., and Wilk, S. (1980) N-Acyl-gamma-glutamyl derivatives of sulfamethoxazole as models of kidney-selective prodrugs. *The Journal of Pharmacology and Experimental Therapeutics*, **212**, 167–172.

**83** Drieman, J.C. and Thijssen, H.H. (1991) Renal selective *N*-acetyl-L-gamma-glutamyl prodrugs. III. *N*-Acetyl-L-gamma-glutamyl-4′-aminowarfarin is not targeted to the kidney but is selectively excreted into the bile. *The Journal of Pharmacology and Experimental Therapeutics*, **259**, 766–771.

**84** Drieman, J.C., Thijssen, H.H., and Struyker-Boudier, H.A. (1993) Renal selective *N*-acetyl-L-gamma-glutamyl prodrugs: studies on the selectivity of some model prodrugs. *British Journal of Pharmacology*, **108**, 204–208.

**85** Elfarra, A.A., Duescher, R.J., Hwang, I.Y., Sicuri, A.R., and Nelson, J.A. (1995) Targeting 6-thioguanine to the kidney with *S*-(guanin-6-yl)-L-cysteine. *The Journal of Pharmacology and Experimental Therapeutics*, **274**, 1298–1304.

**86** Elfarra, A.A. and Hwang, I.Y. (1993) Targeting of 6-mercaptopurine to the kidneys. Metabolism and kidney-selectivity of *S*-(6-purinyl)-L-cysteine analogs in rats. *Drug Metabolism and Disposition: The Biological Fate of Chemicals*, **21**, 841–845.

**87** Hwang, I.Y., and Elfarra, A.A. (1989) Cysteine *S*-conjugates may act as kidney-selective prodrugs: formation of 6-mercaptopurine by the renal metabolism of *S*-(6-purinyl)-L-cysteine. *The Journal of Pharmacology and Experimental Therapeutics*, **251**, 448–454.

**88** Hwang, I.Y. and Elfarra, A.A. (1991) Kidney-selective prodrugs of 6-mercaptopurine: biochemical basis of the kidney selectivity of *S*-(6-purinyl)-L-cysteine and metabolism of new analogs in rats. *The Journal of Pharmacology and Experimental Therapeutics*, **258**, 171–177.

**89** Andreadou, I., Menge, W.M., Commandeur, J.N., Worthington, E.A., and Vermeulen, N.P. (1996) Synthesis of novel Se-substituted selenocysteine derivatives as potential kidney selective prodrugs of biologically active selenol compounds: evaluation of kinetics of beta-elimination reactions in rat renal cytosol. *Journal of Medicinal Chemistry*, **39**, 2040–2046.

90 Commandeur, J.N. *et al.* (2000) Bioactivation of selenocysteine Se-conjugates by a highly purified rat renal cysteine conjugate beta-lyase/glutamine transaminase K. *The Journal of Pharmacology and Experimental Therapeutics*, **294**, 753–761.

91 Rooseboom, M., Vermeulen, N.P., Andreadou, I., and Commandeur, J.N. (2000) Evaluation of the kinetics of beta-elimination reactions of selenocysteine Se conjugates in human renal cytosol: possible implications for the use as kidney selective prodrugs. *The Journal of Pharmacology and Experimental Therapeutics*, **294**, 762–769.

92 Zonderman, J. and Vender, R. (2000) *Understanding Crohn Disease and Ulcerative Colitis*, University Press of Mississippi, Jackson, MS.

93 Adrouny, A.R. (2002) *Understanding Colon Cancer*, University Press of Mississippi, Jackson, MS.

94 Chourasia, M.K. and Jain, S.K. (2003) Pharmaceutical approaches to colon targeted drug delivery systems. *Journal of Pharmacy & Pharmaceutical Sciences*, **6**, 33–66.

95 Friend, D.R. (2005) New oral delivery systems for treatment of inflammatory bowel disease. *Advanced Drug Delivery Reviews*, **57**, 247–265.

96 Scheline, R.R. (1973) Metabolism of foreign compounds by gastrointestinal microorganisms. *Pharmacological Reviews*, **25**, 451–523.

97 Azadkhan, A.K., Truelove, S.C., and Aronson, J.K. (1982) The disposition and metabolism of sulphasalazine (salicylazosulphapyridine) in man. *British Journal of Clinical Pharmacology*, **13**, 523–528.

98 Van Hees, P.A. *et al.* (1981) Effect of sulphasalazine in patients with active Crohn's disease: a controlled double-blind study. *Gut*, **22**, 404–409.

99 Willoughby, C.P., Aronson, J.K., Agback, H., Bodin, N.O., and Truelove, S.C. (1982) Distribution and metabolism in healthy volunteers of disodium azodisalicylate, a potential therapeutic agent for ulcerative colitis. *Gut*, **23**, 1081–1087.

100 van Hogezand, R.A., van Hees, P.A., Zwanenburg, B., van Rossum, J.M., and van Tongeren, J.H. (1985) Disposition of disodium azodisalicylate in healthy subjects. A possible new drug for inflammatory bowel disease. *Gastroenterology*, **88**, 717–722.

101 McIntyre, P.B. *et al.* (1988) Balsalazide in the maintenance treatment of patients with ulcerative colitis, a double-blind comparison with sulphasalazine. *Alimentary Pharmacology & Therapeutics*, **2**, 237–243.

102 Friend, D.R. and Chang, G.W. (1984) A colon-specific drug-delivery system based on drug glycosides and the glycosidases of colonic bacteria. *Journal of Medicinal Chemistry*, **27**, 261–266.

103 Haeberlin, B., Rubas, W., Nolen, H.W., and 3rd & Friend, D.R. (1993) *In vitro* evaluation of dexamethasone-beta-D-glucuronide for colon-specific drug delivery. *Pharmaceutical Research*, **10**, 1553–1562.

104 Ruiz, J.F. *et al.* (2009) Design, synthesis, and pharmacological effects of a cyclization-activated steroid prodrug for colon targeting in inflammatory bowel disease. *Journal of Medicinal Chemistry*, **52**, 3205–3211.

105 El-Kamel, A.H., Abdel-Aziz, A.A., Fatani, A.J., and El-Subbagh, H.I. (2008) Oral colon targeted delivery systems for treatment of inflammatory bowel diseases: synthesis, *in vitro* and *in vivo* assessment. *International Journal of Pharmaceutics*, **358**, 248–255.

106 Jung, Y.J., Lee, J.S., and Kim, Y.M. (2001) Colon-specific prodrugs of 5-aminosalicylic acid: synthesis and *in vitro*/*in vivo* properties of acidic amino acid derivatives of 5-aminosalicylic acid. *Journal of Pharmaceutical Sciences*, **90**, 1767–1775.

**107** Koonin, E.V., Senkevich, T.G., and Dolja, V.V. (2006) The ancient Virus World and evolution of cells. *Biology Direct*, **1**, 29.

**108** Mackman, R.L. *et al.* (2007) Synthesis, anti-HIV activity, and resistance profile of thymidine phosphonomethoxy nucleosides and their bis-isopropyloxymethylcarbonyl (bisPOC) prodrugs. *Bioorganic and Medicinal Chemistry*, **15**, 5519–5528.

**109** Rossi, L. *et al.* (2005) Targeting nucleotide dimers containing antiviral nucleosides. *Current Medicinal Chemistry*, **4**, 37–54.

**110** Elion, G.B. *et al.* (1977) Selectivity of action of an antiherpetic agent, 9-(2-hydroxyethoxymethyl) guanine. *Proceedings of the National Academy of Sciences of the United States of America*, **74**, 5716–5720.

**111** Cai, T.B., Lu, D., Landerholm, M., and Wang, P.G. (2004) Sialated diazeniumdiolate: a new sialidase-activated nitric oxide donor. *Organic Letters*, **6**, 4203–4205.

**112** Torre, D., Pugliese, A., and Speranza, F. (2002) Role of nitric oxide in HIV-1 infection: friend or foe? *Lancet Infectious Diseases*, **2**, 273–280.

**113** Stella, V.J. (2004) Prodrugs as therapeutics. *Expert Opinion on Therapeutic Patents*, **14**, 277–280.

**114** Deryugina, E.I., and Quigley, J.P. (2006) Matrix metalloproteinases and tumor metastasis. *Cancer Metastasis Reviews*, **25**, 9–34.

**115** Takahashi, H. *et al.* (2007) Antiproteases in preventing the invasive potential of pancreatic cancer cells. *Journal of Pancreas*, **8**, 501–508.

# 11
# Prodrug Approaches for Central Nervous System Delivery

*Quentin R. Smith and Paul R. Lockman*

## 11.1
## Blood–Brain Barrier in CNS Drug Development

The central nervous system (CNS) offers special opportunities and challenges for prodrug design and development. Critical among the opportunities is the wide range of neurotransmitter and neuromodulator systems in the CNS that provide attractive targets for drug therapy. Some of these systems are present in different extents in the peripheral nervous system and other organs; hence, selective targeting to the CNS is beneficial. Further, the brain is the site of a broad range of psychiatric, neurologic, and or neurodegenerative disorders, many of which are chronic, have a component that is genetic or inheritable, and currently have no curative therapy with treatment mainly palliative to control symptoms. Based upon figures published by the National Institutes of Health, one of three individuals suffers from a diagnosable CNS disorder in any given year. CNS disorders represent 5 of the top 10 causes of disability and constitute >20% of total health care spending in the United States. Further, the number of individuals with CNS disorders is increasing in many countries as populations age [1]. The CNS drug market (>\$55 U.S. billion in 2005) is second only to the cardiovascular drug market in total drug sales [2]. However, CNS drugs take longer on average to get to market and have lower success rates relative to other drug classes.

Many factors contribute to the challenge of CNS drug development. Included among these are the unique properties of the "blood–brain barrier" (BBB). The brain, unlike most organs, has a highly selective and restrictive molecular permeability interface between the circulation and the brain interstitial space, which impedes the exchange of most solutes between the blood and the CNS [3]. The BBB is formed at the cellular level by the cerebral vascular endothelium that is joined together by high resistance tight junctions (>1500 ohm $cm^2$) [4]. These tight junctions, formed by the proteins occludin and claudin, effectively seal off the aqueous paracellular channels between brain endothelial cells, forcing most drugs and other solutes to cross by the transcellular route [5, 6]. Thus, for a drug to pass readily into brain from the

*Prodrugs and Targeted Delivery: Towards Better ADME Properties.* Edited by Jarkko Rautio

ISBN: 978-3-527-32603-7

circulation, it must either have the appropriate physiochemical properties related to lipid solubility, polarity, ionic charge, and size to readily dissolve and diffuse across the lipophilic cell membranes of the brain vasculature [7] or be transported across the endothelium by one of >20 or more active or facilitated carrier systems that are expressed in brain endothelial cells at high levels [8]. Diazepam is one drug that readily crosses the BBB by passive lipid diffusion across brain vascular endothelial cells. It has moderate lipophilicity (log $D_{\text{octanol/saline pH 7.4}} = 3$), neutral charge, and low molecular weight (<400), all factors favoring good BBB penetration [9]. Further, it does not appear to be a substrate of an active BBB drug efflux carrier, such as P-glycoprotein (Pgp), breast cancer resistance protein (BCRP), or multidrug associate resistance proteins (MRP 1–7) or organic anion transporter 3 (OAT3). All of these transporters have been shown to mediate active drug efflux out of the CNS, leading to lower free drug levels in brain interstitial fluid than serum free drug concentration. As a consequence, diazepam equilibrates in brain rapidly (<15 min) after systemic administration at brain free levels equivalent to serum free drug concentration [10]. The total brain concentration exceeds that free in serum at steady state by about 20-fold due to diazepam binding to CNS protein and membranes. Overall, from comparison of common properties of CNS active drugs, Lipinski recommended the "rule of five" for good CNS exposure [7]:

- 3 or fewer H-bond donors (OHs, NHs)
- 6 or fewer H-bond acceptors (Os and Ns)
- Molecular weight is <400
- c log $P < 5$
- Low active efflux transporter affinity

Other drugs with good BBB penetration and distribution properties include ethanol (alcohol), nicotine, caffeine, antipyrine, chlorpromazine, imipramine, propranolol, naproxen, paroxetine, flunitrazepam, and valproate [9]. Most of these drugs have moderate lipophilicity (log $D_{\text{octanol/saline pH 7.4}} = 0\text{–}3$) and are either neutral or reversible anions or cations (with a measurable neutral fraction).

Drugs with limited brain distribution often exhibit one or more of the following properties:

- High molecular weight (>1000–1 000 000 Da)
- Permanent charge (e.g., quaternary nitrogen)
- Polar with reduced lipophilicity and enhanced hydrogen bonding (e.g., sucrose)
- Substrate for one or more active efflux transporters

Strongly polar compounds, such as sucrose, inulin (3–5 kDa) or dextrans (3–2000 kDa), cross the BBB to only a limited degree and are rapidly removed from brain interstitial fluid by the CSF sink effect [11]. Therefore, their brain levels fail to reach that of plasma even after long exposure periods. Among active efflux transporters, Pgp, BCRP, MRP4, and OAT3 all have been shown to be expressed at high levels at the BBB [12] and to have critical roles in limiting brain exposure for many agents [8]. For example, BBB active efflux transport has been shown to restrict brain exposure of cardiovascular (e.g., digoxin, quinidine, verapamil, and lovastatin), immunologic (e.g., cortisol, dexamethasone, and cyclosporine), anticancer (e.g., paclitaxel, methotrexate, vinblastine, doxorubicin, and lapatinib), anti-infective (ivermectin, erythromycin, and aprenavir), opioid (morphine, methadone, fentanyl, and loperamide), and antiepileptic (phenytoin) compounds [13]. Pgp transports a broad array of compounds, favoring agents with $>8$ (N + O)s, $>400$ MW, and $pK_a > 4$ [14]. The MRPs are a family of transporters that mediate an equally broad array of substrates, including anions, drug conjugates (with glutathione, glucuronic acid, or sulfate), and nucleosides. For Pgp, BCRP, and MRP, active efflux is driven by hydrolysis of ATP to form ADP, whereas for other transporters (e.g., OAT3) net transport is driven by exchange with ions or other compounds.

As a result of low passive permeability and active efflux transport at the BBB >98% of new chemical entities have been reported to show poor penetration into brain [15]. Among critical new biologic agents (i.e., new therapeutic proteins, peptides, and nucleic acids with MW > 10 kDa), the percentage that shows poor delivery to brain is even higher (>99%). As a result, the BBB has been referred to as "the problem lurking behind the problem of CNS drug delivery" [16].

## 11.2 Prodrug Strategies

A primary focus of CNS prodrug strategies has been to improve drug uptake and targeting across the BBB followed by spontaneous or metabolic breakdown to release active agent that is preferentially retained in brain (Figure 11.1). In this manner, drug exposure of active agent is enhanced in the CNS and reduced in other organs that may be susceptible to toxic effects. In some instances, the primary problem has been getting active drug to the site of action within the CNS across the BBB. In other cases, selective expression of CNS or disease state enzymes has been utilized to catalyze local release of active agent.

Prodrugs are common in some fields, such as oncology, where a number of the key drugs are antimetabolites. These agents are taken up into cells and converted to active species by enzymes within the cytoplasm and nucleus. Classic examples include 5-fluorouracil, 6-mercaptopurine, and 6-thioguanine, which are converted within cells to antimetabolite nucleosides and nucleotides that interfere with nucleic acid and protein synthesis and function. They target cancer cells with elevated rates of protein synthesis and mitosis. Capecitabine is a more recently developed prodrug of 5-fluorouracil, which relies on two additional steps, one of which is preferentially upregulated in tumor cells, to target 5-fluorouracil formation in cancer cells and limit exposure to normal cells.

Anticancer drug delivery is a particular problem for therapy of primary brain tumors and for brain metastases of systemic tumors, as the BBB expresses multiple efflux transporters that limit CNS exposure of nucleobases, nucleosides, and nucleotides used in cancer therapy, as well as most natural product chemotherapeutic agents, such as paclitaxel, doxorubicin, vincristine, methotrexate, and etoposide. Therefore, creative prodrug strategies are being explored to improve brain delivery of

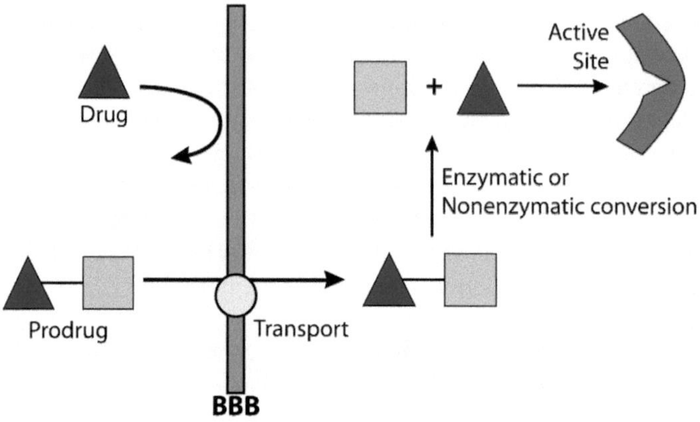


**Figure 11.1** Schematic model of prodrug strategy for drug delivery to the CNS utilizing a prodrug structure to facilitate transfer across the BBB. Once within the CNS compartment, the prodrug is then either enzymatically or nonenzymatically converted to active drug species that interacts at the active site.

chemotherapeutic drugs, as well as drugs from other classes, which show restricted delivery to the CNS. Included within this are antibiotic and antiviral agents, many of which show restricted distribution to brain for the treatment of CNS and meningeal infections.

A number of reviews have covered lipophilic CNS prodrugs that are converted preferentially within the CNS into trapped or active species based upon oxidation/reduction, esterase, or other enzymatic mechanisms [17–20]. Such approaches have some potential for targeting as the brain receives 15% of the cardiac output even though it comprises only 2% of body weight in humans. Thus, if the compound has high CNS extraction (>75% per single pass through the vascular bed) followed by rapid conversion to trapped or active species, the potential exists for selective CNS accumulation above that expected for distribution based upon organ size. However, enhanced lipophilicity, although it may improve passage across the BBB, is also associated with other problems, including rapid metabolic clearance, enhanced binding to plasma and tissue proteins, elevated volume of distribution, and increased affinity for active efflux transporters. Hence, in many cases, it may not improve the fraction of drug that distributes to brain, and in some cases, may actually be associated with marked reductions.

Therefore, this chapter will focus on newer prodrug strategies focused on preferential brain targeting based upon BBB carrier- or receptor-mediated transport. Over 20 carrier transporters have been identified at the cerebral capillaries of the BBB that mediate the brain uptake of various essential nutrients, vitamins, peptides, and hormones. This includes GLUT1 that transports D-glucose into brain for cerebral energy metabolism, as well as LAT1 and CAT1, which, respectively, transport essential large neutral and basic (cationic) amino acids into brain for protein synthesis and neurotransmitter (e.g., serotonin, dopamine, norepinephrine, and histamine) formation [8]. Further, the low-affinity choline transporter is also highly expressed at the BBB and mediates brain entry of the quarternary amine, choline, into brain for phospholipid and acetylcholine synthesis. Similarly, the BBB also expresses a large number of protein receptors, including low-density lipoprotein receptor-related protein (LRP1), insulin receptor, transferrin receptor, and diphtheria toxin receptor [21]. Drug delivery vectors have been created for each of these receptors using antibodies or selective substrates that bind and are transcytosed into brain across the BBB. Due to preferential BBB expression of these receptors and transporters, the potential exists for enhanced drug delivery and trapping by brain with reduced exposure and toxicity to other organs.

## 11.3 Prodrug Strategies Based Upon BBB Nutrient Transporters

Most plasma large neutral amino acids are taken up into brain by the sodium-independent, System LAT1 exchange transporter. This carrier was characterized initially by Oxender and Christensen [22] and was subsequently cloned by Kanai [23]. It mediates the brain uptake of >10 primary neutral amino acids in plasma [24] via saturable, stereospecific (preferring L > D), bidirectional and sodium/energy independent transport. Of the carriers at the BBB, System LAT1 displays several properties that make it well suited as a brain drug delivery vector. First, it has both a large maximal transport capacity ($V_{max}$ ~40–60 nmol/min/g) and an appreciable binding affinity (affinity ≈ $1/K_m$; $K_m$ = 10–200 μM) [25] so that rapid rates of blood–brain barrier exchange can be obtained ($K_{in} > 10^{-3}$ ml/s/g) with half times for brain equilibration of <15 min for high-affinity substrates. Second, it possesses fairly simple structural requirements for binding and accepts a wide variety of amino acid substrates [26]. And third, although the carrier mediates the brain uptake of essential amino acids that are required for brain metabolism, transient disruption in brain supply, as might occur with drug overdose, does not produce irreversible brain damage. This latter possibility may limit use of the cerebrovascular glucose transporter (GLUT1) as a drug delivery vector because of the critical need of the brain for a continuous supply of D-glucose for brain energy metabolism.

BBB System LAT1 has been shown to mediate brain delivery of L-DOPA as a dopamine precursor for the treatment of Parkinson's disease [27]. Dopamine normally exhibits very low uptake into brain across the BBB. The dopamine deficiency that occurs in Parkinson's disease can be treated with dopamine agonists that cross the BBB, but not with dopamine itself due to restricted diffusion of dopamine across the BBB. This dilemma was solved by administration of L-DOPA, which is shuttled across the BBB by System LAT1 and subsequently decarboxylated into dopamine by aromatic amino acid decarboxylase to create a successful therapy. Subsequently, this same carrier has been used for brain delivery of gabapentin and pregabalin.

System LAT1 offers special promise as a brain delivery vector for chemotherapeutic drugs as it is upregulated at the BBB in brain tumors [28, 29]. One prodrug therapy initially targeted in this direction is L-melphalan, the *para*-nitrogen mustard

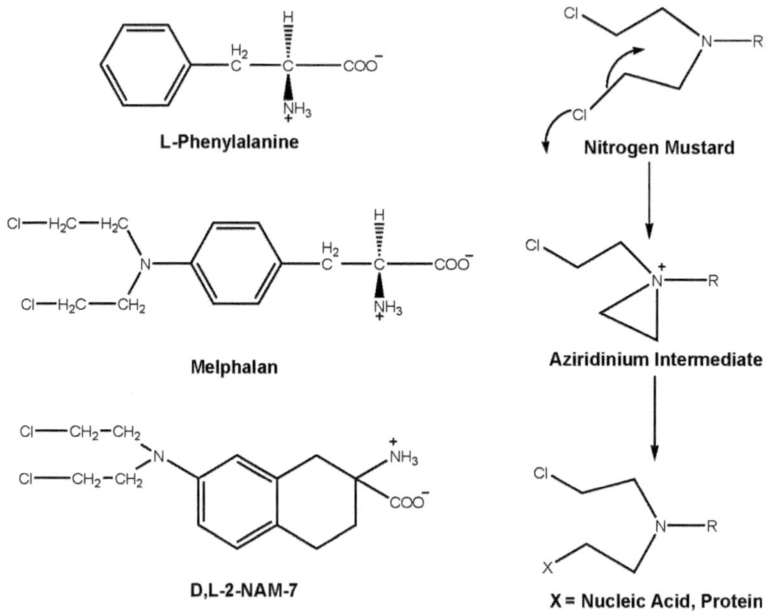


**Figure 11.2** Left: Structure of L-phenylalanine and L-phenylalanine nitrogen mustard analogues, melphalan and DL-2-NAM-7. Right: Schematic showing conversion of the nitrogen mustard to the active azridinium ions intermediate that alkylates electron-rich species including proteins and nucleic acids.

analogue of L-phenylalanine (Figure 11.2). L-Phenylalanine is an excellent substrate for BBB System LAT1 with a $K_m = 11 \pm 1\,\mu M$ and a $V_{max}$ of $41 \pm 2$ nmol/min/g [25, 30]. However, melphalan is a weak substrate for System LAT1, with >10-fold-reduced affinity and 8-fold lower $V_{max}$ than L-phenylalanine. As a consequence, BBB "permeability" to melphalan is only 1% that of L-phenylalanine, leading to reduced brain accumulation and anticancer drug exposure [31].

Various strategies have been explored to enhance BBB melphalan transport across the BBB, including intra-arterial administration and amino acid lowering diets and enzymes [32, 33]. However, the poor transport affinity and capacity of System LAT1 for melphalan have proved limiting. In contrast, Haines *et al.* [34] proposed a tetralin analogue of melphalan with improved affinity for System LAT1. This compound, DL-2-NAM-7 (Figure 11.2), has 50-fold greater affinity ($K_m = 0.2 \pm 0.02\,\mu M$) for System LAT1 than melphalan with an effective BBB "permeability" within 2–3-fold of that of L-phenylalanine. It equilibrates in brain in 8–10 min, as compared to a 2 h $t_{1/2}$ for melphalan [30, 31].

Both melphalan and DL-2-NAM-7 are prodrugs, which enter brain and are converted sequentially into azridinium and carbonium ions on the nitrogen mustard that alkylate nucleic acids and proteins (Figure 11.2). Similarly, Gynther *et al.* [35] created a LAT1 prodrug of the NSAID ketoprofen (Figure 11.3) based upon L-tyrosine with a BBB $K_m$ of $22 \pm 9\,\mu M$ and a $V_{max}$ of $1.4 \pm 0.15$ nmol/min/g. The compound was transported into rat brain by System LAT1 and subsequently

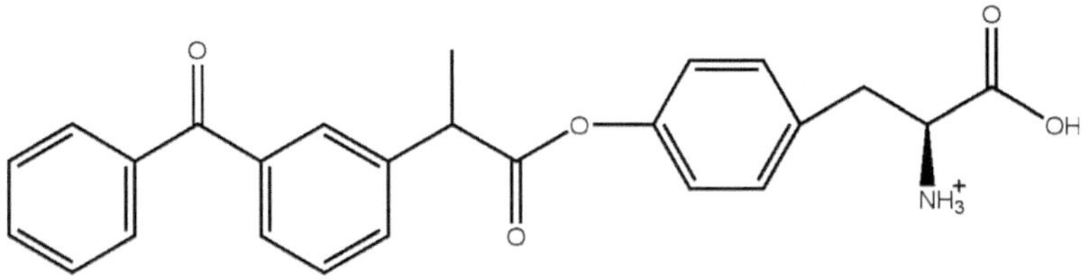


**Ketoprofen Tyrosine Prodrug**

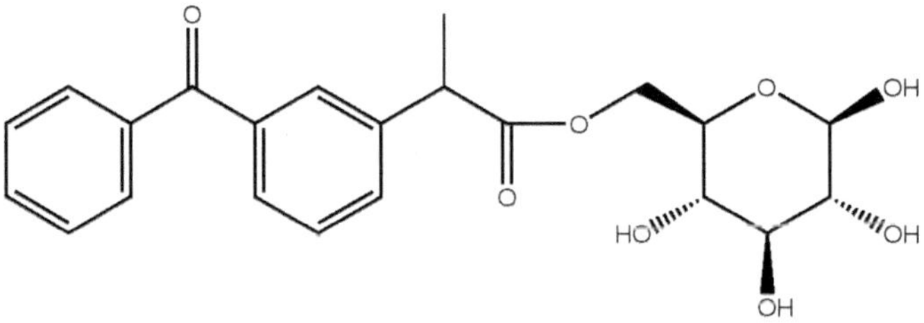


**Ketoprofen Glucose Prodrug**

**Figure 11.3** L-Tyrosine and D-glucose analogues of ketoprofen.

hydrolyzed in brain. The enzymatic hydrolysis followed an *in vitro* half-life of $4.4 \pm 1.8$ min in brain homogenate and $10.2 \pm 0.4$ min in serum. Similarly, Gynther *et al.* [36] prepared glucose analogues of ketoprofen and indomethacin that competitively reduced brain D-glucose uptake by GLUT1 and showed measurable uptake into brain.

BBB System LAT1 has also been used to achieve brain delivery of *N*-methyl-D-aspartate (NMDA) receptor antagonists, 7-chlorokynurenic acid and 5,7-dichlorokynurenic acid (Figure 11.4) [37]. These agents are the prototypic antagonists that helped define the glycine coagonist site of the NMDA receptor and show $\geq$ two orders of magnitude better potency and affinity ($1/K_i$) for the receptor than the nonspecific excitatory amino acid antagonist kynurenic acid [38, 39]. NMDA receptors play important roles in neuronal damage induced by excitatory amino acids following stroke, head injuries, and seizures, and have been suggested to contribute to cell death in several neurodegenerative diseases [40]. When administered directly into the CNS, 7-chlorokynurenic acid and 5,7-dichlorokynurenic acid are neuroprotective in models of excitotoxic injury and neurodegeneration. However, due to poor transport across the BBB, they show minimal passage into brain following systemic administration. Hokari *et al.* [41] demonstrated that systemic administration of kynurenic acid precursors, 4-chlorokynurenine and 4,6-dichlorokynurenine resulted in System LAT1 transport into brain followed by enzymatic conversion to the kynurenic acid products (Figure 11.5). Previous studies by the same group had shown saturable transport of L-kynurenine across the BBB [42]. Similar studies showed that transport of the chlorokynurenine precursors was self-saturable and inhibitable by L-leucine, characteristics consistent with BBB System LAT1 transport

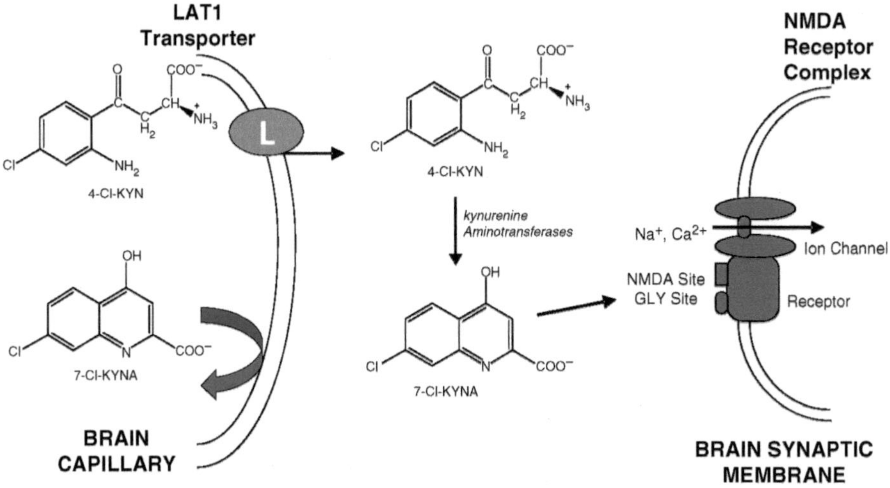


**Figure 11.4** Schematic model of L-kynurenine prodrug strategy showing 4-Cl-kynurenine transport across the BBB by system LAT1 and conversion within brain by the enzyme kynurenine aminotransferase to the active, neuroprotective species, 7-Cl-kynurenic acid.

(Figure 11.6). Best-fit kinetic estimates of BBB transport for 4-chlorokynurenine were $K_m = 105 \pm 14\,\mu M$ and $V_{max} = 17 \pm 2$ nmol/min/g [41]. 4,6-Dichlorokynurenine also showed concentration dependent inhibition of BBB System LAT1 L-leucine transport with a $K_i = 410 \pm 18\,\mu M$. Systemic administration of 4-chlorokynurenine resulted in measurable brain levels of both 4-chlorokynurenine and its metabolic product, 7-chlorokynurenic acid [41] (Figure 11.6). Subsequent studies have confirmed these findings under disease conditions, which augment the quantity of kynurenic acid product formed [43, 44].

Thus, these studies have demonstrated the efficacy of System LAT1 prodrug delivery across the BBB for the treatment of CNS diseases. Beyond L-DOPA, the strategy has been utilized for anticancer amino acid prodrugs (e.g., melphalan/NAM), and amino acid-NSAID conjugates, and precursors of neuroprotective kynurenic acids. Battaglia *et al.* [45] explored brain delivery of 7-chlorokynurenic acid using systemically administered 7-chlorokynurenic acid-D-glucose conjugates targeted toward the BBB GLUT1 transporter This strategy avoided CNS conversion of chlorokynurenine to the kynurenic acid active species. Further, the BBB GLUT1 transporter has greater capacity by >30-fold than the BBB LAT1 carrier. The authors demonstrated uptake of the prodrug and release of the free drug using the GLUT1 targeted strategy. However, as previously noted, the BBB GLUT1 transport system plays a critical role in brain delivery of glucose for cerebral energy metabolism. Therefore, this may not be the best BBB transport system to target for brain delivery, as overdose of the prodrug agent may compromise brain glucose supply, leading to cerebral hypoglycemia, seizures, or coma.

Similar to LAT1, the BBB choline transporter (CHT) has the ability to deliver both cationic prodrugs and its primary substrate choline to the CNS concurrently.

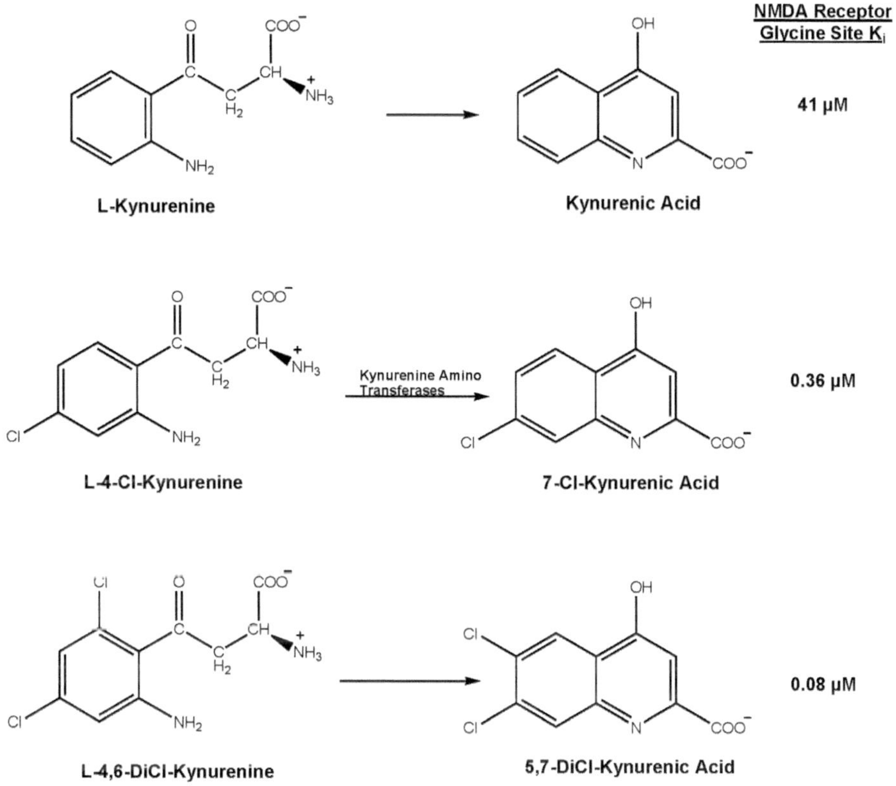


**Figure 11.5** Structures of kynurenine, 4-chlorokynurenine and 4,6-dichlorokynurenine together with matching neuroprotective metabolites, kynurenic acid, 7-chlorokynurenic acid and 5,7-dichlorokynurenic acid. $K_i$ values [38, 39] represent the inhibition constant at the glycine binding site of the NMDA receptor.

This is possible since endogenous choline plasma concentrations are only ~25% of the $K_m$ of the CHT [46, 47] and that the CHT is rather promiscuous in binding molecules that bear cationic charges. It was shown the BBB CHT translocated two nicotinic antagonists, which are preclinical leads for smoking cessation therapy, across the BBB to achieve 10-fold greater brain distribution than that predicted by passive permeation. These compounds are the *bis*-quaternary ammonium, *N*,*N′* dodecyl-bis-picolinium bromide [48] and the *N*-*n*-alkylnicotinium analogue, *N*-*n*-octylnicotinium iodide (NONI)(Figure 11.7) [46]. Further work demonstrated that after crossing the BBB, these two nicotinic antagonists inhibit nAChR-mediated nicotine-evoked [$^3$H]-dopamine release with an $IC_{50}$ of 2–5 nM [49]. While the CHT transporter may have a unique ability to distribute a wide variety of charged cations into brain [50], unlike LAT1, it has not been cloned, which limits drug design and discovery. To overcome this deficit, molecular modeling has been used to outline structural binding and transport requirements (Figure 11.7) [50], which include (1) a significant need for the presence of a cationic nitrogen center in the

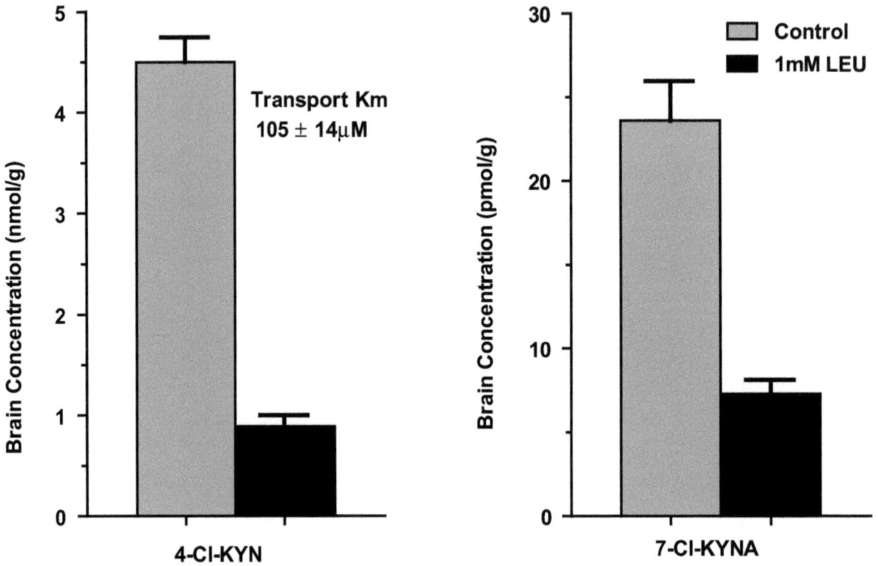


**Figure 11.6** Graphs showing reduction in brain uptake of 4-chlorokynurenine by competition from L-leucine (1 mM) and matching reduction in amounts of 7-chlorokynurenic acid formed within the CNS. Data are from Ref. [41].

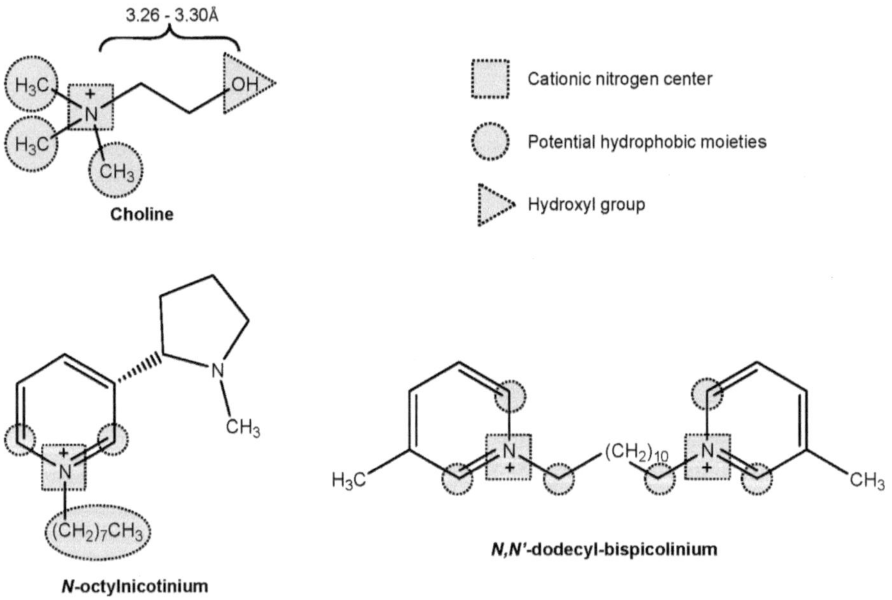


**Figure 11.7** Structures of choline (endogenous substrate) and the two nicotinic antagonists *N*,*N*′-dodecyl-bis-picolinium, and *N*-*n*-octylnicotinium, which are shuttled from blood to brain via the BBB CHT. Structural requirements of a molecule to use this transporter include a requisite cationic nitrogen (square); a hydrophobic interaction adjacent to the quaternary ammonium center (circle); and, less significantly, a hydroxyl group approximately from 3.26 to 3.30 Å away from the cationic nitrogen (triangle).

molecule [51], (2) a molecule that provides a hydrophobic interaction around the anionic binding site that accommodates the quaternary ammonium center, and (3) to a lesser degree the presence of at least one hydroxyl group located approximately from 3.26 to 3.30 Å away from the cationic nitrogen center [52–54]. Further work on utilizing this nutrient transporter as a vector for the delivery of cationic prodrugs may be beneficial since it may improve the less than 1% blood-to-brain extraction (related to diffusion) normally observed at the BBB with charged cations [53, 55, 56].

## 11.4
## Prodrug Strategies Based Upon BBB Receptors

In a manner comparable to the BBB carrier-mediated approach, significant work has also focused on brain drug delivery using BBB receptor-mediated transport strategies. Pardridge [57] has pioneered BBB transcytosis of antibodies to the transferrin and insulin receptors for brain delivery of small drugs, peptides, proteins, nanoparticles and liposomes. Similarly, Karkan *et al.* [58] have explored brain delivery using drug conjugates of the iron transport protein, melanotransferrin. With this approach, they found enhanced survival in mice bearing intracranial mammary tumors or gliomas after treatment with the melanotransferrin-doxorubicin conjugate than with free doxorubicin alone.

In similar manner, a number of investigators have explored BBB prodrug delivery using absorptive-mediated transcytosis strategies based upon cationic peptides and proteins – that is, "cell-penetrating peptides" such as penetratin, transportan, HIV Tat peptide and homoarginine peptides (Arg 7 and 9) [59]. For example, Tanabe *et al.* [60] found 3–4-fold enhanced brain uptake of a cationic arginine-vasopressin peptide via absorptive-mediated endocytosis than of the matching parent peptide. The cationic peptide was specifically tailored with additional arginine, histidine, and proline residues that would be cleaved off by postproline cleaving enzyme once peptide entry was gained to the CNS. Similarly, Rousselle *et al.* [61] showed markedly enhanced (30-fold) brain delivery of the anticancer drug doxorubicin into brain following conjugation to the cationic peptides, penetratin and SynB using the *in situ* brain perfusion technique. BBB transport matched that expected for an absorptive-mediated transport process, showing inhibition with added cationic peptide or polylysine. However, following intravenous administration, brain uptake of the doxorubicin-SynB conjugate only exceeded that of matching free doxorubicin for 10–30 min and at the highest point only achieved a 2.5-fold gradient, suggesting that the conjugate may efflux out of brain rapidly or that other factors conspire to limit brain accumulation via this strategy. One hypothesis put forward to explain this discrepancy is that, because cationic peptides increase uptake into most cells, there is little preferential increase in individual tissues, such as the percent injected dose that goes to brain.

A matching prodrug strategy based upon BBB receptor-mediated transport uses LRP1. LRP1 is one member of a family of LDL receptor proteins [62]. It is preferentially expressed at the endothelial cells of the BBB and mediates rapid cell uptake of a wide variety of ligands, including RAP, $\alpha_2$-macroglobulin, aprotinin, lactoferrin, and tPA, among others. LRP transport has been utilized to deliver cyanoacrylate nanoparticles bearing drugs to the CNS [63]. More recently, LRP1 has been targeted via the 19 amino acid AngioPep peptides (e.g., AngioPep-2) that bind to LRP1 and are transcytosed across the BBB *in vitro* and *in vivo* [64]. Transport via this pathway is competitively reduced by self-peptide as well as LRP1 ligands, including RAP. Further, LRP1 mediated transport of RAP and $\alpha_2$-macroglobulin is inhibited by coadministration of AngioPep-2 [65].

The AngioPep-2 peptide has been conjugated to anticancer drugs, including paclitaxel, doxorubicin, and etoposide [66, 67]. Figure 11.8 illustrates the AngioPep-2 prodrug strategy for paclitaxel. Paclitaxel is a large, highly hydrophobic natural product anticancer compound that normally crosses the BBB very poorly due to BBB active efflux transport. Conjugation of three paclitaxel residues to AngioPep-2 leads to the ANG1005 prodrug that shows 100-fold greater brain accumulation than paclitaxel by *in situ* rat brain perfusion (Figure 11.8) [68]. ANG1005 is taken up into brain and is not simply bound to the vascular luminal membrane, as it cannot be washed out of the vasculature by short perfusion with drug free saline and is present mostly in the brain parenchyma fraction after removal of cerebral endothelial cells by capillary depletion. ANG1005 exhibits 4–50-fold improved delivery to brain and brain metastases of breast cancer when administered *in vivo* to mice [68]. Conjugation of paclitaxel to AngioPep-2 not only allows receptor-mediated transcytosis of the conjugate prodrug across the BBB but also avoids active efflux drug transport of paclitaxel back across the BBB into the circulation. Experiments by Regina *et al.* [67] showed markedly enhanced brain paclitaxel accumulation after IV administration of paclitaxel in Pgp knockout mice, whereas brain ANG1005 uptake is unaffected in matching Pgp transporter knockout animals. For anticancer activity, ANG1005 must be cleaved by esterases to release free paclitaxel. Consistent with improved brain accumulation, the ANG1005 conjugate demonstrated improved *in vivo* anticancer activity against primary brain tumors and against brain metastases in mice [67]). ANG1005 is currently in Phase 1 clinical trials in humans as a new brain tumor anticancer agent with improved delivery across the BBB. The AngioPep-2 peptide has also shown promise for promoting brain uptake of biodegradable nanoparticles, as demonstrated by Ke *et al.* [69].

## 11.5
## CNS Prodrug Summary

In conclusion, a number of prodrug vectors have been developed to promote drug distribution to the CNS to achieve therapeutic concentrations at key brain sites. Most studies have recently focused upon carrier-mediated and receptor-mediated BBB transport strategies to promote selective brain targeting and retention, based upon the concept that the BBB shows enhanced levels of critical nutrient

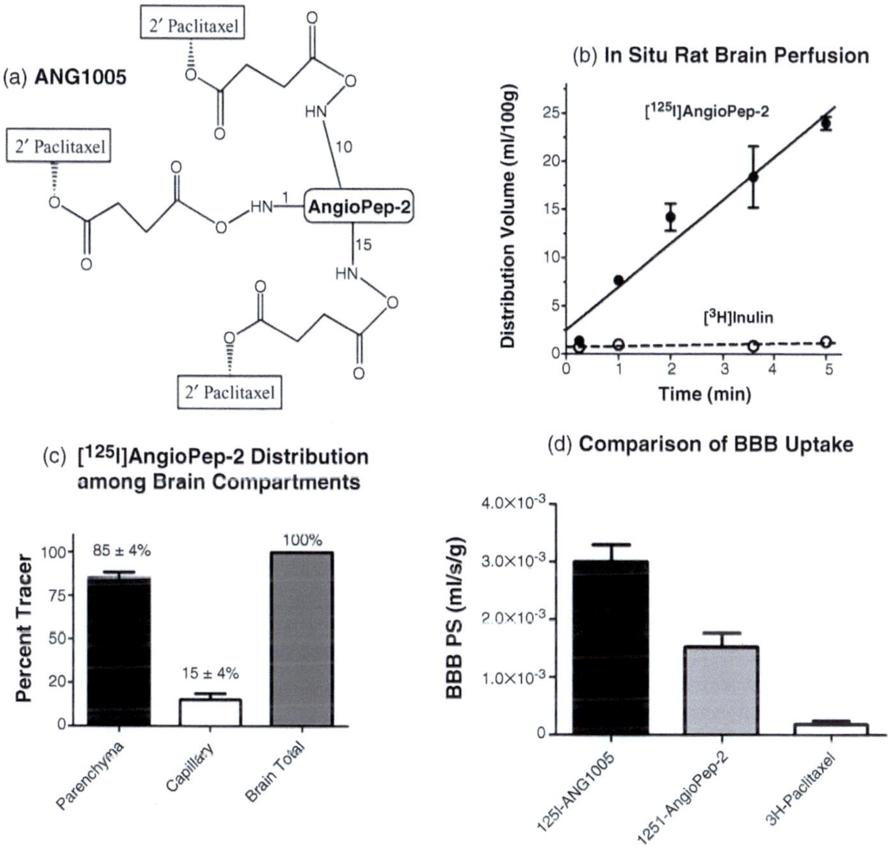


**Figure 11.8** (a) Schematic showing the structure of ANG1005, the 3 paclitaxel + 1 AngioPep-2 peptide conjugate. (b) Time course of AngioPep-2 uptake into brain by *in situ* rat brain perfusion. Inulin is a marker of vascular volume, which normally does not cross in short experiments (<15 min). The low values for inulin space (~1%) indicate that AngioPep-2 does not alter the passive permeability of the BBB. (c) Capillary depletion experiment showing that the majority of ANG1005 tracer is found in the vascular-free, parenchymal fraction. AngioPep-2 was perfused through the brain vasculature for 2 min prior to post perfusion washout followed by capillary depletion using dextran. (d) Mean BBB permeability–surface area product (PS) values for initial brain uptake of ANG1005, AngioPep-2, and paclitaxel during *in situ* brain perfusion. Points and bars equal mean ± SD or SEM for $n = 3$–12 perfusions. Data are from Ref. [68].

transporters (e.g., LAT1 and GLUT1) and receptors (e.g., insulin receptor and LRP1) than other organs. Given that the brain represents 1–3% of body weight in animals, brain distribution for a drug that shows equal distribution among tissues would be expected to be only 1–3%. In fact, most drugs show much less brain distribution than 1–3% of injected dose by one to three orders of magnitude because of the presence of BBB. The hope is that with selective prodrug targeting and retention, this percentage can be increased above 1–3% to achieve true preferential distribution to the CNS.

## Acknowledgments

We would like to acknowledge the contributions of Chris Adkins and Rajender Mittapalli to the preparation of this paper. This research was supported by grant 5R01NS52484 from NIH/NINDS and grant W81XWH-062-0033 from the Department of Defense Breast Cancer Research Program.

## References

1 Alavijeh, M.S., Chishty, M., Qaiser, M.Z., and Palmer, A.M. (2005) Drug metabolism and pharmacokinetics, the blood–brain barrier, and central nervous system drug discovery. *NeuroRx*, **2**, 554–571.

2 Pangalos, M.N., Schechter, L.E., and Hurko, O. (2007) Drug development for CNS disorders: strategies for balancing risk and reducing attrition. *Nature Reviews. Drug Discovery*, **6**, 521–532.

3 Deeken, J.F. and Loscher, W. (2007) The blood–brain barrier and cancer: transporters, treatment, and Trojan horses. *Clinical Cancer Research*, **13**, 1663–1674.

4 Hawkins, B.T. and Davis, T.P. (2005) The blood–brain barrier/neurovascular unit in health and disease. *Pharmacological Reviews*, **57**, 173–185.

5 Ohno, K., Pettigrew, K.D., and Rapoport, S.I. (1978) Lower limits of cerebrovascular permeability to nonelectrolytes in the conscious rat. *The American Journal of Physiology*, **235**, H299–H307.

6 Rapoport, S.I., Ohno, K., and Pettigrew, K.D. (1979) Drug entry into the brain. *Brain Research*, **172**, 354–359.

7 Pajouhesh, H. and Lenz, G.R. (2005) Medicinal chemical properties of successful central nervous system drugs. *NeuroRx*, **2**, 541–553.

8 Ohtsuki, S. and Terasaki, T. (2007) Contribution of carrier-mediated transport systems to the blood–brain barrier as a supporting and protecting interface for the brain; importance for CNS drug discovery and development. *Pharmaceutical Research*, **24**, 1745–1758.

9 Smith, Q.R. (2003) A review of blood–brain barrier transport techniques. *Methods in Molecular Medicine*, **89**, 193–208.

10 Dubey, R.K., McAllister, C.B., Inoue, M., and Wilkinson, G.R. (1989) Plasma binding and transport of diazepam across the blood–brain barrier. No evidence for *in vivo* enhanced dissociation. *The Journal of Clinical Investigation*, **84**, 1155–1159.

11 Sisson, W.B. and Oldendorf, W.H. (1971) Brain distribution spaces of mannitol-$^{3}$H, inulin-$^{14}$C, and dextran-$^{14}$C in the rat. *The American Journal of Physiology*, **221**, 214–217.

12 Kamiie, J., Ohtsuki, S., Iwase, R., Ohmine, K., Katsukura, Y., Yanai, K., Sekine, Y., Uchida, Y., Ito, S., and Terasaki, T. (2008) Quantitative atlas of membrane transporter proteins: development and application of a highly sensitive simultaneous LC/MS/MS method combined with novel *in-silico* peptide selection criteria. *Pharmaceutical Research*, **25**, 1469–1483.

13 Kalvass, J.C., Maurer, T.S., and Pollack, G.M. (2007) Use of plasma and brain unbound fractions to assess the extent of brain distribution of 34 drugs: comparison of unbound concentration ratios to *in vivo* P-glycoprotein efflux ratios. *Drug Metabolism and Disposition: The Biological Fate of Chemicals*, **35**, 660–666.

14 Raub, T.J. (2006) P-glycoprotein recognition of substrates and

circumvention through rational drug design. *Molecular Pharmacology*, **3**, 3–25.
15 Pardridge, W.M. (2005) The blood–brain barrier: bottleneck in brain drug development. *NeuroRx*, **2**, 3–14.
16 Harbaugh, R.E. (1989) Novel CNS-directed drug delivery systems in Alzheimer's disease and other neurological disorders. *Neurobiology of Aging*, **10**, 623–629.
17 Bodor, N. and Buchwald, P. (2002) Barriers to remember: brain-targeting chemical delivery systems and Alzheimer's disease. *Drug Discovery Today*, **7**, 766–774.
18 Chen, Y., Dalwadi, G., and Benson, H.A. (2004) Drug delivery across the blood–brain barrier. *Current Drug Delivery*, **1**, 361–376.
19 Patel, M.M., Goyal, B.R., Bhadada, S.V., Bhatt, J.S., and Amin, A.F. (2009) Getting into the brain: approaches to enhance brain drug delivery. *CNS Drugs*, **23**, 35–58.
20 Rautio, J., Kumpulainen, H., Heimbach, T., Oliyai, R., Oh, D., Jarvinen, T., and Savolainen, J. (2008) Prodrugs: design and clinical applications. *Nature Reviews. Drug Discovery*, **7**, 255–270.
21 Jones, A.R. and Shusta, E.V. (2007) Blood–brain barrier transport of therapeutics via receptor-mediation. *Pharmaceutical Research*, **24**, 1759–1771.
22 Oxender, D.L. and Christensen, H.N. (1963) Distinct mediating systems for the transport of neutral amino acids by the Ehrlich cell. *The Journal of Biological Chemistry*, **238**, 3686–3699.
23 Kanai, Y., Segawa, H., Miyamoto, K., Uchino, H., Takeda, E., and Endou, H. (1998) Expression cloning and characterization of a transporter for large neutral amino acids activated by the heavy chain of 4F2 antigen (CD98). *The Journal of Biological Chemistry*, **273**, 23629–23632.
24 Smith, Q.R., Momma, S., Aoyagi, M., and Rapoport, S.I. (1987) Kinetics of neutral amino acid transport across the blood–brain barrier. *Journal of Neurochemistry*, **49**, 1651–1658.
25 Smith, Q.R. (2000) Transport of glutamate and other amino acids at the blood–brain barrier. *The Journal of Nutrition*, **130**, S1016–S1022.
26 Uchino, H., Kanai, Y., Kim, D.K., Wempe, M.F., Chairoungdua, A., Morimoto, E., Anders, M.W., and Endou, H. (2002) Transport of amino acid-related compounds mediated by L-type amino acid transporter 1 (LAT1): insights into the mechanisms of substrate recognition. *Molecular Pharmacology*, **61**, 729–737.
27 Kageyama, T., Nakamura, M., Matsuo, A., Yamasaki, Y., Takakura, Y., Hashida, M., Kanai, Y., Naito, M., Tsuruo, T., Minato, N., and Shimohama, S. (2000) The 4F2hc/LAT1 complex transports L-DOPA across the blood–brain barrier. *Brain Research*, **879**, 115–121.
28 Miyagawa, T., Oku, T., Uehara, H., Desai, R., Beattie, B., Tjuvajev, J., and Blasberg, R. (1998) "Facilitated" amino acid transport is upregulated in brain tumors. *Journal of Cerebral Blood Flow and Metabolism*, **18**, 500–509.
29 Nawashiro, H., Otani, N., Shinomiya, N., Fukui, S., Ooigawa, H., Shima, K., Matsuo, H., Kanai, Y., and Endou, H. (2006) l-type amino acid transporter 1 as a potential molecular target in human astrocytic tumors. *International Journal of Cancer*, **119**, 484–492.
30 Takada, Y., Vistica, D.T., Greig, N.H., Purdon, D., Rapoport, S.I., and Smith, Q.R. (1992) Rapid high-affinity transport of a chemotherapeutic amino acid across the blood–brain barrier. *Cancer Research*, **52**, 2191–2196.
31 Greig, N.H., Momma, S., Sweeney, D.J., Smith, Q.R., and Rapoport, S.I. (1987) Facilitated transport of melphalan at the rat blood–brain barrier by the large neutral amino acid carrier system. *Cancer Research*, **47**, 1571–1576.
32 Groothuis, D.R., Lippitz, B.E., Fekete, I., Schlageter, K.E., Molnar, P., Colvin, O.M., Roe, C.R., Bigner, D.D., and Friedman, H.S. (1992) The effect of an amino acid-lowering diet on the rate of melphalan entry into brain and xenotransplanted glioma. *Cancer Research*, **52**, 5590–5596.
33 Kurpad, S.N., Friedman, H.S., Archer, G.E., McLendon, R.E., Petros, W.M., Fuchs, H.E., Guaspari, A., and Bigner, D.D. (1995) Intraarterial administration of melphalan for treatment of intracranial

human glioma xenografts in athymic rats. *Cancer Research*, **55**, 3803–3809.

34 Haines, D.R., Fuller, R.W., Ahmad, S., Vistica, D.T., and Marquez, V.E. (1987) Selective cytotoxicity of a system L specific amino acid nitrogen mustard. *Journal of Medicinal Chemistry*, **30**, 542–547.

35 Gynther, M., Laine, K., Ropponen, J., Leppanen, J., Mannila, A., Nevalainen, T., Savolainen, J., Jarvinen, T., and Rautio, J. (2008) Large neutral amino acid transporter enables brain drug delivery via prodrugs. *Journal of Medicinal Chemistry*, **51**, 932–936.

36 Gynther, M., Ropponen, J., Laine, K., Leppanen, J., Haapakoski, P., Peura, L., Jarvinen, T., and Rautio, J. (2009) Glucose promoiety enables glucose transporter mediated brain uptake of ketoprofen and indomethacin prodrugs in rats. *Journal of Medicinal Chemistry*, **52**, 3348–3353.

37 Erhardt, S., Olsson, S.K., and Engberg, G. (2009) Pharmacological manipulation of kynurenic acid: potential in the treatment of psychiatric disorders. *CNS Drugs*, **23**, 91–101.

38 Baron, B.M., Harrison, B.L., McDonald, I.A., Meldrum, B.S., Palfreyman, M.G., Salituro, F.G., Siegel, B.W., Slone, A.L., Turner, J.P., and White, H.S. (1992) Potent indole- and quinoline-containing *N*-methyl-D-aspartate antagonists acting at the strychnine-insensitive glycine binding site. *The Journal of Pharmacology and Experimental Therapeutics*, **262**, 947–956.

39 Kemp, J.A., Foster, A.C., Leeson, P.D., Priestley, T., Tridgett, R., Iversen, L.L., and Woodruff, G.N. (1988) 7-Chlorokynurenic acid is a selective antagonist at the glycine modulatory site of the *N*-methyl-D-aspartate receptor complex. *Proceedings of the National Academy of Sciences of the United States of America*, **85**, 6547–6550.

40 Nemeth, H., Toldi, J., and Vecsei, L. (2005) Role of kynurenines in the central and peripheral nervous systems. *Current Neurovascular Research*, **2**, 249–260.

41 Hokari, M., Wu, H.Q., Schwarcz, R., and Smith, Q.R. (1996) Facilitated brain uptake of 4-chlorokynurenine and conversion to 7-chlorokynurenic acid. *Neuroreport*, **8**, 15–18.

42 Fukui, S., Schwarcz, R., Rapoport, S.I., Takada, Y., and Smith, Q.R. (1991) Blood–brain barrier transport of kynurenines: implications for brain synthesis and metabolism. *Journal of Neurochemistry*, **56**, 2007–2017.

43 Lee, S.C. and Schwarcz, R. (2001) Excitotoxic injury stimulates pro-drug-induced 7-chlorokynurenate formation in the rat striatum *in vivo*. *Neuroscience Letters*, **304**, 185–188.

44 Wu, H.Q., Lee, S.C., Scharfman, H.E., and Schwarcz, R. (2002) l-4-Chlorokynurenine attenuates kainate-induced seizures and lesions in the rat. *Experimental Neurology*, **177**, 222–232.

45 Battaglia, G., La Russa, M., Bruno, V., Arenare, L., Ippolito, R., Copani, A., Bonina, F., and Nicoletti, F. (2000) Systemically administered D-glucose conjugates of 7-chlorokynurenic acid are centrally available and exert anticonvulsant activity in rodents. *Brain Research*, **860**, 149–156.

46 Allen, D.D., Lockman, P.R., Roder, K.E., Dwoskin, L.P., and Crooks, P.A. (2003) Active transport of high-affinity choline and nicotine analogs into the central nervous system by the blood–brain barrier choline transporter. *The Journal of Pharmacology and Experimental Therapeutics*, **304**, 1268–1274.

47 Allen, D.D. and Smith, Q.R. (2001) Characterization of the blood–brain barrier choline transporter using the *in situ* rat brain perfusion technique. *Journal of Neurochemistry*, **76**, 1032–1041.

48 Lockman, P.R., Manda, V.K., Geldenhuys, W.J., Mittapalli, R.K., Thomas, F., Albayati, Z.F., Crooks, P.A., Dwoskin, L.P., and Allen, D.D. (2008) Carrier-mediated transport of the quaternary ammonium neuronal nicotinic receptor antagonist *N,N′*-dodecylbispicolinium dibromide at the blood–brain barrier. *The Journal of Pharmacology and Experimental Therapeutics*, **324**, 244–250.

49 Dwoskin, L.P., Sumithran, S.P., Zhu, J., Deaciuc, A.G., Ayers, J.T., and Crooks, P.A. (2004) Subtype-selective nicotinic receptor antagonists: potential as tobacco use cessation agents. *Bioorganic &*

*Medicinal Chemistry Letters*, **14**, 1863–1867.

50 Geldenhuys, W.J., Manda, V.K., Mittapalli, R.K., Van der Schyf, C.J., Crooks, P.A., Dwoskin, L.P., Allen, D.D., and Lockman, P.R. (2010) Predictive screening model for potential vector-mediated transport of cationic substrates at the blood–brain barrier choline transporter. *Bioorganic & Medicinal Chemistry Letters*, **20**, 870–877.

51 Geldenhuys, W.J., Lockman, P.R., McAfee, J.H., Fitzpatrick, K.T., Van der Schyf, C.J., and Allen, D.D. (2004) Molecular modeling studies on the active binding site of the blood–brain barrier choline transporter. *Bioorganic & Medicinal Chemistry Letters*, **14**, 3085–3092.

52 Allen, D.D. and Lockman, P.R. (2003) The blood–brain barrier choline transporter as a brain drug delivery vector. *Life Sciences*, **73**, 1609–1615.

53 Lockman, P.R. and Allen, D.D. (2002) The transport of choline. *Drug Development and Industrial Pharmacy*, **28**, 749–771.

54 Lerner, J. (1989) Choline transport specificity in animal cells and tissues. *Comparative Biochemistry and Physiology C*, **93**, 1–9.

55 Clark, D.E. (2003) *In silico* prediction of blood–brain barrier permeation. *Drug Discovery Today*, **8**, 927–933.

56 Pardridge, W.M. (2002) Drug and gene targeting to the brain with molecular Trojan horses. *Nature Reviews Drug Discovery*, **1**, 131–139.

57 Pardridge, W.M. (2008) Re-engineering biopharmaceuticals for delivery to brain with molecular Trojan horses. *Bioconjugate Chemistry*, **19**, 1327–1338.

58 Karkan, D., Pfeifer, C., Vitalis, T.Z., Arthur, G., Ujiie, M., Chen, Q., Tsai, S., Koliatis, G., Gabathuler, R., and Jefferies, W.A. (2008) A unique carrier for delivery of therapeutic compounds beyond the blood–brain barrier. *PLoS One*, **3**, e2469.

59 Herve, F., Ghinea, N., and Scherrmann, J.M. (2008) CNS delivery via adsorptive transcytosis. *AAPS Journal*, **10**, 455–472.

60 Tanabe, S., Shimohigashi, Y., Nakayama, Y., Makino, T., Fujita, T., Nose, T., Tsujimoto, G., Yokokura, T., Naito, M., Tsuruo, T., and Terasaki, T. (1999) *In vivo* and *in vitro* evidence of blood–brain barrier transport of a novel cationic arginine-vasopressin fragment 4–9 analog. *The Journal of Pharmacology and Experimental Therapeutics*, **290**, 561–568.

61 Rousselle, C., Smirnova, M., Clair, P., Lefauconnier, J.M., Chavanieu, A., Calas, B., Scherrmann, J.M., and Temsamani, J. (2001) Enhanced delivery of doxorubicin into the brain via a peptide-vector-mediated strategy: saturation kinetics and specificity. *The Journal of Pharmacology and Experimental Therapeutics*, **296**, 124–131.

62 Lillis, A.P., Van Duyn, L.B., Murphy-Ullrich, J.E., and Strickland, D.K. (2008) LDL receptor-related protein 1: unique tissue-specific functions revealed by selective gene knockout studies. *Physiological Reviews*, **88**, 887–918.

63 Ulbrich, K., Hekmatara, T., Herbert, E., and Kreuter, J. (2009) Transferrin- and transferrin–receptor–antibody-modified nanoparticles enable drug delivery across the blood–brain barrier (BBB). *European Journal of Pharmaceutics and Biopharmaceutics*, **71**, 251–256.

64 Demeule, M., Regina, A., Che, C., Poirier, J., Nguyen, T., Gabathuler, R., Castaigne, J.P., and Beliveau, R. (2008) Identification and design of peptides as a new drug delivery system for the brain. *The Journal of Pharmacology and Experimental Therapeutics*, **324**, 1064–1072.

65 Demeule, M., Currie, J.C., Bertrand, Y., Che, C., Nguyen, T., Regina, A., Gabathuler, R., Castaigne, J.P., and Beliveau, R. (2008) Involvement of the low-density lipoprotein receptor-related protein in the transcytosis of the brain delivery vector AngioPep-2. *Journal of Neurochemistry*, **106**, 1534–1544.

66 Che, C., Yang, G., Thiot, C., Lacoste, M.C., Currie, J.C., Demeule, M., Regina, A., Beliveau, R., and Castaigne, J.P. (2010) New AngioPep-modified doxorubicin (ANG1007) and etoposide (ANG1009) chemotherapeutics with increased brain penetration. *Journal of Medicinal Chemistry*, **53**, 2814–2824.

67 Regina, A., Demeule, M., Che, C., Lavallee, I., Poirier, J., Gabathuler, R., Beliveau, R., and Castaigne, J.P. (2008) Antitumour activity of ANG1005, a

conjugate between paclitaxel and the new brain delivery vector AngioPep-2. *British Journal of Pharmacology*, **155**, 185–197.

68 Thomas, F.C., Taskar, K., Rudraraju, V., Goda, S., Thorsheim, H.R., Gaasch, J.A., Mittapalli, R.K., Palmieri, D., Steeg, P.S., Lockman, P.R., and Smith, Q.R. (2009) Uptake of ANG1005, a novel paclitaxel derivative, through the blood-brain barrier into brain and experimental brain metastases of breast cancer. *Pharmaceutical Research*, **26**, 2486–2494.

69 Ke, W., Shao, K., Huang, R., Han, L., Liu, Y., Li, J., Kuang, Y., Ye, L., Lou, J., and Jiang, C. (2009) Gene delivery targeted to the brain using an AngioPep-conjugated polyethyleneglycol-modified polyamidoamine dendrimer. *Biomaterials*, **30**, 6976–6985.

# 12
# Directed Enzyme Prodrug Therapies

*Dan Niculescu-Duvaz, Gabriel Negoita-Giras, Ion Niculescu-Duvaz, Douglas Hedley, and Caroline J. Springer*

## 12.1
## Introduction

The goal for successful anticancer agents has been to design drugs with intrinsic specificity for specific types of cancer cells. Unfortunately, their efficacy is often hampered by an insufficient therapeutic index, lack of specificity, and the emergence of drug-resistant cell subpopulations. Emerging technologies such as genomics and proteomics discovering proteins specific for various types of cancer cells that may be used as target are ways to address these hurdles [1]. An important concept is the design of technologies that target cancer cells without major side effects. Alternatives aimed at enhancing the selectivity of cancer chemotherapy for solid tumors rely on targeting cancer cells and include enzyme-directed prodrug therapies, examples of which are antibody-directed enzyme prodrug therapy (ADEPT) [2, 3] or gene-directed enzyme prodrug therapy (GDEPT or suicide gene therapy) [4–6].

In this chapter, we focus on ADEPT and GDEPT and some derived strategies, described using the term of directed enzyme prodrug therapies (DEPTs), as well as on the design of prodrugs for both technologies.

## 12.2
## Theoretical Background of DEPT

The general principle of DEPT is the conversion of a nontoxic prodrug to a cytotoxic drug by an enzyme expressed selectively in the malignant tissue. The variants of DEPT (ADEPT, GDEPT, bacteria enzyme-directed prodrug therapies (BDEPT) [7, 8], polymer-directed enzyme prodrug therapies (PDEPTs), or ligand-directed enzyme prodrug therapies (LIDEPTs) [9]) describe the different ways in which the prodrug-activating enzyme is delivered to the tumor. The enzyme may be conjugated to a vehicle that is capable of selective tumor delivery (such as an antibody in ADEPT, a ligand in LIDEPT), be produced in the tumor by expression of the gene encoding

*Prodrugs and Targeted Delivery: Towards Better ADME Properties.* Edited by Jarkko Rautio

ISBN: 978-3-527-32603-7

the enzyme (for example, in GDEPT) or be expressed inside bacteria that accumulate in tumors (BDEPT). In order to achieve selective delivery of the enzyme to the tumor, several strategies have been used: targeting of overexpressed receptors/antigens, transcriptional selectivity based on tumor-specific promoters, favorable tropism of the vector carrying the gene for the enzyme and passive accumulation due to leaky tumor vasculature.

### 12.2.1
### ADEPT and Other Enzyme–Conjugates Approaches

Monoclonal antibodies have been used to deliver [10, 11] potent plant and bacterial toxins [12] and radionuclides [13] to tumors. A number of successful conjugates such as Mylotarg [14] (anti-CD33-calicheamicin for the treatment of acute myeloid leukemia), Zevalin and Bexxar [15, 16] (for the treatment of B-cell lymphomas), have been developed. However, there are no clinically approved immunoconjugates for the treatment of solid tumors. The chemoimmunoconjugates suffer from the drawback that the antigens on the malignant cell surface are insufficiently dense and have an irregular distribution, meaning that not all areas of the tumor can bind the conjugate. Also, there is requirement for the internalization of the antibody conjugates, which is often unmet. There are also potential problems linked to the release of the drugs from the conjugates and the absence of bystander effects (BE) [17]. The BE occurs when not only the tumor cells that are bound to the antibody–enzyme conjugate but also the neighboring cells devoid of the targeted antigen are killed.

ADEPT, in which antibody–enzyme conjugates are used to activate subsequently administered prodrugs [18–21] represents an alternative. ADEPT is a two-step procedure for targeted drug delivery in which monoclonal antibodies (mAbs) target the enzyme to tumor cell surfaces. The enzymes were selected for their ability to convert subsequently administered anticancer prodrugs into active antitumor agents. ADEPT is illustrated in Figure 12.1.

The first step involves systemic administration of the mAb–enzyme conjugate. It may take from several hours to several days for localization to take place within the tumor and the clearance from the nontarget tissues to occur depending on the pharmacokinetic properties of the conjugate. The second step involves the systemic prodrug administration. This approach offers two advantages over chemoimmunoconjugates. The first is the amplification effect since one molecule of enzyme–antibody conjugate, acting as a catalyst, is able to activate a large number of prodrug molecules. The second is the induction of a BE, which was observed in ADEPT experiments both *in vitro* and *in vivo*. Tumor-targeting immunoliposomes bearing enzymes on their surface (immunoenzymosomes) have been investigated as a modification of ADEPT. As opposed to the antibody–enzyme conjugate, immunoenzymosomes can carry more than one enzyme molecule per carrier unit [22].

PDEPT is a two-step antitumor approach in which both the enzyme and the prodrugs are targeted to the tumor site using a polymer molecule. The polymeric conjugates accumulate in the tumor due to the increased vascular permeability and the lack of effective tumor drainage (enhanced permeability and retention (EPR)

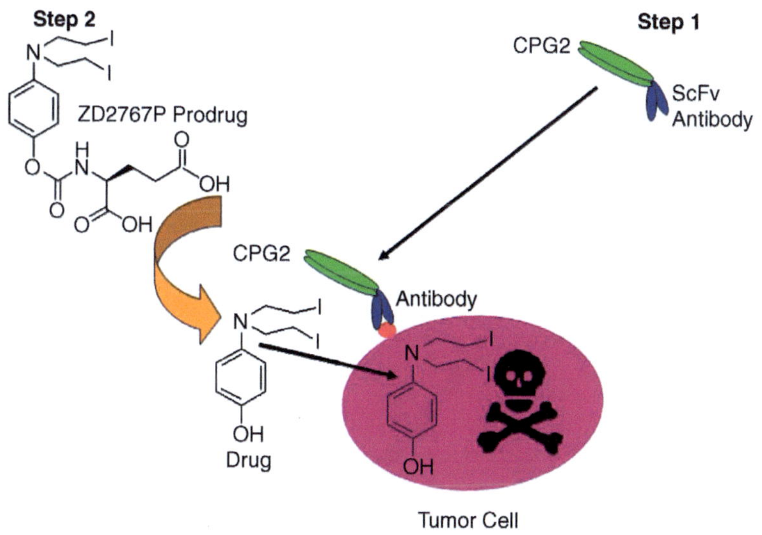


**Figure 12.1** General Principles of ADEPT.

effect). So far, three enzymes (cathepsin B, β lactamase, and a catalytic antibody) have been used in PDEPT [8, 23, 24].

### 12.2.2 LIDEPT

Fusion of a tumor-targeting ligand with an enzyme was proposed as a novel DEPT strategy. This approach, namely, LIDEPT was demonstrated using a VEGF-carboxypeptidase G2 (CPG2) fusion protein. This construct targets the prodrug-activating CPG2 enzyme to the VEGF receptors overexpressed on the endothelial cells of the tumor vasculature [9].

### 12.2.3 GDEPT and Other Gene Delivery Approaches

Gene therapy may be broadly defined as a technology aimed at modifying the genetic component of cells in order to obtain therapeutic benefits. In cancer gene therapy, both malignant and nonmalignant cells can be targeted for therapeutic gain. Two approaches targeting malignant cells are toxin gene therapy (by transfecting genes that express toxic molecules) and enzyme-activating prodrug therapy, by transfecting genes able to express enzymes that can activate specific prodrugs selectively. The latter approach is known as suicide gene therapy (SGT), GDEPT [25, 26], virus-directed enzyme prodrug therapy (VDEPT) [27], or genetic prodrug-activating therapy (GPAT) [28].

GDEPT is a two-step treatment for solid tumors. In the first step, the gene for a foreign enzyme (bacterial, viral, or yeast) is administered and targeted in a variety

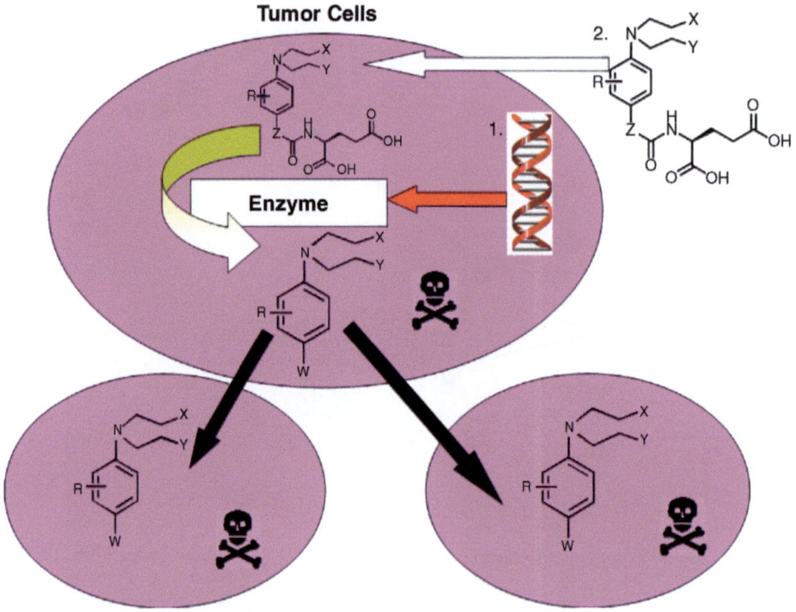


**Figure 12.2** General principles of GDEPT.

of ways to the tumor for expression. In the second step, a prodrug is administered that is activated to the cytotoxic drug selectively by the foreign enzyme expressed in the tumor. Ideally, the enzyme gene should be expressed exclusively, or with a relatively high ratio in the tumor cells compared to normal tissues and blood, and should achieve a concentration to activate prodrug for clinical benefit. The catalytic activity of the expressed protein must be sufficient for activation of the prodrug under physiological conditions.

These general principles of GDEPT are illustrated in Figure 12.2.

Since expression of the foreign enzymes will not occur in all cells of a targeted tumor *in vivo*, a BE is required, whereby the prodrug is cleaved to an active drug that kills not only the tumor cells in which it is formed but also the neighboring tumor cells that do not express the foreign enzyme. Mechanisms of BE in GDEPT have not been fully elucidated but include the generation and export of cytotoxic metabolites able to kill nontransfected neighboring cells and induction of an additional immune response in *in vivo* models.

In GDEPT, the gene must be "carried" in a vehicle or vectors, which is also responsible for the specificity of targeting and for the efficient transfection of the therapeutic genes into cancer cells. The vectors for gene therapy can be divided in two major classes: viral and nonviral.

The viral vectors are the main vehicles used in GDEPT for therapeutic gene transfer. A number of reviews describe their applications in gene therapy [29–32]. Retroviral vectors are most widely used in GDEPT due to their low immunogenicity and high gene delivery efficiency. A tmpk/AZT enzyme prodrug combination has been shown to induce cell death in transduced cells using a lentiviral vector [33]. Adenoviral vectors can be used as well, but with the risk of high immunogenicity. Recently, it has been reported that an adenoviral vector (AdV.hTERT-CPG2) combined with the ZD2767P mustard prodrug can significantly reduce or eradicate xenografts of colorectal carcinoma [34].

Nonviral vector advantages are that they are safer, with a reduced chance of eliciting immunogenic effect and low toxicity. These vectors use the property of DNA to bind positively charged lipid bilayers [35], cationic polymers, and certain cell penetrating peptides. Much effort has been made in the development of alternative nonviral vectors, including naked DNA, liposomes, polymers, peptides, and proteins [36–39].

In GDEPT, the tumor cells become the producers of the activating enzymes. Alternative vehicles for the gene of the expressed enzyme have been investigated. Mammalian tissue culture cells, microencapsulated in cellulose sulfate, have been engineered to express cytochrome P450 (CYP). These microencapsulated cells were then delivered by direct injection in the tumor mass or by using the tumor vasculature. Once delivered, prodrugs are activated locally by the CYP to cytotoxic drugs [40, 41].

Human macrophages have been transfected *ex vivo* with hypoxia-regulated adenoviruses carrying the CYP2B6 gene. These macrophages infiltrated the hypoxic region of the tumors, leading to expression of the CYP2B6 enzyme, which can activate suitably designed prodrugs [42].

### 12.2.4
### BDEPT

Bacteria that selectively colonize cancerous tissues have become the subject of much recent interest. Apart from the intrinsic tumoricidal effect of some of these microorganisms (for example, *Salmonella typhimurium*) they were used as the carrier for suicide genes. The use of bacteria carrying suicide genes has become known as BDEPT (bacteria-directed enzyme prodrug therapy). Three bacterial systems have been studied so far: *Salmonella*, *Clostridium*, and *Bifidobacterium* [43–45]. An alternative area is called CDEPT (clostridial-directed enzyme prodrug therapy) [43, 44]. In this approach, the enzyme is expressed in a clostridial expression plasmid. So far, cytosine deaminase (CD) and nitroreductase (NR) have been applied in CDEPT [45]. Since many clostridia naturally possess β-lactamase genes, a β-lactamase-based anticancer system was proposed in which a cephalosporin is cleaved to release two cytotoxic active metabolites. *Clostridium butyricum*, for example, is nonpathogenic and has a stable β-lactamase encoded in its genes [16].

## 12.3
## Comparison of ADEPT and GDEPT

Suicide gene therapy has some of the same advantages as ADEPT. A comparison between these two systems is summarized in Table 12.1. The main difference is that

**Table 12.1** Comparison between ADEPT and GDEPT systems.

| Parameters | ADEPT | GDEPT | |
|---|---|---|---|
| | | Internal expression | External expression |
| 1. Selectivity | Determined by antigen expression and density on the cell surface, the affinity and the avidity of Ab | Determined by the delivery system and the translational specificity | |
| 2. Targeting | Based on antigen–antibody interactions | Can be achieved with viruses, bacteria, or nonviral vectors | |
| 3. Amplification effect | | Properties of ADEPT and GDEPT systems | |
| | | Intracellular expression | Surface-tethered expression |
| 4. Bystander effect | Prodrugs activated extracellularly. Comparable with enzyme surface-tethered expression in GDEPT. | Export outside the cells of the active drugs is required to achieve the BE. | Presumed to be better compared to GDEPT intracellular expression as no export of drug from the cell is required. |
| 5. Prodrug design | Prodrugs with suitable pharmacokinetic properties have been designed to achieve sufficient tumor concentration. Internalization of the released drugs is necessary for cell killing. | Internalization of the prodrugs is required for activation | As that of ADEPT since internalization of the prodrug is not required |
| 6. Immunogenicity | Immunogenicity is described as a negative factor in clinical trials since it precludes antibody-conjugate repeated treatments. May be overcome by the use of human fusion proteins of antibody with enzyme. | Immunogenicity described as positive factor in experimental protocols since it may result in an immune response against the tumor. | |
| 7. Potential leakage of the drug outside the tumor | Potential risk depending on the nature of the active drugs and their half-lives. | Minimal risks because of an extra barrier to be crossed by the active drug. | Potential risk depending on the nature of the active drugs and their half-lives. |

| | | | |
|---|---|---|---|
| 8. Efficacy of the system in clinical trials | Four Phase I clinical trials, to date. | Encouraging results have been obtained in glioma, head and neck, and ovarian cancers; 34 clinical trials ongoing. | Not performed to date. |
| 9. Miscellaneous | Clearance of antibody–enzyme conjugate from normal body tissues can be achieved by using a second clearing antibody prior to administration of the prodrug and efficacy can be enhanced with an antiangiogenic agent. | The therapeutic effect can be enhanced by combining two suicide genes, adding immunostimulatory genes, or mutating the active site of the enzyme to obtain greater specificity for the substrate prodrug. | |

the vector, which delivers the therapeutic enzyme gene, provides the targeting to cancer cells and the length of time the therapeutic enzyme resides at the tumor is likely to be longer than with ADEPT.

In ADEPT, the activating enzymes are linked to an antibody, which is bound to the cell surface. In GDEPT, the genes can be engineered for expression of their product either intracellularly or extracellularly. With extracellular expression, the enzyme can be tethered to the outer cell surface or secreted from the recipient cells [25, 47–49]. There are advantages for each approach. Where the enzyme is intracellularly expressed the prodrug must enter the cell for activation and subsequently the active drug must diffuse through the interstitium across the cell membrane to elicit a BE. Cells in which the enzyme is expressed in a secretory form or tethered to their outer surface are able to activate the prodrug extracellularly. A more substantial BE could in theory be generated in the latter systems since the prodrug does not have to enter cells for activation. A leak-back of the active drug to the general circulation is a possible disadvantage of extracellular expression.

The factors important for efficacy both in ADEPT and in GDEPT are listed in Table 12.2.

## 12.4
## Enzymes in ADEPT and GDEPT

In ADEPT and GDEPT, there are many enzymes used to activate prodrugs and release drugs (see Table 12.3).

The enzymes must meet specific requirements, whereby they must catalyze scission or other types of reactions such as phosphorylation, ribosyl transfer, redox reactions, or β-elimination that lead to prodrug formation. The reaction catalyzed should be different from those of any circulating endogenous enzymes. The enzymes should be expressed in sufficient concentrations and have high catalytic activity to provide efficient prodrug conversion for extended periods of time, preferably without the need for cofactors. They must be selectively expressed only in tumor cells.

The enzymes that have been proposed for ADEPT and GDEPT can be characterized into two broad categories. The first comprises "foreign" exogenous enzymes with or without human analogues, for example, viral tyrosine kinase (TK), bacterial cytosine deaminase (bCD), carboxylpeptidase (CPG2), purine nucleotide phosphorylase (PNP), D-amino acid oxidase (DAAO), α- and β-galactosidase (α- and β-Gal), β-lactamase (β-L), methionine-α,γ-lyase (MET), NR, rabbit cytochrome P450 (CYP4B1), canine cytochrome P450 (CYP4B11), deoxyribonucleoside kinase (dNK), and xanthine-guanine phosphoribosyl transferase (XGPT). Where there are human analogues of these enzymes, they are significantly different in terms of substrate structural requirements. The main disadvantage of the foreign enzymes is their potential to elicit an immune response in humans although this could provide benefits to therapy. Fused protein constructs consisting of the enzyme and humanized mAbs could be used in ADEPT to overcome this drawback [121, 158, 159].

Table 12.2 Requirements for ADEPT/GDEPT systems.

| | ADEPT | GDEPT |
|---|---|---|
| Enzymes | No human analogues with the same substrate requirement or the same kinetics; Low immunogenicity; High catalytic activity | |
| Prodrugs | Low cytotoxicity; Good substrates with suitable $K_m$ and $k_{cat}$ parameters; Good pharmacokinetic properties; Not substrates for endogenous enzymes; Good physiological stability. | |
| Released active drugs | High cytotoxicity; Diffusible across cell membranes; Suitable half-life, to minimize leakage outside the tumor, but to allow tumor diffusion; Active against dividing and quiescent cells; Linear dose-dependent cell killing profile. | |
| Vectors | — | Specificity for tumor cells; Carrier capacity large enough to allow the insertion of 1–3 therapeutic genes; Good transfection efficiency; Low toxicity; Low immunogenicity. |
| Antibodies enzyme conjugates | High specificity for tumor cells; Good clearance from body fluids; Good pharmacokinetic parameters; High catalytic activity. | — |

Table 12.3 Enzymes used in ADEPT and GDEPT systems.

| Enzymes | Released active drug | | References |
|---|---|---|---|
| | ADEPT | GDEPT | |
| DAAO | | Hydrogen peroxide | [50] |
| Alkaline phosphatase | Doxorubicin | — | [19] |
| | Etoposide | — | [51] |
| | Mitomycin | — | [52] |
| | Phenol mustard | — | [53] |
| Acid phosphatase (human, prostatic) | FudR and Ara-C | FudR and Ara-C | [54] |
| Aminopeptidase | Melphalan | — | [55] |

(*Continued*)

**Table 12.3** (*Continued*)

| Enzymes | Released active drug | | References |
|---|---|---|---|
| | ADEPT | GDEPT | |
| Aryl sulfatase | Etoposide | — | [56] |
| | Phenol mustard | — | [56] |
| Carboxyl Esterase | — | SN38 | [57, 58] |
| Carboxypeptidase A | Methotrexate | Methotrexate | [59, 60] |
| | Antifolates | — | [61–63] |
| Carboxypeptidase G2 | Nitrogen mustards | Nitrogen mustards | [64–73] |
| | | Anthracyclines | [74] |
| | | Tyrphostins | |
| Catalytic antibodies | Cloramphenicol | — | [75] |
| | 5-Fluorodeoxyuridine | — | [76] |
| | Phenol mustard | — | [77] |
| | Campthotecin | — | [78] |
| | — | Phosphoramidic nitrogen mustards | [79–82] |
| | — | *N*-acetyl benzoquinone imine | [82] |
| Cytochromes P450 | — | Toxic metabolites from ipomeanol and 2-aminoanthracene. | [83] |
| | — | Anthracyclines | [84, 85] |
| | — | AQ4 | [82, 86] |
| Cytochrome c P450 reductase | | α-[(1-Aziridinyl)methyl]-2-nitro-1*H*-imidazole-1-ethanol | [87] |
| CD | 5-Fluorouracil | 5-Fluorouracil | [88–94] |
| Deoxycytidine kinase | — | Cytosine arabinoside monophosphate | [95, 96] |
| DT-Diaphorase | — | Reduced forms of EO9 | |
| α-Galactosidase | Doxorubicin | ? | [97] |
| β-Galactosidase | Anthracyclines | Anthracyclines | [98–100] |
| | Amino-CBI derivatives | — | [101, 102] |
| | Geldamycin | — | [103] |
| | 5-Fluorouridine | — | [104] |
| Glucose oxidase | Peroxides, reactive oxygen, and iodine | — | [105] |
| β-Glucosidase | Cyanide | | [106] |
| β-Glucuronidase | Anthracyclines | Anthracyclines | [107–110] |
| | Phenol mustards | — | [111] |
| | 5-Fluorouracil | 5-Fluorouracil | [110, 112] |
| | 9-Aminocampthotecin | 9-Aminocampthotecin | [110, 113] |
| | Verapamil | — | [114] |
| | Quinine | — | [114] |
| | Dipyridamole | — | [114] |
| | $O^6$-Benzylguanine and $O^6$-benzyl-2′-deoxyguanosine | — | [115] |

Table 12.3 (*Continued*)

| Enzymes | Released active drug | | References |
|---|---|---|---|
| | ADEPT | GDEPT | |
| Horseradish peroxidase | — | Reactive species of indole-3-acetic acid | [116, 117] |
| | — | *N*-acetyl-p-benzoquinone imine | [118] |
| β-Lactamase | Nitrogen mustards | Nitrogen mustards | [119] |
| | Doxorubicin | Anthracyclines | [120, 121] |
| | Mitomycin | — | [122] |
| | Vinca derivatives | Vinca derivatives | [123] |
| | Paclitaxel | — | [124] |
| | Platinum reagents | — | [125] |
| Methionine-α,γ-liase | — | Methylselenol | [126, 127] |
| Multiple drug-activating enzyme (MDAE) | — | 6-Thioguanine | [128] |
| | — | Methotrexate | [128] |
| | — | Cytotoxic purines | [128] |
| Nitroreductase | Benzodiazepines | | [129] |
| | Amino-CBI derivatives | Amino-CBI derivatives | [130, 131] |
| | Actinomycin D | | [132] |
| | Mitomycin C | | [132] |
| | Doxorubicin | Doxorubicin | [132, 133] |
| | Nitrogen mustards | Nitrogen mustards | [131, 132, 134–136] |
| | Aromatic ethylene imines (CB1954) | Aromatic ethylene imines (CB1954) | [137] |
| | Enediynes | Enediynes | [138] |
| Penicillin amidase | Doxorubicin | | [139] |
| | Melphalan | | [139] |
| | Palytoxin | | [140] |
| Purine nucleotide phosphorylase | — | 6-Methylpurine | [141–143] |
| | — | 2-Fluoroadenine | [143] |
| Thymidine kinase | — | GCV, ACV monophosphate | [144–151] |
| | | Ara-MMP | [152, 153] |
| | — | Nucleotides monophosphate | [154] |
| Thymidine phosphorylase | — | 5-Fluorodeoxyuridine monophosphate | [155, 156] |
| Xanthine-guanine phosphoribosyl transferase | — | 6-Thiopurine monophosphate | [157] |
| Xanthine oxidase | Peroxides and reactive oxygen species | — | [87] |

The second category consists of enzymes of mammalian origin: carboxypeptidase A (CPA), deoxycytidine kinase (dCK), DT-diaphorase, thymidine phosporylase (TP), β-glucuronidase (β-Glu), carboxylesterase (CE), cytochrome c P450 reductase (HRE-P450), and several cytochrome P450 (CYP) isoforms (CYP1A2, CYP3A, CYP2B, CYP2B1, CYP2C, and CYP2D6). Some of these enzymes are absent or are expressed only at low concentrations in tumor cells, for example, dCK, CA, TP, and CYP. The main advantage of the mammalian enzymes resides in their reduced potential for inducing an immune response. However, the presence of these enzymes in normal tissues is likely to preclude specific activation of the prodrugs only in tumors. Intratumoral administration of prodrug in these systems would likely result in less systemic toxicity [160].

## 12.5 Design of Prodrugs

The requirements for the prodrugs and the released active drugs for any DEPT system are summarized in Table 12.2.

The general structure of a prodrug is comprised of a trigger that provides specificity and is converted by the enzyme in DEPT, and an effector that is the active drug or metabolite. These prodrugs that possess the trigger and the effector only are termed direct prodrugs and their activation is achieved in one step. The structure can also contain an additional linker that deactivates the effector until the trigger is released by the enzyme, and transmits the effect of activation from trigger to effector [135, 161]. Prodrugs including a linker are called self-immolative drugs or proprodrugs, and are activated in two or more steps as the activation of the trigger and the release of the drug are distinct steps.

This section will focus on mechanisms of prodrug activation and the structure, role, and SAR of the effector, trigger, and linker.

### 12.5.1 Mechanisms of Prodrug Activation

A fundamental characteristic of the prodrug in DEPT approaches is that the biological activity of the drug is suppressed. The prodrug must be designed or selected in such a way that the cytotoxic activity is unmasked upon activation of the trigger [115, 162]. There are a few general principles that have been applied to convert drugs into prodrugs or to design prodrugs able to release active drugs.

#### 12.5.1.1 Electronic Switch

Reversing or altering the electronic effect of a key functional group, during activation, with consequent increase in the chemical reactivity of the drug. In prodrug activation, the conversion of electron-withdrawing or electron-neutral groups to electron-donating ones has been used. Nitrogen mustard prodrugs are activated by this mechanism. Nitro [163, 164] (Scheme 12.1a), quaternary ammo-

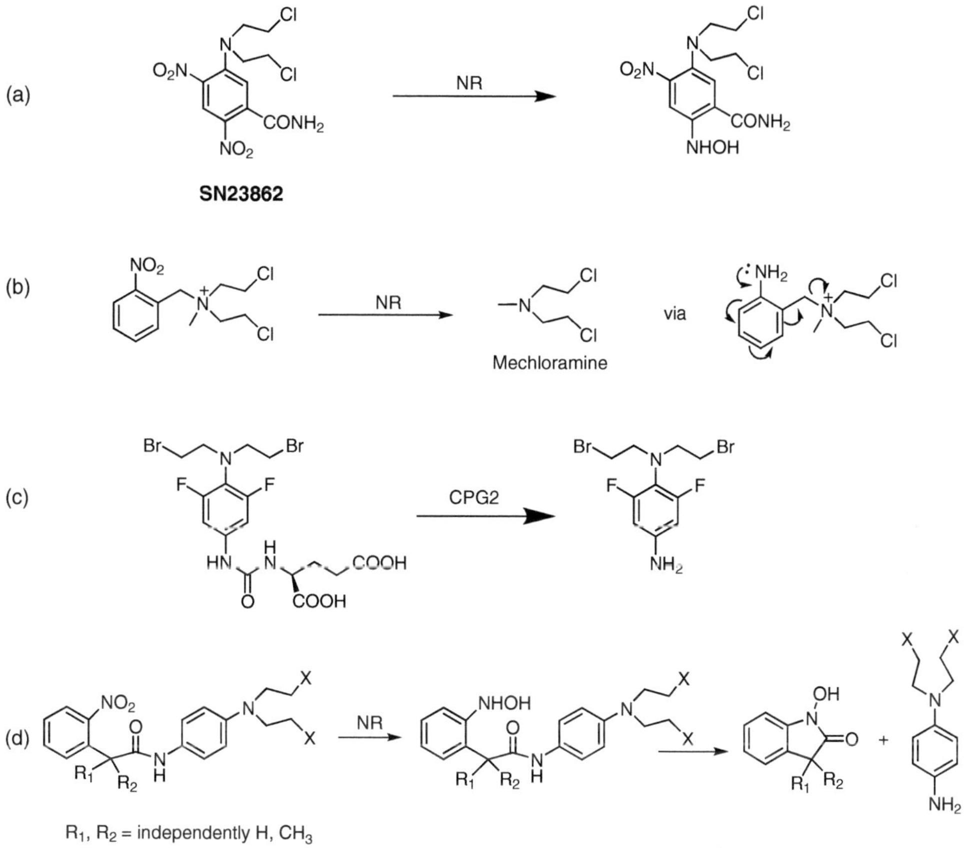


**Scheme 12.1**

nium [165] (Scheme 12.1b), urea [71] (Scheme 12.1c), or amide [166] (Scheme 12.1c) have been converted by DEPT enzymes to strong electron-donating amine or hydroxylamine moieties. Carbamates [67] (Scheme 12.2a), carbonates [70] (Scheme 12.2b, X=O), ethers [167, 168] (Scheme 12.2c), phosphates [53] (Scheme 12.2d), and sulfates [56] (Scheme 12.2e) have been hydrolyzed to phenols. Amides have been converted to charged carboxylic acids [65] (Scheme 12.3a), and neutral phosphoesters to charged phosphoric acid derivatives [54] (Scheme 12.3b). The general effect of these transformations is the release of a newly available pair of electrons, which increases the chemical reactivity of the aromatic mustard and subsequently the rate of DNA alkylation [169]. For seco-CC1065 analogues (Scheme 12.4a), the release of the free amino or hydroxy group trigger the expulsion of chloride and allow the formation of the key alkylating spiro-[cyclopropane-cyclohexadienone] moiety [102, 170]. In enediyne carbamate prodrugs (Scheme 12.4b), liberation of the free amine increases electron density promoting opening of the epoxide with change of conformation of the enediyne macrocycle. This triggers the Bergman cyclization, with formation of a diradical species and

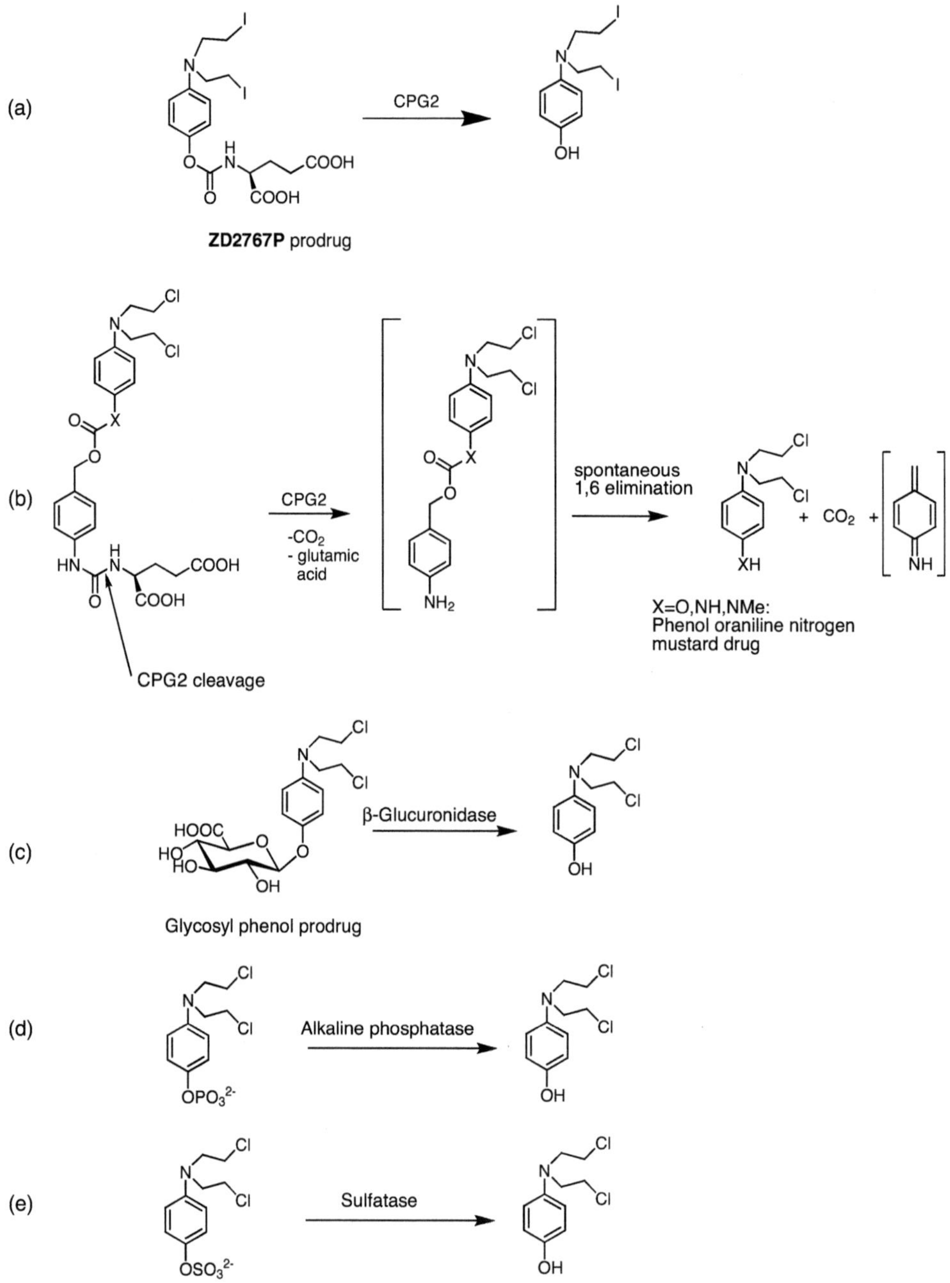
(a)
CPG2
ZD2767P prodrug
(b)
CPG2
-CO2
- glutamic acid
spontaneous 1,6 elimination
+ CO2 +
X=O,NH,NMe:
Phenol oraniline nitrogen mustard drug
CPG2 cleavage
(c)
β-Glucuronidase
Glycosyl phenol prodrug
(d)
Alkaline phosphatase
(e)
Sulfatase

Scheme 12.2

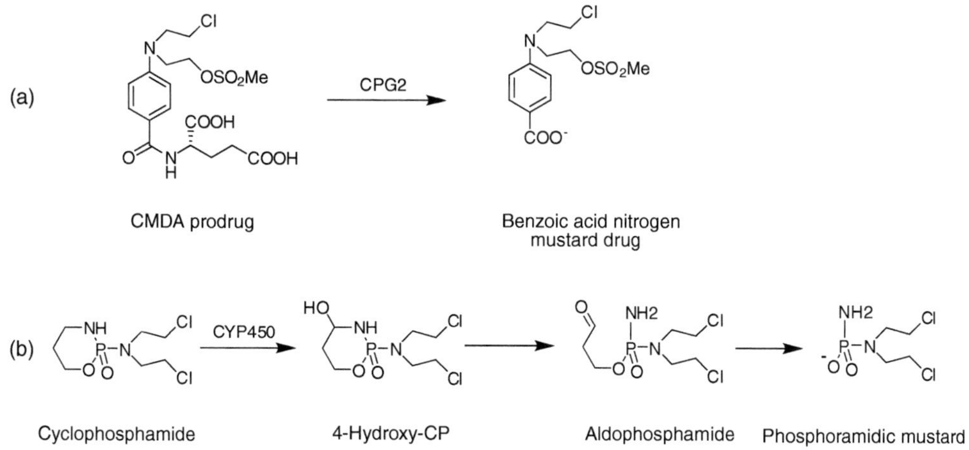


**Scheme 12.3**

induction of DNA double-strand breaks. The electronic switch mechanism was also employed to induce 1,4-elimination, 1,6-elimination, and cyclization in the case of self-immolative prodrugs (see below).

#### 12.5.1.2 **Cell Exclusion**

Prodrugs that are charged or very hydrophilic cannot penetrate the cell membrane to reach its cellular target. Upon cleavage of the charged/hydrophilic moiety, the released drug becomes more lipophilic and cell permeable. Typical examples are phosphate prodrugs [171] (activated by phosphatases, Scheme 12.2d), sulfate prodrugs, (activated by aryl sulfatases, Scheme 12.2e) [56], and some of the prodrugs for glycosidases and carboxypeptidases. This mechanism is relevant for enzymes that are expressed extracellularly (ADEPT and GDEPT with surface-tethered or secreted enzymes) [47, 48, 172, 173].

#### 12.5.1.3 **Blockage of the Pharmacophore**

Steric hindrance of key functional groups responsible for the interaction of a drug with the active site of its target renders the respective drug inactive. Conjugation of taxol at the critical 2′-OH decreases the cytotoxicity by two to three orders of magnitude in prodrugs for β-lactamase (Scheme 12.5) or β glucuronidase [124, 174, 175]. Incubation with these enzymes restore completely or partially the cytotoxicity. In cephalosporin-vinblastine prodrug, some deactivation of the drug is achieved, presumably by steric hindrance of tubulin binding by the cephalosporin side chain [103, 123, 176].

For irinotecan (CPT-11), activation by carboxylesterases unmasks an OH group that has an important role in the interaction with topoisomerase 1 (Scheme 12.6) [57, 177].

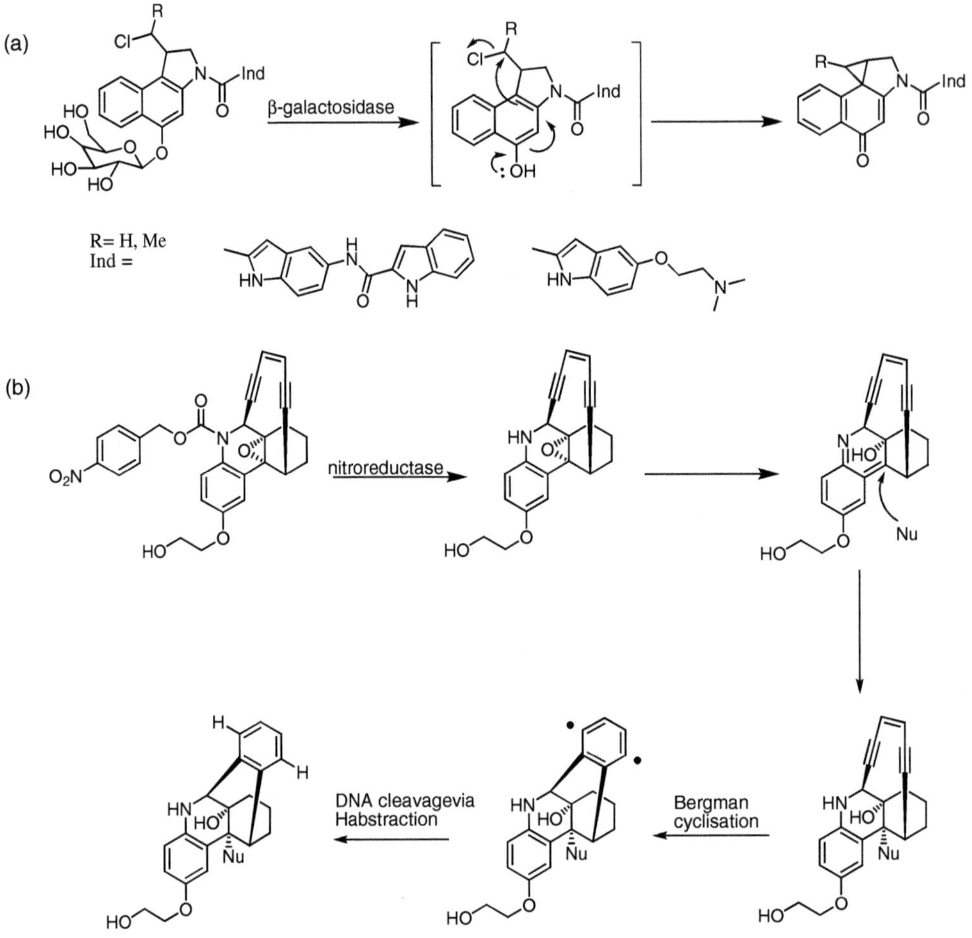


Scheme 12.4

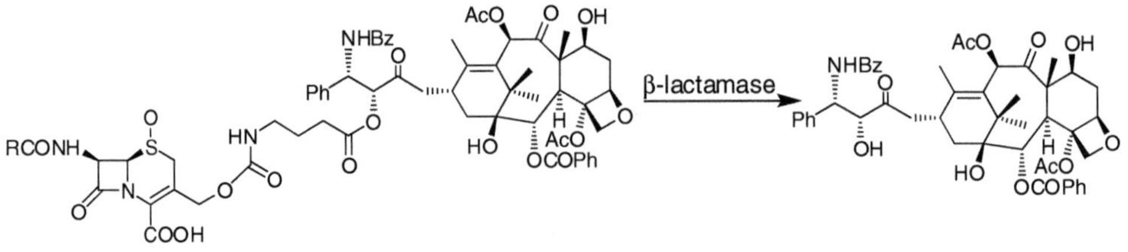


Scheme 12.5

Methotrexate (MTX) and other antifolates have been used as prodrugs for CPA, by blocking the key α-carboxylate of the glutamic acid as an amide, preventing interaction with the reduced folate carrier (RFC) and cellular uptake [63, 172].

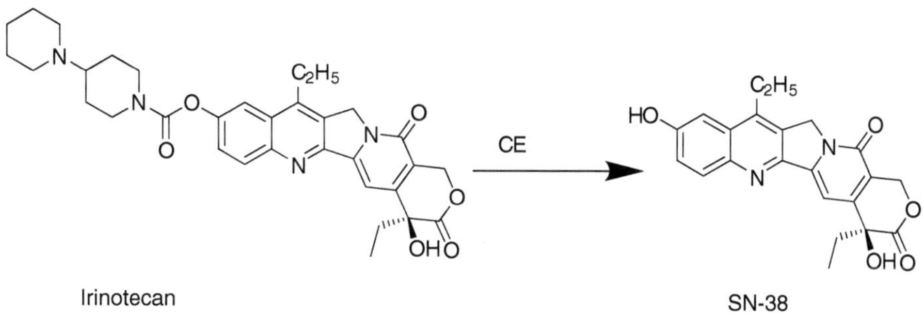


Scheme 12.6

#### 12.5.1.4 Conversion to Substrate for Endogenous Enzymes

Nucleoside-like prodrugs can be phosphorylated to nucleotides by kinases such as herpes simplex virus tk (HSV-TK for example, ganciclovir (GCV) Scheme 12.7) [154, 178, 179], varicella zoster virus tk (VZV-TK) [152], and dCK [96].

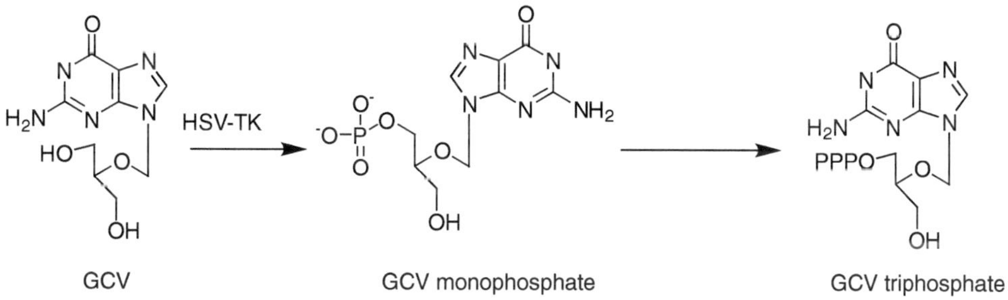


Scheme 12.7

The monophosphates thus formed are phosphorylated further to triphosphates by endogenous enzymes. The triphosphates are substrates for DNA polymerases and generate stunted DNA. The prodrug itself is a poor substrate for endogenous enzymes prior to conversion to the monophosphate.

5-Fluorocytosine (5-FC) is converted by cytosine deaminase to 5 fluorouracil (5-FU) [92], a further substrate for UPRT to generate a thymidine synthase inhibitor.

#### 12.5.1.5 Formation of a Reactive Moiety

Prodrugs that contain no obvious chemically reactive functionality can be converted by activating enzymes to compounds containing a very reactive moiety, such as an epoxide (conversion of 4-ipomeanol by CYP450, Scheme 12.8) [180], Michael acceptor (conversion of paracetamol by CYP450) [181], cyanide (released from amygdalin by β-glucosidase) [182] (Scheme 12.9), or methylselenol (released from selenomethionine by methioninase) [127].

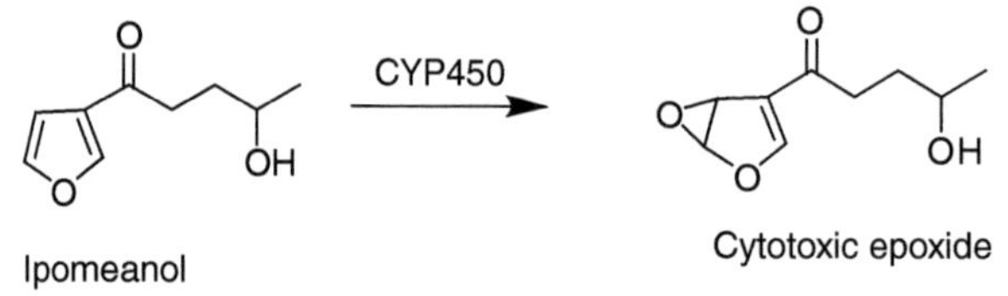


**Scheme 12.8**

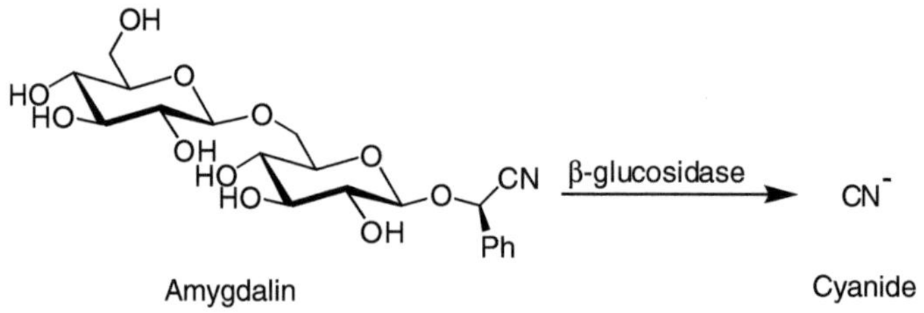


**Scheme 12.9**

12.5.1.6 **Formation of a Second Interactive Group**

Prodrugs containing one DNA-interacting group become more cytotoxic when a second DNA-reactive group is formed, allowing formation of interstrand cross-links. Activation of 2,4-dinitro-5-aziridinyl-benzamide (CB1954) by NR transforms a weak DNA monoalkylator into a bifunctional DNA cross-linking compound. The first alkylating group is the aziridine. The second alkylating group is generated from the conversion of the 2(4)-nitro group to hydroxylamine, acetylation of hydroxylamine by CoA transferases, and acetate elimination. The nitrenium intermediate formed is very reactive toward DNA nucleophiles (Scheme 12.10a) [183–185].

*N*-(4-Ethoxy-4-β-glucuronyl)butyl-doxorubicin is a prodrug for β-glucuronidase, with potency similar to doxorubicin. Upon activation, the *N*-(4-ethoxy-4-hydroxybutyl) group is converted spontaneously to a cyclic carbinolamine, which ultimately generates a very reactive iminium ion (Scheme 12.10). The drug formed possesses two DNA-interacting groups, the aglycon and the daunosamine moiety, with up to 10 000-fold increase in cytotoxicity [98, 186].

### 12.5.2
### Enzymatic Reactions Activating the Prodrug. The Trigger

The trigger provides a recognition motif for the expressed enzyme responsible for prodrug activation, either directly or via a cascade of further steps (fragmentation in self-immolative prodrugs or further endogenous enzymatic steps) to generate the ultimate cytotoxic agent. The activating enzymes and the corresponding triggers used in ADEPT and GDEPT approaches are presented below.

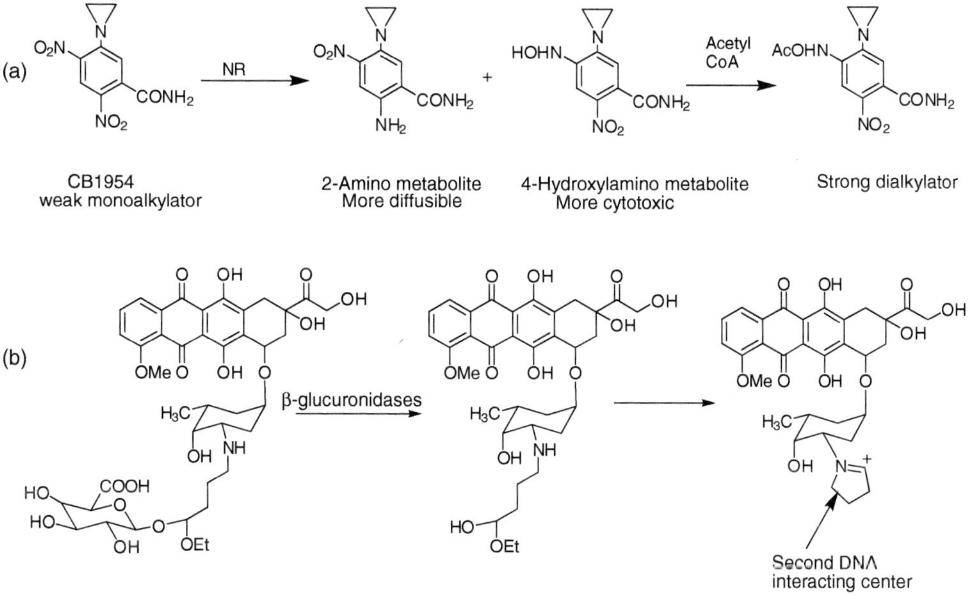


**Scheme 12.10**

#### 12.5.2.1 **Reactions Catalyzed by Hydrolases: Hydrolytic Cleavage**

Hydrolysis of amides, carbamates, ureas, glycosidic ethers, sulfuric esters, or phosphoric esters has been used to release cytotoxic drugs from prodrugs.

Hydrolysis of amide bonds has been applied to activate prodrugs by enzymes such as carboxypeptidases (CPG2, Scheme 12.3a), penicillin amidase, prolyl endopeptidase, and β-lactamase. CPG2 is a bacterial enzyme, which specifically cleaves the terminal glutamates of molecules, such as natural or synthetic folates. A number of alkylating prodrugs for CPG2 were synthesized, for example, 4-[(2-chloroethyl)(2-mesyloxyethyl)amino]benzoyl-L-glutamic acid, also known as CMDA. The recognition motif for CPG2 is a glutamic acid linked to an aromatic nucleus via an amide (Scheme 12.3a), a urea (Scheme 12.2b), or a carbamate bond (Scheme 12.2a). Following activation by CPG2, the electron withdrawing amide ($\sigma_p = 0.38$) of the 4-[(2-chloroethyl)(2-mesyloxyethyl)amino]benzoyl-L-glutamate (CMDA prodrug) is converted to the electron-donating negatively charged carboxylate ($\sigma_p = -0.20$), increasing the electron density at the *para*-nitrogen and consequently activating the nitrogen mustard [60, 63, 65]. Penicillin amidase specifically removes phenylacetyl groups from amides. Prodrugs of melphalan, doxorubicin [139], and palytoxin [140] are deactivated by acylation of the crucial amino group with a phenylacetyl moiety and were investigated as prodrugs for ADEPT with penicillin amidase. An engineered human prolylpeptidase has been shown to cleave a prolyl amide bond, releasing melphalan [187].

A urea or a carbamate linkage between the glutamic acid and an aromatic nucleus can also be cleaved by CPG2 [188]. This property has been used to generate prodrugs from the more potent 4-amino and 4-hydroxy nitrogen mustards (Schemes 12.1c and 12.2a) [67]. Phosphate esters are frequently used to increase the solubility of phenol and alcohol drugs. Cleavage by various phosphatases regenerates the active drugs. This strategy was used in one of the first examples of ADEPT. Phosphate prodrugs releasing doxorubicin, etoposide, and phenol mustard (Scheme 12.2d) were synthesized and cleaved with alkaline phosphatase [51, 189]. Etoposide phosphate was also proposed for GDEPT [171].

Cleavage of sulfate esters to release phenols (such as phenol mustard, Scheme 12.2e) was investigated as an ADEPT strategy with *Streptomyces* aryl sulfatase [56].

Prodrugs for glycosidases such as β-glucuronidase, α-galactosidase, β-galactosidase, linamarase, and β-glucosidase have been synthesized for ADEPT and GDEPT. The carbohydrate forms the recognition moiety, and is linked directly or via a linker to the hydroxy or amino group of the drug. Glycosidic carbamates have been used as specifiers for prodrugs of amine-containing drugs, linked directly or via a self-immolative linker [97, 190].

#### 12.5.2.2 **Activation by Nucleotide Phosphorylation**

Viral kinases (HSV-TK and VZV-TK) are more efficient in phosphorylating nucleotide prodrugs (such as GCV) than human kinases (Scheme 12.7). HSV/TK is one of the first GDEPT systems [178].

The activity of human kinases such as dCK is insufficient to activate the prodrug cytosine arabinoside (araC), and overexpression using a GDEPT approach increases the therapeutic efficacy of this prodrug in glioma [96]. Monophosphorylated nucleotides (NMP) are further converted by endogenous enzymes to nucleotide triphosphates (NTP) (see above). Due to the requirement for further endogenous enzymes for activation and the charged nature of the monophosphate intermediate that precludes cell permeation, this type of enzyme/prodrug system has been used only in GDEPT.

#### 12.5.2.3 **Activation by Reductases**

Reductases accept a broad range of substrates. Apart from a few structural restrictions that can be rationalized in terms of the crystal structure of NR [137], the recognition motifs for the prodrugs activated by reductases are functional groups with high reduction potential such as nitroaromatics, quinones, and *N*-oxides [131, 191]. Reduction of an electron-withdrawing aromatic nitro group to electron-donating hydroxylamino is performed efficiently by *Escherichia* coli NR, much faster than by the human DT-diaphorase (DT-d) [192]. This electronic switch activates effectors such as nitrogen mustards (Scheme 12.1a) [163] seco-CC1065 analogues (Scheme 12.4a) [193], or triggers fragmentation of self-immolative prodrugs (see, for example, Schemes 1d or 4b). Another role of the NHOH group formed is to generate the second alkylating moiety, converting a weakly monoalkylating prodrug such as CB1954 to a potent difunctional metabolite (Scheme 12.10a).

*N*-Oxides can also be reduced to reactive intermediates or active drugs. One-electron reduction of tirapazamine by DT-d or P450 reductase generates a TPZ radical, which abstracts hydrogen atoms from DNA, inducing single- and double-strand breaks [194, 195]. Another *N*-oxide prodrug, AQ4N, has a different mechanism of activation. The *N*-oxide in AQ4N serves both to ablate the basicity of the two tertiary amino groups, potential sites of interaction with DNA, and to ensure exclusion of prodrug from cells. Following four-electron reduction, the drug AQ4 becomes a potent topoisomerase II inhibitor (Scheme 12.11) [86, 196]. Both TPZ [194, 197] and AQ4N [86, 198] have been proposed as prodrugs for cytochrome P450/P450 reductase in GDEPT.

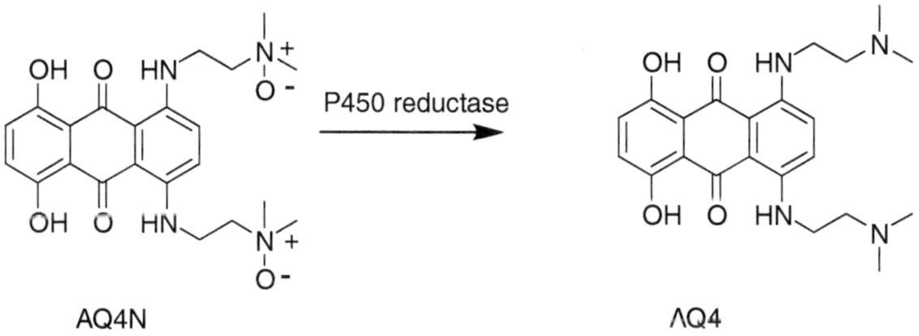


**Scheme 12.11**

#### 12.5.2.4 **Activation by Oxidases**

The oxidative enzymes investigated most for GDEPT are various cytochrome P450 isoforms and horseradish peroxidase (HRP).

Cyclophosphamide (CP) and ifosfamide (IF) are activated by C-hydroxylation. The 4-hydroxy-CP or -IF are unstable and fragment with formation of acrolein and phosphoramide mustard, a DNA alkylating agent (Scheme 12.3b) [79]. Other substrates for CYP450 proposed as prodrugs for GDEPT include 4-ipomeanol (Scheme 12.0), 2-aminoanthracene [83], paracetamol [181], and methoxymorpholinyl doxorubicin [84, 85].

A plant hormone (2-indoleacetic acid (IAA)) and a number of its analogues were found to generate a toxic species when activated by HRP (radicals under anoxic conditions, or α,β-unsaturated Michael acceptors in oxic conditions) [116, 117]. Paracetamol [118] and acetylacetone [199] were also metabolized to more toxic compounds by HRP.

Other oxidative enzymes that have been investigated for ADEPT or GDEPT include DAAO, which produces $H_2O_2$ by oxidation of D-aminoacids (e.g., D-alanine) [50], glucose oxidase [200], and xanthine oxidase.

#### 12.5.2.5 **(Deoxy)Ribosyl Transfer**

This reversible reaction has been employed in GDEPT in two ways. Transfer of ribosyl to 6-thioguanine has been achieved by XGPRT to generate a toxic nucleotide (Scheme 12.12a) [157]. Removal of ribosyl from relatively nontoxic nucleosides by purine nucleotide phosphorylases generates toxic purines (2-Me-purine, 2-F-adenine, Scheme 12.12b) [201]. Human thymidine phosphorylase catalyses a similar

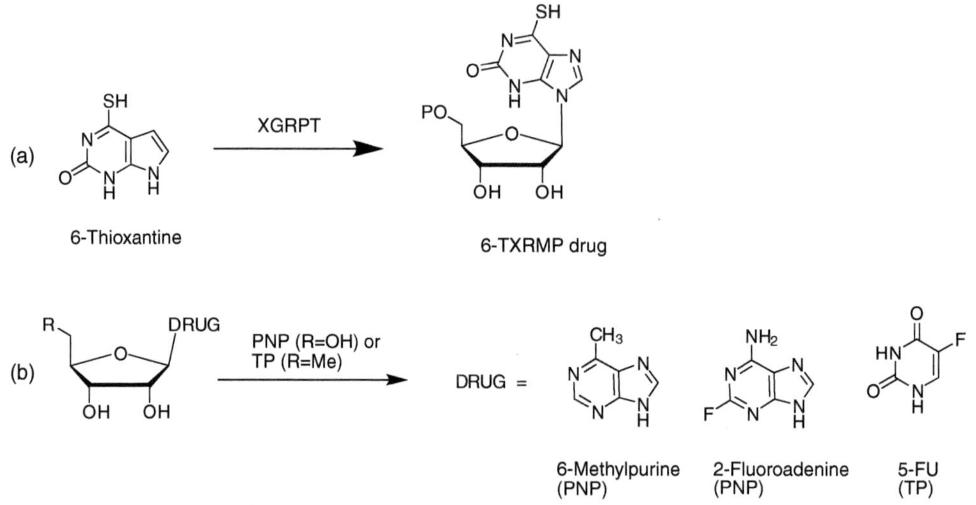


Scheme 12.12

reaction: the removal of 5′-deoxyribosyl from 5′-deoxy-5-fluorouridine to release 5-FU [155].

### 12.5.3
### The Linker. Self-Immolative Prodrugs

Drugs incorporating linkers are known under the name of self-immolative prodrugs, proprodrugs, or tripartite prodrugs [202].

In a number of prodrugs developed for DEPT, the trigger and the effector are joined together by a linker. The linker separates the activation motif from the point of drug release in order to make the activation step less dependent upon structural features of the drug. The main function of the linker is to rapidly release the active drug in a spontaneous fragmentation process following enzymatic activation. The design of the linker is very important for the kinetics of activation and for the cytotoxicity differential. It can affect the stability of the prodrug, the selectivity for the target enzyme and the pharmacokinetic properties [203].

There are several potential advantages of self-immolative prodrugs: (i) prodrugs delivering a wide range of drugs can be designed for an activating enzyme, unrestricted by the structural substrate requirement of the enzyme; (ii) poor kinetics of enzymatic activation of a prodrug due to electronic or steric effects of the drug can be improved by setting the specifier and the drug apart through the linker; (iii) several important properties of the prodrug, such as stability, pharmacokinetic profile, and physicochemical properties can be modulated by structural modifications of the linker; and (iv) additional functionalities (for example, targeting moieties) can be added to the prodrug using the linker as a handle [204].

Two main mechanisms of fragmentation of self-immolative prodrugs have been employed: elimination and cyclization. Both are triggered by an electronic switch – the generation or unmasking of an electron-donating group/nucleophile.

#### 12.5.3.1 **Self-Immolative Prodrugs Fragmenting by Elimination**

1,6-, 1,4- and 1,2-Elimination mechanisms have been exploited for the design of self-immolative prodrugs.

1,6-Elimination linkers are aromatic or heteroaromatic benzylic compounds, bearing a leaving group on the benzylic position (the effector or the drug) and a substituent in *para*-position with respect to the benzylic moiety that can be converted to an electron-donating group (the trigger). The most common electron-donating groups that initiate the 1,6-elimination process are hydroxylamine, amine, and hydroxy. Delocalization of the lone pair of electrons induces the self-immolation process, with extrusion of the drug and formation of *para*-quinomethide or *para*-iminoquinomethide (Scheme 12.2b, Scheme 12.13).

Hydroxylamine and amine can be formed by reduction of the nitro group in prodrugs by NR, and is used as the trigger for fragmentation of many self-immolative prodrugs (for example, see Scheme 12.13) [131, 133, 136, 183, 203, 205].

The hydroxy trigger can be formed by hydrolysis of an ester, a carbamate (by CPG2, Scheme 12.2a) [69, 70, 74], or a glycosyl ether (by β-glucuronidase, β-galactosidase, and α-galactosidase, Scheme 12.13b) [79, 142, 178–181], or by oxidation of the unsubstituted 4-position of the linker (by tyrosine hydroxylase) [206].

Three chemical classes of 1,4-elimination linkers have been described for DEPT prodrugs: 2-amino- or 2-hydroxy-benzylic compounds, cephalosporins, and enols.

The mechanism of elimination and the type of triggers used for the 2-substituted benzylic linkers is very similar to those discussed for their 4-substituted analogues activated by 1,6-elimination, for example, prodrugs of anthracyclins activated by β-glucuronidase (Scheme 12.14a) and β-galactosidase [100, 107].

Cephalosporins are substrates for β-lactamase. Following cleavage of the lactam bond, the pair of electrons on the nitrogen is released, and delocalization through the conjugated double-bond leads to the expulsion of the drug from the exocyclic methylene (Scheme 12.14b) [8, 119, 123, 125, 203, 207–209].

Self-immolative doxorubicin prodrugs based on a glycosidic enol and activated by β-glucuronidase via 1,4-elimination have also been described [210].

1,2-Elimination mechanism is encountered in the fragmentation of aminomethyl carbamate linkers, and the first step of the activation of CP by cytochrome P450 (Scheme 12.3b) [211].

#### 12.5.3.2 **Linker–Drug Connection**

For the fragmentation of the linker to proceed, the drug attached to the benzylic position (or the equivalent methylene group for the other types of linkers) should behave as a leaving group. The connection between the linker and the drug thus has a dual role: (a) to deactivate the drug and (b) to provide a good leaving group. The propensity of the drug to be extruded increases with the leaving group ability. The

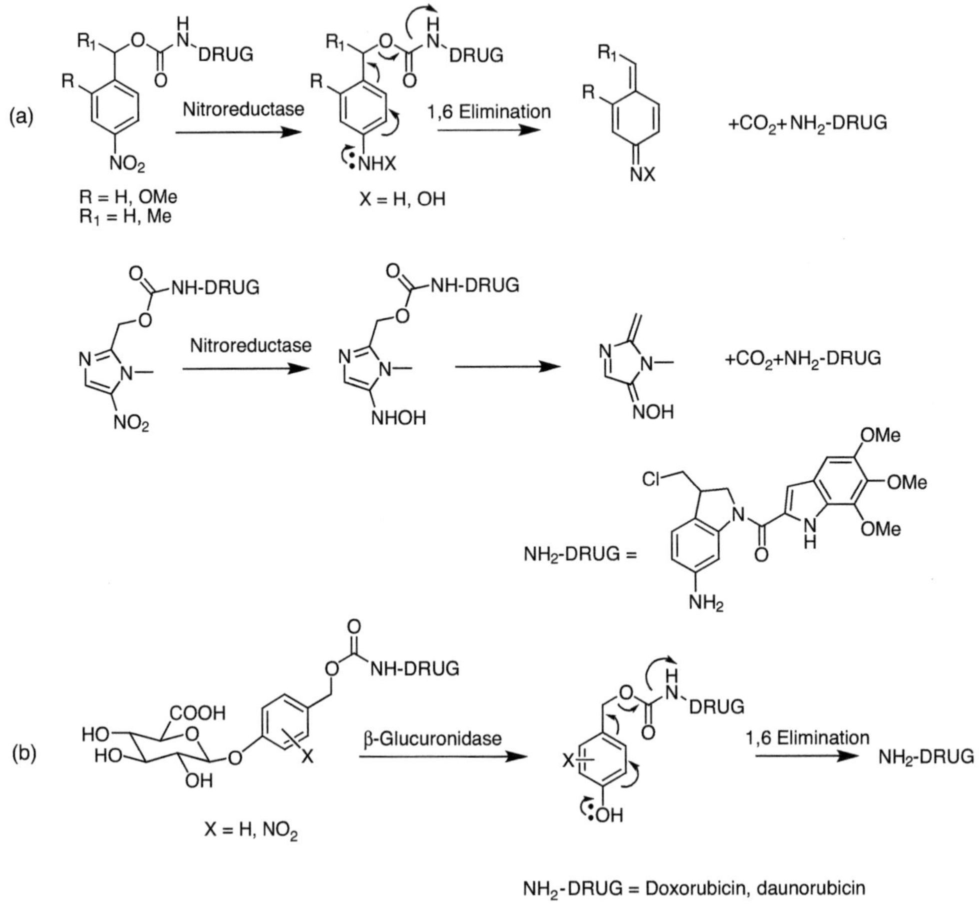


**Scheme 12.13**

most common handle to deactivate and conjugate a drug is via an amino group. However the amine in itself is not a good leaving group, and will not be deactivated by simple alkyl connection with the linker (at least not by lowering of electron density) [176]. The most common strategy to connect the amine drug to the linker is to convert it into a carbamate linkage. The process is irreversible due to the decomposition of the unstable carbamic acid to amine and carbon dioxide. Examples of amino-containing drugs that were deactivated as carbamates in self-immolative prodrugs include aniline mustards (Scheme 12.2b, X = NH, $NMe_2$) [70], anthracyclines (Scheme 12.13b) [100, 212], duocarmycin analogues (Scheme 12.13a) [100, 212], and enediyne [100, 212] (Scheme 12.4a).

Another option for amino-containing drugs is conversion to quaternary ammonium prodrugs that are a good leaving group and can release tertiary amine drugs in an elimination process (Scheme 12.1b) [165].

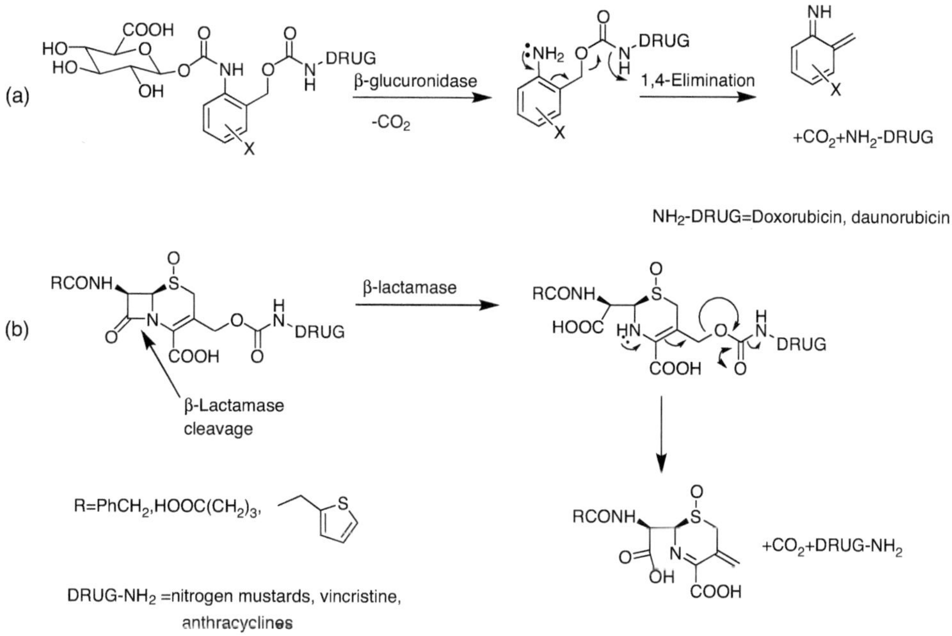


**Scheme 12.14**

Phenol drugs can be connected to the linker via the hydroxy group, either as carbonates (Scheme 12.2b) [70] or as ethers [168, 213].

Aliphatic ethers would normally be too stable to release an alcohol drug in a self-immolative mechanism. However, this case has been described in the activation of a prodrug of 3-amino-4-hydroxymethylacridine by nitroreductase, where the 4-hydroxymethyl group is masked as an ether part of an oxazolidine ring. The initial 1,6-elimination triggered by the nitro group reduction expels the 4-hydroxymethyl group and forms an intermediate imine, which is hydrolytically decomposed to aldehyde with release of the 3-amino-4-hydroxymethylacridine drug [214].

Other functional groups on drugs that were masked by the linker and form a leaving group are phosphoramide (of a phosphoramide mustard, deactivated as phosphoric ester, such as cyclophosphamide shown in Scheme 12.3b) [136]; carboxylic acid (of a platinum drug, linked as ester) [125]; and thiol (of a vincristine derivative, masked as thioether) [215].

One concern with self-immolative systems activated by elimination is that the quinonemethide formed will react with the activating enzyme and induce suicide inhibition. Two studies have shown that this is not the case, and that water addition to the quinomethide with formation of benzylic alcohol is the main reaction [216, 217].

#### 12.5.3.3 Self-Immolative Prodrugs Fragmenting Following Cyclization

Self-immolative prodrugs activated by cyclization contain a latent nucleophilic group that become available for reaction following activation. The nucleophile (such as amino, hydroxylamino, and hydroxy) is situated in a constrained and entropically favorable position with respect to the carboxylic or the carbonic acid derivative of the drug. Nucleophilic attack on the carbonyl with elimination of the drug generates a stable five- or six-membered ring in an intramolecular process. A combination of entropic and energetic factors concurs to drive the process toward drug elimination, once the required starting nucleophile is formed and cyclization takes place.

The rate of cyclization can be increased by designing more sterically constrained linkers, such as geminal dimethyl substitution of the linker [218] or locking the geometry in the *cis* conformation (coumarin-based linkers) [219]. An example is shown in Scheme 12.15: the cleavage of β-glucuronic acid releases the phenolate group, which generate the stable cyclic carbamate with expulsion of the phenol mustard drug [220].

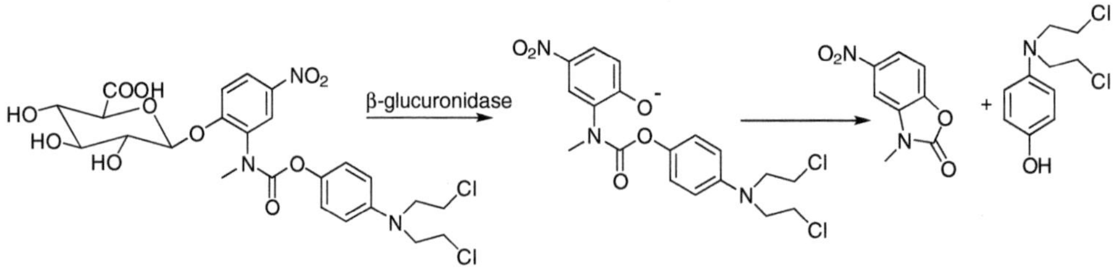


Scheme 12.15

The linkage between the drug and the linker is complementary to that used in the elimination linkers. More stable linkers such as amides (Scheme 12.1b) can be used for drugs possessing amino functionalities. For phenolic drugs, carbamate linkages can be used (Scheme 12.15), which are more stable than the carbonate linkage.

## 12.6 Strategies Used for the Improvement of DEPT Systems

### 12.6.1 Improvement of the Prodrug

In order to achieve success in DEPT, the prodrug, enzyme, and delivery vehicle need to be optimized. Cytotoxicity differential, stability, kinetics of activation, BE, pharmacokinetic properties are prodrug characteristics that require optimization. This is achieved by (i) chemical modification of a lead prodrug (for example, the synthesis of SN23 862, Scheme 12.1a, based on the structure of CB1954, Scheme 12.10a);

(ii) rationale prodrug design based on known substrate requirement of a specific enzyme (for example, the development of prodrugs for CPG2, glycosidases, or self-immolative prodrugs for NR); crystallographic data are available for some of the important enzymes for ADEPT and GDEPT and should assist in the rational and structure-based design of improved prodrugs [154, 221–229]; and (iii) screening of drugs/compounds similar to a lead prodrug as potential substrates for the activating enzyme with improved prodrug profile (e.g., new nucleotides for HSV-TK [230] or PNP [201]).

The important characteristics of prodrugs in DEPT, as well as strategies to improve them, are discussed in this section.

#### 12.6.1.1 **Cytotoxicity Differential**

Two parameters are important in describing the cytotoxicity differential of a prodrug. One is the potential for activation, measured by the $IC_{50}$ ratio between prodrug and drug in cells in the absence of activating enzyme. This parameter describes how much the drug has been deactivated by conversion to prodrug. Low potential of activation can indicate inefficient deactivation of prodrug or premature release of the drug (for example, a seco-duocarmycin prodrug was found to be as toxic as the drug, presumably due to active uptake in cells and lysosomal cleavage [101] (Scheme 12.4a). The other is the degree of activation, measuring the prodrug $IC_{50}$ ratio between the same cell line expressing the activating enzyme and the nonexpressing counterpart. This parameter describes the efficiency of the enzyme–prodrug system. In many cases, the degree of activation is lower than the potential of activation due to incomplete release of the parent drug, slow kinetics of activation, side reactions or poor access of the prodrug to the enzyme.

More than 100-fold differential (in terms of degree of activation) is considered as a necessary therapeutic window [231, 232], although lower values have been reported to produce good biological effect [47, 233, 234]. Differentials upto 1000-fold have also been suggested as suitable thresholds for useful therapeutic effect [235]. Several GDEPT systems achieve more than 100-fold cytotoxicity differential.

For prodrugs activated by an electronic switch, the magnitude of the shift in electronic effect frequently parallels the cytotoxicity differential, especially for nitrogen mustard prodrugs. The mustard moiety reactivity correlates strongly with the basicity of the nitrogen atom. For *para*-substituted aromatic nitrogen mustards, this basicity is determined by the electronic effect of the *para*-substituent, expressed by the Hammett constant $\sigma_p$. Differentials of up to 200-fold have been obtained with 4-aminoaniline mustards deactivated as carbamates or ureas (the differences in Hammett constants $\Delta\sigma_p = 0.42$ between amine and urea and 0.49 between amine and carbamate) [67]. *N*-Methylation of the carbamate nitrogen tends to increase the differential (Scheme 12.2b, X = NMe versus X = NH) [69, 236]. For aromatic mustard prodrugs activated by reduction of nitro group to hydroxylamine ($\Delta\sigma_p = 1.12$), differentials from 100 to 2500 have been achieved (Scheme 12.1a) [163]. For quaternary ammonium prodrugs of mechloramine (that would correspond to $\Delta\sigma_p = 1.64$), a 3000-fold degree of activation was observed (Scheme 12.1b) [165]. For a self-immolative 4-nitrobenzyl phosphoramide mustard prodrug, a huge degree of activation of 170 000-fold was reported between V79 cells expressing versus non-expressing nitroreductase [237].

Up to 4500-fold activation has been shown for carbohydrate prodrugs of (1*S*,10*R*)-methyl-seco-CBI-DMAI analogues in the presence of the corresponding glycosidase [238].

Other activation strategies that were particularly effective in achieving high differentials are conversion to substrate for endogenous enzymes (for example, 44 000-fold activation of GCV by HSV-TK (Scheme 12.7) in osteosarcoma [179]) and formation of a second interactive group (up to 2000-fold differential for CB1954 activation by NR, Scheme 12.10a, 10 000-fold for activation of *N*-(4-ethoxy-4-β-glucuronyl)butyl-anthracyclins by β-glucuronidase [98, 186], Scheme 12.10b).

#### 12.6.1.2 **Stability of Prodrugs**

A requirement for prodrugs for DEPT is stability in physiological conditions. Instability of prodrugs can lead to early release of drugs, with associated side effects, or inactivation of prodrugs before reaching the target enzyme.

Premature drug release can result from chemical or catalytic hydrolysis (by plasma esterases) of the bonds between the trigger/specifier, the linker, and the drug.

In self-immolative PEG-doxorubicin conjugates, the ester linkage is more sensitive to plasma hydrolysis than the carbonate ($t_{1/2}$: 1 h versus 2.9 h). Improved stability can be achieved by increasing the steric hindrance around the ester bond on the *ortho*-positions of the phenol or the α-position of the ester [239, 240]. The instability of the carbonate linkage for many phenol drugs in self-immolative prodrugs was greatly improved by using a stable ether link instead [213]. Self-immolative carbonate prodrugs of phenol mustards were unstable at physiological pH (Scheme 12.2b, X = O), whereas carbamate prodrugs of aniline mustards were stable (Scheme 12.2b, X = NH, NMe) [70]. A similar behavior was observed comparing the carbonate and ether prodrugs of 10-hydroxycamptothecin [168]. A comparison of model prodrugs found that esters are hydrolyzed fast in plasma whereas carbamates are stable [241, 242]. Similar results were obtained with paclitaxel prodrugs containing an ester or carbamate link [174, 175]. Therefore, for prodrugs releasing phenol drugs (or linkers), the order of stability to plasma esterases is ester < carbonate < carbamate < ether.

In general, prodrugs of amine drugs are more stable than prodrugs of phenol drugs. The amide linkage in prodrugs is usually stable *in vivo* although surprising instability can be observed if the amide is substrate for endopeptidases [172]. Carbamate prodrugs of secondary amines tend to be more stable than those of primary amines [69, 243].

Premature deactivation of the prodrug by hydrolysis is an issue with nitrogen mustard prodrugs. The rate of hydrolysis increases with the leaving group ability of the mustard halogen (mesyl ≫ I > Br > Cl). *Ortho*-NH and *para*-NMe aniline mustard prodrugs are two to three times more stable than *para*-NH aniline mustards [69]. A comparison between similar prodrugs of aniline mustard and amine-containing CC1065 analogue shows the former to be deactivated by hydrolysis of the mustard group ($t_{1/2} = 1$ h), whereas the latter was stable ($t_{1/2} > 24$ h) [131].

#### 12.6.1.3 Cytotoxicity and Mechanism of Action of the Released Drug

An important factor in designing prodrugs for GDEPT is the potency of the released drug. Their cytotoxicity should be as high as possible, in order to overcome potential limitations in prodrug penetration of tumors and in the capacity of the activation mechanism [244]. The less cytotoxic drugs usually fail to achieve total cell killing. Also, in order to improve the activation potential, prodrugs with lower cytotoxicity should be designed, which release very cytotoxic drugs. An example of very potent cytotoxic drug is the CC-1065 analogue seco-CBI-Q-galactoside, with $IC_{50}$ 0.13 nM (in PancTu 1 cell line) and cytotoxicity differential of 3400-fold (Scheme 12.4a).

A QSAR based on nitrogen mustard self-immolative prodrugs showed a direct correlation between the potency of the released drugs and the logarithm of differential in a GDEPT system with CPG2 [69]. For CB1954 and the mustard SN23 682 metabolites, the alkylating reactivity correlates with the electron-donating properties of the *ortho*- and *para*-substituents. This correlation holds provided the mechanism of activation is the same for all compounds. There is one interesting exception, the 4-hydroxylamino (4-NHOH) metabolite of CB1954, which is 300-fold more cytotoxic than predicted, in agreement with the different mechanism of activation based on the formation of a second reactive group (Scheme 12.10a) [184].

Ideally, the cytotoxicity induced by the released drug should be cell cycle phase or proliferation independent, to kill a wide range of tumor cell population [5, 117, 231, 245]. Examples of drugs from this category are nitrogen mustards (Scheme 12.3a), 6-methylpurine, flutarabine, and CB1954 (Scheme 12.10a).

#### 12.6.1.4 Stability of the Released Drug

Another important parameter for the released drug in DEPT is the half-life in physiological conditions. The half-life of the drug should be optimized, in order to achieve the right compromise between tumor diffusion and prevention of systemic escape [68, 231, 232]. If a drug is too stable and highly diffusible, leakage into the general circulation will occur, with corresponding systemic toxicity. If the half-life is too short, the drug cannot reach the neighboring cells to mount a BE. For aromatic nitrogen mustard drugs, the cytotoxicity and half-life of released drugs are correlated (drugs with shorter half-lives are usually more cytotoxic), and are very dependent on the substituents on the aromatic ring. The reactivity varies linearly with $\sigma_p$ of the substituent. Electron-donating groups in *para*-position increase the reactivity of the mustard and decrease its $t_{1/2}$. *Ortho*-substituents produce steric hindrance of resonance, twisting the nitrogen mustard moiety and disrupting the conjugation with the aromatic nucleus, with consequent increase in reactivity of the mustard. This effect increases with the bulkiness of the *ortho*-substituent. The nature of the leaving group on the mustard also has a large effect on $t_{1/2}$ of the drug, better leaving groups meaning shorter half-life (F $\gg$ Cl > Br > I > mesyloxy in the order of half-lives) [68]. CMDA (Scheme 12.3a), the compound that reached clinical Phase I trial in ADEPT with CPG2 [246] has a $t_{1/2}$ of the released drug of 48 min (in physiological buffer), long enough to allow leak-back from the tumor and to elicit systemic side effects. Therefore, prodrug ZD2767P was designed, releasing a more potent drug, the phenol mustard drug (4-[bis-(2-iodoethyl)amino]phenol) (Scheme 12.2a), with a shorter $t_{1/2}$ of <1 min and superior therapeutic index [67]. The higher reactivity of the phenol mustard drug compared to the benzoic mustard drug released from CMDA can be attributed to the better leaving group in the mustard moiety (bis-iodo versus chloro-mesyl) and the stronger electron-donating ability of the *para*-activating group (phenol versus carboxylate).

The BE is affected by the $t_{1/2}$ of the released drug. For SN23 682 analogues, the more reactive mustards (bis-bromo and bis-iodo) have the best BE effect [163]. However, prodrugs generating less reactive benzoic acid mustards show a superior BE and efficacy at 50 and 10% cells expressing CPG2 than the more potent 4-[bis(2-iodoethyl)amino]phenyloxy carbonyl-L-glutamate, (ZD2767P) (Scheme 12.2a), which shows instead better therapeutic efficacy in xenografts where 100% of cells express CPG2 [73]. This suggests there is an optimal $t_{1/2}$ of drugs for BE. A suggested range of suitable $t_{1/2}$ is from many seconds to several minutes [245]. Based on a diffusion radius in the tumor of 100–200 μm, the optimum $t_{1/2}$ of the drug should be about 1 min [247].

Prodrugs generating short-lived species such as radicals are expected to produce a poor BE. IAA is a substrate for HRP. The first intermediates in the oxidation are radicals, with very short $t_{1/2}$, and unlikely to explain the BE observed. A later intermediate, 3-methylene-2-oxindole, a Michael acceptor, has a longer $t_{1/2}$ and was suggested as the actual active species [116]. Surprising BE was obtained in hypoxic conditions with CYP2B6/P450R and tirapazamine (TPZ), given the short $t_{1/2}$ and high reactivity of the radical intermediate considered to be the active species of TPZ [197].

#### 12.6.1.5 **Resistance (Prodrug Related)**

Little is known about resistance to DEPT. Drugs that act directly without requirement for extra endogenous enzymatic activation steps have an advantage in circumventing potential resistance due to low expression of endogenous enzyme. A strategy to address this issue is cotransfection of the activating enzyme and the enzyme responsible for further metabolism of the released drug. Examples of this double enzyme approach are HSV-TK with guanylate cyclase and CD/UPRT [248, 249].

The ATP-dependent drug transporter ABCG2 confers resistance to camptothecin. Expression of ABCG2 confers resistance to CPT-11 (releasing SN38, Scheme 12.6) in cells transfected with the activating enzyme CE. Resistance to this DEPT system is likely to be an issue in tumors overexpressing this transporter [250].

#### 12.6.1.6 **Kinetics of Activation**

The kinetics of prodrug activation determines the rate of drug formation at the tumor site, the concentration of released drug and therefore the concentration of prodrug required to reach therapeutically significant active drug level. The parameters $K_m$ (measuring the affinity of the substrate for the enzyme) and $k_{cat}$ or $V_{max}$ (measuring the rate of substrate conversion) are used to describe the kinetics of enzymatic conversion of substrates to products. Efficient prodrug activation even at low concentration of prodrug (low $K_m$) and rapid conversion of the prodrug to the active drug (high $k_{cat}$) are generally considered desirable features of a prodrug/enzyme system [231, 232, 251, 252]. For example, comparing canine P450 isoform 2B11 with human P450 isoform 2B6, in a GDEPT system with CP and IF prodrugs, the former isoform has better efficacy *in vitro* and *in vivo* and in terms of BE. The advantage of the 2B11 isoform was attributed to its 10–20-fold lower $K_m$ for CP and IF [253].

Enzyme/substrate systems with slow kinetics of activation (for example, human carboxylesterase hCE2 with prodrug CPT11) cannot reach high enough drug concentration [57]. There are, however, a few caveats. Very low $K_m$ values can be unfavorable for selectivity in systems using human enzymes or enzymes with human homologues, as even low level of the endogenous enzyme in normal tissues can induce prodrug activation [110]. Fast release of drug can be more effective against proliferating cells, whereas a slow constant release might be more efficient against quiescent cells.

The optimal prodrug is not necessarily the one with the fastest kinetics of activation. Slower kinetics are acceptable if offset by improvement in other properties. 5-Fluoroindole-3-acetic acid is oxidized slower than indoleacetic acid by HRP but shows more cytotoxicity in cell lines [254]. Prodrug ZD2767P (Scheme 12.2a), despite poorer kinetics ($k_{cat} = 29.5\ s^{-1}$) compared to CMDA ($k_{cat} = 583\ s^{-1}$) (Scheme 12.3a), is the compound of choice for clinical trials due to the higher potency, shorter half life of the released drug and better cytotoxicity differential [73].

In a series of prodrugs, the kinetics of activation can be altered by structural modifications. CB1954 prodrug for NR has $k_{cat} = 360\ min^{-1}$ (Scheme 12.10a). Replacement of the aziridine moiety with nitrogen mustard in prodrug SN23 862 led to a better substrate for NR ($k_{cat} = 1580\ min^{-1}$). The 2-amino-3,5-dinitrobenzamide isomer of SN23 862 is an even better substrate ($k_{cat} = 4540\ min^{-1}$) [134].

For self-immolative prodrugs, the kinetics of activation and the kinetics of fragmentation are both relevant for the overall rate of drug release, the slower step being rate limiting.

The kinetics of activation of a prodrug is dependent upon the structure of the specifier. The linkers can improve the kinetics by separating the specifier and the bulky drug. For example, the galactose self-immolative prodrug of doxorubicin, containing a *p*-aminobenzyl linker, is a better substrate for α-galactosidase than the direct prodrug [97, 190].

Usually, substitutions that introduce steric hindrance reduce the rate of activation. Whereas unsubstituted nitrobenzyl carbamates have a relatively fast kinetics of activation [136], the presence of bulky substituents on the aromatic ring (Scheme 12.13a) or *ortho*-effects can greatly reduce the rate of activation [236]. Anthracyclins-spacer-β-glucuronyl prodrugs containing the *ortho*-benzylic linker have a slower rate of activation than those containing the *para*-benzylic linkers (900 min versus 100 min, respectively). This difference is most likely due to slower enzymatic activation rather than slower fragmentation [107]. For self-immolative nitrogen mustard prodrugs for CPG2, the specifier–linker fragments are good substrates for the enzyme ($k_{cat} = 65–140\ s^{-1}$) (Scheme 12.16). The self-immolative prodrugs, additionally containing the drug fragment (Scheme 12.2b) are poorer substrates ($k_{cat} = 3–5\ s^{-1}$) than the specifier–linkers, and poorer than the corresponding direct prodrug ($k_{cat} = 30\ s^{-1}$) (Schemes 12.1c and 12.2a), despite similar $K_m$ values [69].

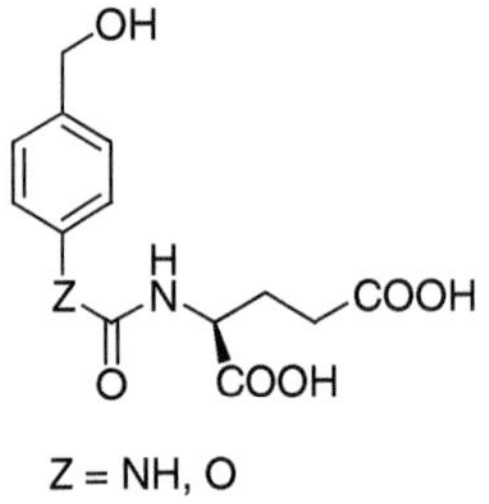

Scheme 12.16

The kinetics of fragmentation of the unstable linker–drug intermediate formed following enzymatic activation can be modulated by structural modifications of the linker. Electron-withdrawing substituents on the aromatic ring (such as Cl and $NO_2$) decrease the rate of elimination from aminobenzylic linkers, in contrast with electron-donating ones. Alkylation of the benzylic position also increases the rate of fragmentation [255]. For hydroxybenzylic linkers, the strong electron-withdrawing substituents ($NO_2$) actually increase the elimination, due to the formation of the strong electron-donating phenolate anion instead of the phenol (Scheme 12.16) [100, 212]. This pattern of structure–activity relationship is consistent with the stabilization of the positive charge on the benzylic position.

#### 12.6.1.7 **Physicochemical Properties**

Lipophilicity and water solubility are important properties of prodrugs and released drugs. Lipophilicity determines the cell permeability of prodrugs by passive diffusion and their ability to mount a BE. Increasing the lipophilicity of prodrugs enhances their cell permeability. GCV elaidic acid ester ($c\log P + 0.7$) is more potent than GCV ($c\log P - 2.07$) in cell culture, due to better cell penetration and longer retention of the active mono-, di-, and triphosphate metabolites [256].

There are two mechanisms for BE, depending on the charge and lipohilicity of the active drugs. For prodrugs releasing charged drugs that are unable to cross cell membranes (such as GCV, Scheme 12.7), cell–cell contact and gap junctions are required for BE. Prodrugs releasing neutral drugs rely on passive diffusion to achieve BE. In general, prodrugs releasing more diffusible drugs produce a better BE. A comparisons of several GDEPT systems has shown that CD/5-FC and NR/CB1954 (Scheme 12.10a), which generate lipophilic diffusible metabolites, have a higher BE than HSV-TK/GCV (Scheme 12.7) and dCK/ara-C, which generate phosphate metabolites and rely on gap junctions to kill neighboring cells [257, 258]. In a multilayer cells model, the BE of dinitrobenzamide aziridine and nitrogen mustard prodrugs for NR (Scheme 12.1a) correlate well with their lipophilicity [164]. Among the metabolites of CB1954, the more diffusible 2-amino metabolite is responsible for most of the activity of the prodrug, despite being less potent than the 4-hydroxylamine metabolite (Scheme 12.10a) [185]. A review compiling $c\log P$ data for the most common prodrugs used in GDEPT and discussing the influence of this parameter on BE and cellular activity of prodrug has been published [161]. The conclusion of the review is that more lipophilic neutral prodrugs tend to have improved cellular activity and bystander effect. This correlation is based on the assumption that the drug lipophilicity parallels the prodrug lipophilicity, and that passive transport of prodrug and released drug occurs. When active transport is involved the same rules do not apply. For example, MTX released from Met-Phe prodrug by CA is a substrate for the reduced folate carrier. The transport of its analogues is structure dependent rather than lipophilicity dependent [172, 259].

#### 12.6.1.8 Pharmacokinetics

Prodrug pharmacokinetic is very important for *in vivo* tumor efficacy. A prodrug with good *in vitro* profile can fail *in vivo* due to pharmacokinetic issues. A doxorubicin prodrug has cytotoxicity differential of >370 between EMT6 cells expressing and nonexpressing NR, but unfavorable physicochemical properties (MW about 900 Da, 7 HBD, and 20 HBA). Unsurprisingly, it lacks *in vivo* activity, which was attributed to poor plasma pharmacokinetics or poor tumor accumulation [133].

Increased plasma retention can be achieved by plasma albumin binding of the prodrug. Self-immolative prodrugs of glycosylases were substituted with Cl or aliphatic chains to increase this albumin binding [107]. Nitrogen mustard prodrugs for CPG2 are stabilized by plasma protein binding (as reflected by their longer half-life) without adverse effect on activation.

In a GDEPT approach, tumors transfected with the P450 enzyme were found to have increased sensitivity to treatment with CP, despite the high level of circulating 4-hydroxy-CP (the activated metabolite) generated by the high CYP activity of the liver (proximity effect) [82]. Several strategies were suggested to increase the tumor: liver partition rate: (i) increasing the CYP activity of the tumor by coexpression of the P450 reductase, required for reactivation of CYP. A 10-fold increase in tumor cells killing *in vivo* was obtained with this strategy [260]; (ii) implanting intratumorally controlled release polymer pellets containing CP – a 250 fold increase in the 4-hydroxy-CP compared to IP injection was observed [261]; (iii) improving the kinetics of enzyme activation by selecting a more active CYP isoform or by site-directed mutagenesis of the enzyme; (iv) selective inhibition of the liver P450R or of other CYP liver isoforms except the one used for GDEPT [262, 263]; and (v) choosing the suitable schedule of prodrug administration. It was found that continuous administration of CP at 0.125 mM for 3 days decreases the CYP activity due to killing of the cells expressing the activating enzyme. Bolus administration of prodrug for 8 h at 1 mM concentration followed by a drug free period until day three administrations of another 8 h at 1 mM does not diminish the capacity of CYP activation, presumably due to the recovery of cells expressing CYP. The same overall dose is achieved in the tumor. Comparing the continuous administration without GDEPT of high 1 mM dose in patients, the AUC of toxic metabolite in blood is three times higher than the 8 h bolus administration combined with GDEPT, and the tumor concentration of the toxic metabolite is similar. Therefore, the same efficacy can be obtained with bolus treatment and GDEPT as with continuous infusion without GDEPT but with three times less toxic side effects [264].

#### 12.6.1.9 **Specificity of Enzyme Activation**

The prodrug should be activated only by the enzyme expressed in tumor; otherwise, general toxicity will ensue. This is a potential risk when using endogenous enzyme for DEPT systems. Even for foreign enzymes, for example, of bacterial origin, the prodrug can be activated nonselectively by the enzymes in the gut flora [265].

Two analogues of the natural nucleotide dT, the (North)metanocarbathymidine and (South)metanocarbathymidine, were tested as prodrugs for HSV-tk. Both compounds are good substrates for HSV-tk. In addition, the (North) derivative is a weak substrate for the human thymidine kinase (hTK1), whereas the (South) analogue is not a substrate for hTK1. Therefore, the (South)metanocarbathymidine is considered a safer prodrug for GDEPT with HSV-tk [154].

For prodrugs activated by NR, the selectivity for NR against other reductases (for example, DT-diaphorase) is dependent on the reduction potential of the prodrug. Optimal selectivity is achieved for prodrugs with redox potential in the range of 400–500 mV [131, 137].

### 12.6.2
### **Improving the Enzymes**

New techniques are available to increase the efficacy of enzymes to activate prodrugs for ADEPT and GDEPT [266]. There are three ways of improving the efficacy of enzymes: (i) Using orthologous enzymes or enzymes with similar profiles of activity from different species; (ii) Crystallographic investigation of the active site of the enzymes that allows the rational synthesis of better substrates using molecular modeling and computer-aided techniques; and (iii) modification of the active site of the enzyme by site-directed mutagenesis, in order to increase its catalytic efficiency toward a given substrate, or to allow the design of better modified substrates.

Enzymes from different origins can have very different kinetics with the same substrate. The rat DT-diaphorase is a more effective activating enzyme compared to the human one for CB1954, with a $k_{cat}$ sevenfold higher. The *E.* coli NR exhibits a $k_{cat}$, which is higher (360 $min^{-1}$ compared to 4.1 for rat and 0.64 $min^{-1}$ for the human enzyme) for the reduction of the nitro group, making it the enzyme of choice for GDEPT with NR [192].

A new NR has been identified from a different bacterium: *Bacillus amyloliquefaciens* that metabolizes the prodrug CB1954 only to its cytotoxic drug, 4-hydroxylamine (Scheme 12.10a), compared with the previously used enzyme that formed an additional secondary inactive metabolite, 2-hydroxylamine [267].

The rabbit carboxylesterase is 100–1000-fold more efficient in activating the prodrug CPT-11 than the human homologue [177]. *Drosophila melanogaster* deoxyribonucleoside kinase (Dm-dNK) exhibits a catalytic rate that is 10- to 100-fold higher than that reported of previously studied deoxyribonucleoside kinases [268]. The yeast CD is also more effective in activating the 5-FC prodrug compared to the bacterial CD [94].

Crystallographic data are now available for a number of GDEPT enzymes: HRP [269], CYP2C [82], HSV-TK [154], CPG2 [226], yeast CD [223], and

NR [221, 222, 270], which aid in the design of better substrates and guiding mutagenesis assays.

Another way to modify the enzyme is by protein engineering and site-directed mutagenesis. An example was the engineering of HSV-TK producing mutants with increased sensitivity to both GCV and acyclovir (ACV). Compared to wild type, the $K_m$ was slightly higher for GCV and ACV in the mutant, but much higher (35-fold) for the endogenous thymidine substrate competing for the same site. The $k_{cat}$ for thymidine was significantly reduced (88-fold) compared to the $k_{cat}$ for GCV and ACV (6- and 8-fold, respectively). As a consequence, the mutant displayed greatly reduced competition for the active site and better selectivity for the prodrug substrates than for endogenous thymidine [271]. Three HSV-TK mutants were selected (obtained by introducing a restricted set of semirandom sequences in the active site), which conferred a substantial increase in $IC_{50}$ of GCV and ACV (of 39–294-fold and 3–182-fold, respectively) with respect to the wild-type enzyme [272, 273]. At a dose of 5 mg/kg GCV the growth of the xenograft expressing the SR39 mutant enzyme was completely prevented while the tumors expressing the wild-type TK grew [272].

Based on the NR cocrystal structure with nicotinic acid [270], nine aminoacid residues around the active site of the enzyme suspected of being involved in substrate binding have been mutated. From these, a number of mutant enzymes have been isolated with an increased sensitivity to CB1954. Kinetic and structural characterization of these mutants was carried out [274]. One of these, F124K, was shown to increase fivefold the sensitivity to the prodrug in human ovarian carcinoma SKOV3 cells [275]. A double mutant was also created (N71S/F124K), combining the most beneficial single mutations, and it was shown that this has the highest specificity constant for CB1954 of all the mutants studied [274].

An adenoviral vector encoding a mutant bacterial cytosine deaminase bCD-D314A gene has been developed (harboring a substitution of an alanine for the aspartic acid at position 314 in the CD protein), which is up to 206-fold more active than the wild-type CD for a multiplicity of infection of 2 [276].

Until recently, only nonhuman enzymes have been used in ADEPT, but due to their immunogenicity, their use has been restricted to Phase I clinical trials [277, 278]. However, in 2009, a double mutant human (E201Q : N243D) purine nucleoside phosphorylase (hDM) has been reported, which unlike the wild-type enzyme (hPNP) can use (deoxy)adenosine prodrugs as substrates [279].

### 12.6.3 The Multigene Approach

A different strategy to develop more efficient suicide gene therapy systems uses transgenes with more than one gene. Several different approaches based either on transfection of multiple suicide genes or on a combination of suicide gene(s) with cytokine or other genes have been reported. A typical example is the combination of HSV-TK and endostatin (angiogenesis inhibitor) genes followed by treatment with GCV, which is capable of eradicating orthotopic human renal cell carcinomas (Caki-1) in nude mice [280].

A double gene transfer is able to enhance the efficacy of a GDEPT system. By transfecting target cells with two different suicide gene, the expressed enzymes are able to activate two distinct types of prodrugs releasing anticancer drugs with different mechanisms of action and therefore making the system more effective.

The first attempt concerned the association between CD and TK genes followed by 5-FC and GCV administrations. The rationale behind this is that the permeable toxic metabolites resulting from the CD/5-FC system will enhance the overall BE and therefore a synergic antitumoral effect can be achieved [281–283]. Examples were reported in which cells were infected with CYP + CD or TK + CD genes. In each case, the "double suicide gene" systems proved to be more effective both *in vitro* and *in vivo* compared to each single system alone [284, 285].

If a metabolic cascade is to be considered in the activation of a prodrug that requires more than one enzyme, (for example, in the activation of GCV to GCVTP), then the cotransfection of genes expressing the enzymes catalyzing each intermediate step of this pathway is expected to increase the overall yield of the desired final cytotoxic metabolite. The enhancement of GCV and ACV activation using the simultaneous transfection of HSV-TK, guanylate kinase (GMPK), and nucleoside diphosphate kinase (NDPK) responsible for the mono-, di-, and triphosphorylation of these substrates allows more than 90% of the GCV to be converted to GCVTP [286]. An attempt was made to overcome resistance to 5-FU by modification of 5-FU phosphorylation. A recombinant adenovirus containing both the UPRT and HSV-TK was engineered and the dual system assayed on esophageal carcinoma cells. A significantly enhanced antitumor activity was reported [287].

The kinases needed for the first two phosphorylation steps of gemcitabine (dCK and uridine monophosphate kinase) were introduced in pancreatic carcinoma PC1.0 cell line (using a fusion gene combining dCK and UMK), which showed sensitization to gemcitabine by reducing dramatically both *in vitro* cell viability and *in vivo* tumor volume [288].

The same strategy was applied to the CD/5-FC system that showed poor results in cancer cell lines (such as breast and pancreatic carcinoma cell lines) resistant to 5-FU, due to defects in the downstream metabolism of 5-FU. Transduction of a bicistronic fusion gene encoding CD and uracil phosphotransferase was superior to the CD system alone both *in vitro* and *in vivo* [289]. A fusion bifunctional gene incorporated in an adenovirus, AdCDUPRT, increases sensitization to 5-FC by 80–168-fold compared to AdCD vector and by 2800–9600-fold compared to uninfected cells [290].

The cotransfection of cyt-P450 gene with the P450 reductase, results in a significant increase in the conversion of CP to their toxic metabolites and therefore in the overall increase of the efficiency of the cyt P450/CP system up to 10-fold [82, 260].

An alternative approach consisted of the transduction of two (or more) copies of the same gene in the target cells. It was demonstrated that the UMSCC29 and T98G human cancer cell lines containing two copies of the TK gene led to more effective metabolism of GCV and therefore exhibited enhanced sensitivity to the prodrug [291].

### 12.6.4
### Enhancing the Immune Response

Enhancing the immune response can increase the effectivity of a GDEPT system (see below), which may be done by cotransfecting a suicide gene with one or more cytokine genes. The role of IL-2 in these systems has been investigated. Cells grown as xenografts in BALB/c syngeneic mice were injected with an adenoviral vector containing the HSV-TK gene or the IL-2 gene, followed by treatment with GCV [292]. While the tumors continued to grow in the animals injected with a control vector or the vector carrying the IL-2 gene, those treated with HSV-TK with or without coadministration of the IL-2, exhibited tumor necrosis and regressions. However, only animals treated with both the HSV-TK and the IL-2 genes developed effective systemic antitumor immunity against tumorigenic rechallenges. The antitumor immunity was associated with the presence of tumor-specific cytolytic CD8+ T lymphocytes. In order to enhance and prolong the antitumor immunity, a third vector containing the mouse granulocyte macrophage colony stimulating factor (mGM-CSF) gene was employed. The animals treated simultaneously with HSV-TK + IL-2 + mGM-CSF vectors followed by administration of GCV, developed long-term antitumor immunity and survived for more than 4 months without recurrence [292].

IL-12 also plays a multifunctional role in controlling the immune system, augmenting the proliferation of T and NK cells. In a suicide gene strategy, both HSV-TK and IL-12 genes were incorporated in replication-defective vectors. Following CT26 murine colon adenocarcinoma infection, treatment with GCV was significantly more effective than in gene therapy using IL-12 or HSV-TK alone [293]. The combined treatment with AdHSV-TK/GCV and AdmIL-12 also resulted in enhanced tumor inhibition and improved antimetastatic activity [294].

Finally, combining strategies is another way to improve DEPT. For instance, combining an antiapoptotic approach (by using inhibitory caspase baculovirus protein p35 with GDEPT CYP450/CP system) prolongs intratumoral production of the active drug without inducing resistance [295].

## 12.7
## Biological Data for ADEPT and GDEPT

Stage 1 of a GDEPT or ADEPT therapy requires a vector to deliver the therapeutic gene. In GDEPT, the vector is usually a virus or a bacterium that expresses a prodrug-activating enzyme. In ADEPT, the vector is either a monoclonal antibody covalently bound to the enzyme or a fusion protein with both antibody and enzymic characteristics.

Efficient tumor targeting of all vectors is important to reduce nonspecific toxicity of the prodrugs generated by these techniques.

### 12.7.1 Bacteria

The most prevalent bacteria in GDEPT are reduced pathogenicity auxotrophs of *S. typhimurium* [296–299] and species of *Clostridium* [300, 301] but others, such as *Bifidobacterium* sp. [302–304] and recently, a nonpathogenic, nonreplicating strain of *E. coli* [305] have been investigated. The latter two species have the advantage of being potentially less toxic to the host than either *Salmonella* or *Clostridium*. Tumor targeting, however, remains problematical with these bacteria, relying on the presence of a hypoxic microenvironment or specific cell-surface receptors. Systemically administered *Salmonellae* have been demonstrated noninvasively in xenograft tumors in mice by imaging with green fluorescent protein [306] and by PET scanning [307], showing the capability of these organisms to target the intended tissue. An oncolytic *S. typhimurium*-derived bacterium has been engineered to selectively express CPG2 in tumors [308]. The bacteria multiply within in the tumor cells; thus, the concentration of CPG2 is higher in these cells compared to others. It was reported that these bacteria are not killed by the activated drug. Treatment with nitrogen mustard prodrugs caused shrinkage of the tumors, showing that bacterial oncolytic therapy combined with CPG2-mediated prodrug activation has great potential in the treatment of tumors.

### 12.7.2 Viruses

The use of viruses as gene vectors (VDEPT) is well established. Viruses may be modified to target specific cell-surface receptors [309, 310] and hence specific tumor types, but unlike bacteria, they cannot be controlled by antibiotics.

### 12.7.3 Adenoviral Vectors

The adenovirus is a double-stranded DNA virus. There are 42 serotypes of adenovirus known to infect humans, but the majority of VDEPT studies currently use conditionally replicative adenoviral vectors of serogroups 2 and 5 that have been modified to target and reproduce exclusively in tumor cells, using the host to express prodrug-activating enzymes instead of viral proteins. However, the infection of cells by adenovirus relies to a large extent on the presence of the coxsackievirus and adenovirus receptor (CAR) [311], a cell-surface protein that is not expressed by all cancer cell types. Moreover, unless viruses are surface modified to protect them from the host's immune system, they can quickly give rise to an immune response, which limits their repeated administration unless tested in immunocompromised animals such as SCID or athymic mice. Several methods have been used to reduce viral immunogenicity such as cationic liposome conjugation [312] or coupling with polyethylene glycol ("PEGylation"). Tumor cell infectivity has been modulated by modification of the structure of the capsid fibers to target receptors other than CAR [313] and tumor-specific replication, which has been enhanced by replacing the E1 promoter with the human telomerase reverse transcriptase (hTERT) [314–316].

One of the challenges in using the adenoviral vector is to reduce the level of uptake by the reticuloendothelial system (RES) so that the engineered vector can reach its new target. Strategies for temporarily blocking the function of RES cells and hepatic uptake during intravascular administration of vectors have been reported by the laboratories of Seymour *et al.* [317, 318] and Gerritsen *et al.* [319]. These include bisphosphonates and gadolinium to inhibit the function of the RES cells, reactive polymers to cover the charges of the adenoviral vector [317, 318], and mutational change of the adenoviral vector fiber protein and the penton base proteins, to decrease uptake into the hepatocytes [319].

### 12.7.4
### Pox Vival Vectors

Yang *et al.* [320] have developed a new oncolytic vaccinia virus, the targeted deletions of three viral genes encoding thymidine kinase and antiapoptotic/host range proteins SPI-1 and SPI-2 (vSPT). Systemic delivery of vSPT showed significant tumor inhibition in subcutaneous MC38 tumor, human ovarian A2780, and murine ovarian MOSEC carcinomatosis models. However, the tumor inhibition by vSPTwas reduced compared with the parental viruses. These results demonstrate that deletion of these three viral genes not only further enhanced tumor selectivity but also weakened the oncolytic potency.

### 12.7.5
### Adeno-Associated Viral Vectors

The adeno-associated virus (AAV) is a replication defective, single-strand DNA virus. In the absence of a helper virus, the wild-type AAV genome can integrate into the host cell chromosomal DNA to maintain a latent state. In the presence of a helper virus (adenovirus), the AAV viral genome replicates episomally, followed by viral protein synthesis. AAV generates a very low or undetectable level of immune response. Disadvantages of using AAV are the small capacity (5 kb) and the difficulties encountered in production of the vector for clinical trial.

### 12.7.6
### Retroviral Vectors

The retrovirus buds from the plasma membrane of infected cells and contains a lipid coat within which is found homodimers of linear single-stranded RNA. The infection of cells by retrovirus is mediated by attachment of the viral envelope glycoprotein to the target cell-surface receptors. Once entry into the cytoplasm is completed, viral RNA is reverse transcribed into DNA and then randomly integrated into the host–cell genome.

Most of the retroviral vectors are based on the murine leukemia virus. Their cDNA can be integrated into the DNA of dividing cells with high efficiency. However, this process of random integration may also cause leukemia. The long-time interval between transplantation with the retrovirally modified bone marrow cells and the emergence of leukemia has suggested that the factors in addition to integration mutagenesis are involved. One of these may be that some preparations of retroviral vectors may carry "passenger" noncoding regulatory RNAs that can upregulate genes involved in cellular proliferation [321]. Retroviral vectors are suitable for targeting endothelial cells in the tumor neovasculature because of their intrinsic selectivity for proliferating cells. Several specific promoters, such as Flt-1, ICAM-2, and KDR have been used in the development of transcriptionally targeted retroviral vectors to tumor endothelial cells [322]. Hiraoka *et al.* [323] have showed that by combining optical imaging, flow cytometry, and molecular analysis they could monitor replication-competent retrovirus (RCR) vector spread after administration in hepatic metastasis model of colorectal cancer. RCR replication was confirmed, transduction levels reaching >90% in <12 days *in vitro*. *In vivo*, infusion of RCR supernatant into the portal circulation resulted in significant transduction of CT26 tumors in syngenic mice. Also, immunohistochemistry and quantitative PCR analysis showed no evidence of RCR spread to adjacent normal liver or to any other normal tissues.

### 12.7.7 Lentiviral Vectors

The lentivirus is a subclass of retroviruses. Lentiviral vectors are derived from the human immunodeficiency virus (HIV) by removal of the nonessential regulatory genes and sequences through which homologous recombination could lead to the recombination of therapeutic vector with HIV. Unlike retroviral vectors, lentiviral vectors can integrate their cDNA into both dividing and nondividing cells. Thus, they can also transduce terminally differentiated cells such as neurons, macrophages, and hematopoietic stem cells [324].

### 12.7.8 Measles Viral Vectors

The measles virus is an enveloped negative-strand RNA virus. The Edmonston vaccine strain of measles viruses (MV-Edm) has oncolytic effects against Hodgkin and non-Hodgekin lymphomas [325].

There are two proteins that project from the measles virus envelope: the fusion protein (F) and the attachment protein (H). Both the H and the F proteins are required for infection and subsequent cell-to-cell fusion. The MV-Edm infects cells through the CD46 or CDw150 receptor [326, 327].

The great advantage of the measles virus is that the tumor cells have no defense against the mechanism through which it destroys cells, and that the measles virus can be easily engineered to target tumor vasculature by inserting single-chain antibodies (scFv) into the coat protein. The Russel laboratory has developed an Echistatin-targeted measles virus vector (MV-ERV), which binds the $\alpha_v\beta_3$ integrin receptor with a high affinity [328]. The MV-ERV vector can target the activated endothelial cells in tumor tissue by Echistatin binding to the $\alpha_v\beta_3$ integrin, and it can also target to tumor cells by the H protein binding to the native CD46 receptor, thus making the vector of potential use in gene therapy.

### 12.7.9 Herpes Simplex Viral Vectors

The herpes simplex virus (HSV) is an enveloped, double-strand DNA virus. The envelope glycoproteins gB and gC of HSV bind to the HSV receptor heparin sulfate molecules or nectin-1 [329]. Internalization of the virus involves the viral envelope gD protein and the cellular FGF receptor [330]. HSV can infect lytically or can establish latency. However, the toxicity of the vector limits its use.

### 12.7.10 Neural Stem Cells/Progenitor Cells

Neural stem cells (NSC), neural progenitor cells (NPC), and mesenchymal stem cells from bone marrow or adipose tissue migrate *in vivo* to tumor sites. It has been shown that these cells migrate to multiple tumor types including glioblastoma, prostate and breast carcinoma, melanoma, and neuroblastoma in immunocompromised mouse models [331–336]. Recently, the preferential migration of HB1.F3.C1 cells to SK-N-AS, NB-1643, and NB-1691 neuroblastoma tumors has been documented. Efficacy has been reported in mice bearing these tumors following treatment with HB1.F3.C1 cells expressing a secreted form of rabbit carboxyesterase (rCE) in combination with CPT-11 [332, 337–340]. For this approach, it has been shown that 90% of mice treated rCE expressing HB1.F3.C1 cells and 15 mg/kg CPT-11 survived for 1 year without detactable tumors [341].

### 12.7.11 Liposomes

Nonviral vectors have emerged as attractive alternatives to recombinant viruses for gene therapy. Synthetic gene delivery systems are free of the problems associated with the use of recombinant viruses, including safety concerns and practical issues relating to bulk production and quality control. Cationic lipids are particularly attractive as it is possible to synthesize a wide variety of well-characterized reagents with favorable features such as biodegradability and low toxicity. Accordingly, various cationic lipid-based gene delivery systems have been developed over the past years and used for cancer gene therapy. Among these, cholesterol derivatives are characterized by polar head groups with guanidinium functions [342]. Bis-guanidinium-tren-cholesterol (BGTC) is a multivalent T-shaped lipid with two guanidinium groups (providing DNA binding strength) and a carbomyl linker. It was found that BGTC/DOPE liposomes are highly efficient for gene transfection *in vitro* into a variety of mammalian cell lines, and it mediates efficient gene transfection into the mouse respiratory epithelium *in vivo* [343]. Hajri *et al.* [344] reported that BGTC/DOPE liposomes can efficiently mediate gene transfection into peritoneal tumor nodules. The liposomes were complexed with plasmids encoding HSV-TK and bCD, and their administration was followed by treatment with the corresponding prodrugs GCV and 5-FC. Expression analysis showed that transgene expression lasted for about 2 weeks and was preferential for the tumor nodules [344].

This proves BGTC-based prodrug-activating gene therapy may constitute a potential treatment modality for peritoneal carcinomatosis.

### 12.7.12
### ADEPT Vectors

Monoclonal antibodies and fusion proteins against carcinoembryonic antigen for colorectal adenocarcinoma, c-erbB2 for breast cancer and melanotransferrin for melanomas and some carcinomas have been used as vectors [17, 345, 346]. Enzymes/prodrug combinations include a number of systems (see Section 12.3 and Table 12.3 and the references therein). Biopsies of xenograft LS174T colorectal tumor cells in mice treated with an antibody-CPG2 followed by nitrogen mustard prodrug ZD2767P have revealed evidence in comet assays of extensive DNA interstrand cross-linking, the toxic mechanism of the parent drug [347]. Thus, it has been demonstrated that the ADEPT concept can be correlated with a therapeutic effect. Derivatization of these vectors may be necessary to reduce a patient's immune reaction against them [348] and the timing of the vector and prodrug must be controlled to allow optimum drug delivery [349]. Recently, the successful production of a human anti-γ-seminoprotein Fab antibody has been reported [350]. Being a humanized antibody, this is less likely to cause an immunogenic response.

Examples of *in vivo* studies using GDEPT and ADEPT paradigms are listed in Table 12.4.

### 12.7.13
### Vectors for Prodrugs

Generally, little or no attention is paid to the way the prodrug is delivered to solid tumors. However, it is known that in some cases the delivery of such prodrugs to the tumor is quite low because of their insufficient transfer from the blood.

It has been shown that in the case of *E. coli* CD/5-FC therapy, prolonged time of prodrug administration combined with its high doses can cause significant side effects. One way to limit the side effects is to encapsulate the high concentration prodrug solutions in liposomes (polar lipid bilayer entrapping a central aqueous space) [377, 378]. The main benefits of such approaches are limited side effects, increased drug circulation time, passive or active drug targeting, and possibility of site-specific and time-specific drug release [379].

**Table 12.4** *In vivo* studies using GDEPT and ADEPT.

| Enzyme | Vector | Prodrug | Cells/Tumor | Cell type | References |
|---|---|---|---|---|---|
| HSV-TK | *Salmonella* | Ganciclovir (GCV) | B16-F10 | Murine melanoma | [296, 351] |
| | Retrovirus | | Peritoneal carcinomatosis | | [352] |
| | Adenovirus | | DHDK | Rat colon carcinoma | |
| | | | B16-F10 | | [353, 354] |
| | | | CMT93 | | [355] |
| | | | Hurthle | Human thyroid carcinoma | |
| | | | Ov-ca-2774 | CELO avian adenovirus | [356] |
| | | | SW620 | Human colorectal carcinoma | |
| | | | HUH7 | Hepatocellular carcinoma | [357] |
| | | | FCT113 | Human thyroid carcinoma | |
| | | | ARO | | |
| | RGD fiber-mutated adenovirus | | B16BL6 | Murine melanoma | [358] |
| | CELO avian adenovirus | | B16F1 | Murine melanoma | [359] |
| | Sendai virus | | HUH7 | | [360] |
| | Vesicular stomatitis virus | | B16-F10 | | [361] |
| | Herpes simplex virus | GCV/mutant IκBα | NXS2 | Murine neuroblastoma | |
| CD | *Salmonella* | 5-FC | C38 | Murine colon carcinoma | [362] |
| | | | LoVo | Human colon carcinoma | |
| | | | WiDr | Human colorectal carcinoma | |
| | | | B16-F10 | | [363, 364] |
| | Sendai virus | | BXPC3 | Human pancreatic carcinoma | [366] |
| | *Clostridium* | | SCCVII | Murine squamous cell | [365] |

*(Continued)*

**Table 12.4** (*Continued*)

| Enzyme | Vector | Prodrug | Cells/Tumor | Cell type | References |
|---|---|---|---|---|---|
| CD/UPRT | Vesicular stomatitis virus | | A20 | Murine B-cell lymphoma | [249] |
| | Adenovirus | | SW480 | Human colorectal carcinoma | |
| *E. coli* purine nucleoside reductase | Adenovirus | Flutarabine | RM1 | Human prostate | [367] |
| | | 6MPDR | PC-3 | Human prostate carcinoma | [368] |
| Rabbit carboxyl-esterase | Adenovirus | CPT-11 | MDA-MB231 | Human breast | [369] |
| | | | A549 | Human nonsmall cell lung | |
| | | | C33a | Human cervical carcinoma | |
| *E. coli* nitro-reductase | *Clostridium* | CB1954 | EMT6 | Human breast | [301, 370] |
| | Adenovirus | | HepG2 | Human hepatocarcinoma | |
| | | | HNX14C | Human squamous cell carcinoma | [316] |
| | | | WiDr | | |
| | | | PC-3 | | |
| | | | C33a | | |
| | | | DU145 | | |
| | | | A2780 | Human prostate carcinoma | |
| | | | CP70 | Human ovarian carcinoma | |
| | | | ADR | A2780 variant | |
| | | | UVW | A2780 variant | |
| | | | 5627 | Human malignant glioma | |
| | | | SW480 | Human bladder carcinoma | [371] |
| | | | WiDr | | |
| Cytochrome P450/ | Retrovirus | Cyclo-phosphamide | HT29 | Human colon carcinoma | [372] |
| Methionase | Adenovirus | Seleno-methionine | N1S1 | Rat hepatoma | [127] |
| CPG2 | Adenovirus | | Hep3B | Human hepatocarcinoma | [373] |
| | | | HepG2 | | |

| | | | | | |
|---|---|---|---|---|---|
| | | | SW620 | Human colorectal carcinoma | [34] |
| | A5B7F$(ab')_2$ antibody–enzyme conjugate | Mustard prodrug ZD2767P | LS174T | Human colorectal carcinoma | [374] |
| | | | LoVo | | [72] |
| | MFE-CP fusion protein | | LS174T<br>SW1222 | | [375] |
| Beta-lactamase | L49-Fab'-bL antibody–enzyme conjugate and L49-sFv-bL fusion protein | Cephalosporin-based mustard prodrug | SN12P | Human renal cell carcinoma | [376] |

It has been reported that in a CD/5-FC therapy, 5-FC encapsulated in dipalmitoylphosphatidylcholine (DPPC) and cholesterol 1: 1 composed liposomes administered IV to mice in the second step showed complete regression of tumors in colon carcinoma xenografts in comparison with the free prodrug where only a 50% tumor regression was observed [380].

### 12.7.14
### Clinical Studies

In a Phase I study with intravenous *S. typhimurium* in patients with metastatic melanoma, fever, hypotension, thrombocytopenia, and anemia was observed despite low levels of bacteria being found in tumor biopsies and the attenuated nature of the organism [381]. All the patients eventually developed progressive disease. Pilot clinical trials of intratumoral TAPET-CD and oral 5-FC have been carried out [382, 383] and showed bacterial colonization and tumor conversion of 5-FC to 5FU. Some toxicity was observed although some of this may have been due to disease progression. Results were mixed, with some patients showing a positive response and others not. Whether higher levels or more prolonged dose schedules would have made a difference is unknown.

Adenoviral vectors in VDEPT clinical trials for malignant glioma [384, 385], ovarian cancer [386], colorectal adenocarcinoma [387], and prostate cancer [388, 389] have been found to be in general well tolerated, even with repeated administration [390], although the clinical benefit has so far been modest.

ADEPT CPG2/ZD2767P has been used in the clinic to treat colorectal tumors [278, 374, 391] A Phase I ADEPT trial in advanced colorectal carcinoma patients using CPG2- mouse anti-CEA monoclonal antibody $F(ab)_2$/ZD2767P found that the treatment was well tolerated but that the antibody–enzyme complex did not target the tumors exclusively [392]. Likewise, in the study of [347] only one in three patients in a Phase I trial showed liver tumor DNA interstrand cross-links on biopsy.

Although these studies are mostly at a very early stage and will undergo refinement in the future, their general lack of the expected pharmacodynamic end points illustrates the difficulties that may be encountered in extrapolating from animal models to human patients and from xenograft tumors to neoplasia.

Data on both ADEPT and GDEPT are summarized in Table 12.5.

## 12.8
## Conclusions

Suicide gene therapy for cancer represents 8% of the 113 protocols for cancer gene therapy listed by the U.S. Recombinant Advisory Committee [401]. Most of these used HSV-TK/GCV system and were Phase I/Phase II trials [402, 403]. One Phase III trial using a retroviral vector has been completed and showed no benefit, in terms of survival for the patients [398]. A trial that used an adenoviral vector by direct intratumoral injection (into brain tumors) showed improved survival [404].

**Table 12.5** Suicide gene therapy clinical trials.

| Enzyme | Vector | Prodrug | Tumor | Phase | Reference |
|---|---|---|---|---|---|
| HSV-TK | Adenovirus | Acyclovir<br>Valacyclovir | Ovarian | I | [393] |
| | Adenovirus<br>Retrovirus | Ganciclovir | Malignant glioma | I | [394] |
| | Adenovirus | Ganciclovir | Metastatic colrectal adenocarcinoma | I | [387] |
| | Retrovirus | | Ovarian | I | [386] |
| | Adenovirus | | Malignant glioma | III | [385] |
| | Adenovirus | | Malignant glioma | I | [384] |
| | Retrovirus expressing interleukin-2 | | Relapsed malignant glioma | I | [395] |
| | Retrovirus | | End-stage anaplastic thyroid carcinoma | I | [396] |
| | | | Melanoma, breast, nonsmall-cell lung, osteogenic sarcoma | I | [397] |
| | | | Glioblastoma mutiforme | III | [398] |
| CD/HSV-TK | Adenovirus (Replication competent) | 5-FC and gancyclovir | Locally recurrent prostate | I | [388] |
| | | | Intermediate-to-high-risk prostate | I | [389] |
| | | | Localized prostate | I | [390] |
| Nitro-reductase | Adenovirus | CB1954 | Hepatic metastatic colorectal cancer or primary hepatocellular carcinoma | I | [399] |
| CD | *Salmonella* | 5-FC | Metastatic cancer | I | [382] |
| | | | Head and neck | I | [383] |
| | Direct plasmid injection | | Breast | I | [400] |
| CPG2 | A5CP antibody–enzyme conjugate | ZD2767P | Human colorectal carcinoma (HCC) | I | [392] |
| | | | | I | [278] |
| | A5B7 $F(ab')_2$ antibody–enzyme conjugate | | HCC liver metastases | I | [347] |

Phase I/II clinical trials have been reported with CD/5-FC [400] and CYP450/CP or IF [82]. In the United Kingdom, a retroviral vector expressing CYP2B6 (MetXia) is currently been assessed in patients with advanced breast and ovarian cancers. In Germany, microencapsulated mammalian cells expressing CYP2B1 and IF were tested on 14 patients with inoperable pancreatic carcinoma. The follow-up showed that the 1-year survival was increased to threefold [41]. Suicide gene therapy has proved to be safe, with only minor side effects being reported.

In summary, there are still hurdles to be overcome before GDEPT will become a clinically accepted treatment of cancers. The domain in need of more improvements is vectors compared to selective targeting and delivery of suicide genes. Multiple options are becoming clinically available, from nonviral vectors to a variety of different viral vectors.

## Acknowledgments

Our work was funded by the Cancer Research Campaign (grant numbers SP2330/0201 and SP2330/0102) and the Institute of Cancer Research.

## References

1 Workman, P. (2000) Editorial overview. Toward genomic cancer pharmacology: innovative drugs for the new millennium. *Current Opinion in Oncologic, Endocrine & Metabolic Investigational Drugs*, **2**, 21–25.

2 Niculescu-Duvaz, I. and Springer, C.J. (1995) Antibody-directed enzyme prodrug therapy (ADEPT): a targeting strategy in cancer chemotherapy. *Current Medicinal Chemistry*, **2**, 687–706.

3 Melton, R.G. and Knox, R. (1999) *Enzyme–Prodrug Strategies for Cancer Therapy*, Kluwer Academic/Plenum Publishers, New York.

4 Roth, J.A. and Cristiano, R.G. (1997) Gene therapy for cancer: what have we done and where are we going? *Journal of the National Cancer Institute*, **89**, 21–30.

5 Niculescu-Duvaz, I., Spooner, R., Marais, R., and Springer, C.J. (1998) Gene-directed enzyme prodrug therapy. *Bioconjugate Chemistry*, **9**, 4–22.

6 Springer, C.J. and Niculescu-Duvaz, I. (2001) Gene-directed enzyme prodrug therapy, in *Anticancer Drug Development* (ed. B. Baguley), Academic Press, pp. 137–152.

7 Duncan, R., Gac-Breton, S., Keane, R., Musila, R., Sat, Y., Satchi, R., and Searle, P. (2001) Polymer–drug conjugates, PDEPT and PELT: basic principles for design and transfer from the laboratory to clinic. *Journal of Controlled Release*, **74**, 135–146.

8 Satchi-Fainaro, R., Hailu, H., Davies, J., Summerford, C., and Duncan, R. (2003) PDEPT: polymer-directed enzyme prodrug therapy. 2. HPMA copolymer-β-lactamase and HPMA copolymer-C-Dox as a model combination. *Bioconjugate Chemistry*, **14**, 797–804.

9 Spooner, R.A., Friedlos, F., Maycroft, K., Stribbling, S.M., Roussel, J., Brueggen, J., Stolz, B., O'Reilly, T., Wood, J., Matter, A., Marais, R., and Spooner, C.J. (2003) A novel vascular endothelial growth factor-directed therapy that selectively activates cytotoxic prodrugs. *British Journal of Cancer*, **88**, 1622–1630.

10 Dubowchik, G.M. and Walker, M.A. (1999) Receptor-mediated and enzyme-dependent targeting of cytotoxic

anticancer drugs. *Pharmacological Therapy*, **83**, 67–123.
11 Chari, R.V. (1998) Targeted delivery of therapeutics: tumor activated prodrug therapy. *Advanced Drug Delivery Reviews*, **31**, 89–104.
12 Brinkmann, U. (2000) Recombinant antibody fragments and immunitoxin fusions for cancer therapy. *In Vivo*, **14**, 21–27.
13 Illidge, T.M. and Johnson, P.W. (2000) The emerging role of radioimmunotherapy in haematological malignancies. *British Journal of Haematology*, **108**, 679–688.
14 Sievers, E.L. (2000) Targeted therapy of acute myeloid leukemia with monoclonal antibodies and immunoconjugates. *Cancer Therapy and Pharmacology*, **26**, 18–22.
15 Wiseman, G.A., White, C.A., Stabin, M., Dunn, W.L., Erwin, W., Dahlbom, M., Raubitschek, A., Karvelis, K., Schultheiss, T., Witzig, T.E., Belanger, R., Spies, S., Silverman, D.H., Berlfein, J.R., Ding, E., and Grillo-Lopez, A.G. (2000) PhaseI/II 90-Y Zevalin (ytrium-90 ibritumomab tiuxentan, IDEC-Y2B8) radioimmunotherapy dosimetry results in relapsed or refractory non-Hodgkin's lymphoma. *European Journal of Nuclear Medicine*, **27**, 766–777.
16 Hainsworth, J.D. (2000) Monoclonal antibody therapy in lymphoid malignancies. *Oncologist*, **5**, 376–384.
17 Niculescu-Duvaz, I. and Springer, C.J. (1995) Antibody-directed enzyme prodrug therapy (ADEPT): a targeting strategy in cancer chemotherapy. *Current Medicinal Chemistry*, **2**, 687–706.
18 Bagshawe, K.D. (1989) Toward generating cytotoxic agents at cancer sites. *British Journal of Cancer*, **60**, 275–281.
19 Senter, P.D. (1990) Activation of prodrugs by antibody–enzyme conjugates: a new approach to cancer therapy. *FASEB Journal*, **4**, 188–193.
20 Bagshawe, K.D., Rogers, G.T., Sharma, S.K., Antoniw, P., Sherwood, R.F., Springer, C.J., Searle, F., Burke, P., Melton, R., Boden, J., and Green, A. (1990) Antibody-directed enzyme prodrug therapy (ADEPT), in *Monoclonal Antibodies and Immunoconjugates* (eds R.W. Baldwin, V.S. Byers, and R.D. Mann), Parthenon Publishing, UK, pp. 95–102.
21 Senter, P.D. and Springer, C.J. (2001) Selective activation of anticancer prodrugs by monoclonal antibody–enzyme conjugates. *Advanced Drug Delivery Reviews*, **53**, 247–264.
22 Fonseca, M., Jagtenberg, J., Haisma, H., and Storm, G. (2003) Liposome-mediated targeting of enzymes to cancer cells for site-specific activation of prodrugs: comparison with the corresponding antibody–enzyme conjugate. *Pharmaceutical Research*, **20**, 423–428.
23 Satchi, R., Connors, T.A., and Duncan, R. (2001) PDEPT: polymer-directed enzyme prodrug therapy I. HPMA copolymer–cathepsin B and PK1 as a model combination. *British Journal of Cancer*, **85**, 1070–1076.
24 Satchi-Fainaro, R., Wrasidlo, W., Lode, H., and Shabat, D. (2002) Synthesis and characterisation of a catalytic antibody-HPMA copolymer conjugate as a tool for tumor selective prodrug activation. *Bioorganic & Medicinal Chemistry*, **10**, 3023–3029.
25 Marais, R., Spooner, R.A., Light, Y., Martin, J., and Springer, C.J. (1996) Gene-directed enzyme prodrug therapy with a mustard prodrug/carboxypeptidase G2 combination. *Cancer Research*, **56**, 4735–4742.
26 Bridgewater, G., Springer, C.J., Knox, R., Minton, N., Michael, P., and Collins, M. (1995) Expression of the bacterial nitroreductase enzyme in mammalian cells renders them selectively sensitive to killing by the prodrug CB1954. *European Journal of Cancer*, **31**, 2362–2370.
27 Huber, B.E., Richards, C.A., and Austin, E.A. (1995) VDEPT: an enzyme/prodrug gene therapy approach for the treatment of metastatic colorectal cancer. *Advanced Drug Delivery Reviews*, **17**, 279–292.
28 Eaton, J.L., Perry, M.J.A., Todryk, S.M., Mazucco, R.A., Kirby, R.S., Griffiths, G.R., and Dalgleish, A.G. (2001) Genetic prodrug activation therapy (GPAT) in two rat prostate models generates an immune

bystander effect and can be monitored by magnetic resonance techniques. *Gene Therapy*, **8**, 557–567.
29 Springer, C.J. (2004) Introduction to vectors in suicide gene therapy, in *Suicide Gene Therapy* (ed. C.J. Springer), Humana Press, Inc., pp. 29–47.
30 Yamamoto, M. and Curiel, D.T. (2004) Nonreplicating DNA viral vectors for suicide gene therapy: the adenoviral vectors, in *Suicide Gene Therapy* (ed. C.J. Springer), Humana Press, Inc., pp. 61–71.
31 Hallden, G., Thorne, S.H., Yang, G., and Kirn, D.H. (2004) Replication-selective oncolytic adenoviruses, in *Suicide Gene Therapy* (ed. C.J. Springer), Humana Press, Inc., pp. 71–91.
32 Porter, C. (2004) Retroviral vectors for suicide gene therapy, in *Suicide Gene Therapy* (ed. C.J. Springer), Humana Press, Inc., pp. 91–107.
33 Sato, T., Neschadim, A., Konrad, M., Fowler, D.H., Lavie, A., and Medin, J.A. (2007) Engineered human tmpk/AZT as a novel enzyme/prodrug axis for suicide gene therapy. *Molecular Therapy: The Journal of the American Society of Gene Therapy*, **15**, 962–70.
34 Schepelmann, S., Ogilvie, L.M., Hedley, D., Friedlos, F., Martin, J., Scanlon, I., Chen, P., Marais, R., and Springer, C.J. (2007) Suicide gene therapy of human colon carcinoma xenografts using an armed oncolytic adenovirus expressing carboxypeptidase G2. *Cancer Research*, **67**, 4949–55.
35 Kostarelos, K., Emfietzoglou, D., Papakostas, A., Yang, W.H., Ballangrud, A.M., and Sgouros, G. (2005) Engineering lipid vesicles of enhanced intratumoral transport capabilities: correlating liposome characteristics with penetration into human prostate tumor spheroids. *Journal of Liposome Research*, **15**, 15–27.
36 Miller, A.D. (1998) Cationic liposomes for gene therapy. *Angewandte Chemistry International Edition*, **37**, 1768–1785.
37 Schatzlein, A.G. (2001) Non-viral vectors in cancer gene therapy: principles and progress. *Anti-Cancer Drug Design*, **12**, 275–304.
38 Ilies, M.A., Seitz, M.A., and Balaban, A.T. (2002) Cationic lipids in gene delivery: principles, vector design and therapeutical application. *Current Pharmaceutical Design*, **8**, 2441–2474.
39 Niculescu-Duvaz, D., Heyes, J., and Springer, C.J. (2003) Structure–activity relationship in cationic lipid mediated gene transfection. *Current Medicinal Chemistry*, **10**, 1233–1261.
40 Löhr, M., Müller, P., Karle, P., Stange, J., Mitzner, S., Jesnowski, R., Nizze, H., Nebe, B., Liebe, S., Salmons, B., and Günzburg, W.H. (1998) Targeted chemotherapy by intratumoral injection of encapsulated cells engineered to produce CYP2B1, an ifosfamide activating cytochrome P450. *Gene Therapy*, **5**, 1070–1078.
41 Lohr, M., Hoffmeyer, A., Kroeger, j., Freund, M., Hain, J., Holle, A., Karle, P., Knofel, W.T., Liebe, S., Muller, P., Nizze, H., Renner, M., Saller, R.M., Wagner, T., Hauenstein, K., Gunzburg, W.H., and Salmons, B. (2001) Microencapsulated cell-mediated treatment of inoperable pancreatic carcinoma. *Lancet*, **357**, 1591–1592.
42 Griffiths, L., Binley, K., Iqball, S., Kan, O., Maxwell, P., Ratcliffe, P., Lewis, C., Harris, A., Kingsman, S., and Naylor, S. (2000) The macrophage: a novel system to deliver gene therapy to pathological hypoxia. *Gene Therapy*, **7**, 255–262.
43 Minton, N.P., Mauchline, M.L., Lemmon, M.J., Brehm, J.K., Fox, M., Michael, N.P., Giaccia, A., and Brown, J.M. (1995) Chemotherapeutic tumour targeting using clostridial spores. *FEMS Microbiology Reviews*, **17**, 357–64.
44 Nuyts, S., Van Mellaert, L., Theys, J., Landuyt, W., Lambin, P., and Anne, J. (2002) Clostridium spores for tumor-specific drug delivery. *Anticancer Drugs*, **13**, 115–25.
45 Minton, N.P. (2003) Clostridia in cancer therapy. *Nature Reviews Microbiology*, **1**, 237–42.
46 Bush, K., Jacoby, G.A., and Medeiros, A.A. (1995) A functional classification scheme for beta-lactamases and its correlation with molecular structure.

*Antimicrobial Agents and Chemotherapy*, **39**, 1211–33.

**47** Marais, R., Spooner, R.A., Stribbling, S.M., Light, Y., Martin, J., and Springer, C.J. (1997) A cell surface tethered enzyme improves efficiency in gene-directed enzyme prodrug therapy. *Nature Biotechnology*, **15**, 1373–1377.

**48** Heine, D., Muller, R., and Brusselbach, S. (2001) Cell surface display of a lysosomal enzyme for extra-cellular gene-directed enzyme prodrug therapy. *Gene Therapy*, **8**, 1005–1010.

**49** Cowen, R.L., Williams, J.C., Emery, S., Blakey, D., Darling, J.L., Lowenstein, P.R., and Castro, M.G. (2002) Adenovirus vector-mediated delivery of the prodrug-converting enzyme carboxypeptidase G2 secreted or GPI-anchored form: high level expression of this active conditional cytotoxic enzyme at the plasma membrane. *Cancer Gene Therapy*, **9**, 897–907.

**50** Stegman, L.D., Zheng, H., Neal, E.R., Ben-Yoseph, O., Pollegioni, L., Pillone., M.S., and Ross, B.D. (1998) Induction of cytotoxic oxidative stress by D-alanine in brain tumor cells expressing *Rhodotorula gracilis* D-amino acid oxidase: a cancer gene therapy strategy. *Human Gene Therapy*, **9**, 185–193.

**51** Senter, P.D., Saulnier, M.G., Schreiber, G.J., Hirshberg, D.L., Brown, J.P., Hellström, I., and Hellström, K.E. (1988) Anti-tumor effects of antibody–alkaline phosphatase conjugates in combination with etoposide phosphate. *Proceedings of the National Academy of Sciences of the United States of America*, **85**, 4842–4846.

**52** Senter, P.D., Saulnier, M.G., Schreiber, G.J., Hirschberg, D.L., Brown, J.P., Hellström, I., and Hellström, K.E. (1989) Antitumor effect of antibody–alkaline phosphatase conjugates in combination with etoposide phosphate. *Chemtracts Organic Chemistry*, **2**, 1–4.

**53** Wallace, P.M. and Senter, P.D. (1991) *In vitro* and *in vivo* activities of monoclonal antibody–alkaline phosphatase conjugates in combination with phenol mustard phosphate. *Bioconjugate Chemistry*, **2**, 349–352.

**54** McIntee, E.J. and Wagner, C.R. (2001) Amino acid phophoramidate nucleosides: potential ADEPT/GDEPT substrates. *Bioorganic & Medicinal Chemistry*, **11**, 2803–2805.

**55** Larden, D.W. and Cheung, H.T.A. (1999) Synthesis of α-aminoacyl derivatives of melphalan for use in antibody directed enzyme prodrug therapy. *Tetrahedron*, **55**, 3265–3276.

**56** Senter, P.D., Vrudhula, V., Wallace, P.M., Somerville, J.E., Wang, I.K., and Lowe, D.A. (1995) Sulfated etoposide and nitrogen mustard prodrugs and their activation by *Streptomyces* arylsulfatase. *Drug Delivery*, **2**, 110–116.

**57** Senter, P.D., Beam, K.S., Mixan, B., and Wahl, A.F. (2001) Identification and activities of human carboxylesterases for the activation of CPT11, a clinically approved anticancer drug. *Bioconjugate Chemistry*, **12**, 1074–1080.

**58** Oosterhoff, D., Pinedo, H.M., van der Meulen, I.H., de Graaf, M., Sone, T., Kruyt, F.A., van Beusekem, V.W., Haisma, H.J., and Gerritsen, W.R. (2002) Secreted and tumor targeted human carboxyl esterase for activation of irinotecan. *British Journal of Cancer*, **87**, 659–664.

**59** Vitols, K.S., Haag-Zeino, B., Baer, T., Montejano, Y.D., and Huennekens, F.M. (1995) Methotrexate-α-phenylalanine: optimization of methotrexate prodrug for activation by carboxypeptidase A-monoclonal antibody. *Cancer Research*, **55**, 478–481.

**60** Smith, G.K., Banks, S., Blumenkopf, T.A., Cory, M., Humphreys, J., Laethem, A.M., Miller, G., Moxham, C.P., Mullin, R., Ray, P.H., Walton, L.M., and Wolfe, L.A. III (1997) Toward antibody-directed enzyme prodrug therapy with the T268G mutant of human carboxypeptidase A1 and novel *in vivo* stable prodrugs of methotrexate. *Journal of Biological Chemistry*, **272**, 15804–15816.

**61** Springer, C.J., Bavetsias, V., Jackman, A.L., Boyle, T.F., Marshall, D., Pedley, R.B., and Bisset, G.M.F. (1996) Prodrugs of thymidylate synthase inhibitors: potential for antibody-directed enzyme prodrug therapy (ADEPT). *Anti-Cancer Drug Design*, **11**, 625.

62 Wolfe, L.A., Mullin, R.J., Laethum, R., Blumenkopf, T.A., Cory, M., Miller, J.F., Keth, B.R., Humphreys, G., and Smith, G.K. (1999) Antibody-directed enzyme prodrug therapy with the T268G mutant of carboxipeptidase A1: *in vitro* and *in vivo* studies with prodrugs of methotrexateand the thymidilate synthase inhibitorsGW1031 and GW1843. *Bioconjugate Chemistry*, **10**, 38–48.

63 Wright, J.E. and Rosowski, A. (2002) Synthesis and enzymatic activation of *N*-[$N^{\alpha}$-(4-amino-4-deoxypteroyl)-$N^{\delta}$-hemiphthaloyl-L-ornithinyl]-L-phenylalanine, a candidate for antibody-directed enzyme prodrug therapy (ADEPT). *Bioorganic & Medicinal Chemistry*, **10**, 493–500.

64 Bagshawe, K.D., Springer, C.J., Searle, F., Antoniw, P., Sharma, S.K., Melton, R.G., and Sherwood, R.F. (1988) A cytotoxic agent can be generated selectively at cancer sites. *British Journal of Cancer*, **58**, 700–703.

65 Springer, C.J., Antoniw, P., Bagshawe, K.D., Searle, F., Bisset, G.M.F., and Jarman, M. (1990) Novel prodrugs which are activated to cytotoxic alkylating agents by carboxypeptidase G2. *Journal of Medicinal Chemistry*, **33**, 677–681.

66 Mann, J., Haase-Held, M., Springer, C.J., and Bagshawe, K.D. (1990) Synthesis of an N-mustard prodrug. *Tetrahedron*, **46**, 5377–5382.

67 Springer, C.J., Dowell, R., Burke, P.J., Hadley, E., Davies, D.H., Blakey, D.C., Melton, R.G., and Niculescu-Duvaz, I. (1995) Optimization of alkylating agent prodrug derived from phenol and aniline mustards: a new clinical candidates prodrug (ZD2767) for antibody-directed prodrug therapy (ADEPT). *Journal of Medicinal Chemistry*, **38**, 5051–5065.

68 Springer, C.J. and Niculescu-Duvaz, I. (1995) Antibody-directed enzyme prodrug therapy (ADEPT) with mustard prodrugs. *Anti-Cancer Drug Design*, **10**, 361–372.

69 Niculescu-Duvaz, D., Niculescu-Duvaz, I., Friedlos, F., Martin, J., Lehouritis, P., Marais, R., and Springer, C.J. (2003) Self-immolative nitrogen mustards prodrugs cleavable by carboxypeptidase G2 (CPG2) showing large cytotoxicity differential in GDEPT. *Journal of Medicinal Chemistry*, **46**, 1690–1705.

70 Niculescu-Duvaz, D., Niculescu-Duvaz, I., Friedlos, F., Martin, J., Spooner, R., Davies, L., Marais, R., and Springer, C.J. (1998) Self-immolative nitrogen mustard prodrugs for suicide gene therapy. *Journal of Medicinal Chemistry*, **41**, 5297–5309.

71 Niculescu-Duvaz, I., Scanlon, I., Niculescu-Duvaz, D., Friedlos, F., Martin, J., Marais, R., and Springer, C.J. (2004) Significant differences in biological parameters between prodrugs cleavable by carboxypeptidase G2 that generate 3,5- difluoro-phenol and -aniline nitrogen mustards in gene-directed enzyme prodrug therapy systems. *Journal of Medicinal Chemistry*, **47**, 2651–2658.

72 Blakey, D.C., Burke, P.J., Davies, D.H., Dowell, R.I., East, S.J., Eckersley, K.P., Fitton, J.E., McDaid, J., Melton, R.G., Niculescu-Duvaz, I.A., Pinder, P.E., Sharmer, S.K., Wright, A.F., and Springer, C.J. (1996) ZD2767, an improved system for antibody-directed enzyme prodrug therapy that results in tumor regressions in colorectal tumor xenografts. *Cancer Research*, **56**, 3278–3292.

73 Friedlos, F., Davies, L., Scanlon, I., Ogilvie, L.M., Martin, J., Stribbling, S.M., Spooner, R.A., Niculescu-Duvaz, I., Marais, R., and Springer, C.J. (2002) Three new prodrugs for suicide gene therapy using carboxypeptidase G2 elicit bystander efficay in two xenograft models. *Cancer Research*, **62**, 1724–1729.

74 Niculescu-Duvaz, I., Niculescu-Duvaz, D., Friedlos, F., Spooner, R., Martin, J., Marais, R., and Springer, C.J. (1999) Self-immolative anthracycline prodrugs for suicide gene therapy. *Journal of Medicinal Chemistry*, **42**, 2485–2489.

75 Miyashita, H., Karaki, Y., Kinichi, M., and Fujii, I. (1993) Prodrug activation via catalytic antibodies. *Proceeding of the*

*National Academy of Sciences of the United States of America*, **90**, 5337–5340.

76 Campbell, D.A., Gong, B., Kochersperger, L.M., Yonkovich, S., Gallop, M.A., and Schultz, P.G. (1994) Antibody-catalyzed prodrug activation. *Journal American Chemical Society*, **116**, 2165–2166.

77 Wentworth, P., Datta, A., Blackey, D., Boyle, T., Partridge, L.D., and Blackburn, G.M. (1996) Toward antibody-directed "abzyme" prodrug therapy, ADAPT: carbamate prodrug activation by a catalytic antibody and its *in vitro* application to human tumor cell killing. *Proceedings of the National Academy of Sciences of the United States of America*, **93**, 799–803.

78 Shabat, D., Rader, C., List, B., Lerner, R.A., and Barbas, C.F. III (1999) Multiple event activation of a generic prodrug trigger by antibody catalysis. *Proceedings of the National Academy of Sciences of the United States of America*, **96**, 6925–6930.

79 Chang, T.K.H., Weber, G.F., Crespi, C.L., and Waxman, D.J. (1993) Differential activation of cyclophosphamide and ifosphamide by cytochromes P450 2B and 3A in human liver microsomes. *Cancer Research*, **53**, 5629–5637.

80 Manome, Y., Wen, P.Y., Chen, L., Tanaka, T., Dong, Y., Yamazoe, M., Hirshowitz, A., Kufe, D.W., and Fine, H.A. (1996) Gene therapy for malignant gliomas using replication incompetent retroviral and adenoviral vectors encoding the cytochrome P-450 2B1 gene together with cyclophosphamide. *Gene Therapy*, **3**, 513–520.

81 Chiocca, E.A. and Waxman, D.J. (2004) Cytochrome P-450-based gene therapies for cancer, in *Suicide Gene Therapies* (ed. C.J. Springer), Humana Press, Inc., pp. 203–233.

82 Chen, L. and Waxman, D.J. (2002) Cytochrome P-450 gene-directed enzyme prodrug therapy (GDEPT) for cancer. *Current Pharmaceutical Design*, **8**, 1405–1416.

83 Rainov, N.G., Dobberstein, K.-U., Sena-Estevez, M., Herlinger, U., Kramm, C.M., Philpot, R.M., Hilton, J., Chiocca, E.A., and Breakefield, X.O. (1998) New prodrug activation gene therapy for cancer using cytochrome P450 4B1 and 2-aminoanthracene/4-ipomeanol. *Human Gene Therapy*, **9**, 1261–1273.

84 Lu, H. and Waxman, D.J. (2005) Antitumor activity of methoxymorpholinyl doxorubicin: potentiation by cytochrome P450 3A metabolism. *Molecular Pharmacology*, **67**, 212–219.

85 Baldwin, A., Huang, Z., Jounaidi, Y., and Waxman, D.J. (2003) Identification of novel enzyme–prodrug combinations for use in cytochrome P450-based gene therapy for cancer. *Archives of Biochemistry and Biophysics*, **409**, 197–206.

86 McCarthy, H.O., Ykkundi, A., McErlane, V., Hughes, C.M., Keilty, G., Murray, M., Patterson, L.H., Hirst, D.G., McKeown, S.R., and Robson, T. (2003) Bioreductive GDEPT using cytochrome P450 3A4 in combination with AQ4N. *Cancer Gene Therapy*, **10**, 40–48.

87 Patterson, A.V., Williams, K.J., Coven, R.L., Jaffar, M., Telfer, B.A., Saunders, M., Honess, D., Van der Koegel, A.J., Wolf, C.R., and Stratford, I.J. (2002) Oxygen-sensitive enzyme–prodrug gene therapy for the eradication of radiation-resistant solid tumors. *Gene Therapy*, **9**, 946–954.

88 Senter, P.D., Su, P.C.D., Katsuragi, T., Sakai, T., Cosand, W.L., Hellström, I., and Hellström, K.E. (1991) Generation of 5-fluorouracil from 5-fluorocytosine by monoclonal antibody–cytosine deaminase conjugates. *Bioconjugate Chemistry*, **2**, 447–451.

89 Wallace, P.M., MacMaster, J.F., Smith, V.F., Kerr, D.E., Senter, P.D., and Cosand, W.L. (1994) Intratumoral generation of 5-fluorouracil mediated by an antibody–cytosine deaminase conjugate in combination with 5-fluorocytosine. *Cancer Research*, **54**, 2719–2723.

90 Aboagye, E.O., Artemov, D., Senter, P.D., and Bhujwalla, Z.M. (1998) Intratumoral conversion of 5-fluorocytosine to 5-fluorouracilby monoclonal antibody–cytosine deaminase conjugates: non-invasive detection of prodrug activation by magnetic

resonance spectroscopic imaging. *Cancer Research*, **58**, 4075–4078.

91 Huber, B.E., Austin, E.A., Good, V.C., Knick, V.C., Tibbels, S., and Richards, C.A. (1993) *In vivo* antitumor activity of 5-fluorocytosine on human colorectal carcinoma cells genetically modified to express cytosine deaminase. *Cancer Research*, **53**, 4619–4626.

92 Huber, B.E., Austin, E.A., Richards, C.A., Davis, S.T., and Good, S.S. (1994) Metabolism of 5-fluorocytidine to 5-fluorouracil in human colorectal tumor cells transduced with the cytosine deaminase gene: significant antitumor effects when only a small percentage of tumor cells express cytosine deaminase. *Proceedings of the National Academy of Sciences of the United States of America*, **91**, 8302–8306.

93 Ohwada, A., Hirschowitz, E.A., and Crystal, R.G. (1996) Regional delivery of an adenovirus vector containing the *Escherichia coli* cytosine deaminase gene to provide local activation of 5-fluorocytosine to suppress the growth of colon carcinoma metastatic to liver. *Human Gene Therapy*, **7**, 1567–1576.

94 Kievit, E., Bershad, E., Ng, E., Sethna, P., Dev, I., Lawrence, T.S., and Rehemtulla, A. (1999) Superiority of yeast over bacterial cytosine deaminase for enzyme/prodrug gene therapy in colon cancer. *Cancer Research*, **59**, 1417–1421.

95 Hapke, D.M., Stegmann, A.P.A., and Mitchell, B.S. (1996) Retroviral transfer of deoxycytidine kinase into tumor cell lines enhances nucleoside toxicity. *Cancer Research*, **56**, 2343–2347.

96 Manome, Y., Wen, P.Y., Dong, Y., Tanaka, T., Mitchell, B.S., Kufe, D.W., and Fine, H.A. (1996) Viral vector transduction of the human deoxycytidine kinase cDNA sensitizes glioma cells to the cytotoxic effects of cytosine arabinoside *in vitro* and *in vivo*. *Nature Medicine*, **2**, 567–573.

97 Azoulay, M., Florent, J.-C., Monneret, C., Gesson, J.P., Jacquessy, J.-C., Tillequin, F., Koch, M., Bosslet, K., Czech, J., and Hoffman, D. (1995) Prodrugs of anthracycline antibiotics suited for tumor specific activation. *Anti-Cancer Drug Design*, **10**, 441–450.

98 Bakina, E., Wu, Z., Rosenblum, M., and Farquhar, D. (1997) Intensely cytotoxic anthracycline prodrugs: glucuronides. *Journal of Medicinal Chemistry*, **40**, 4013–4018.

99 Bakina, E. and Farquhar, D. (1999) Intensely cytotoxic anthracycline prodrugs: galactosides. *Anti-Cancer Drug Design*, **14**, 507–515.

100 Gesson, J.P., Jacquesy, J.C., Mondon, M., Petit, P., Renoux, B., Andrianomenjanahary, S., Dufat-Trinh Van, H., Koch, M., Michel, S., Tillequin, F., Florent, J.C., Monneret, C., Bosslet, K., Czech, J., and Hoffmann, D. (1994) Prodrugs of anthracyclines for chemotherapy via enzyme–monoclonal antibody conjugates. *Anti-Cancer Drug Design*, **9**, 409–423.

101 Tietze, L.F., Lieb, M., Herzig, T., Haunert, F., and Schuberth, I. (2001) A strategy for tumor-selective chemotherapy by enzymatic liberation of seco-duocarmycin SA-derivatives from nontoxic prodrugs. *Bioorganic & Medicinal Chemistry*, **9**, 1929–1393.

102 Tietze, L.F., Feuerstein, T., Fecher, A., Haunbert, F., Pranknin, O., Borchers, U., Schuberth, I., and Alves, F. (2002) Proof of principle in the selective treatment of cancer by antibody-directed enzyme prodrug therapy: the development of a highly potent prodrug. *Angewante Chemie International Edition*, **41**, 759–761.

103 Cheng, H., Cao, X., Xian, M., Fang, L., Cai, T.B., Ji, J.J., Tunac, J.B., Sun, D., and Wang, P.G. (2005) Synthesis and enzyme-specific activation of carbohydrate–geldanamycin conjugates with potent anticancer activity. *Journal of Medicinal Chemistry*, **48**, 645–652.

104 Abraham, R., Aman, N., Von Borstel, R., Darsley, M., Kamireddy, B., Kenten, J., Morris, G., and Titmas, R. (1994) Conjugates of COL-1 monoclonal antibody and β-galactosidase can specifically kill tumor cells by generation of 5-flourouridine from the prodrug β-D-galactosyl-5-fluorouridine. *Cell Biophysics*, **24/25**, 127–133.

105 Philpott, G.W., Bower, R.G., and Parker, C.W. (1973) Selective iodination and cytotoxicity of tumor cells with

an antibody–enzyme conjugate. *Surgery*, 74, 51.

106 Rowlinson-Busza, G., Bamias, A., Krausz, T., and Epenetos, A.A. (1992) Antibody-guided enzyme nitrile therapy (Agent): *in vitro* cytotoxicity and *in vivo* tumor localisation, in *Monoclonal Antibodies. Application in Clinical Oncology*, vol. 2 (ed. A.A. Epenetos), Chapmann and Hall, London, pp. 111–118.

107 Leenders, R.C.G., Damen, E.W.P., Bijterveld, E.J.A., Scheeren, H.W., Houba, P.H.J., Van der Meulen-Muileman, I.H., Boven, E., and Haisma, H.J. (1999) Novel anthracycline-spacer-β-glucuronide, -β-glucoside and -β-galactoside podrugs for application in selective chemotherapy. *Bioorganic & Medicinal Chemistry*, **7**, 1597–1610.

108 Bosslet, K., Czech, J., Seeman, G., Monneret, C., and Hoffmann, D. (1994) Fusion protein mediated prodrug activation (FMPA) *in vivo*. *Cell Biophysics*, **24/25**, 51–63.

109 Florent, G.C., Dong, X., Gaudel, G., Gesson, J.-P., Jacquesy, J.C., Mondon, M., Renoux, S., Adrianomenjanahary, S., Michel, S., Koch, M., Tillequin, F., Gerken, M., Czech, J., Straub, R., and Bosslet, K. (1998) Prodrugs of anthracyclines for use in antibody-directed enzyme prodrug therapy. *Journal of Medicinal Chemistry*, **41**, 3572–3581.

110 de Graaf, M., Boven, E., Scheeren, H., Haisma, H.J., and Pinedo, H.M. (2002) Beta-glucuronidase-mediated drug release. *Current Pharmaceutical Design*, **8**, 1391–1403.

111 Lougerstay-Madec, R., Florent, G.C., Monneret, C., Nemati, F., and Poupon, M.F. (1998) Synthesis of self-immolative glucuronide-based prodrugs of a phenol mustard. *Anti-Cancer Drug Design*, **13**, 995–1007.

112 Guerquin Kern, J.L., Volk, A., Chenu, A., Lougerstay-Madec, R., Monneret, C., Florent, G.C., Carrez, D., and Croisy, A. (2000) Direct *in vivo* observation of 5-fluorouracil release from a prodrug in human tumors heterotransplanted in nude mice: a magnetic resonance study. *NMR in Biomedicine*, **13**, 306–310.

113 Leu, Y., Roffler, S., and Chern, J. (1999) Design and synthesis of water-soluble glucuronide derivatives of camptothecin for cancer prodrug monotherapy and antibody-directed enzyme prodrug therapy (ADEPT). *Journal of Medicinal Chemistry*, **42**, 3623–3628.

114 Debene, S., Van, H.D., Tillequin, F., Koch, M., Schmidt, F., Florent, G.C., Monneret, C., Straub, R., Czech, J., Gerken, M., and Bosslet, K. (1999) Application of the ADEPT strategy to the MDR resistance in cancer chemotherapy. *Anti-Cancer Drug Design*, **14**, 93–106.

115 Wei, G., Loktionova, N.A., Pegg, A.E., and Moschel, R.C. (2005) β-Glucuronidase-cleavable prodrugs of $O^6$-benzylguanine and $O^6$-benzyl-2′-deoxyguanosine. *Journal of Medicinal Chemistry*, **48**, 256–261.

116 Greco, O., Folkes, L.K., Wardman, P., Tozer, G.M., and Dachs, G.U. (2000) Development of a novel enzyme/prodrug combination for gene therapy of cancer: horseradish peroxidase/indole-3-acetic acid. *Cancer Gene Therapy*, **7**, 1414–1420.

117 Greco, O., Rossiter, S., Kanthou, C., Wardman, P., Tozer, G., and Dachs, G.U. (2001) Horseradish peroxidase-mediated gene therapy: choice of prodrugs in oxic and anoxic conditions. *Molecular Cancer Therapeutics*, **1**, 151–160.

118 Tupper, J., Tozer, G.M., and Dachs, G.U. (2004) Use of horseradish peroxidase for gene-directed enzyme prodrug therapy wih paracetamol. *British Journal of Cancer*, **90**, 1858–1862.

119 Alexander, R.P., Beeley, N.R.A., O'Driscoll, M., O'Neil, F.P., Millican, T.A., Pratt, A.J., and Willenbrock, F.W. (1991) Cephalosporin nitrogen mustard carbamate prodrugs for "ADEPT". *Tetrahedron Letters*, **32**, 3269–3272.

120 Vrudhula, V., Svensson, H.P., and Senter, P.D. (1995) Cephalosporin derivatives of doxorubicin as prodrugs for activation by monoclonal antibody-β-lactamase conjugates. *Journal of Medicinal Chemistry*, **38**, 1380–1385.

121 Rodrigues, M.L., Presta, L.G., Kotts, C.E., Wirth, C., Mordenti, C., Osaka, G., Wong, W.T., Nuijens, A., Blackburn, B., and

Carter, P. (1995) Development of a humanized disulfide-stabilized anti-p185HER Fv-β-lactamase fusion protein for activation of a cephalosporin doxorubicin prodrug. *Cancer Research*, **55**, 63–70.

**122** Vrudhula, V., Svensson, H.P., and Senter, P.D. (1997) Immunologically specific cephalosporin derivative of mitomycin C by monoclonal antibody-β-lactamase conjugates. *Journal of Medicinal Chemistry*, **40**, 2788–2792.

**123** Meyer, D.L., Jungheim, L.N., Law, K.L., Mikolajczyk, S.D., Shepherd, T.A., Mackensen, D.G., Briggs, S.L., and Starling, J.J. (1993) Site-specific prodrug activation by antibody-β-lactamase conjugates: regression and long-term growth inhibition by human colon carcinoma xenograft models. *Cancer Research*, **53**, 3956–3963.

**124** Rodrigues, M., Carter, P., Wirth, C., Mullins, S., Lee, A., and Blackburn, B. (1995) Synthesis and β-lactamase-mediated activation of cephalosporin-taxol prodrug. *Chemical Biology*, **2**, 223–227.

**125** Hanessian, S. and Wang, J. (1993) Design and synthesis of a cephalosporin-carboplatinum prodrug activatable by a β-lactamase. *Canadian Journal of Chemistry*, **71**, 896–906.

**126** Miki, K., Xu., M., An, Z., Wang, X., Yang, M., Al-Refaie, W., Sun, X., Baranov, E., Tan, Y., Chishima, T., Shimada, H., Moossa, A.R., and Hoffman, R.M. (2000) Survival efficacy of the combination of the methioninase gene and methioninase in a lung cancer orthotopic model. *Cancer Gene Therapy*, **7**, 332–338.

**127** Miki, K., Xu, M., Gupta, A., Ba, Y., Tan, Y., Al-Refaie, W., Bouvet, M., Makuuchi, M., Moossa, A.R., and Hoffman, R.M. (2001) Methionine cancer gene therapy with selenomethionine as suicide prodrug substrate. *Cancer Research*, **61**, 6805–6810.

**128** Sethna, P., Talarico, T., Merrill, B., Moore, J., Davis, S., Dikerson, S., and Dev, I. (1997) Cloning of the gene of a multiple drug activation enzyme from tomato for viral-directed enzyme prodrug therapy (VDEPT) for cancer. *Proceedings of the American Association for Cancer Research*, **38**, 381, Abstract 2554.

**129** Sagnou, M.J., Howard, P.W., Gregson, S.J., Eno-Amooquaye, E., Burke, P.J., and Thurston, D.E. (2000) Design and synthesis of novel pyrrolobenzodiazepine (PBD) prodrugs for ADEPT and GDEPT. *Bioorganic & Medicinal Chemistry Letters*, **10**, 2083–2086.

**130** Hay, M.P., Sykes, B.M., Denny, W.A., and Wilson, W.R. (1999) A 2-nitroimidazole carbamate prodrug of 5-amino-1-(chloromethyl)-3-[(5,6,7-trimethoxyindol-2-yl)carbonyl]-1,2-dihydro-3*H*-benz[*e*]indole (amino-seco-CBI-TMI) for use with ADEPT and GDEPT. *Bioorganic & Medicinal Chemistry Letters*, **9**, 2237–2242.

**131** Hay, M.P., Anderson, R.F., Ferry, D.M., Wilson, W.R., and Denny, W.A. (2003) Synthesis and evaluation of nitroheterocyclic carbamate prodrugs for use with nitroreductase-mediated gene-directed enzyme prodrug therapy. *Journal of Medicinal Chemistry*, **46**, 5533–5545.

**132** Mauger, A.B., Burke, P.J., Somani, H.H., Friedlos, F., and Knox, R.J. (1994) Self-immolative prodrugs: candidates for antibody-directed enzyme prodrug therapy in conjunction with a nitroreductase enzyme. *Journal of Medicinal Chemistry*, **37**, 3452–3458.

**133** Hay, M.P., Wilson, W.R., and Denny, W.A. (2005) Nitroarylmethyl carbamate prodrugs of doxorubicin for use with nitroreductase gene-directed enzyme prodrug therapy. *Bioorganic & Medicinal Chemistry*, **13**, 4043–4045.

**134** Anlezark, G.M., Melton, R.G., Sherwood, R.F., Wilson, W.R., Denny, W.A., Palmer, B.D., Knox, R.G., Friedlos, F., and Williams, A. (1995) Bioactivation of dinitrobenzamide mustards by an *E. coli* B nitroreductase. *Biochemical Pharmacology*, **50**, 609–618.

**135** Atwell, G.J., Boyd, M., Palmer, B.D., Anderson, R.F., Pullen, S.M., Wilson, R.W., and Denny, W.A. (1996) Synthesis and evaluation of 4-substituted analogues of 5-[*N*,*N*-bis-(2-chloroethyl)amino]-2-nitrobenzamide as bioreductively activated prodrugs using an *Escherichia coli* nitroreductase. *Anti-Cancer Drug Design*, **11**, 553–567.

136 Hu, L., Yu, C., Jiang, Y., Han, J., Li, Z., Browne, P., Race, P.R., Knox, R.J., Searle, P.F., and Hyde, E.I. (2003) Nitroaryl phosphoramide as novel prodrugs for *E. coli* nitroreductase activation in enzyme prodrug therapy. *Journal of Medicinal Chemistry*, **46**, 4818–4821.

137 Helsby, N.A., Atwell, G.J., Yang, S., Palmer, B.D., Anderson, R.F., Pullen, S.M., Ferry, D.M., Hogg, A., Wilson, W.R., and Denny, W.A. (2004) Aziridinyldinitrobenzamides: synthesis and structure–activity relationships for activation by *E. coli* nitroreductase. *Journal of Medicinal Chemistry*, **47**, 3295–3307.

138 Hay, M.P., Wilson, W.R., and Denny, W.R. (1999) Nitrobenzyl carbamate prodrugs of enediynes for nitroreductase gene-directed enzyme prodrug therapy. *Bioorganic & Medicinal Chemistry Letters*, **9**, 3417–3422.

139 Vrudhula, M.V., Senter, P.D., Fischer, K., and Wallace, P.M. (1993) Prodrugs of doxorubicin and melphalan and their activation by a monoclonal antibody-penicillin-G amidase conjugate. *Journal of Medicinal Chemistry*, **36**, 919–923.

140 Bignami, G.S., Senter, P.D., Grothaus, P.G., Fischer, K.J., Humphreys, T., and Wallace, P.M. (1992) N-(4′-Hydroxyphenylacetyl)palytoxin: a palytoxin prodrug that can be activated by a monoclonal antibody-penicillin-G amidase conjugate. *Cancer Research*, **52**, 5759–5764.

141 Hughes, B.W., Wells, A.H., Bebock, Z., Gadi, V.K., Garver, R.I. Jr., Parker, W.B., and Sorscher, E.J. (1995) Bystander killing of melanoma cells using the human tyrosinase promoter to express the *E. coli* purine nucleoside phosphorylase gene. *Cancer Research*, **55**, 3339–3345.

142 Sorscher, E.J., Peng, S., Bebock, Z., Allan, P.W., Bennett, L.L. Jr., and Parker, W.B. (1994) Tumor cell bystander killing in colonic carcinoma utilizing the *Escherichia coli* deo-D gene to generate toxic purines. *Gene Therapy*, **1**, 233–238.

143 Curlee, K.V., Parker, W.B., and Sorscher, E.J. (eds) (2004) Tumor sensitisation to purine analogs by *E. Coli* PNP, in *Suicide Gene Therapy* (ed. C.J. Springer), Humana Press, Inc., pp. 223–247.

144 Moolten, F.L., Vonderhaar, B.K., and Mroz, P.J. (1996) Transduction of the herpes thymidine kinase gene into premalignant murine mammary epithelial cells renders subsequent breast cancers responsive to ganciclovir therapy. *Human Gene Therapy*, **7**, 1197–1204.

145 Moolten, F.L. and Wells, J.M. (1990) Curability of tumors bearing Herpes virus thymidine kinase genes transferred by retroviral vectors. *Journal National Cancer Institute*, **82**, 297–300.

146 Vile, R.G. and Hart, I.R. (1993) Use of tissue-specific expression of the herpes simplex virus thymidine kinase gene to inhibit growth of established murine melanomas following direct intratumoral injection of DNA. *Cancer Research*, **53**, 3860–3864.

147 Wallace, H., Clarke, A.R., Harrison, D.J., Hooper, M.L., and Bishop, J.O. (1996) Ganciclovir-induced ablation of non-proliferating thyrocytes expressing herpes virus thymidine kinase occurs by p53-independent apoptosis. *Oncogene*, **13**, 55–61.

148 Kuriyama, S., Nakatani, T., Masui, K., Sakamoto, T., Tominaga, K., Yoshikawa, M., Fukui, H., Ikenaka, K., and Tsujii, T. (1996) Evaluation of prodrugs ability to induce effective ablation of cells transduced with viral thymidine kinase gene. *Anticancer Research*, **16**, 2623–2628.

149 Culver, K.W. (1996) The role of herpes simplex thymidine kinase gene transfer in the drug treatment of brain tumors. *CNS Drugs*, **6**, 1–11.

150 Culver, K.W., Ram, Z., Wallbridge, S., Oldfield, H.E.H., and Blaese, M.R. (1992) *In vivo* gene transfer with retroviral vector-producer cells for treatment of experimental brain tumors. *Science*, **256**, 1550–1552.

151 Rosenfeld, M.E., Wang, M., Siegal, G.P., Alvarez, R.D., Mikheeva, G., Krasnykh, V., and Curiel, D.T. (1996) Adenoviral-mediated delivery of herpes simplex virus thymidine kinase results in tumor reduction and prolonged survival in SCID

mouse model of human ovarian carcinoma. *Journal of Molecular Medicine*, **74**, 455–462.

**152** Huber, B.A., Richards, C.A., and Krenitsky, T.A. (1991) Retroviral-mediated gene therapy for the treatment of hepatocellular carcinoma: an innovative approach for cancer therapy. *Proceedings of the National Academy of Sciences of the United States of America*, **88**, 8039–8043.

**153** Averett, D.R., Koszalka, G.W., Fyfe, J.A., Roberts, G.B., Purifoy, D.J.M., and Krenitsky, T.A. (1991) 6-Methoxypurine arabinoside as a selective and potent inhibitor of varicella-zoster virus. *Antimicrobial Agents and Chemotherapy*, **35**, 851–857.

**154** Schelling, P., Claus, M., Johner, R., Marquez, V.E., Schulz, G.E., and Scapozza, l. (2004) Biochemical and structural characterization of (South)-methanocarbathymidine that specifically inhibits growth of Herpes simplex virus type 1 thymidine kinase-transduced osteosarcoma cells. *Journal of Biological Chemistry*, **279**, 32832–32838.

**155** Patterson, A.V., Zhang, H., Moghaddam, A., Bicknell, R., Talbot, D.C., Stratford, I.J., and Harris, A.L. (1995) Increased sensitivity to the prodrug 5′-deoxy-5-fluorouridine and modulation of 5-fluoro-2′-deoxyuridine sensitivity in MCF-7 cells transfected with thymidine phosphorylase. *British Journal of Cancer*, **72**, 669–675.

**156** Evrard, A., Ciccolini, G., Cuq, P., and Cano, J.-P. (2004) Enzyme–prodrug systems: thymidine phosphorylase/5′-deoxy-5-fluorouridine, in *Suicide Gene Therapy* (ed. C.J. Springer), Humana Press, Inc., pp. 263–279.

**157** Tamiya, T., Ono, Y., Wei, M.X., Mroz, P.J., Moolten, F.L., and Chiocca, E.A. (1996) Escherichia *coli* gpt gene sensitizes rat glioma cells to killing by 6-thioxanthine or 6-thioguanine. *Cancer Gene Therapy*, **3**, 155–162.

**158** Goshorn, S.C., Svensson, H.P., Kerr, D.E., Somerville, J.E., Senter, P.D., and Fell, H.P. (1993) Genetic construction, expression and characterisation of a single chain anti-carcinoma antibody fused to β-lactamase. *Cancer Research*, **53**, 2123–2127.

**159** Siemers, N.O., Kerr, D.E., Yarnold, S., Stebbins, M.R., Vrudhula, V.M., Hellstrom, I., Hellstrom, K.E., and Senter, P.D. (1997) Construction, expression and activities of L49-sFv-β-lactamase, as a single chain antibody fusion protein for anticancer prodrug activation. *Bioconjugate Chemistry*, **8**, 510–519.

**160** Lu, H., Chen, C.-S., and Waxman, D.J. (2009) Potentiation of methoxymorpholinyl doxorubicin antitumor activity by P450 3A4 gene transfer. *Cancer Gene Therapy*, **16**, 393–404.

**161** Denny, W.A. (2003) Prodrugs for gene-directed enzyme prodrug therapy (GDEPT). *Journal of Biomedicine and Biotechnology*, **2003**, 48–70.

**162** Desbene, S., Dufat-Trinh Van, H., Michel, S., Tillequin, F., Koch, M., Schmidt, F., Florent, J.-C., Monneret, C., Straub, R., Czech, J., Gerken, M., and Bosslet, K. (1999) Application of the ADEPT strategy to the MDR resistance in cancer chemotherapy. *Anti-Cancer Drug Design*, **14**, 93–106.

**163** Friedlos, F., Denny, W.A., Palmer, B.D., and Springer, C.J. (1997) Mustard prodrugs for activation by *Escherichia coli* nitroreductase in gene-directed enzyme prodrug therapy. *Journal of Medicinal Chemistry*, **40**, 1270–1275.

**164** Wilson, R.W., Pullen, S.M., Hogg, A., Helsby, N.A., Hichs, K.O., and Denny, W.A. (2002) Quantitation of the bystander effects in nitroreductase suicide gene therapy using three-dimensional cell cultures. *Cancer Research*, **62**, 1425–1432.

**165** Tercel, M., Wilson, R.W., Anderson, R.F., and Denny, W.A. (1996) Hypoxia selective antitumor agents. 12. Nitrobenzyl quaternary ammonium salts as bioreductive prodrugs of the alkylating agent mechloramine. *Journal of Medicinal Chemistry*, **39**, 1084–1094.

**166** Atwell, G.J., Sykes, B.M., O'Connor, C.J., and Denny, W.A. (1994) Relationships between structure and kinetics of cyclisation of 2-aminoaryl amides: potential prodrugs of cyclisation-activated aromatic mustards. *Journal of Medicinal Chemistry*, **37**, 371–380.

**167** Roffler, S.R., Wang, S.M., Chern, J.W., Yeh, M.Y., and Tung, E. (1991) Anti-neoplastic glucuronide prodrug treatment of human tumor cells targeted with a monoclonal antibody–enzyme conjugate. *Biochemical Pharmacology*, **42**, 2062–2065.

**168** Leu, Y.L., Chen, C.S., Wu, Y.J., and Chern, J.W. (2008) Benzyl ether-linked glucuronide derivative of 10-hydroxycamptothecin designed for selective camptothecin-based anticancer therapy. *Journal of Medicinal Chemistry*, **51**, 1740–1746.

**169** Voiculetz, N. and Niculescu-Duvaz, I. (1990) General mechanisms of carcinogenesis and anticarcinogenesis. *Archives roumaines de pathologie expérimentales et de microbiologie*, **49**, 105–17.

**170** Tietze, L., Hannemann, R., Buhr, W., Lögers, M., Menningen, P., Lieb, M., Starck, D., Grote, T., Döring, A., and Schuberth, I. (1996) Prodrugs of the cytostatic CC-1065 that can be activated in a tumor-selective manner. *Angewante Chemie International Edition*, **35**, 2674–2677.

**171** Hayes, G.M., Carpenito, C., Davis, P.D., Dougherty, S.T., Dirks, G.F., and Dougherty, G.H. (2002) Alternative splicing as a novel means of regulating the expression of therapeutic genes. *Cancer Gene Therapy*, **9**, 133–141.

**172** Hamstra, D.A., Page, M., Maybaum, J., and Rehemtulla, A. (2000) Expression of endogenously activated secreted or cell surface carboxypeptidase A sensitizes tumor cells to methotrexate-β-peptide prodrugs. *Cancer Research*, **60**, 657–665.

**173** Weyel, D., Sedlacek, H.H., Muller, R., and Brusselbach, S. (2000) Secreted human β-glucuronidase: a novel tool for gene-directed enzyme prodrug therapy. *Gene therapy*, **7**, 224–231.

**174** de Bont, D.B.A., Leenderens, R.G.G., Haisma, H.J., van der Meulen-Muileman, I., and Scheeren, H.W. (1997) Synthesis and biological activity of β-glucuronyl carbamate-based prodrugs of paclitaxel as potential candidates for ADEPT. *Bioorganic & Medicinal Chemistry*, **5**, 405–414.

**175** Schmidt, F., Ungureanu, I., Duval, R., Pompon, A., and Monneret, C. (2001) Cancer chemotherapy: a paclitaxel prodrug for ADEPT (antibody-directed enzyme prodrug therapy). *European Journal of Organic Chemistry*, **11**, 2129–2134.

**176** Shepherd, T., Junghein, L., and Meyer, D. (1992) Synthesis of acylhydrazido-substituted cephems. Design of cephalosporin-vinca alkaloid prodrugs: substrates for an antibody targeted enzyme. *Journal of Organic Chemistry*, **57**, 2334.

**177** Wierdl, M., Morton, C.L., Weeks, J.K., Danks, M.K., Harris, L.C., and Potter, P.M. (2001) Sensitization of human tumor cells to CPT-11 via adenoviral-mediated delivery of a rabbit liver carboxylesterase. *Cancer Research*, **61**, 5078–5082.

**178** Moolten, F.L. (1986) Tumor chemosensitivity conferred by inserted Herpes thymidine kinase genes: paradigm for a prospective cancer control strategy. *Cancer Research*, **46**, 5276–5281.

**179** Degreve, B., DeClerq, E., and Balzarini, J. (1999) Bystander effect of purine nucleoside analogues in HSV-tk suicide gene therapy is superior to that of pyrimidine nucleoside analogues. *Gene Therapy*, **6**, 162–170.

**180** Mohr, L., Rainov, M.G., Mohr, U.G., and Wands, G.R. (2000) Rabbit cytochrome P450 4B1: a novel prodrug activating gene for pharmacogene therapy of hepatocellular carcinoma. *Cancer Gene Therapy*, **7**, 1008–1014.

**181** Thatcher, N.J., Edwards, R.J., Lemoine, N.R., Doehmer, J., and Davies, D.S. (2000) The potential of acetaminophen as a prodrug in gene-directed enzyme prodrug therapy. *Cancer Gene Therapy*, **7**, 521–525.

**182** Syrigos, K., Rowlinson-Busza, G., and Epenetos, A. (1998) *In vitro* cytotoxicity following specific activation of amygdalin by beta-glucosidase conjugated to a bladder cancer-associated monoclonal antibody. *International Journal of Cancer*, **78**, 712–719.

183 Denny, A.W. (2002) Nitroreductase-based GDEPT. *Current Pharmaceutical Design*, **8**, 1349–1361.

184 Helsby, N., Wheeler, J., Pruijn, F., Palmer, B., Yang, S., Denny, W., and Wilson, W. (2003) Effect of nitroreduction on the alkylating reactivity and cytotoxicity of the 2,4-dinitrobenzamide-5-aziridine CB1954 and the corresponding nitrogen mustard SN23 862: a distinct mechanism of bioreductive activation. *Chemical Research in Toxicology*, **16**, 469–478.

185 Helsby, N., Ferry, D., Patterson, A., Pullen, S., and Wilson, W. (2004) 2-Amino metabolites are key mediators of CB1954 and SN23 862 bystander effects in nitroreductase GDEPT. *British Journal of Cancer*, **90**, 1084–1092.

186 Farquhar, D., Cherif, A., Bakina, E., and Nelson, G.A. (1998) Intensely potent doxorubicin analogues: structure–activity relationships. *Journal Medicinal Chemistry*, **41**, 965–972.

187 Heinis, C., Alessi, P., and Neri, D. (2004) Engineering a thermostable human prolyl endopeptidase for antibody-directed enzyme prodrug therapy. *Biochemistry*, **43**, 6293–6303.

188 Dowell, R.I., Springer, C.J., Davies, D.H., Hadley, E.M., Burke, P.J., Boyle, F.T., Melton, R.G., Connors, T.A., Blakey, D.C., and Mauger, A.B. (1996) New mustard prodrug for antibody-directed enzyme prodrug therapy: alternative to amide link. *Journal of Medicinal Chemistry*, **39**, 1100–1105.

189 Senter, P.D., Schreiber, G.J., Hirshberg, D.L., Ashe, S.A., Hellström, K.E., and Hellström, I. (1989) Enhancement of the *in vitro* and *in vivo* antitumor activities of phosphorylated mitomycin C and etoposide derivatives by monoclonal antibody-alkaline phosphatase conjugates. *Cancer Research*, **49**, 5789–5792.

190 Devalapally, H., Navath, R.S., Yenamandra, V., Akkinepally, R.R., and Devarakonda, R.K. (2007) Beta-galactoside prodrugs of doxorubicin for application in antibody directed enzyme prodrug therapy/prodrug monotherapy. *Archives of Pharmacal Research*, **30**, 723–32.

191 Wardman, P. (2001) Electron transfer and oxidative stress as key factors in the design of drugs selectively active in hypoxia. *Current Medicinal Chemistry*, **8**, 739–761.

192 Grove, J.I., Searle, P.F., Weedon, S.J., Green, N.K., McNeish, I.A., and Kerr, D.J. (1999) Virus-directed enzyme prodrug therapy using CB1954. *Anti-Cancer Drug Design*, **14**, 461–472.

193 Tercel, M., Denny, W., and Wilson, W. (1996) A novel nitro-substituted seco-CI: application as a reductively activated adept prodrug. *Bioorganic & Medicinal Chemistry Letters*, **6**, 2741–2744.

194 Cowen, R., Williams, K., Chinje, E., Jaffar, M., Sheppard, F., Telfer, B., Wind, N., and Stratford, I. (2004) Hypoxia targeted gene therapy to increase the efficacy of tirapazamine as an adjuvant to radiotherapy: reversing tumor radioresistance and effecting cure. *Cancer Research*, **64**, 1396–1402.

195 Rauth, A.M., Melo, T., and Misra, V. (1998) Bioreductive therapies: an overview of drugs and their mechanisms of action. *International Journal of Radiation Oncology, Biology and Physics*, **42**, 755–762.

196 Denny, W.A. (2001) Prodrug strategies in cancer therapy. *European Journal of Medicinal Chemistry*, **36**, 577–595.

197 Jounaidi, Y. and Waxman, D.J. (2000) Combination of the bioreductive drug tirapazamine with the chemotherapeutic prodrug cyclophosphamide for P450/P450-reductase-based cancer gene therapy. *Cancer Research*, **60**, 3761–3769.

198 Patterson, L.H. and Raleigh, S.M. (1998) *Reductive Metabolism: Its Application in Prodrug Activation.*, IOS Press, pp. 72–79.

199 Rodrigues, A.P., da Fonseca, L.M., de Faria Oliveira, O.M., Brunetti, I.L., and Ximenes, V.F. (2006) Oxidation of acetylacetone catalysed by horseradish peroxidase in the absence of hydrogen peroxide. *Biochimica et Biophysica Acta*, **1760**, 1755–1761.

200 Philpott, G.W., Shearer, W.T., Bower, R.W., and Parker, C.W. (1973) Selective cytotoxicity of hapten-substituted cells with an antibody–enzyme conjugate. *Journal of Immunology*, **111**, 921–929.

201 Secrist, J.A. III, Parker, W.B., Allan, P.W., Bennett, L.L., Waud, W.R., Truss, J.W., Fowler, A.T., Montgomery, J.A., Ealick, S.E., Gillepsie, G.Y., Gadi, V.K., and Sorscher, E.J. (1999) Gene therapy of cancer: activation of nucleoside prodrugs with *E. coli* purine nucleoside phosphorylase. *Nucleosides & Nucleotides*, **18**, 745–757.

202 Carl, P.L., Chakravarty, P.K., and Katzenellenbogen, J.A. (1981) A novel connector linkage applicable in prodrug design. *Journal of Medicinal Chemistry*, **24**, 479–480.

203 Papot, S., Tranoy, I., Tillequin, F., Florent, J.-C., and Gesson, J.-P. (2002) Design of selectively activated anticancer prodrugs: elimination and cyclization strategies. *Current Medicinal Chemistry. Anti-Cancer Agents*, **2**, 155–185.

204 Shabat, D., Amir, R., Gopin, A., Pessah, N., and Shamis, M. (2004) Chemical adaptors systems. *Chemistry, An European Journal*, **10**, 2626–2634.

205 Niculescu-Duvaz, D., Niculescu-Duvaz, I., and Springer, C.J. (2004) Design of prodrugs for suicide gene therapy, in *Suicide Gene Therapy*, vol. 90 (ed. C.J. Springer), Humana Press, Inc., pp. 161–202.

206 Jikai, J., Shamis, M., Huebener, N., Schroeder, U., Wrasidlo, W., Wenkel, J., Lange, B., Gaedicke, G., Shabat, D., and Lode, H. (2003) Neuroblastoma directed therapy by a rational prodrug design of etoposide as a substrate for tyrosine hydroxylase. *Cancer Letters*, **197**, 219–224.

207 Svensson, H.P., Kadow, J.F., Vrudhula, V.M., Wallace, P.M., and Senter, P.D. (1992) Monoclonal antibody-β-lactamase conjugates for the activation of a cephalosporin mustard prodrug. *Bioconjugate Chemistry*, **3**, 176–181.

208 Jungheim, L.N., Shepherd, T.A., and Kling, J.K. (1993) Synthesis of a cephalosporin-doxorubicin antitumor prodrug: a substrate for an antibody-targeted enzyme. *Heterocycles*, **35**, 339–348.

209 Wang, Y., Yuan, H., Wright, S., Wang, H., and Larrick, J. (2001) Synthesis and preliminary cytotoxicity study of a cephalosporin-CC-1065 analogue prodrug. *BMC Chemical Biology*, **1**, 4.

210 Papot, S., Combaud, D., and Gesson, J.-P. (1998) A new spacer group derived from arylmalonaldehydes for glucuronylated prodrugs. *Bioorganic & Medicinal Chemistry Letters*, **8**, 2545.

211 Sladek, N.E. (1987) Oxazaphosphorines, in *Metabolism and Action of Anti-Cancer Drugs* (eds G. Powis, and R.A. Prough), Taylor & Francis, London, pp. 48–89.

212 Ghosh, A.K., Khan, S., Marini, F., Nelson, J.A., and Farquhar, D. (2000) A daunorubicin β-galactoside prodrug for use in conjunction with gene-directed enzyme prodrug therapy. *Tetrahedron Letters*, **41**, 4871–4874.

213 Toki, B.E., Cerveny, C.G., Wahl, A.F., and Senter, P.D. (2002) Protease-mediated fragmentation of *p*-amidobenzyl ethers: a new strategy for the activation of anticancer prodrugs. *Journal of Organic Chemistry*, **67**, 1866–1872.

214 Ouberai, M., Asche, C., Carrez, D., Croisy, A., Dumy, P., and Demeunynck, M. (2006) 3,4-Dihydro-1*H*-[1,3]oxazino [4,5-*c*]acridines as a new family of cytotoxic drugs. *Bioorganic & Medicinal Chemistry Letters*, **16**, 4641–4643.

215 Shepherd, T.A., Jungheim, L.N., Meyer, D.L., and Starling, J.J. (1991) A novel targeted delivery system utilizing a cephalosporin oncolytic prodrug activated by an antibody β-lactamase conjugate for the treatment of cancer. *Bioorganic & Medicinal Chemistry Letters*, **1**, 21–26.

216 Bosslet, K., Czech, J., and Hoffmann, D. (1994) Tumor-selective prodrug activation by fusion protein-mediated catalysis. *Cancer Research*, **54**, 2151–2159.

217 Azoulay, M., Chalard, F., Gesson, J.-P., Florent, J.-C., and Monneret, C. (2001) 2-Nitro and 4-nitro-quinone-methides are not irreversible inhibitors of bovine β-glucuronidase. *Carbohydrate Research*, **332**, 151–156.

218 Dillon, M.P., Cai, H., and Maag, H. (1996) Application of the "trimethyl lock" to ganciclovir, a pro-prodrug with increased oral bioavailability. *Bioorganic & Medicinal Chemistry Letters*, **6**, 1653–1656.

219 Wang, B., Zhang, H., and Wang, W. (1996) Chemical feasibility studies of a potential coumarin-based prodrug system. *Bioorganic & Medicinal Chemistry Letters*, **6**, 945–950.

220 Schmidt, F., Florent, J.-C., Monneret, C., Straub, R., Czech, J., Gerken, M., and Bosslet, K. (1997) Glucuronide prodrugs of hydroxy compounds for antibody directed enzyme prodrug therapy (ADEPT): a phenol nitrogen mustard carbamate. *Bioorganic & Medicinal Chemistry Letters*, **7**, 1071–1076.

221 Johansson, E., Parkinson, G., Denny, W., and Neidle, S. (2003) Studies on the nitroreductase prodrug-activating system. Crystal structures of complexes with the inhibitor dicoumarol and dinitrobenzamide prodrugs and of the enzyme active form. *Journal of Medicinal Chemistry*, **46**, 4009–4020.

222 Johansson, E., Parkinson, G., Read, M., Denny, B., and Neidle, S. (2001) The crystal structure of a complex between the prodrug CB1954 and the enzyme nitroreductase. *Clinical Cancer Research*, **7**, 368.

223 Ko, T., Lin, J., Hu, C., Hsu, Y., Wang, A., and Liaw, S. (2003) Crystal structure of yeast cytosine deaminase: insights into enzyme mechanism and evolution. *Journal of Biological Chemistry*, **278**, 19111–19117.

224 Ostermann, N., Lavie, A., Padiyar, S., Brundiers, R., Veit, T., Reinstein, J., Goody, R., Konrad, M., and Schlichting, I. (2000) Potentiating AZT activation: structures of wild-type and mutant human thymidylate kinase suggest reasons for the mutants' improved kinetics with the HIV prodrug metabolite AZTMP. *Journal of Molecular Biology*, **304**, 43–53.

225 Parkinson, G., Skelly, J., and Neidle, S. (2000) Crystal structure of FMN-dependent nitroreductase from *Escherichia coli* B: a prodrug-activating enzyme. *Journal of Medicinal Chemistry*, **43**, 3624–3631.

226 Rowsell, S., Pauptit, R.A., Tucker, A.D., Melton, R.G., Blow, D.M., and Brick, P. (1997) Crystal structure of carboxypeptidase G(2), a bacterial enzyme with applications in cancer therapy. *Structure*, **5**, 337–347.

227 Sabini, E., Ort, S., Monnerjahn, C., Konrad, M., and Lavie, A. (2003) Structure of human dCK suggests strategies to improve anticancer and antiviral therapy. *Nature Structural Biology*, **10**, 513–519.

228 Zhang, Y., Secrist, J.A. 3rd, and Ealick, S.E. (2006) The structure of human deoxycytidine kinase in complex with clofarabine reveals key interactions for prodrug activation. *Acta Crystallographica. Section D, Biological Crystallography*, **62**, 133–9.

229 Sabini, E., Hazra, S., Konrad, M., Burley, S.K., and Lavie, A. (2007) Structural basis for activation of the therapeutic L-nucleoside analogs 3TC and troxacitabine by human deoxycytidine kinase. *Nucleic Acids Research*, **35**, 186–92.

230 De Clercq, E., Andrei, G., De Bolle, L., Naesens, L., Degreve, B., Balzarini, J., Zhang, Y., Schols, D., Leyssen, P., Ying, C., and Neyts, J. (2001) Acyclic/carbocyclic guanosine analogues as anti-herpesvirus agents. *Nucleosides, Nucleotides & Nucleic Acids*, **20**, 271–285.

231 Connors, T.A. (1995) The choice of prodrugs for gene directed enzyme prodrug therapy of cancer. *Gene Therapy*, **2**, 702–709.

232 Greco, O. and Dachs, G.U. (2001) Gene directed enzyme/prodrug therapy of cancer: hystorical appraisal and future prospectives. *Journal of Cellular Physiology*, **187**, 22–36.

233 Chen, L., Waxman, D.J., Chen, D., and Kufe, D.C. (1996) Sensitization of human breast cancer cells to cyclophosphamide and ifosfamide by transfer of a liver cytochrome P-450 gene. *Cancer Research*, **56**, 1331–1340.

234 Kojima, A., Hackett, N.R., Ohwada, A., and Crystal, R.G. (1998) *In vivo* human carboxylesterase cDNA gene transfer to activate the prodrug CPT-11 for local treatment of solid tumors. *Journal Clinical Investigation*, **101**, 1789–1796.

235 Tietze, L.F., Major, F., and Schuberth, I. (2006) Antitumor agents: development of highly potent glycosidic duocarmycin analogues for selective cancer therapy.

*Angewante Chemistry International Edition*, **45**, 6574–6577.

236 Hay, M.P., Atwell, G.J., Wilson, W.R., Pullen, S.M., and Denny, W.A. (2003) Structure–activity relationships for 4-nitrobenzyl carbamates of 5-aminobenz [*e*]indoline minor groove alkylating agents as prodrugs for GDEPT in conjunction with *E. coli* nitroreductase. *Journal of Medicinal Chemistry*, **46**, 2456–2466.

237 Jiang, Y., Han, J., Yu, C., Vass, S.O., Searle, P.F., Browne, P., Knox, R.J., and Hu, L. (2006) Design, synthesis and biological evaluation of cyclic and acyclic nitrobenzylphosphoramide mustards for *E. coli* nitroreductase activation. *Journal of Medicinal Chemistry*, **49**, 4333–4343.

238 Tietze, L.F., Schuster, H.J., Krewer, B., and Schuberth, I. (2009) Synthesis and biological studies of different duocarmycin based glycosidic prodrugs for their use in the antibody-directed enzyme prodrug therapy. *Journal of Medicinal Chemistry*, **52**, 537–43.

239 Greenwald, R.B., Pendri, A., Conover, C.D., Zhao, H., Choe, Y.H., Martinez, A., Shum, K., and Guan, S. (1999) Drug delivery systems employing 1,4-or 1,6-elimination: poly(ethylene glycol) prodrugs of amine-containing compounds. *Journal of Medicinal Chemistry*, **42**, 3657–3667.

240 Greenwald, R.B., Choe, Y.H., Conover, C.D., Shum, K., Wu, D., and Roysen, M. (2000) Drug delivery systems based on trimethyl lock lactonization: poly (ethylene glycol) prodrugs of amino-containing compounds. *Journal of Medicinal Chemistry*, **43**, 475–487.

241 Saari, W.S., Schwering, J., Lyle, P., Smith, S., and Engelhardt, E. (1990) Cyclization-activated prodrugs-basic esters of 5 bromo-2-deoxiuridine. *Journal of Medicinal Chemistry*, **33**, 2590.

242 Saari, W.S., Schwering, J.E., Lyle, P.A., Smith, S.J., and Engelhardt, E.D. (1990) Cyclization-activated prodrugs-basic carbamates of 4-hydroxyanisole. *Journal of Medicinal Chemistry*, **33**, 97.

243 Nicolaou, M.G., Wolfe, J.L., Schowen, R.L., and Borchardt, R.T. (1996) Facilitated intramolecular conjugate addition of amides of 3-(3′,6′-dioxo-2′,4′-dimethyl-1′,4′-cyclohexadienyl)-3,3-dimethylpropionic acid. 2. Kinetics of degradation. *Journal of Organic Chemistry*, **61**, 6633.

244 Denny, W.A. (1996) The design of selectively-activated prodrugs for cancer chemotherapy. *Current Pharmaceutical Design*, **2**, 281–294.

245 Denny, W.A. and Wilson, W.R. (1998) The design of selectively-activated anti-cancer prodrugs for use in antibody-directed and gene-directed enzyme prodrugs therapies. *Journal of Pharmaceutical Pharmacology*, **50**, 387–394.

246 Bagshawe, K.D., Sharma, S.K., Springer, C.J., Antoniw, P., Boden, J.A., Rogers, G.T., Burke, P.J., Melton, R.G., and Sherwood, R.F. (1991) Antibody-directed enzyme prodrug therapy (ADEPT): clinical report. *Disease Markers*, **9**, 233–238.

247 Patterson, A.V. and Harris, A.L. (1999) Molecular chemotherapy for breast cancer. *Drugs & Aging*, **14**, 75–90.

248 Akyurek, L.M., Nallamshetty, S., Aoki, K., Yang, Z.-Y., Nabel, G.J., and Nabel, E.G. (2001) Coexpression of guanylate kinase with thymidine kinase enhances prodrug cell killing *in vitro* and suppresses vascular cell proliferation *in vivo*. *Molecular Therapy*, **3**, 779–786.

249 Chung-Faye, G., Chen, M., Green, N., Burton, A., Anderson, D., Mautner, V., Searle, P., and Kerr, D. (2001) *In vivo* gene therapy for colon cancer using adenovirus-mediated, transfer of the fusion gene cytosine deaminase and uracil phosphoribosyltransferase. *Gene Therapy*, **8**, 1547–1554.

250 Wierdl, M., Wall, A., Morton, C., Sampath, J., Danks, M., Schuetz, J., and Potter, P. (2003) Carboxylesterase-mediated sensitization of human tumor cells to CPT-11 cannot override ABCG2-mediated drug resistance. *Molecular Pharmacology*, **64**, 279–288.

251 Springer, C.J. and Niculescu-Duvaz, I. (2000) Prodrug-activating systems in suicide gene therapy. *The Journal of Clinical Investigation*, **105**, 1161–1167.

252 Niculescu-Duvaz, I. and Springer, C.J. (2004) Introduction to the background,

principles and state of the art in suicide gene therapy, in *Suicide Gene Therapy*, vol. **90** (ed. C.J. Springer), Humana Press, Inc., pp. 1–28.

253 Jounaidi, Y., Chen, C.-S., Veal, G.J., and Waxman, D.J. (2006) Enhanced antitumor activity of P450 prodrug-based gene therapy using the low Km cyclophosphamide 4-hydroxylase P450 2B11. *Molecular Cancer Therapeutics*, **5**, 541–555.

254 Folkes, L., Greco, O., Dachs, G., Stratford, M., and Wardman, P. (2002) 5-Fluoroindole-3-acetic acid: a prodrug activated by a peroxidase with potential for use in targeted cancer therapy. *Biochemical Pharmacology*, **63**, 265–272.

255 Hay, M.P., Sykes, B.M., Denny, W.A., and O'Connor, C.J. (1999) Substituents effect of the kinetics of reductively-initiated fragmentation of nitrobenzylcarbamates designed as triggers for prodrugs. *Journal of the Chemical Society, Perkin Transactions 1*, 2759–2770.

256 Balzarini, G., Degreve, B., Andrei, G., Neyst, J., Sandvold, M., Myhren, F., and de Clerq, E. (1998) Superior cytostatic activity of the ganciclovir elaidic acid ester due to the prolonged intracellular retention of ganciclovir anabolites in herpes simplex virus type 1 thymidine kinase gene-transfected tumor cells. *Gene Therapy*, **5**, 419–426.

257 Hoganson, D.K., Batra, R.K., Olsen, J.C., and Boucher, R.C. (1996) Comparison of the effect of three different toxin genes and their levels of expression on cell growth and bystander effect in lung adenocarcinoma. *Cancer Research*, **56**, 1315–1323.

258 Nishihara, E., Nagayama, Y., Narimatsu, M., Namba, H., Watanabe, M., Niwa, M., and Yamashita, S. (1998) Treatment of thyroid carcinoma cells with four different suicide gene/prodrug combinations *in vitro*. *Anticancer Research*, **18**, 1521–1526.

259 Hamstra, D.A. and Rehemtulla, A. (1999) Toward an enzyme/prodrug strategy for cancer gene therapy: endogenous activation of carboxypeptidase A mutants by the PACE/Furin family of propeptidases. *Human Gene Therapy*, **10**, 235–248.

260 Chen, L., Yu, L.J., and Waxman, D.J. (1997) Potentiation of cytochrome P450/cyclophosphamide-based cancer gene therapy by coexpression of the P450 reductase gene. *Cancer Research*, **57**, 4830–4837.

261 Ichikawa, T., Petros, W.P., Ludeman, S.M., Fangmeier, J., Hochberg, W.H., Colvin, M.O., and Chiocca, A. (2001) Intraneoplastic polymer-based delivery of cyclophosphamide for intratumoral bioconversion by a replicating oncolytic viral vector. *Cancer Research*, **61**, 864–868.

262 Huang, Z., Raychowdhury, K., and Waxman, D.J. (2000) Impact of liver P450 reductase suppression on cyclophosphamide activation, pharmacokinetics and antitumoral activity in a cytochrom P450-based cancer gene therapy model. *Cancer Gene Therapy*, **7**, 1034–1042.

263 Huang, Z. and Waxman, D.J. (2001) Modulation of cyclophosphamide-based cytochrome p450 gene therapy using liver P450 inhibitors. *Cancer Gene Therapy*, **8**, 450–458.

264 Schwartz, P., Chen, C., and Waxman, D. (2003) Sustained P450 expression and prodrug activation in bolus cyclophosphamide-treated cultured tumor cells. Impact of prodrug schedule on P450 gene-directed enzyme prodrug therapy. *Cancer Gene Therapy*, **10**, 571–582.

265 van der Eb, M., de Leeuw, B., van der Eb, A., and Hoeben, R. (2004) Side effects of suicide gene therapy, in *Suicide Gene Therapy* (ed. C. Springer), Humana Press, Inc., pp. 479–490.

266 Encell, L.P., Landis, D.M., and Loeb, L.A. (1999) Improving enzymes for gene therapy. *Nature Biotechnology*, **17**, 143–147.

267 Anlezark, G.M., Vaughan, T., Fashola-Stone, E., Michael, N.P., Murdoch, H., Sims, M.A., Stubbs, S., Wigley, S., and Minton, N.P. (2002) Bacillus *amyloliquefaciens* orthologue of *Bacillus subtilis* ywrO encodes a nitroreductase enzyme which activates the prodrug CB 1954. *Microbiology*, **148**, 297–306.

268 Kamiya, H., Ochiai, H., Harashima, H., Ito, M., and Matsuda, A. (2006) Transient expression of *Drosophila melanogaster* deoxynucleoside kinase gene enhances cytotoxicity of nucleoside analogs. *Nucleosides Nucleotides Nucleic Acids*, **25**, 553–60.

269 Wardman, P. (2002) Indole-3-acetic acid and horseradish peroxidase: a new prodrug/enzyme combination for targeted cancer therapy. *Current Pharmaceutical Design*, **8**, 1363–1374.

270 Lovering, A.L., Hyde, E.I., Searle, P.F., and White, S.A. (2001) The structure of *Escherichia coli* nitroreductase complexed with nicotinic acid: three crystal forms at 1.7 Å, 1. 8 Å and 2. 4 Å resolution. *Journal of Molecular Biology*, **309**, 203–13.

271 Kokoris, M.S., Sabo, P., Adman, E.T., and Black, M.E. (1999) Enhancement of tumor ablation by a selected HSV-1 thymidine kinase mutants. *Gene Therapy*, **6**, 1415–1426.

272 Black, M., Kokoris, M.S., and Sabo, P. (2001) Herpes simplex virus-1 thymidine kinase mutants created by semi-random sequence mutagenesis improve prodrug-mediated tumor cell killing. *Cancer Research*, **61**, 3022–3026.

273 Kokoris, M.S. and Black, M.E. (2002) Characterization of herpes simplex virus type 1 kinase mutants engineered for improved ganciclovir and acyclovir activity. *Protein Science*, **11**, 2267–2272.

274 Race, P.R., Lovering, A.L., White, S.A., Grove, J.I., Searle, P.F., Wrighton, C.W., and Hyde, E.I. (2007) Kinetic and structural characterisation of *Escherichia coli* nitroreductase mutants showing improved efficacy for the prodrug substrate CB1954. *Journal of Molecular Biology*, **368**, 481–92.

275 Grove, J.I., Lovering, A.L., Guise, C., Race, P.R., Wrighton, C.J., White, S.A., Hyde, E.I., and Searle, P.F. (2003) Generation of *Escherichia coli* nitroreductase mutants conferring improved cell sensitization to the prodrug CB1954. *Cancer Research*, **63**, 5532–7.

276 Kaliberov, S.A., Market, J.M., Gillespie, G.Y., Krendelchtchikova, V., Della Manna, D., Sellers, J.C., Kaliberova, L.N., Black, M.E., and Buchsbaum, D.J. (2007) Mutation of *Escherichia coli* cytosine deaminase significantly enhances molecular chemotherapy of human glioma. *Gene Therapy*, **14**, 1111–9.

277 Francis, R.J., Sharma, S.K., Springer, C.J., Green, A.J., Hope-Stone, L.D., Sena, L., Martin, J., Adamson, K.L., Robbins, A., Gumbrell, L., O'Malley, D., Tsiompanou, E., Shahbakhti, H., Webley, S.D., Hochhauser, D., Hilson, A.J., Blakey, D., and Begent, R.H. (2002) A Phase I trial of antibody directed enzyme prodrug therapy (ADEPT) in patients with advanced colorectal carcinoma or other CEA producing tumours. *British Journal of Cancer*, **87**, 600–607.

278 Napier, M., Sharma, S.K., Springer, C.J., Bagshawe, K.B., Green, A.J., Martin, J., Stribbling, S.M., Cushen, N., O'Malley, D., and Begent, R.H.J. (2000) Antibody-directed enzyme prodrug therapy: efficacy and mechanism of action in colorectal carcinoma. *Clinical Cancer Research*, **6**, 765–772.

279 Afshar, S., Asai, T., and Morrison, S.L. (2009) Humanized ADEPT comprised of an engineered human purine nucleoside phosphorylase and a tumor targeting peptide for treatment of cancer. *Molecular Cancer Therapeutics*, **8**, 185–93.

280 Pulkanen, K.J., Laukanen, J.M., Fuxe, J., Kettunen, M.I., Rehn, M., Kannasto, J.M., Parkkinen, J.J., Kaupinen, R.A., Pettersson, R.F., and Yla-Herttuala, S. (2002) The combination of HSV-tk and endostatin gene therapy eradicates orthotopic human renal cell carcinomas in nude mice. *Cancer Gene Therapy*, **9**, 908–916.

281 Rogulski, K.R., Zhang, K., Kolozsvary, A., Kim, J.H., and Freitag, S.O. (1997) Pronounced antitumor effect and tumor radiosensitization of double suicide gene therapy. *Clinical Cancer Research*, **3**, 2081–2088.

282 Uckert, W., Kammertons, T., Haack, K., Qin, Z., Gebert, J., Schendel, D.J., and Blankenstein, T. (1998) Double suicide gene (cytosine deaminase and herpes simplex virus thymidine kinase) but not single gene transfer allows reliable elimination of tumor cells *in vivo*. *Human Gene Therapy*, **9**, 855–865.

283 Blackburn, R.V., Galoforo, S.S., Corry, P.M., and Lee, Y.J. (1998) Adenoviral-mediated transfer of a heat-inducible double suicide gene into prostate carcinoma cells. *Cancer Research*, **58**, 1358–1362.

284 Kammertoens, T., Gelbmann, W., Karle, P., Alton, K., Saller, R., Salmons, B., Gunzburg, W.h., and Uckert, W. (2000) Combined chemotherapy of murine mammary tumors by local activationof the prodrug ifosfamide and 5-fluorocytosine. *Cancer Gene Therapy*, **7**, 629–636.

285 Rogulski, K.R., Wing, M.S., Paielli, D.L., Gilbert, J.D., Kim, J.H., and Freytag, S.O. (2000) Double suicide gene therapy augments the antitumor activity of a replication-competent lytic adenovirus through enhanced cytotoxicity and radiosensitization. *Human Gene Therapy*, **11**, 67–76.

286 Blanche, F., Cameron, B., Couder, M., and Crouzet, J. (1997.) Enzymes combinations for destroying proliferative cells. WO 9735024.

287 Shimizu, T., Shimada, H., Ochiai, T., and Hamada, H. (2001) Enhanced growth suppression in esophageal carcinoma cells using adenovirus-mediated fusion gene transfer uracil phosphoryl transferase and herpes simplex virus thymidine kinase. *Cancer Gene Therapy*, **8**, 512–521.

288 Vernejoul, F., Ghenassia, L., Souque, A., Lulka, H., Drocourt, D., Cordelier, P., Pradayrol, L., Pyronnet, S., Buscail, L., and Tiraby, G. (2006) Gene therapy based on gemcitabine chemosensitization suppresses pancreatic tumor growth. *Molecular Therapy: The Journal of the American Society of Gene Therapy*, **14**, 758–67.

289 Erbs, P., Regulier, E., Kintz, J., Leroy, P., Poitevin, Y., Exinger, F., Jund, R., and Mehtali, M. (2000) *In vivo* cancer gene therapy by adenovirus-mediated transfer of a bifunctional yeast cytosine deaminase/uracil phosphoribosyltransferase fusion gene. *Cancer Research*, **60**, 3813–3822.

290 Chung-Faye, G.A., Chen, M.J., Green, N.K., Burton, A., Anderson, D., Mautner, V., Searle, P.F., and Kerr, D.J. (2001) *In vivo* gene therapy for colon cancer using adenovirus-mediated transfer of the fusion gene cytosine deaminase and uracil phosphoribosyltransferase. *Gene Therapy*, **8**, 1547–1554.

291 Kim, Y.G., Bi, W., Feliciano, E.S., Drake, R.R., and Stambrook, P.J. (2000) Ganciclovir-mediated cell killing and bystander effect is enhanced in cells with two copies of the herpes simplex virus thymidine kinase. *Cancer Gene Therapy*, **7**, 240–246.

292 Chen, S.H., Kosai, K., Xu, B., Pham-Nguyen, K., Contant, C., Finegold, M.J., and Woo, S.L.C. (1996) Combination suicide and cytokine gene therapy for hepatic metastases of colon carcinoma: sustained antitumor immunity prolongs animal survival. *Cancer Research*, **56**, 3758–3762.

293 Toda, M., Martuza, R.L., and Rabkin, S.D. (2001) Combination suicide/cytokine gene therapy as adjuvants to a defective herpes simplex virus-based cancer vaccine. *Gene Therapy*, **8**, 332–339.

294 Hall, S.J., Sanford, M.A., Atkinson, G., and Chen, S.-H. (1998) Induction of potent antitumor natural killer cell activity by herpes simplex virus-thymidine kinase and ganciclovir therapy in an orthotopic mouse model of prostate cancer. *Cancer Research*, **58**, 3221–3225.

295 Schwartz, P., Chen, C., and Waxman, D. (2002) Enhanced bystander cytotoxicity of P450 gene-directed enzyme prodrug therapy by expression of the antiapoptotic factor p35. *Cancer Research*, **62**, 6928–6937.

296 Pawelek, J.M., Low, K.B., and Bermudes, D. (1997) Tumor-targeted *Salmonella* as a novel anticancer vector. *Cancer Research*, **57**, 4537–4544.

297 Clairmont, C., Lee, K.C., Pike, J., Ittensohn, M., Low, K.B., Pawelek, J.M., Bermudes, D., Brecher, S.M., Margitich, D., Turnier, J., Li, Z., Luo, X., King, I., and Zheng, L.M. (2000) Biodistribution and genetic stability of the novel antitumor agent VNP20009, a genetically modified strain of *Salmonella typhimurium*. *The*

*Journal of Infectious Diseases*, **181**, 1996–2002.

298 Lee, K.C., Zheng, L.-M., Luo, X., Clairmont, C., Fischer, J., Margitich, D., Turnier, J., Almassian, B., Bermudes, D., and King, I. (2000) Comparative evaluation of the acute toxic effects in monkeys, pigs and mice of a genetically engineered *Salmonella* strain (VNP20009) being developed as an antitumor agent. *International Journal of Toxicology*, **19**, 19–25.

299 Low, K.B., Ittensohn, M., Le, T., Platt, J., Sodi, S., Amoss, M., Ash, O., Carmichael, E., Chakraborty, A., Fischer, J., Lin, S.L., Luo, X., Miller, S.I., Zheng, L.-M., King, I., Pawelek, J.M., and Bermudes, D. (1998) Lipid A mutant *Salmonella* with suppressed virulence and TNFα induction retail tumor-targeting *in vivo*. *Nature Biotechnology*, **17**, 37–41.

300 Fox, M.E., Lemmon, M.J., Mauchline, M.L., Davis, T.O., Giaccia, A.J., Minton, N.P., and Brown, J.M. (1996) Anaerobic bacteria as a delivery system for cancer gene therapy: *in vitro* activation of 5-fluorocytosine by genetically engineered clostridia. *Gene Therapy*, **3**, 173–178.

301 Lemmon, M.J., van Zijl, P., Fox, M.E., Mauchline, M.L., Giaccia, A.J., Minton, N.P., and Brown, J.M. (1997) Anaerobic bacteria as a gene delivery system that is controlled by the tumor microenvironment. *Gene Therapy*, **4**, 791–796.

302 Nakamura, T., Sasaki, T., Fujimori, M., Yazawa, K., Kano, Y., Amano, J, and Taniguchi, S. (2002) Cloned cytosine deaminase gene expression of *Bifidobacterium longum* and application to enzyme/pro-drug therapy of hypoxic solid tumors. *Bioscience, Biotechnology and Biochemistry*, **66**, 2362–2366.

303 Yazawa, K., Fujimori, M., Amano, J., Kano, Y., and Taniguchi, S. (2000) Bifidobacterium *longum* as a delivery system for cancer gene therapy: selective localization and growth in hypoxic tumors. *Cancer Gene Therapy*, **7**, 269–274.

304 Yazawa, K., Fujimori, M., Nakamura, T., Sasaki, T., Amano, J., Kano, Y., and Taniguchi, S. (2001) Bifidobacterium *longum* as a delivery system for gene therapy of chemically induced rat mammary tumors. *Breast Cancer Research and Treatment*, **66**, 165–170.

305 Critchley, R.J., Jezzard, S., Radford, K., Goussard, S., Lemoine, N.R., Grillot-Courvalin, C., and Vassaux, G. (2004) Potential, therapeutic applications of recombinant, invasive *E. coli*. *Gene Therapy*, **11**, 1224–1233.

306 Zhao, M., Yang, M., Li, X.-M., Jiang, P., Baranov, E., Li, S., Xu, M., Penman, S., and Hoffman, R.M. (2005) Tumor-targeting bacterial therapy with amino acid auxotrophs of GFP-expressing *Salmonella typhimurium*. *Proceedings of the National Academy of Sciences of the United States of America*, **102**, 755–760.

307 Soghomonyan, S.A., Doubrovin, M., Pike, J., Luo, X., Ittensohn, M., Runyan, J.D., Balatoni, J., Finn, R., Tjuvajev, J.G., Blasberg, R., and Bermudes, D. (2005) Positron emission tomography (PET) imaging of tumor-localized *Salmonella* expressing HSV1-TK. *Cancer Gene Therapy*, **12**, 101–108.

308 Friedlos, F., Lehouritis, P., Ogilvie, L., Hedley, D., Davies, L., Bermudes, D., King, I., Martin, J., Marais, R., and Springer, C.J. (2008) Attenuated *Salmonella* targets prodrug activating enzyme carboxypeptidase G2 to mouse melanoma and human breast and colon carcinomas for effective suicide gene therapy. *Clinical Cancer Research*, **14**, 4259–66.

309 Liu, Y. and Deisseroth, A. (2006) Tumor vascular targeting therapy with viral vectors. *Blood*, **107**, 3027–33.

310 Alemany, R. (2007) Cancer selective adenoviruses. *Molecular Aspects of Medicine*, **28**, 42–58.

311 Bergelson, J.M., Cunningham, J.A., Droguett, G., Kurt-Jones, E.A., Krithivas, A., Hong, J.S., Horwitz, M.S., Crowell, R.L., and Finberg, R.W. (1997) Isolation of a common receptor for Coxsackie B viruses and adenoviruses 2 and 5. *Science*, **275**, 1320–3.

312 Fukuhara, H., Hayashi, Y., Yamamoto, N., Fukui, T., Nishikawa, M., Mitsudo, K., Tohnai, I., Ueda, M., Mizuno, M., and Yoshida, J. (2003) Improvement of

transduction efficiency of recombinant adenovirus vector conjugated with cationic liposome for human oral squamous cell carcinoma cell lines. *Oral Oncology*, **39**, 601–609.

313 Xu, Z.-L., Mizuguchi, H., Sakurai, F., Koizumi, N., Hosono, T., Kawabata, K., Watanabe, Y., Yamaguchi, T., and Hayakawa, T. (2005) Approaches to improving the kinetics of adenovirus-delivered genes and gene products. *Advanced Drug Delivery Reviews*, **57**, 781–802.

314 Lanson, N.A. Jr., Friedlander, P.A., Schwartzenberger, P., Kolls, J.K., and Wang, G. (2003) Replication of an adenoviral vector controlled by the human telomerase reverse transcriptase promotor causes tumor-selective tumor lysis. *Cancer Research*, **63**, 7936–7941.

315 Irving, J., Wang, Z., Powell, S., O'Sullivan, C., Mok, M., Murphy, B., Cardoza, L., Lebkoxski, J.S., and Majumdar, A.S. (2004) Conditionally replicative adenovirus driven by the human telomerase promoter provides broad-spectrum antitumor activity without liver toxicity. *Cancer Gene Therapy*, **11**, 174–185.

316 Bisland, A.F., Anderson, C.J., Fletcher-Monaghan, A., McGregor, F., Evans, T.R.J., Ganly, I., Knox, R.J., Plumb, J.A., and Keith, W.N. (2003) Selective ablation of human cancer cells by telomerase-specific adenoviral suicide gene therapy vectors expressing bacterial nitroreductase. *Oncogene*, **22**, 370–380.

317 Fisher, K.D., Ulbrich, K., Subr, V., Ward, C.M., Mautner, V., Blakey, D., and Seymour, L.W. (2000) A versatile system for receptor-mediated gene delivery permits increased entry of DNA into target cells, enhanced delivery to the nucleus and elevated rates of transgene expression. *Gene Therapy*, **7**, 1337–43.

318 Green, N.K., Herbert, C.W., Hale, S.J., Hale, A.B., Mautner, V., Harkins, R., Hermiston, T., Ulbrich, K., Fisher, K.D., and Seymour, L.W. (2004) Extended plasma circulation time and decreased toxicity of polymer-coated adenovirus. *Gene Therapy*, **11**, 1256–63.

319 van Beusechem, V.W., van den Doel, P.B., and Gerritsen, W.R. (2005) Conditionally replicative adenovirus expressing degradation-resistant p53 for enhanced oncolysis of human cancer cells overexpressing murine double minute 2. *Molecular Cancer Therapeutics*, **4**, 1013–1018.

320 Yang, S., Guo, Z.S., O'Malley, M.E., Yin, X., Zeh, H.J., and Bartlett, D.L. (2007) A new recombinant vaccinia with targeted deletion of three viral genes: its safety and efficacy as an oncolytic virus. *Gene Therapy*, **14**, 638–47.

321 Deisseroth, A. (2005) Normal and pathological functions of mammalian retroelements. *Proceedings of the National Academy of Sciences of the United States of America*, **102**, 12292–3.

322 Richardson, T.B., Kaspers, J., and Porter, C.D. (2004) Retroviral hybrid LTR vector strategy: functional analysis of LTR elements and generation of endothelial cell specificity. *Gene Therapy*, **11**, 775–83.

323 Hiraoka, K., Kimura, T., Logg, C.R., and Kasahara, N. (2006) Tumor-selective gene expression in a hepatic metastasis model after locoregional delivery of a replication-competent retrovirus vector. *Clinical Cancer Research*, **12**, 7108–16.

324 Barker, E. and Planelles, V. (2003) Vectors derived from the human immunodeficiency virus, HIV-1. *Frontiers in Bioscience: A Journal and Virtual Library*, **8**, d491–510.

325 Grote, D., Russell, S.J., Cornu, T.I., Cattaneo, R., Vile, R., Poland, G.A., and Fielding, A.K. (2001) Live attenuated measles virus induces regression of human lymphoma xenografts in immunodeficient mice. *Blood*, **97**, 3746–54.

326 Dorig, R.E., Marcil, A., and Richardson, C.D. (1994) CD46, a primate-specific receptor for measles virus. *Trends in Microbiology*, **2**, 312–8.

327 Tatsuo, H., Ono, N., Tanaka, K., and Yanagi, Y. (2000) The cellular receptor for measles virus: SLAM (CDw 150). *Uirusu*, **50**, 289–96.

328 Hallak, L.K., Merchan, J.R., Storgard, C.M., Loftus, J.C., and Russell, S.J. (2005) Targeted measles virus vector displaying

Echistatin infects endothelial cells via alpha(v)beta3 and leads to tumor regression. *Cancer Research*, **65**, 5292–300.

329 Valyi-Nagy, T., Sheth, V., Clement, C., Tiwari, V., Scanlan, P., Kavouras, J.H., Leach, L., Guzman-Hartman, G., Dermody, T.S., and Shukla, D. (2004) Herpes simplex virus entry receptor nectin-1 is widely expressed in the murine eye. *Current Eye Research*, **29**, 303–9.

330 Kaner, R.J., Baird, A., Mansukhani, A., Basilico, C., Summers, B.D., Florkiewicz, R.Z., and Hajjar, D.P. (1990) Fibroblast growth factor receptor is a portal of cellular entry for herpes simplex virus type 1. *Science*, **248**, 1410–3.

331 Aboody, K.S., Brown, A., Rainov, N.G., Bower, K.A., Liu, S., Yang, W., Small, J.E., Herrlinger, U., Ourednik, V., Black, P.M., Breakefield, X.O., and Snyder, E.Y. (2000) Neural stem cells display extensive tropism for pathology in adult brain: evidence from intracranial gliomas. *Proceedings of the National Academy of Sciences of the United States of America*, **97**, 12846–51.

332 Aboody, K.S., Bush, R.A., Garcia, E., Metz, M.Z., Najbauer, J., Justus, K.A., Phelps, D.A., Remack, J.S., Yoon, K.J., Gillespie, S., Kim, S.U., Glackin, C.A., Potter, P.M., and Danks, M.K. (2006) Development of a tumor-selective approach to treat metastatic cancer. *PLoS One*, **1**, e23.

333 Aboody, K.S., Najbauer, J., Schmidt, N.O., Yang, W., Wu, J.K., Zhuge, Y., Przylecki, W., Carroll, R., Black, P.M., and Perides, G. (2006) Targeting of melanoma brain metastases using engineered neural stem/progenitor cells. *Neuro-Oncology*, **8**, 119–26.

334 Brown, A.B., Yang, W., Schmidt, N.O., Carroll, R., Leishear, K.K., Rainov, N.G., Black, P.M., Breakefield, X.O., and Aboody, K.S. (2003) Intravascular delivery of neural stem cell lines to target intracranial and extracranial tumors of neural and non-neural origin. *Human Gene Therapy*, **14**, 1777–85.

335 Kabos, P., Ehtesham, M., Black, K.L., and Yu, J.S. (2003) Neural stem cells as delivery vehicles. *Expert Opinion on Biological Therapy*, **3**, 759–70.

336 Studeny, M., Marini, F.C., Dembinski, J.L., Zompetta, C., Cabreira-Hansen, M., Bekele, B.N., Champlin, R.E., and Andreeff, M. (2004) Mesenchymal stem cells: potential precursors for tumor stroma and targeted-delivery vehicles for anticancer agents. *Journal of the National Cancer Institute*, **96**, 1593–603.

337 Dickson, P.V., Hamner, J.B., Burger, R.A., Garcia, E., Ouma, A.A., Kim, S.U., Ng, C.Y., Gray, J.T., Aboody, K.S., Danks, M.K., and Davidoff, A.M. (2007) Intravascular administration of tumor tropic neural progenitor cells permits targeted delivery of interferon-beta and restricts tumor growth in a murine model of disseminated neuroblastoma. *Journal of Pediatric Surgery*, **42**, 48–53.

338 Potter, P.M., Wolverton, J.S., Morton, C.L., Whipple, D.O., and Danks, M.K. (1998) *In situ* subcellular localization of epitope-tagged human and rabbit carboxylesterases. *Cytometry*, **32**, 223–32.

339 Danks, M.K., Morton, C.L., Krull, E.J., Cheshire, P.J., Richmond, L.B., Naeve, C.W., Pawlik, C.A., Houghton, P.J., and Potter, P.M. (1999) Comparison of activation of CPT-11 by rabbit and human carboxylesterases for use in enzyme/prodrug therapy. *Clinical Cancer Research*, **5**, 917–24.

340 Khanna, R., Morton, C.L., Danks, M.K., and Potter, P.M. (2000) Proficient metabolism of irinotecan by a human intestinal carboxylesterase. *Cancer Research*, **60**, 4725–8.

341 Danks, M.K., Yoon, K.J., Bush, R.A., Remack, J.S., Wierdl, M., Tsurkan, L., Kim, S.U., Garcia, E., Metz, M.Z., Najbauer, J., Potter, P.M., and Aboody, K.S. (2007) Tumor-targeted enzyme/prodrug therapy mediates long-term disease-free survival of mice bearing disseminated neuroblastoma. *Cancer Research*, **67**, 22–5.

342 Aissaoui, A., Oudrhiri, N., Petit, L., Hauchecorne, M., Kan, E., Sainlos, M., Julia, S., Navarro, J., Vigneron, J.P., Lehn, J.M., and Lehn, P. (2002) Progress in gene delivery by cationic lipids: guanidinium–cholesterol-based systems

as an example. *Current Drug Targets*, **3**, 1–16.
343 Pitard, B., Oudrhiri, N., Lambert, O., Vivien, E., Masson, C., Wetzer, B., Hauchecorne, M., Scherman, D., Rigaud, J.L., Vigneron, J.P., Lehn, J.M., and Lehn, P. (2001) Sterically stabilized BGTC-based lipoplexes: structural features and gene transfection into the mouse airways *in vivo*. *The Journal of Gene Medicine*, **3**, 478–87.
344 Hajri, A., Wack, S., Lehn, P., Vigneron, J.P., Lehn, J.M., Marescaux, J., and Aprahamian, M. (2004) Combined suicide gene therapy for pancreatic peritoneal carcinomatosis using BGTC liposomes. *Cancer Gene Therapy*, **11**, 16–27.
345 Kerr, D.E., Schreiber, G.L., Vrudhula, V.M., Svensson, H.P., Hellstrom, I., Hellstrom, K.E., and Senter, P.D. (1995) Regressions and cures of melanoma xenografts following treatment with monoclonal antibody beta-lactamase conjugates in combination with anticancer prodrugs. *Cancer Research*, **55**, 3558–3563.
346 Eccles, S., Court, W.J., Box, G.A., Dean, C.J., Melton, R.G., and Springer, C.J. (1994) Regression of established breast carcinoma xenografts with antibody-directed enzyme prodrug therapy against C-erbB2 p185. *Cancer Research*, **54**, 5171–5177.
347 Webley, S.D., Francis, R.J., Pedley, R.B., Sharma, S.K., Begent, R.H.J., Hartley, J.R., and Hochhauser, D. (2001) Measurement of the critical DNA lesions produced by antibody-directed enzyme prodrug therapy (ADEPT) *in vitro*, *in vivo* and in clinical material. *British Journal of Cancer*, **84**, 1671–1676.
348 Mayer, A., Sharma, S.K., Tolner, B., Lowe, H., Minton, N., Purdey, D., Amlot, P., Tharakan, G., Begent, R.H.J., and Chester, K.A. (2004) Modifying an immunogenic epitope on a therapeutic protein: a step towards an improved system for antibody-directed enzyme prodrug therapy (ADEPT). *British Journal of Cancer*, **90**, 2402–2410.
349 Stribbling, S.M., Martin, J., Pedley, R.B., Boden, J.A., Sharma, S.K., and Springer, C.J. (1997) Biodistribution of an antibody–enzyme conjugate for antibody-directed enzyme prodrug therapy in nude mice bearing a human colon adenocarcinoma xenograft. *Cancer Chemotherapeutics and Pharmacology*, **40**, 277–284.
350 Zhang, Q., Zhang, S.H., Su, M.Q., Bao, G.Q., Liu, J.Y., Yi, J., Shen, J.J., and Hao, X.K. (2007) Guided selection of an anti-gamma-seminoprotein human Fab for antibody directed enzyme prodrug therapy of prostate cancer. *Cancer Immunology, Immunotherapy*, **56**, 477–89.
351 Lechanteur, C., Delvenne, P., Princen, F., Lopez, M., Fillet, G., Gielen, J., Merville, M.-P., and Bours, V. (2000) Combined suicide and cytokine gene therapy for peritoneal carcinomatosis. *Gut*, **47**, 343–348.
352 Solly, S.K., Trajcevski, S., Frisen, C., Holzer, G.W., Nelson, E., Clerc, B., Abordo-Adesida, E., Castro, M., Lowenstein, P., and Klatzmann, D. (2003) Replicative retroviral vectors for cancer gene therapy. *Cancer Gene Therapy*, **10**, 30–39.
353 Zhang, W.W. (1999) Development and application of adenoviral vectors for gene therapy of cancer. *Cancer Gene Therapy*, **7**, 113–138.
354 Kieback, D.G., Fischer, D.-C., Engehausen, D.G., Sauerbrei, W., Oehler, M.K., Tong, X.-W., and Aguilar-Cordova, E. (2002) Intraperitoneal adenovirus-mediated suicide gene therapy in combination with either topotecan or paclitaxel in nude mice with human ovarian cancer. *Cancer Gene Therapy*, **9**, 478–481.
355 Boucher, P.D., Ostruszka l.J., MKurphy, P.J.M., and Shewach, D.S. (2002) Hydroxyurea significantly enhances tumor growth delay *in vivo* with herpes simplex virus thymidine kinase/ganciclovir gene therapy. *Gene Therapy*, **9**, 1023–1030.
356 Takeda, T., Inaba, H., Yamazuki, M., Kyo, S., Miyamoto, T., Suzuki, S., Ehara, T., Kakizawa, T., Hara, M., DeGroot, L., and Hashizume, K. (2003) Tumor-specific gene therapy for undifferentiated thyroid

carcinoma utilizing the telomerase reverse transcriptase promoter. *The Journal of Clinical Endocrinology and Metabolism*, **88**, 3531–3538.

**357** Okada, Y., Okada, N., Mizuguchi, H., Hayakawa, T., Nakagawa, S., and Mayumi, T. (2005) Transcriptional targeting of RGD fiber-mutant adenovirus vectors can improve the safety of suicide gene therapy for murine melanoma. *Cancer Gene Therapy*, **12**, 608–616.

**358** Shashkova, E.V., Cherenova, L.V., Kazansky, D.B., and Doronin, K. (2005) Avian adenovirus vector CELO-TK displays anticancer activity in human cancer cells and suppresses established murine melanoma tumors. *Cancer Gene Therapy*, **12**, 617–626.

**359** Hirano, T., Kaneko, S., Kaneda, Y., Saito, I., Tamaoki, T., Furuyama, J., Tamaoki, T., Kobayashi, K., Ueki, T., and Fujimoto, J. (2001) HVJ-liposome-mediated transfection of HSVtk gene driven by AFP promotor inhibits hepatic tumor growth of hepatocellular carcinoma in SCID mice. *Gene Therapy*, **8**, 80–83.

**360** Fernandez, M., Porosnicu, M., Markovic, D., and Barber, G.N. (2002) Genetically engineered vesicular stomatitis virus in gene therapy: application for treatment of malignant disease. *Journal of Virology*, **76**, 895–904.

**361** Qiu, Z., Harms, J.S., Zhu, J., and Splitter, G.A. (2004) Bovine herpesvirus tegument protein VP22 enhances thymidine kinase/ganciclovir suicide gene therapy for neuroblastomas compared to herpes simplex virus VP22. *Journal of Virology*, **78**, 4224–4233.

**362** King, I., Bermudes, D., Lin, S., Belcourt, M., Pike, J., Troy, K., Le, T., Ittensohn, M., Mao, J., Lang, W., Runyan, J.D., Luo, X., li, Z., and Zheng, L. (2002) Tumor-targeted *Salmonella* expressing cytosine deaminase as an anticancer agent. *Human Gene Therapy*, **13**, 1225–1233.

**363** Jazowiecka-Rakus, J. and Szala, S. (2004) Antitumour activity of *Salmonells typhimurium* VNP20047 in B16 (F10) murine melanoma model. *Acta Biochimica polonica*, **51**, 851–856.

**364** Liu, S.-C., Minton, N.P., Giaccia, A.J., and Brown, J.M. (2002) Anticancer efficacy of systemically delivered anaerobic bacteria as gene therapy vectors targeting tumor hypoxia/necrosis. *Gene Therapy*, **9**, 291–296.

**365** Kanayama, H., Tomita, N., Yamano, t., Aihara, T., Miyoshi, Y., Ohue, M., Sekimoto, M., Sakita, I., Tamaki, Y., Kaneda, Y., Senter, P.D., and Monden, M. (2001) Usefulness of repeated intratumoral gene transfer using hemagglutinating virus of Japan-liposome method for cytosine deaminase suicide gene therapy. *Cancer Research*, **61**, 14–18.

**366** Porosnicu, M., Mian, A., and Barber, G.N. (2003) The oncolytic effect of vesicular stomatitis virus is enhanced by expression of the fusion cytosine deaminase/uracil phosphoribosyltransferase suicide gene. *Cancer Research*, **63**, 8366–8376.

**367** Voeks, D., Martiniello-Wilks, R., Madden, V., Smith, K., Bennetts, E., Both, G.W., and Russell, P.J. (2002) Gene therapy for prostate cancer delivered by ovine adenovirus and mediated by purine nucleoside phosphorylase and fludarabine in mouse models. *Gene Therapy*, **9**, 759–68.

**368** Martiniello-Wilks, R., Tsatralis, T., Russell, P., Brookes, D.E., Zandvliet, D., Lockett, L.J., Both, G.W., Molloy, P.L., and Russell, P.J. (2002) Transcription-targeted gene therapy for androgen-independent prostate cancer. *Cancer Gene Therapy*, **9**, 443–452.

**369** Stubdal, H., Perin, N., Lemmon, M., Holman, P., Bauzon, M., Potter, P.M., Danks, M.K., Fattaey, A., Dubensky, T., and Johnson, L. (2003) A prodrug strategy using ONYX-015-based replicating adenovirus to deliver rabbit carboxylesterase to tumor cells for conversion of CPT-11 to SN-38. *Cancer Research*, **63**, 6900–6908.

**370** Djeha, A.H., Thomson, T.A., Leung, H., Searle, P.F., Young, L.S., Kerr, D.J., Harris, P.A., Mountain, A., and Wrighton, C.J. (2001) Combined adenovirus-mediated nitroreductase gene delivery and CB1954 treatment:

a well-tolerated therapy for established solid tumors. *Molecular Therapy*, **3**, 233–240.

**371** Chen, M.J., Green, N.K., Reynolds, G.M., Flavell, J.R., Mautner, V., Kerr, D.J., Young, L.S., and Searle, P.F. (2004) Enhanced efficacy of *Escherichia coli* nitroreductase/CB1954 prodrug activation gene therapy using an E1B-55K-deleted adenovirus vector. *Gene Therapy*, **11**, 1126–1136.

**372** Kan, O., Griffiths, L., Baban, D., Iqbal, S., Uden, M., Spearman, H., Slingsby, J., Price, T., Esapa, M., Kingsman, A., Slade, A., and Naylor, S. (2001) Direct retroviral delivery of human cytochrome P450 2B6 for gene-directed enzyme prodrug therapy of cancer. *Cancer Gene Therapy*, **8**, 473–482.

**373** Schepelmann, S., Hallenbeck, P., Ogilvie, L.M., Hedley, D., Friedlos, F., Martin, J., Scanlon, I., Hay, C., Hawkins, L.K., Marais, R., and Springer, C.J. (2005) Systemic gene-directed enzyme prodrug therapy of hepatocellular carcinoma using a targeted adenovirus armed with carboxypeptidase G2. *Cancer Research*, **65**, 5003–8.

**374** Pedley, R., Sharma, S.K., Boxer, G.M., Boden, R., Stribbling, S.M., Davies, L., Springer, C.J., and Begent, R.H.J. (1999) Enhancement of antibody-directed enzyme prodrug therapy in colorectal xenografts by an antivascular agent. *Cancer Research*, **59**, 3998–4003.

**375** Sharma, S.K., Pedley, R.B., Bhatia, J., Boxer, M., El-Emir, E., Qureshi, U., Tolner, B., Lowe, H., Michael, N.P., Minton, N., Begent, R.H.J., and Chester, K.A. (2005) Sustained tumour regression of human colorectal cancer xenografts using a multifunctional mannosylated fusion protein in antibody-directed enzyme prodrug therapy. *Clinical Cancer Research*, **11**, 814–825.

**376** Kerr, D.E., Vrudhula, V.M., Svensson, H.P., Siemers, N.O., and Senter, P.D. (1999) Comparison of recombinant and synthetically formed monoclonal antibody-beta-lactamase conjugates for anticancer prodrug activation. *Bioconjugate Chemistry*, **10**, 1084–1089.

**377** Gabizon, A. (2003) Emerging role of liposomal drug carrier systems in cancer chemotherapy. *Journal of Liposome Research*, **13**, 17–20.

**378** Harrington, K.J., Syrigos, K.N., and Vile, R.G. (2002) Liposomally targeted cytotoxic drugs for the treatment of cancer. *Journal of Pharmacy and Pharmacology*, **54**, 1573–600.

**379** Torchilin, V.P. (2005) Recent advances with liposomes as pharmaceutical carriers. *Nature Reviews. Drug Discovery*, **4**, 145–60.

**380** Chaszczewska-Markowska, M., Stebelska, K., Sikorski, A., Madej, J., Opolski, A., and Ugorski, M. (2008) Liposomal formulation of 5-fluorocytosine in suicide gene therapy with cytosine deaminase: for colorectal cancer. *Cancer Letters*, **262**, 164–72.

**381** Toso, J.F., Gill, V.J., Hwu, P., Marincola, F.M., Restifo, N.P., Schwartzentruber, D.J., Sherry, R.M., Topalian, S.L., Yang, J.C., Stock, F., Freezer, L.J., Morton, K.E., Seipp, C., Haworth, L., Mavroukakis, S., White, D., MacDonald, S., Mao, J., Sznol, M., and Rosenberg, S.A. (2001) Phase I study of the intravenous administration of attenuated *Salmonella typhimurium* to patients with metastatic melanoma. *Journal of Clinical Oncology*, **20**, 142–152.

**382** Cunningham, C. and Nemunaitis, J. (2001) A Phase I trial of genetically modified *Salmonells typhimurium* expressing cytosine deaminase (TAPET-CD, VNP20029) administered by intratumoral injection in combination with 5-fluorocytosine for patients with advanced metastatic cancer. *Human Gene Therapy*, **12**, 1594–1596.

**383** Nemunaitis, J., Cunningham, C., Tong, A.W., Post, L., Netto, G., Paulson, A.S., Rich, D., Blackburn, A., Gibson, B., Randlev, B., and Freeman, R. (2003) Pilot trial of intravenous infusion of a replication-selective adenovirus (ONYX-015) in combination with chemotherapy or IL-2 treatment in refractory cancer patients. *Cancer Gene Therapy*, **10**, 341–352.

**384** Immonen, A., Vapalahti, M., Tyynela, S., Hurskainen, H., Sandmair, A., Vanninen,

R., Langford, G., Murray, N., and Yla-Herttuala, S. (2004) AdvHSV-TK gene therapy with intravenous ganciclovir improves survival in human malignannt glioma: a randomised, controlled study. *Molecular Therapy*, **10**, 967–972.

385 Floeth, F.W., Shand, N., Bojar, H., Prisack, H.B., Felsberg, J., Neuen-Jacob, E., Aulich, A., Burger, K.J., Bock, W.J., and Weber, F. (2001) Local inflammation and devascularization: *in vivo* mechanisms of the "bystander effect" in VPC-mediated HSV-TK/GCV gene therapy for human malignant glioma. *Cancer Gene Therapy*, **8**, 843–851.

386 Alvarez, R.D., Gomez-Navarro, J., Wang, M., Barnes, M.N., Strong, T.V., Arani, R.B., Arafat, W., Hughes, J.V., Siegal, G.P., and Curiel, D.T. (2000) Adenoviral-mediated suicide gene therapy for ovarian cancer. *Molecular Therapy*, **2**, 524–530.

387 Sung, M.W., Yeh, H.-C., Thung, S.N., Schwartz, M.E., Mandeli, J.P., Chen, S.-H., and Woo, S.L.C. (2001) Intratumoral adenovirus-mediated suicide gene transfer for hepatic metastases from colorectal adenocarcinoma: results of a Phase I clinical trial. *Molecular Therapy*, **4**, 182–191.

388 Freytag, S.O., Khil, M., Stricker, H., Peabody, J., Manon, M., DeParalta-Venturina, M., Nafziger, D., Pegg, J., Paielli, D., Brown, S., Barton, K., Lu, M., Aguilar-Cordova, E., and Kim, J.H. (2002) Phase I study of replication competent adenovirus mediated double suicide-gene therapy for the treatment of locally recurrent prostate cancer. *Cancer Research*, **62**, 4968–4976.

389 Freytag, S.O., Stricker, H., Pegg, J., Paielli, D., Pradhan, D.P., Peabody, J., DeParalta-Venturina, M., Xueqing, X., Brown, S., Lu, M., and Kim, J.H. (2003) Phase I study of replication-competent adenovirus-mediated double-suicide gene therapy in combination with conventional-dose three-dimensional conformal radiation therapy for the treatment of newly diagnosed, intermediate-to-high-risk prostate cancer. *Cancer Research*, **63**, 7497–7506.

390 Shalev, M., Kadmon, D., Teh, B.S., Butler, E.B., Aguilar-Cordova, E., Thompson, T.C., Herman, J.R., Adler, H.L., Scardino, P.T., and Miles, B.J. (2000) Suicide gene therapy toxicity after multiple and repeat injections in patients with localized prostate cancer. *Journal of Urology*, **163**, 1747–1750.

391 Pedley, R.B., El-Amir, E., Flinn, A.A., Boxer, G.M., Dearling, G., Raleigh, G.A., Hill, S.A., Stuart, S., Motha, R., and Begent, R.H.J. (2002) Synergy between vascular targeting agents and antibody-directed therapy. *International Journal of Radiation Oncology, Biology and Physics*, **54**, 1524–1531.

392 Francis, R.J., Sharma, S.K., Springer, C.J., Green, A.J., Hope-Stone, L.D., Sena, L., Martin, J., Adamson, K.L., Robbins, A., Gumbrell, L., O'Malley, D., Tsiompanou, E., Shahbakhti, H., Webley, S., Hochhauser, D., Hilson, A.J., Blakey, D., and Begent, R.H.J. (2002) A Phase I trial of antibody directed enzyme prodrug therapy (ADEPT) in patients with advanced colorectal carcinoma or other CEA producing tumours. *British Journal of Cancer*, **87**, 600–607.

393 Hasenburg, A., Tong, X.W., Rojas-Martinez, A., Nyberg-Hoffman, C., Kieback, C.C., Kaplan, A.L., Kaufman, R.H., Ramzy, I., Aguilar-Cordova, E., and Kieback, D.G. (1999) Thymidine kinase (TK) gene therapy of solid tumors: valacyclovir facilitates outpatients treatment. *Anticancer Research*, **19**, 2163–2166.

394 Sandmair, A.M., Loimas, S., Puranen, P., Immonen, A., Kossila, A., Puranen, M., Hurskainen, H., Tyynela, K., Turunen, M., Vanninen, R., Lehtolainen, P., Paljarvi, L., Johanssen, R., Vapalahti, M., and Yla-Herttuala, S. (2000) Thymidine kinase gene therapy for human malignant glioma, using replication deficient retroviruses or adenoviruses. *Human Gene Therapy*, **11**, 2197–2205.

395 Smitt, P.S., Driesse, M., Wolbers, J., Kros, M., and Avezaat, C. (2003) Treatment of relapsed malignant glioma with an adenoviral vector containing the herpes simplex thymidine kinase gene

followed by ganciclovir. *Molecular Therapy*, 7, 851–858.

396 Barzon, L., Pacenti, M., Taccaliti, A., Franchin, E., Bruglia, M., Boscaro, M., and Palu, G. (2004) A pilot study of combined suicide/cytokine gene therapy in two patients with end-stage anaplastic thyroid carcinoma. *Journal of Clinical Endocrinology and Metabolism*, **90**, 2831–2834.

397 Singh, S., Cummingham, C., Buchanan, A., Jolly, D.J, and Nemunaitis, J. (2001) Toxicity assessment of intratumoreal injection of herpes simplex type 1 thymidine kinase gene delivered by retrovirus in patients with refractory cancer. *Molecular Therapy*, **4**, 157–160.

398 Rainov, N.G. (2000) A Phase III clinical evaluation of herpes simplex virus type 1 thymidine kinase and ganciclovir gene therapy as an adjuvant to surgical resection and radiationin adults with previously untreated glioblastoma multiforme. *Human Gene Therapy*, **11**, 2389–2401.

399 Palmer, D.H., Milner, A.E., Kerr, D.J., and Young, L.S. (2003) Mechanism of cell death induced by the novel enzyme–prodrug combination, nitroreductase/CB1954, and identification of synergism with 5-fluorouracil. *British Journal of Cancer*, **89**, 944–950.

400 Pandha, H.S., Martin, L.A., Rigg, A., Hurst, H.C., Stamp, G.W.H., Sikora, K., and Lemoine, N.R. (1999) Genetic prodrug activation therapy for breast cancer: a Phase I clinical trial of erbB-2-directed suicide gene expression. *Journal of Clinical Oncology*, **17**, 2180–2189.

401 McCormick, F. (2001) Cancer gene therapy: fringe or cutting edge? *Nature Reviews Cancer*, **1**, 130–141.

402 Ganly, I. (1999) Phase II trial of intratumoral infection with an E1B deleted adenovirusin patients with recurrent refractory head and neck cancers. *Human Gene Therapy*, **10**, 844.

403 Sunk, M.W., Yeh, H.C., Thung, S.N., Schwartz, M.E., Mandeli, J.P., Chen, S.H., and Woo, S.L.C. (2001) Intratumoral adenovirus-mediated suicide gene transfer for hepatic metastasis from colorectal carcinoma: results of a Phase I clinical trial. *Molecular Therapy*, **4**, 182–191.

404 Sandmair, A.M. (2000) Thymidine kinase gene therapy for human malignant glioma, using replication deficient retroviruses and adenoviruses. *Human Gene Therapy*, **11**, 2197–2205.

# Part Three
# Codrugs and Soft Drugs

*Prodrugs and Targeted Delivery: Towards Better ADME Properties*. Edited by Jarkko Rautio

ISBN: 978-3-527-32603-7

# 13
# Improving the Use of Drug Combinations Through the Codrug Approach

*Peter A. Crooks, Harpreet K. Dhooper, and Ujjwal Chakraborty*

## 13.1
## Codrugs and Codrug Strategy

There are instances in prodrug design where the prodrug molecule incorporates two identical or nonidentical drugs into a single chemical entity. This is often desirable when two synergistic drugs have different physicochemical and pharmacokinetic properties, and it is desirable to have the parent drugs released concomitantly at the site of action to obtain a synergistic pharmacodynamic effect that is not attainable by delivering a physical mixture of the two drugs. Also, one of the drugs in the codrug structure may be incorporated to counterbalance the known side effects associated with the other parent drug, or may amplify the pharmacodynamic effect of the other parent drug through an action at another biological target. Thus, codrugs can be designed to overcome various barriers to drug formulation and delivery, such as poor aqueous solubility, chemical instability, insufficient oral absorption, rapid presystemic metabolism, inadequate brain penetration, toxicity, and local irritation. Structurally, a codrug (also known as a mutual prodrug or hybrid drug) comprises two or more different drugs within a single chemical entity where the drugs must each contain an appropriate chemical functionality to enable them to be connected together, either directly or by means of a cleavable, biolabile covalent linker [1]. Such codrugs can be either bipartate or tripartate in nature [2] (Figure 13.1) and the design of the linker moiety can be adopted from current linker design strategies and chemistries already established in the broad area of prodrug design.

Thus, a codrug strategy can be useful when

- synergistic drugs need to be given concomitantly to act at the same time, either at the same or different biological targets;
- the physicochemical properties of two synergistic drugs are not favorable for delivery of the two drugs as a physical mixture, but can be improved by chemical combination of the two drugs; and
- improved pharmacokinetics results from a chemical combination of two synergistic drugs compared to those of a physical mixture of the two drugs.

*Prodrugs and Targeted Delivery: Towards Better ADME Properties.* Edited by Jarkko Rautio

ISBN: 978-3-527-32603-7

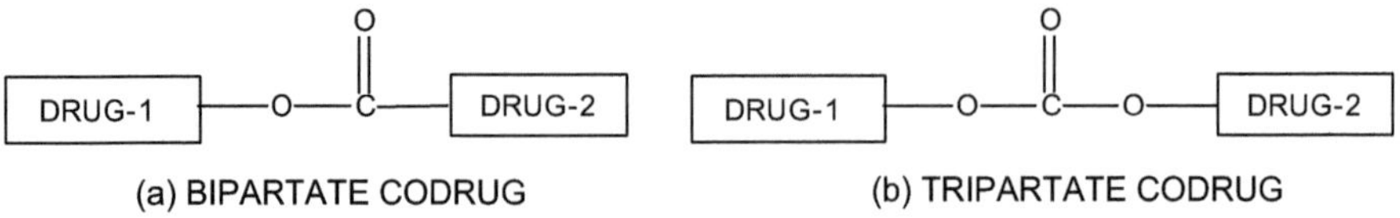


**Figure 13.1** Examples of bipartate and tripartate codrugs: (a) conjugation of a carboxylic drug with an alcoholic drug to form a bipartate codrug where the two drugs are connected by an ester linkage that cleaves *in vivo* to release only the two parent drugs; (b) conjugation of two alcoholic drug molecules via a carbonate ester linker to form a tripartate codrug that cleaves *in vivo* to form the two parent drugs and an equivalent of carbonic acid.

As with prodrugs, the codrug structure can incorporate two drugs joined together by linker moieties such as ester, carbonate, amide, carbamate, and so on, which are then enzymatically cleaved *in vivo* to release the active drugs at a required site in the body. By appropriate structural design of these linkers, it may be possible to control the release kinetics of one or both drugs. When the two drugs are chemically combined together, the resulting codrug will usually have physicochemical properties different from those of the individual parent drugs, which may provide superior properties for delivery of the two drugs compared to the delivery of a physical mixture of the drugs [3].

## 13.2 Ideal Codrug Characteristics

An ideal codrug will generate parent drugs with high recovery rates and will incorporate linkers that give rise to nontoxic linker residues upon cleavage *in vivo*. There may be other advantages in delivering of two drugs as a single chemical entity versus a physical mixture. These include, for example, improved chemical stability of the formulation (i.e., no chemical interaction of the two parent drugs within the formulation), improved metabolic stability (especially with regard to possible protection of either drug from high first-pass metabolism), and improved targeting of drugs to the site of action (e.g., the central nervous system), and more desirable pharmacokinetic properties, in particular for drugs with different physicochemical properties (e.g., differences in lipid solubility or polarity).

There are also certain disadvantages that are associated with a codrug strategy. One disadvantage is that codrugs are usually large molecules with molecular weights that are often greater than 500. Thus, codrugs with large molecular weights may well violate Lipinski's rule of five [4] as unfavorable molecules for oral or topical dosage form development, or for CNS (central nervous system) delivery. In addition, by the very nature of their structural design, these cleavable molecules may possess poor stability profiles for formulation development. Thus, it must be initially established that the codrug is resilient enough to withstand the rigors of formulation development and must not be too stable to not efficiently cleave into the parent drugs *in vivo*.

Another important aspect of codrug design is the toxicological significance of delivering a codrug to an individual. Since codrugs are novel chemical entities (although the parent drugs they generate may or may not be novel), they will have to be treated as new xenobiotics by the FDA, as are all new drugs entities that have never been previously administered to humans. Thus, there are important toxicological and safety issues associated with the development of codrugs, as they move toward clinical status.

Several important criteria are required for codrugs to be effective. A codrug must be well absorbed, and distribution, metabolism, and elimination of the codrug should be superior to the physical mixture of the parent drugs. Both parent drugs should be released concomitantly and quantitatively after absorption, and the maximal effect of the drug combination should occur when a simple molar ratio, that is, 1:1, 2:1, or 3:1, is utilized.

Before designing the codrug, one needs to know the route of administration. Routes of administration can be broadly divided into topical, enteral, and parenteral routes. The topical route involves a local drug effect. The drug is directly applied where the action is desired, for example, asthma medications, eye or eardrops, and decongestant nasal sprays. In the enteral route, drug administration involves any part of the gastrointestinal tract. The effect is nonlocal. Sublingual, oral, and rectal are all enteral routes. In sublingual administration, the drug is placed under the tongue, is rapidly absorbed, and avoids first-pass metabolism. The first-pass effect refers to the hepatic metabolism of a drug when it is absorbed from the gastrointestinal tract and delivered to the liver via the hepatic portal circulation. The greater the first-pass effect, the lower the concentration of drug that reaches the systemic circulation. In the oral route, the drug is swallowed. It passes through the whole gastrointestinal tract. Drugs taken orally are usually less expensive to manufacture than ones administered by any other route and can be easily self-administered (minimal invasiveness) by the patient. The disadvantage of oral delivery is that the drug has to be absorbed from the gastrointestinal tract and experience the first-pass effect. Sometimes this route of administration is inefficient because only part of the drug may be absorbed; also, a significant first-pass effect may occur. In addition, some orally administered drugs can cause irritation of the gastric mucosa and cause nausea and vomiting.

*Note*: Drugs given orally take more time than any other route to show a pharmacological response, but the oral route is considered to be the safest, pain-free, and cheapest method of drug administration. Other routes are used if there is an emergency situation where the effect of the drug is immediately needed [2].

## 13.3 Examples of Marketed Codrugs

A good example of an effective and marketed codrug is the antibiotic sultamicillin (Unasyn Oral), a tripartate codrug of ampicillin and penicillanic acid sulfone (Figure 13.2) [5, 6]. Ampicillin is a well-known β-lactam antibiotic, but it is ineffective against resistant bacteria that excrete high concentrations of the bacterial enzyme,

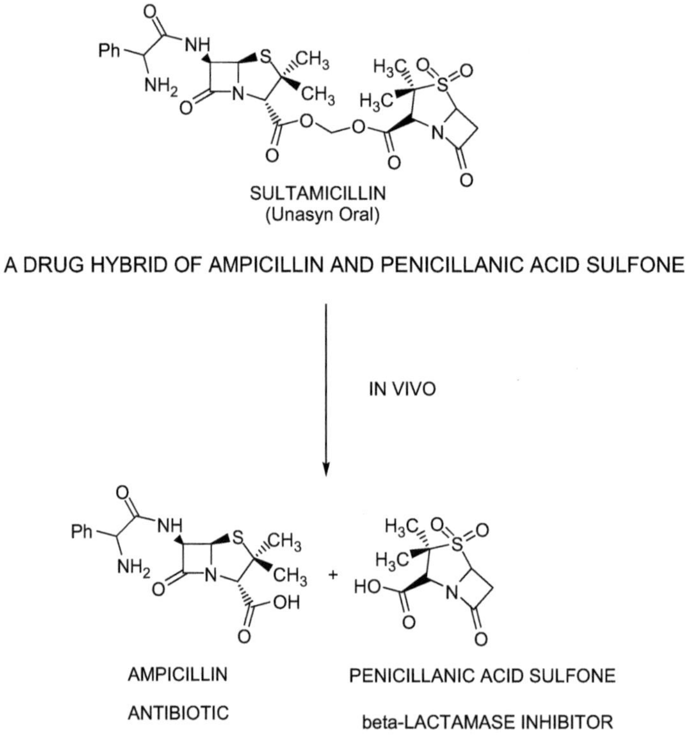


**Figure 13.2** Sultamicillin codrug and the *in vivo* hydrolysis products generated from the codrug.

β-lactamase. β-Lactamase degrades penicillins such as ampicillin by hydrolysis of the β-lactam ring with consequent loss of antibacterial activity. Subsequent coadministration of a β-lactam antibiotic with a β-lactamase inhibitor was utilized as a strategy for treating resistant strains of bacteria. For example, the antibiotic Augmentin is a mixture of the β-lactam penicillin, amoxicillin, and the β-lactamase inhibitor, potassium clavulanate (Figure 13.2). One of the problems of administering the two synergistic drugs together (as a physical mixture) is that they may not have similar pharmacokinetic profiles, and thus may not arrive at the target site at the same time or at the same concentration. The codrug sultamicillin incorporates a labile linker, which upon hydrolysis by a plasma esterase affords the two synergistic parent drugs in equimolar amounts together with a molar equivalent of formaldehyde.

Another example of a marketed codrug is sulfasalazine [7], which is prescribed for the treatment of ulcerative colitis, a chronic inflammatory disease characterized by a diffuse inflammation of the mucosa that is mainly restricted to the colon. Aminosalicylates are the mainstay of treatment in case of active ulcerative colitis. Sulfasalazine is the prototype of this drug class and releases 5-aminosalicylic acid and antibacterial sulfonamide, sulfapyridine, in the colon. After oral administration, 80–90% of the drug is delivered to the colon intact. About 10–20% of the drug is absorbed from small intestine and undergoes enterohepatic circulation without

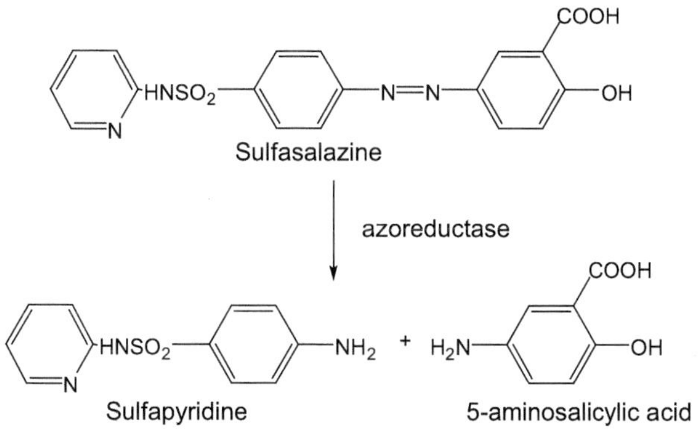


**Figure 13.3** Generation of 5-aminosalicylic acid and sulfapyridine from sulfasalazine codrug.

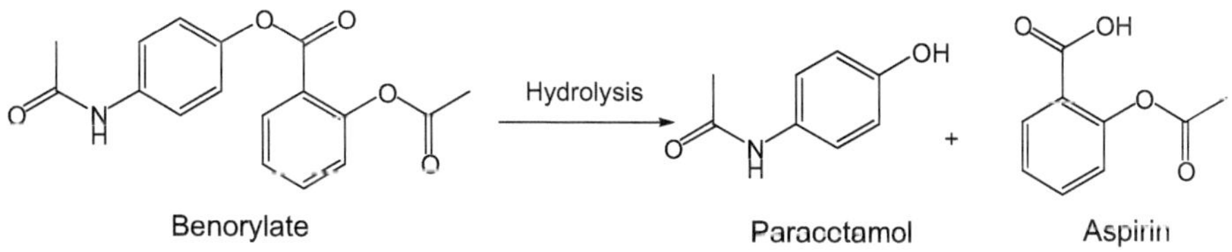


**Figure 13.4** Generation of paracetamol and aspirin from hydrolysis of benorylate.

biotransformation and is excreted in the bile [8]. In the colon, the azo bond in sulfasalazine is cleaved by colonic bacterial azoreductases liberating sulfapyridine and 5-aminosalicylic acid [9, 10] (Figure 13.3).

Benorylate is another good example of a marketed codrug used in the treatment of rheumatoid arthritis. Benorylate is an ester of acetylsalicylic acid and paracetamol and is an effective analgesic and anti-inflammatory drug with less potential for gastric irritation. The antipyretic activity of benorylate is similar to that of acetylsalicylic acid (aspirin) and paracetamol [11]. The pharmacological actions of benorylate are due to the effects of both aspirin and paracetamol released by hydrolytic cleavage. Benorylate is actively hydrolyzed by liver cytosol and plasma to generate the two parent drugs (Figure 13.4). Only paracetamol and salicylate can be detected in plasma after oral administration of benorylate [12].

## 13.4
## Topical Codrug Therapy for the Treatment of Ophthalmic Diseases

### 13.4.1
### Codrugs for the Treatment of Diabetic Retinopathy

The codrug strategy has previously been used when the physicochemical and/or pharmacokinetic properties of two synergistic drugs are not favorable for delivery of the two drugs as a physical mixture, but can be improved by chemical combination of the two drugs. For example, 5-fluorouracil (5-FU) is a polar, water-soluble antiviral, and cytotoxic drug that is rapidly cleared from the vitreous when delivered topically to the eye. In a topical drug combination treatment consisting of 5-FU and the lipophilic, water-insoluble, anti-inflammatory drug, trihydroxy steroid (THS), a codrug strategy was used that provided a superior sustained release delivery of these two synergistic parent drugs for the treatment of diabetic retinopathy [13, 14]. The individual physicochemical properties of 5-FU and THS are not favorable for sustained release of a physical mixture of the two drugs. However, utilizing a codrug approach, the chemical combination of 5-FU and THS in a 2:1 molar ratio (for optimal synergistic activity) afforded a molecule with greatly improved physicochemical characteristics for sustained delivery compared to formulations of the two drugs as a physical mixture [13]. Figure 13.5 shows the structure of THS, 5-FU, and the THS-BIS-5-FU codrug.

The 5-FU-THS codrug was designed as a "chemical delivery" system [13] that joined together the two drugs via a labile linker moiety. The physicochemical properties of the codrug were favorable for formulation as a sutured ophthalmic pellet and for slow dissolution of the codrug pellet in the vitreous humor. The labile linker was specifically designed to undergo rapid hydrolysis once the codrug pellet had dissolved, providing sustained release of the parent drugs, which depended on the rate of dissolution of the codrug pellet. This concept of a chemical delivery system, where the target tissue is never exposed to dissolved codrug, has been patented [15] and represents a unique form of a codrug formulation, which may be considered as just another formulation for delivery of the parent drugs; the important concept is that the body is never exposed to the new codrug entity, and thus issues of codrug toxicity would not be relevant. One molar equivalent of the codrug produces one

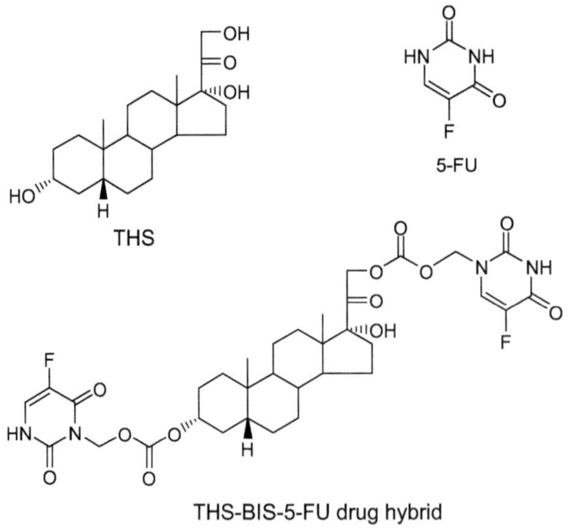


**Figure 13.5** Structures of THS, 5-FU, and the THS-BIS-5-FU codrug.

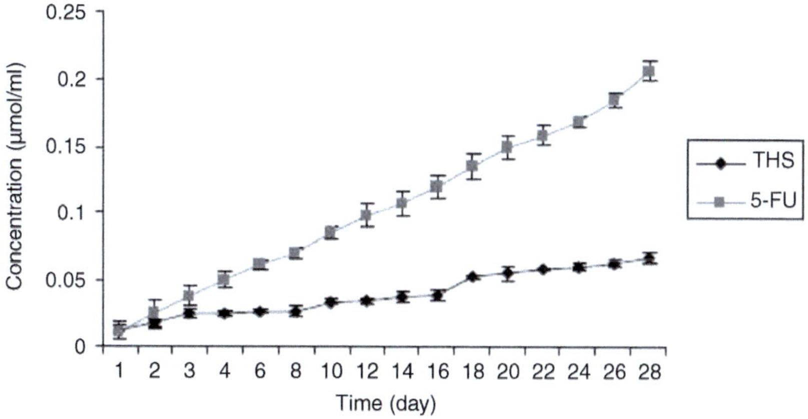


**Figure 13.6** Cumulative release of THS and 5-FU from neat pellets containing 2 mg of the THS-BIS-5-FU codrug in bovine vitreous humor.

molar equivalent of THS, two molar equivalents of 5-FU, and two molar equivalents of both formaldehyde and carbon dioxide after hydrolysis. Another important consideration in the design of the 5-FU-THS codrug was the structure of the labile linker. The two drugs were linked together via a linker that afforded hydrolysis products considered nontoxic. The pellets containing the THS-BIS-5-FU codrug simultaneously released THS and 5-FU in 0.1 M phosphate buffer (pH = 7.4), in human serum and in bovine vitreous humor. Figure 13.6 shows the release of THS and 5-FU from the codrug in bovine vitreous humor. The results demonstrate that a neat pelleted THS-5-FU codrug can be utilized as a sustained release ocular delivery form of the parent compounds and that the unique physicochemical properties of the codrug allow both slow dissolution and rapid release of the two parent drugs (Figure 13.6).

### 13.4.2
### Codrugs Containing Corticosteroids for Proliferative Vitreoretinopathy

Proliferative vitreoretinopathy (PVR) refers to migration and proliferation of cells into the subretinal space, vitreous cavity, and onto the retinal surface and undersurface. Subsequent collagen production and cell-mediated contraction of the resulting collagenous scar leads to retinal detachment and loss of vision [16]. Different pharmacological adjuncts have been examined in animal models and human trials to reduce the formation of fibrocellular membranes in PVR, but due to the short half-lives of these drugs when delivered by intravitreal injection, repeated postoperative intraocular injections are necessary. When administered systemically, toxic effects are observed as a consequence of the high doses needed to achieve therapeutic intraocular drug levels. This also limits the clinical usefulness of these therapeutic agents. An intraocular device providing therapeutic intraocular drug levels for several months via sustained delivery of the drugs is needed for the treatment of PVR since reproliferation and recurrent retinal detachment can occur in the first few months after initial retinal reattachment surgery. An implantable, nonerodible intraocular device has been developed and has shown potential in the treatment of experimental uveitis [17]. Both 5-FU (a cytotoxic agent) and corticosteroids such as dexamethasone (DX) and triamcinolone (TA) are known to be effective in the treatment of experimental PVR. The following are some pros and cons associated with 5-FU and corticosteroids as therapeutic agents for the treatment of PVR:

- Both DX and TA are known to reduce incidents of retinal detachment in a rabbit model of PVR [18, 19].
- Although corticosteroids are advantageous in suppressing the inflammatory arm of the wound-healing response, their weak antiproliferative properties reduce their clinical potential.
- 5-FU is known to be a potent inhibitor of rabbit dermal fibroblast proliferation in cell culture [20].
- 5-FU is also well tolerated in the rabbit when intravitreally administered at high doses.
- Due to a very short half-life and rapid clearance of 5-FU from the eye, repeated injections of 5-FU are required to achieve a clinically significant effect of the drug when given alone.
- Repeated injections of ophthalmic drugs can cause endophthalmitis and retinal detachment, and are inconvenient and uncomfortable for the patient.
- 5-FU is toxic to the cornea and retina when given in high doses [21].

In a recent study, codrugs of 5-FU covalently linked to either DX or TA have been prepared and evaluated in a rabbit model of PVR [22]. The corticosteroid-5-FU codrugs retain the anti-inflammatory properties of the corticosteroids and incorporate the antiproliferative properties of 5-FU.

The codrugs of 5-FU and corticosteroids were designed to take advantage of the best characteristics of the individual drugs and to reduce their individual disadvantages (Figure 13.7). The parent drugs possessed unfavorable physicochemical

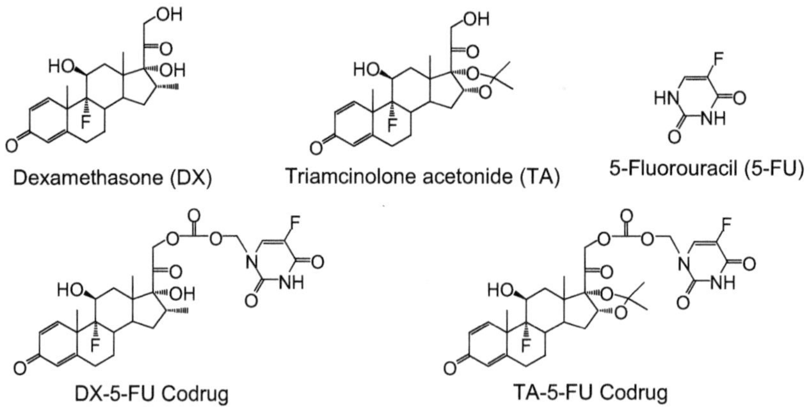


**Figure 13.7** Codrugs of corticosteroids and 5-fluorouracil.

properties for sustained delivery; however, when converted to the codrug form, the molecules were found to possess good characteristics for sustained delivery of the parent drugs. An implantable sustained release formulation containing the DX-5-FU codrug was developed and surgically implanted into the right eyes of New Zealand white rabbits. In separate experiments, as an alternative to DX-5-FU pellets, a suspension of the more insoluble TA-5-FU codrug was injected into the vitreous of the right eye of the rabbits. TA is less soluble than DX and as a result TA-5-FU codrug is less soluble and therefore longer lasting than DX-5-FU codrug. It was observed that the DX-5-FU device fully released the parent drugs after approximately 1 week, whereas the TA-5-FU suspension took an extended period of time (1 month) to release the parent drugs. *In vitro* pharmacokinetic data showed that the DX-5-FU pellet was effective but allowed the disease to progress at later time points due to insufficient amount of the drug left in the pellet as a consequence of high solubility of DX-5-FU pellet. However, the TA-5-FU codrug was much more effective in causing regression of PVR severity especially at later time points. Thus, intravitreal sustained release of the DX-5-FU device and the TA-5-FU suspension were both effective against progression of PVR in the rabbit model.

### 13.4.3
### Codrugs Containing Nonsteroidal Anti-Inflammatory Agents for Treatment of Proliferative Vitreoretinopathy

Although corticosteroids have been used to prevent and treat intraocular inflammation, these therapeutic agents might interfere more severely with wound healing, exacerbate infection, or cause an increase in intraocular pressure. The development of nonsteroidal anti-inflammatory drugs (NSAIDs) provides the ocular surgeon with an alternative way to control inflammation and to avoid the problems associated with corticosteroid therapy. Also, a sustained release of the drug with prolonged effects is expected to be more effective in the treatment of experimental post-traumatic PVR than the transient nature of the free drug form, and it is also known that single intravitreal injections of either 5-FU or the NSAID naproxen have too short a half-life to provide an adequate therapeutic effect [23]. Based on these observations and on the encouraging data from the 5-FU-corticosteroid codrugs, a naproxen-5-FU codrug (Figure 13.8) was synthesized for the treatment of experimental post-traumatic PVR. It was also hypothesized that treatment with a NSAID and 5-FU together might be more effective than either of the drugs alone and that such a drug combination could

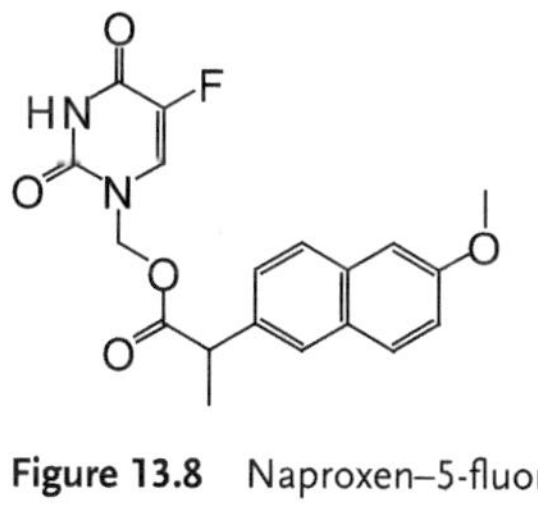


**Figure 13.8** Naproxen–5-fluorouracil codrug.

simultaneously downregulate the inflammatory and proliferative components of the wound healing response. Bioerodible implantable sustained release pellets containing a naproxen-5-FU codrug were developed and tested in a rabbit trauma model of PVR. The naproxen-5-FU pellets were found to release 5-FU and naproxen linearly over a 30-day time course in *in vitro* release experiments. Rabbits administered codrug in sutured corneal pellet implants showed a significant decrease in retinal detachment rate compared to the control group (untreated eye) at almost all time points. The codrug pellet did not exhibit any toxic effect on the retina when examined electrophysiologically or histologically. The overall results of the study showed that the napreoxen-5-FU codrug device effectively inhibited the frequency and severity of PVR in a rabbit trauma model without any observable toxic effects of the codrug on the retina.

### 13.4.4
### Codrugs Containing Ethacrynic Acid for Treatment of Elevated Intraocular Pressure

Elevated intraocular pressure (IOP) is one of the major risk factors leading to glaucomatous damage of the optic nerve and a consequent cause of blindness. It is known that ethacrynic acid (ECA), a diuretic drug, can reduce IOP in rabbit and monkey eyes [24, 25]. Intracameral injection of ECA into the eye can also reduce IOP in humans [26]. These observations suggest ECA as a potential glaucoma drug. However, topical administration of ECA shows many adverse effects and limitations. For example,

- eyelid edema, conjunctival hyperemia, and moderate diffuse superficial corneal erosion are some of the side effects of long-term topical administration of ECA;
- due to the low $pK_a$ (2.8) of ECA, the molecule exists exclusively in the anionic form at physiological pH (pH = 7.4), and the very low lipophilicity of the anionic form of ECA limits its ability to effectively penetrate cornea to provide a therapeutic dose at the site of action; and
- oral administration of ECA does not produce any significant effect on IOP [27].

On the other hand, β-adrenergic receptor antagonists such as atenolol (ATL) and timolol (TML) are effective against a variety of hypertensive disorders, ischemic heart disease, some arrhythmias, and ocular hypertensive effects [28]. Diuretics produce additive antihypertensive effects when coadministered with β-adrenergic receptor antagonists [29]. Thus, ECA delivered together with a β-adrenergic receptor antagonists can act synergistically to lower elevated IOP since these two classes of drugs work via different physiological mechanisms. To overcome the unsuitable physicochemical properties of ECA for ocular delivery and to utilize the synergistic interaction between ECA and β-adrenergic receptor antagonists, codrugs of ECA with ATL and TML have been synthesized and evaluated (Figure 13.9).

ECA was coupled with ATL and TML through an ester linkage using 1,1-carbonyldiimidazole (CDI) as the coupling reagent. The stability of the ECA-ATL codrug was studied in nonenzymatic aqueous buffer at pH 7.4 and enzymatic hydrolysis was studied using human serum. The codrug was hydrolyzed in both buffer

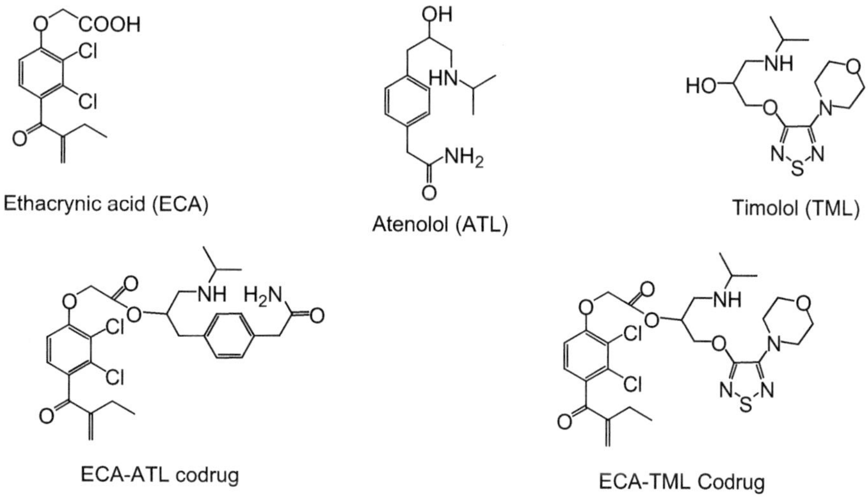


**Figure 13.9** Ethacrynic acid–β-adrenergic receptor antagonist codrugs.

(half-life = 14 h) and human serum (half-life = 30 min) to produce the parent drugs. The stability study confirmed that biotransformation of the codrug would occur after penetration into the vitreous. The main target behind the codrug approach was to overcome the solubility and clearance problems associated with the parent drugs, and thus improve the delivery of the parent drugs through topical membranes.

## 13.5 Codrugs for Transdermal Delivery

Many available drugs do not have suitable physicochemical properties for transdermal delivery. For a drug to permeate across the skin, it must be able to partition into and diffuse across the lipophilic region of stratum corneum, and also the more hydrophilic underlying epidermis. Many different strategies have been utilized to enhance topical drug delivery. One of these strategies is to chemically modify the structure of the penetrant. Prodrug and codrug approaches to drug delivery come under this category.

### 13.5.1 Codrugs for the Treatment of Alcohol Abuse and Tobacco Dependence

Naltrexone (NTX) is an opioid antagonist and useful drug for the treatment of alcohol dependence [30], and cigarette smoking is known to be a social cue for alcoholics. Many alcoholics are also chronic smokers. Naltrexol (NTXOL) is the active metabolite of NTX [31, 32]. At present, NTX is used in the form of an oral tablet for the treatment of the above-mentioned morbidities. It has been shown that alcohol dependence can be reduced by 50% in adult alcoholics after administering NTX orally [33]. However, there are adverse g.i. side effects associated with NTX oral therapy, such as abdominal pain, constipation, nausea, and vomiting. NTX is also a hepatotoxin and can cause dose-related hepatocellular injury. Due to this hepatotoxicity, dosage cannot be increased above 50 mg/day, and patients who need a dosage regimen of more than 50 mg/day cannot benefit from oral NTX therapy. In addition to these adverse effects, NTX undergoes extensive first-pass metabolism in humans, which reduces the oral bioavailability of NTX to about 5–40% [34]. Thus, these adverse effects, along with the low bioavailability, limit the clinical utility of oral NTX therapy, and poor patient compliance is observed. Neither NTX nor NTXOL is deliverable in therapeutic concentrations via the transdermal route [35]. A codrug approach was applied in an attempt to solve these problems. Hydroxybupropion (BUPOH) is the active metabolite of the orally active smoking cessation agent, bupropion (Zyban) [36–39]. A transdermal NTX-BUPOH codrug should have improved transdermal delivery characteristics, lower toxicity, offer patients the freedom from intravenous injections and surgical implantations, and afford better patient compliance. This single codrug entity would have the potential to treat both alcohol and nicotine abusers when delivered transdermally. Figure 13.10 shows the structure of NTX, NTXOL, BUP, BUPOH, and two codrugs of BUPOH covalently linked to either NTX or NTXOL.

In order to determine the stability of the codrugs, hydrolytic studies were carried out in isotonic phosphate buffer at pH 7.4 (physiological pH). The results showed that the codrugs were susceptible to hydrolysis and produced the parent drugs at physiological pH. NTX, NTXOL, and BUPOH were stable in the buffer solution, and NTX-BUPOH and CB-NTXOL-BUPOH codrugs underwent slow hydrolysis in the buffer solution with half-lives of 36.68 and 28.88 h, respectively. The proposed hydrolytic conversion of the NTX-BUPOH codrug to the parent drugs is shown in

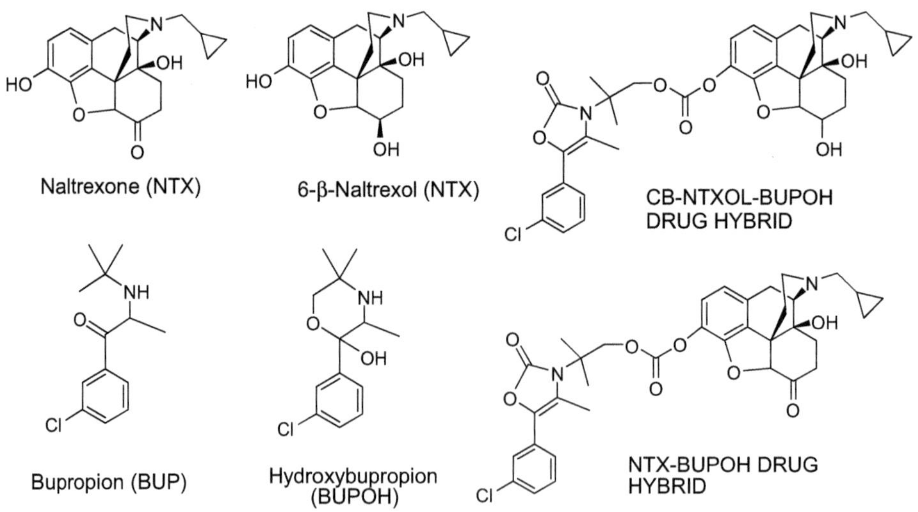


**Figure 13.10** Structures of parent drugs NTX, NTXOL, BUP, and BUPOH and codrugs NTX-BUPOH and CB-NTXOL-BUPOH, which contain a cyclic carbamate prodrug moiety of BUPOH.

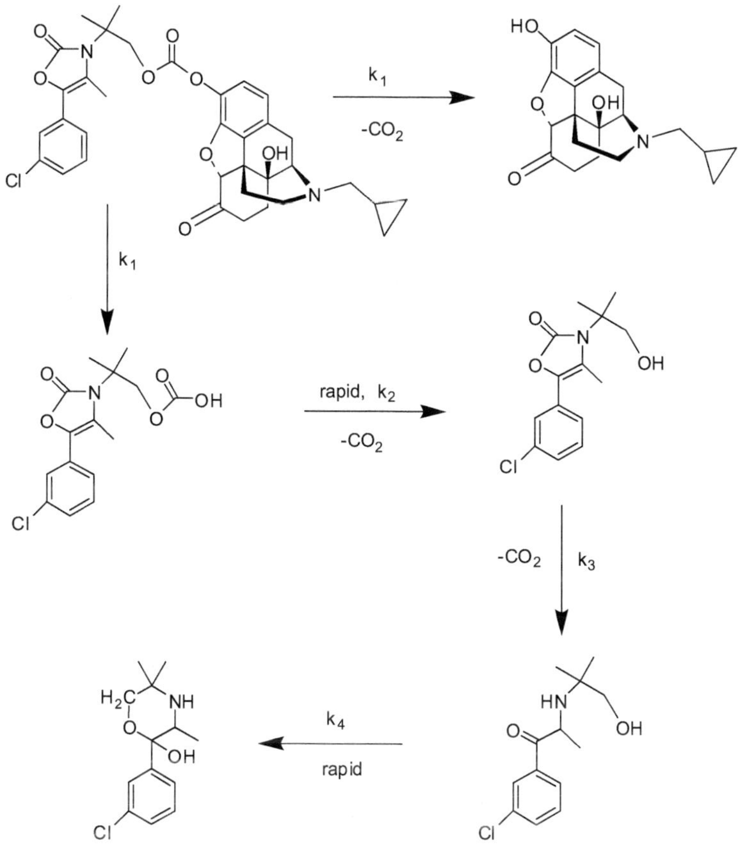


**Figure 13.11** Hydrolytic behavior of the NTX-BUPOH codrug.

detail in Figure 13.11. The NTX-BUPOH codrug undergoes cleavage of the carbonate bond to generate NTX, and a relatively stable cyclic carbamate intermediate of BUPOH, which subsequently undergoes hydrolysis to generate BUPOH. The chemical stability of the NTX-BUPOH codrug was studied in isotonic phosphate buffer at pH 7.4 over 4 days. The disappearance of the codrug and the appearance of the two parent drugs over time are shown in Figure 13.12. The rate of appearance of NTX was identical to the rate of disappearance of the codrug. However, the rate of formation of BUPOH was found to be slower than the rate of disappearance of the codrug, involving the formation of a relatively stable intermediate, which was identified as the five-membered cyclic carbamate analogue of BUPOH [1].

The stability of the carbonate codrug of 6-β-naltrexol and hydroxybupropion (CB-NTXOL-BUPOH) was also evaluated in guinea pig plasma. Figure 13.13 illustrates the hydrolytic profile of the carbonate codrug and the time course of formation of the two active parent drugs in the plasma. The release of 6-β-naltrexol from the codrug was a one-step process, as confirmed by the rate of appearance of 6-β-naltrexol correlating with the rate of disappearance of the carbonate codrug.

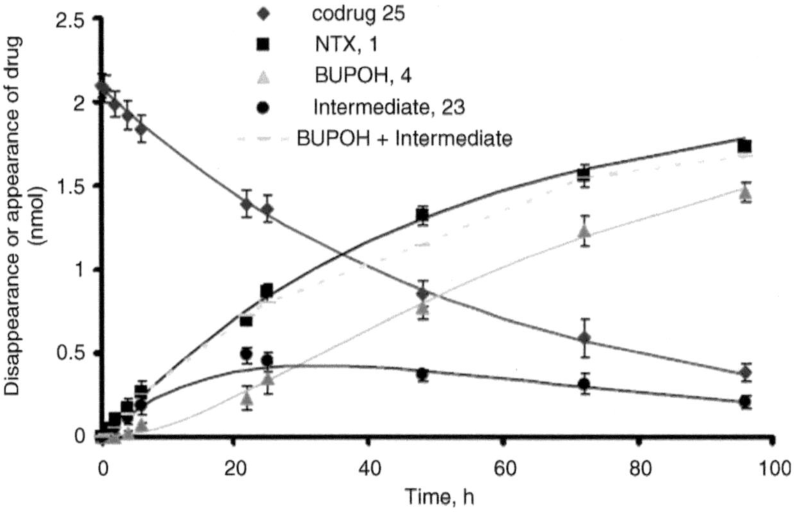


**Figure 13.12** Hydrolysis profile of the carbonate drug hybrid, NTX-BUPOH, in isotonic phosphate buffer at pH 7.4.

The release of BUPOH involved the initial formation of the cyclic carbamate analogue of BUPOH, which was then converted subsequently to the parent drug, BUPOH. The rate of hydrolysis of the CB-NTXOL-BUPOH codrug in plasma was three times faster compared to the rate of hydrolysis in isotonic phosphate buffer at pH 7.4 [40].

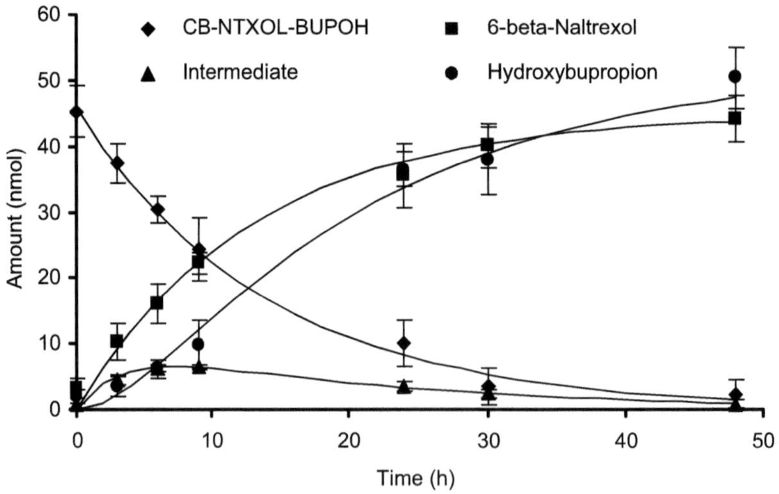


**Figure 13.13** Hydrolysis profile of the carbonate drug hybrid, CB-NTXOL-BUPOH, in guinea pig plasma at 37 °C.

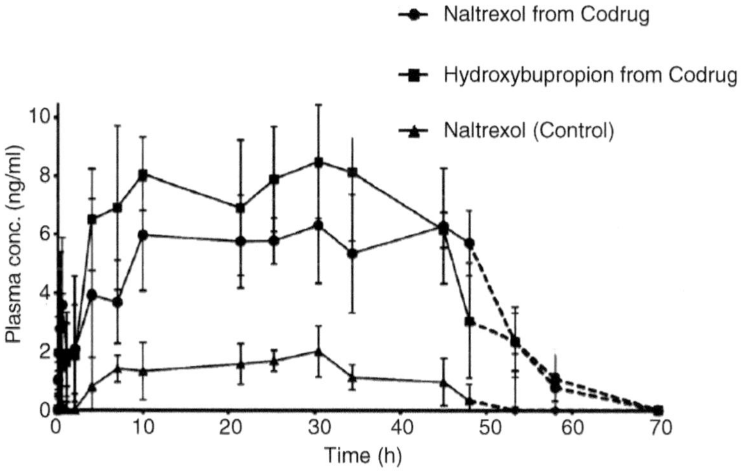


**Figure 13.14** Mean (± SD) plasma concentration profiles in guinea pigs after topical application of a gel formulation containing either CB-NTXOL-BUPOH or 6-β-naltrexol (control). The dotted line (----) indicates the plasma concentration after the removal of the formulation.

The CB-NTXOL-BUPOH codrug and 6-β-naltrexol were transdermally administered to hairless guinea pigs. The plasma concentration profiles of the analytes following topical application of either CB-NTXOL-BUPOH or 6-β-naltrexol are shown in Figure 13.14. The results showed a fivefold enhancement in the transdermal delivery of 6-β-naltrexol when given in the form of the codrug. Also, the codrug delivered a significant amount of BUPOH to the plasma when transdermally administered. The cyclic carbamate intermediate of BUPOH was not detected in the plasma of codrug-treated guinea pigs. The calculated pharmacokinetic parameters for the CB-NTXOL-BUPOH codrug and 6-β-naltrexol are listed in Table 13.1 [40].

**Table 13.1** Pharmacokinetic parameters of NTXOL in the guinea pig after application of a gel formulation containing either CB NTXOL-BUPOH or NTXOL base.

| Parameter | NTXOL | NTXOL from CB-NTXOL-BUPOH |
|---|---|---|
| $AUC_{0\text{-}48}$ (ng/ml h) | 66.4 ± 7.9 | 282.0 ± 14.5 |
| $C_{max}$ (ng/ml) | 1.5 ± 0.2 | 6.6 ± 0.4 |
| $T_{max}$ (h) | 28.1 ± 1.5 | 10.1 ± 0.9 |
| $T_{lag}$ (h) | 5.1 ± 0.7 | 5.0 ± 1.1 |
| Observed $C_{ss}$ (ng/ml) | 1.3 ± 0.5 | 6.4 ± 0.9 |
| Predicted $C_{ss}$ (ng/ml)[a)] | 0.2 ± 0.1 | 0.7 ± 0.3 |
| Enhancement factor | 1 | 5.3 |

Data are represented as mean SD $n = 5$ for NTXOL and $n = 6$ for CB-NTXOL-BUPOH.

a) Predicted from *in vitro* human skin diffusion data.

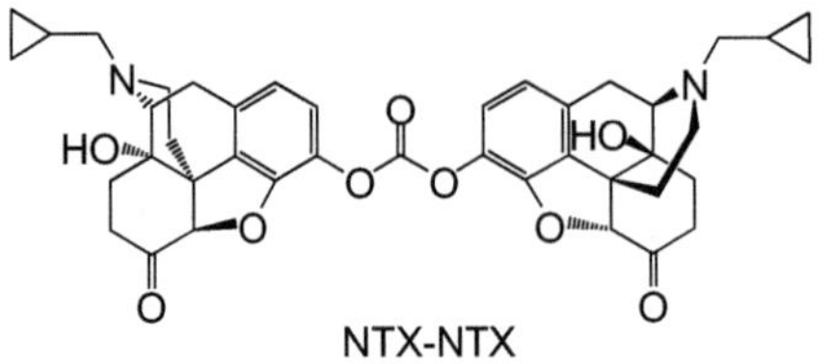


**Figure 13.15** Duplex gemini prodrug of NTX.

### 13.5.2
### Duplex Codrugs of Naltrexone for Transdermal Delivery

The problem of dealing with a released linker moiety was partially solved in the study of an NTX "gemini" or duplex codrug. Although the transdermal patch provides a sustained release of drug, NTX does not have the ideal physicochemical properties that allow delivery of therapeutic doses of the drug across the skin. Stinchcomb and coworkers addressed this problem in a recent study of transdermal delivery of NTX [41]. A synthetic dimer of NTX termed "duplex gemini prodrug" (NTX-NTX) (Figure 13.15) was synthesized and then evaluated in *in vitro* diffusion studies using human cadaver skin samples.

It was observed that NTX-NTX was hydrolyzed in the skin to afford two equivalents of NTX and one equivalent of harmless carbon dioxide (half-life = 31 min), and appeared primarily as NTX in the receiver solution of an *in vitro* Franz cell. It was also observed that the maximum flux from the duplex drug, in terms of NTX equivalents, was twice as high as that from NTX alone (6.2 and 3.0 $nmol/cm^2/h$ from the duplex codrug and NTX, respectively). According to the authors, the main reason for the increased flux from the NTX-NTX duplex was rapid bioconversion causing a difference in the concentration gradient profile for the NTX-NTX codrug.

### 13.5.3
### Codrugs Containing α-Tocopherol for Skin Hydration

Proper hydration conditions of human skin are maintained by natural moisturizing factors, which contain different amino acids, pyroglutamic acid, and some other water-soluble molecules [42]. Water retention inside the stratum corneum is maintained by fatty acids and cholesterol present on the skin surface. α-Tocopherol (VE) is one of the lipophilic antioxidants and carries out several important functions in the skin. Some of the important properties of VE are listed below.

- VE, along with ascorbic acid, forms an antioxidant network in the skin to protect the skin from oxidative damage [43].
- VE also protects polyunsaturated fatty acids (PUFA) and biological membranes against attack by free radicals that initiate lipid peroxidation.
- Biological membranes containing high levels of PUFA are protected against oxidizing radicals by VE as it penetrates into the lipid bilayers and acts as a radical scavenger.
- VE functions as a moisturizer by reducing transepidermal water loss.

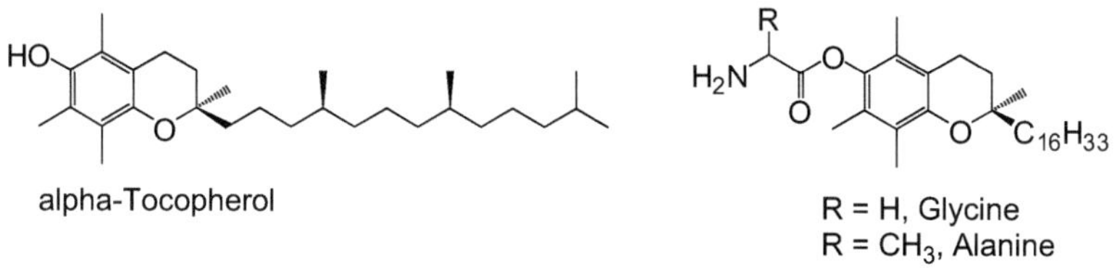


**Figure 13.16** Structures of α-tocopherol and α-tocopherol–amino acid codrugs.

Although possessing many useful properties, the VE molecule has some disadvantages. It is very readily degraded by oxidants, moisture, and UV irradiation. The stability of VE toward oxidation is generally increased by converting it to either an acetate or a succinate ester [44–46]. However, during this process the bioavailability of VE depends on the enzyme-catalyzed hydrolysis of the ester linkage. Bearing in mind that amino acids are components of natural moisturizing factors, Santi and coworkers synthesized ester codrugs of VE with amino acids such as alanine and glycine (Figure 13.16) [47].

As VE is the main active moiety in the codrug, the ester linkage should be cleavable by hydrolytic enzymes to produce the parent compounds. Porcine liver esterase was used to examine the stability of the ester bond between VE and various amino acids; these molecules can also be regarded as prodrugs. Under the experimental conditions, the codrug concentration decayed exponentially and the concentration of the parent compound (VE) increased exponentially. The experimentally determined half-lives of the glycine and alanine codrugs of VE were 49.5 and 142 h, respectively. Skin accumulation and metabolism experiments were performed on freshly excised rabbit ear skin considered to be similar to human skin in terms of drug permeability. The extent of metabolism for the glycine codrug was higher than that of the alanine codrug, a trend that was followed in the *in vitro* stability of the two codrugs. Experiments also showed that the alanine and glycine codrugs accumulated in skin in significant concentrations. The amount of VE found in the dermis after 6 h was almost double compared to the amount in dermis when VE was administered alone.

## 13.6
## Codrugs of L-DOPA for the Treatment of Parkinson's Disease

### 13.6.1
### L-DOPA Codrugs that Incorporate Inhibitors of L-DOPA Metabolism

Dopamine is deficient in the brains of patients suffering from Parkinson's disease. Unfortunately, dopamine cannot be given as a drug for this disease because it cannot cross the blood–brain barrier. L-3,4-Dihydroxyphenylalanine (L-DOPA) is a precursor of dopamine used in the treatment of Parkinson's disease. L-DOPA crosses the blood–brain barrier via facilitated transport, and is then converted to dopamine in the brain by the enzyme DOPA decarboxylase. For the treatment of

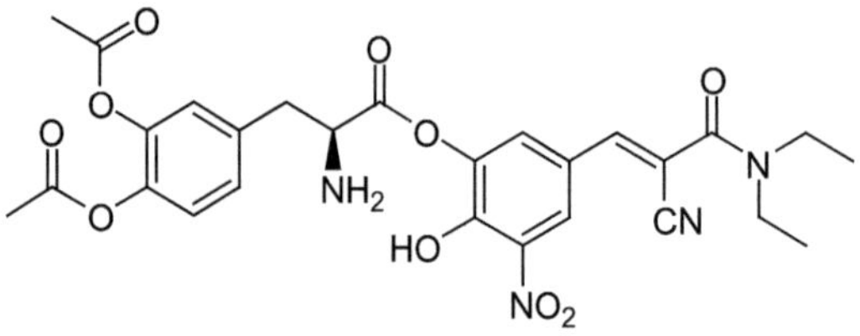


**Figure 13.17** L-DOPA–entacapone codrug.

Parkinson's disease, L-DOPA is given in combination with a peripheral DOPA decarboxylase inhibitor such as carbidopa, to prevent degradation of L-DOPA in the systemic circulation. Entacapone is a catechol-*O*-methyltransferase (COMT) inhibitor, which is also used with L-DOPA to treat Parkinson patients; entacapone inhibits the metabolism of L-DOPA by COMT to afford the inactive O-methylated metabolite. Since oral L-DOPA bioavailability is low, a codrug approach was used, by combining L-DOPA and entacapone via an ester linkage to improve L-DOPA brain delivery (Figure 13.17). The codrug showed stability in aqueous media at different pH levels and was hydrolyzed to the parent drugs in liver homogenate, fulfilling the codrug criteria [48].

Similar to carbidopa, benserazide is a DOPA-decarboxylase inhibitor. An L-DOPA codrug that incorporates benserazide was demonstrated to have good lipophilicity compared to either L-DOPA or benserazide alone (Figure 13.18). The codrug was also stable in aqueous buffer solutions. In plasma, the catechol esters and amide bonds in the codrug structure were efficiently cleaved, releasing the parent drugs in one step [49].

## 13.6.2
## L-DOPA–Antioxidant Codrugs

A series of codrugs have also been designed by linking L-DOPA and dopamine with antioxidant compounds such as α-lipoic acid, glutathione, caffeic acid, carnosine, benserazide, and *N*-acetylcysteine [50–54].

As shown in Figure 13.19, L-DOPA and dopamine can be directly conjugated to α-lipoic acid via an amide linkage [50]. α-Lipoic acid is an effective antioxidant. It exists as dihydrolipoate *in vivo*, which can regenerate (reduce) antioxidants such as glutathione, vitamin C, and vitamin E [55, 56]. The strained five-membered ring conformation of lipoic acid contributes to its good scavenging activity [57]. All the four

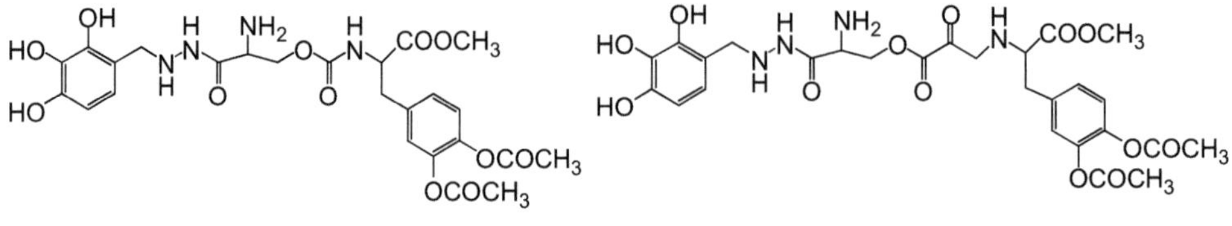


**Figure 13.18** Codrugs of L-DOPA with benserazide.

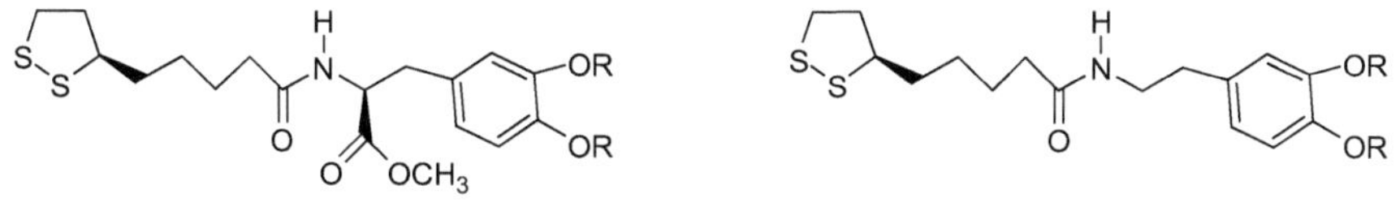

1. R=$COCH_3$
2. R=H

(a)

3. R=$COCH_3$
4. R=H

(b)

**Figure 13.19** (a) L-DOPA and α-lipoic acid codrugs; (b) dopamine and α-lipoic acid codrugs.

codrugs in Figure 13.19 showed good stability in the gastrointestinal tract and are cleaved enzymatically in rat and human plasma to release the parent drugs. The prolonged release of L-DOPA showed the effectiveness of the L-DOPA codrugs. Codrugs 1 and 2 were used to test antioxidant efficacy using superoxide dismutase (SOD) and glutathione peroxidase (GPx) markers. These enzymes have a central role in the control of reactive oxygen species (ROS). SOD dismutates highly reactive superoxide into oxygen and hydrogen peroxide, and GPx reduces hydrogen peroxide to water by oxidizing GSH. The oxidized form of GSH (GSSG) is reduced back to GSH by glutathione reductase, as shown in the equations below:

$$H_2O_2 + 2\,GSH \rightarrow GSSG + 2\,H_2O$$

$$GSSG + NADPH + H^+ \rightarrow 2\,GSH + NADP^+$$

Codrugs 1 and 2 afforded an increase in GPx activity compared to L-DOPA alone, indicating a decreased production of free radicals. Also, these codrugs induced a decrease in the activity of SOD compared to L-DOPA alone, indicating a reduced production of superoxide anions.

Similar results were obtained when codrugs of L-DOPA and glutathione were constructed with amide linkages joining the two drug entities (Figure 13.20) [51]. Glutathione is involved in the decomposition of toxic peroxide molecules, protects enzymes by maintaining their SH groups in a reduced state, and repairs oxidized iron–sulfur centers of the mitochondrial complex. No hydrolysis of the glutathione-L-DOPA codrugs was observed in gastrointestinal fluids and L-DOPA was shown to be released in plasma via enzymatic hydrolysis. The codrugs also exhibited an antioxidant effect as indicated using SOD and GPx markers.

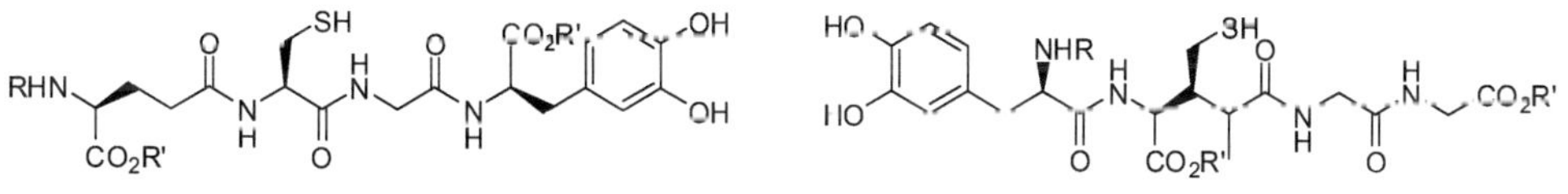

1: R=Ac; R'=Me   2: R=H; R'=H

(a)

3: R=Ac; R'=Me   4: R=H; R'=H

(b)

**Figure 13.20** (a) L-DOPA and glutathione codrugs; (b) dopamine and glutathione codrugs.

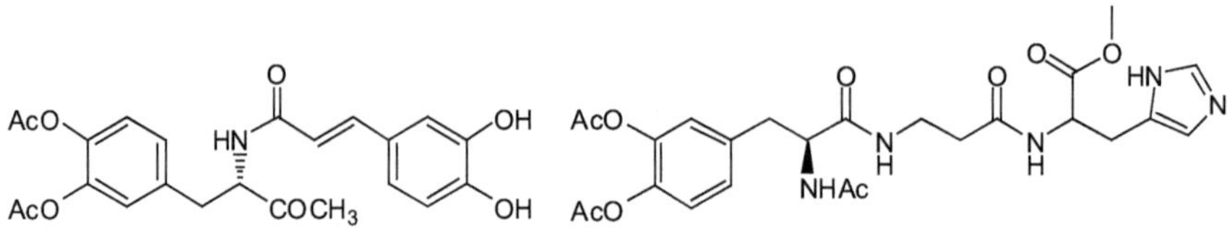


(a) (b)

**Figure 13.21** Structures of (a) a 3,4-diacetyl-L-DOPA methyl ester–caffeic acid codrug and (b) a 3,4-diacetyl-L-DOPA methyl ester–carnosine codrug.

Like glutathione and α-lipoic acid, two other antioxidants, caffeic acid and carnosine, have also been conjugated with L-DOPA (Figure 13.21) and the resulting codrugs assessed by evaluating plasma activities utilizing SOD and GPx markers in rats [52]. These codrugs were devoid of significant antioxidant activity, although the literature lists many reports that caffeic acid and carnosine act as natural antioxidants with hydroxyl radical-scavenging and lipid peroxidase activities.

To overcome the pro-oxidant effects of L-DOPA, other antioxidants utilized in L-DOPA codrug design were sulfur-containing compounds, such as *N*-acetyl cysteine (NAC), methionine, and bucillamine (Figure 13.22). N-Acetylation of cysteine speeds up cysteine absorption and distribution when given orally. NAC helps in increasing the intracellular concentration of glutathione by elevating intracellular cysteine levels. NAC is rapidly absorbed, enters cells, and is rapidly hydrolyzed to cysteine. Methionine is also an intermediate in the synthesis of cysteine and helps PC 12 cells against DA-induced nigral cell loss in Parkinson's disease by binding to oxidative metabolites of dopamine [58–60]. Bucillamine is a synthetic cysteine derivative used for the treatment of rheumatoid arthritis [61]. It contains two thiol groups, which

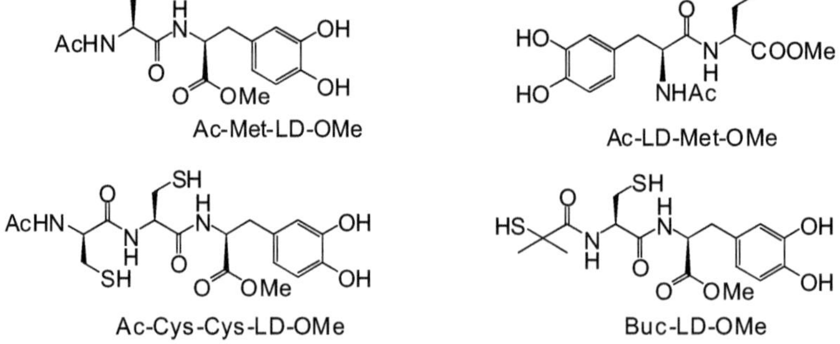


**Figure 13.22** Codrugs of L-DOPA linked to cysteine, methionine, and bucillamine.

makes it a more powerful antioxidant compared to NAC and methionine. It can be easily transported into cells to restore glutathione under conditions of oxidative stress and glutathione depletion [62].

Six codrugs have been constructed using L-DOPA as one of the parent drugs and NAC/methionine/bucillamine as the other parent drug [54]. All the codrugs showed good lipophilicity and water solubility for optimal intestinal absorption. Stability studies at pH 1.3 and in SGF indicated that the codrugs would be stable enough to pass unhydrolyzed through the stomach mucosa after oral administration. At pH 7.4, the codrugs were shown to be stable enough to be absorbed intact from the intestine. In rat and human plasma, the codrugs hydrolyzed to release the parent drugs, although the release of L-DOPA was very slow. The antioxidant efficacy of the codrugs was evaluated using a chemiluminescent assay and compared with NAC; all the codrugs showed a superior antioxidant effect as compared to NAC. The physicochemical and pharmacokinetic data showed high levels of L-DOPA in the plasma and brain, even 12 h after administration. Ac-Met-LD-OMe and Ac-LD-Met-OMe codrugs were able to induce a sustained release of L-DOPA and dopamine in rat striatum with respect to an equimolar dose of L-DOPA. When Ac-LD-Met-OMe codrug was injected intracerebroventricularly, it afforded levels of dopamine in the striatum that were higher than those in L-DOPA-treated rats and indicated that the codrug had a longer half-life in brain than L-DOPA [54].

## 13.7 Analgesic Codrugs Containing Nonsteroidal Anti-Inflammatory Agents

The clinical usefulness of nonsteroidal anti-inflammatory drugs has been documented for decades, and these drugs are the mainstay of the treatment of rheumatic disorders and other degenerative and inflammatory joint diseases, in sports medicine, and as a multipurpose pain killer. However, NSAIDs containing carboxylic acids are known to have g.i. toxicity, causing upper g.i. irritation, bleeding, ulceration, and perforation, due to the presence of a free carboxylic acid group and due to local inhibition of the cytoprotective actions of prostaglandins on gastric mucosa. In addition, NSAIDs may have an indirect effect attributed to their ion-trapping properties. One common way to solve the g.i toxicity problem is to design ester prodrugs of NSAIDs by masking the carboxylic acid group in the molecule. A recent and more effective approach is the design of codrugs of NSAIDs with another drug molecule by forming an ester linkage with the carboxylic acid group of the NSAID.

### 13.7.1 Flurbiprofen–Histamine $H_2$ Antagonist Codrugs

The first codrug of this category was synthesized and examined by Otagiri and Fukuhara [63]. Flurbiprofen (FP) was chosen as a model NSAID and linked to an antiulcer histamine $H_2$ antagonist agent to reduce the gastric mucosal damage

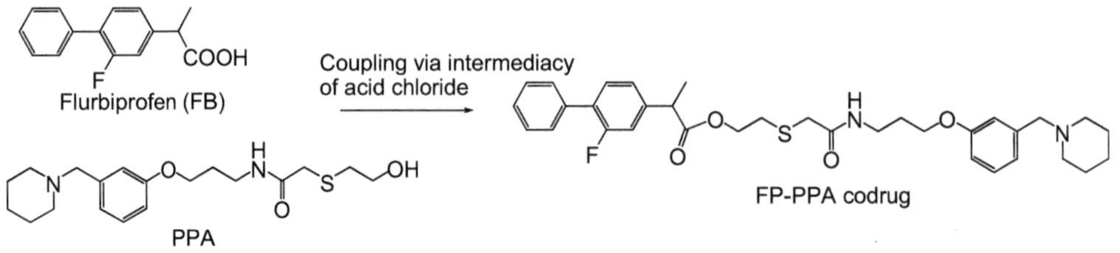


**Figure 13.23** Codrug of flurbiprofen and PPA.

caused by the NSAID. *N*-[3-{3-(1-Piperidinylmethyl)phenoxy}propyl]-2-(2-hydroxyethylthio)acetamide (PPA) was chosen as the histamine $H_2$ antagonist (Figure 13.23). The FP-PPA codrug showed high hydrophilicity and lipophilicity, suggesting that the codrug would not have an adverse effect on FP absorption. The codrug was also stable in the aqueous buffers over the pH range 1–7.4, and was also stable in the presence of the enzymes pepsin and trypsin. The codrug rapidly hydrolyzed in 10% plasma (half-life = 35 s). The pharmacokinetic results showed that the codrug was nearly completely absorbed into systemic circulation after oral delivery and was sufficiently hydrolyzed to produce both the parent drugs. The acute anti-inflammatory effects of both the FP-PPA codrug and the parent drug (FP) were analyzed by measuring the inhibition of carrageenan-induced edema. No difference was observed when the inhibitory effects of FP and the FP-PPA codrug were compared, demonstrating that the codrug had the same anti-inflammatory effect as FP. Pharmacokinetic data in rats also supported this result. However, experimental data showed the occurrence of gastric damage after FP administration; and when PPA was coadministered with FP as a physical mixture, the gastric damage by FP was not reduced. On the other hand, while the FP-PPA codrug inhibited ulcer formation induced by FP, the codrug was effective in reducing the gastric damage caused by FP alone, and this was attributed to the masking of the carboxylic acid group of FP by linking it to the histamine $H_2$ antagonist, PPA.

### 13.7.2
### NSAID–Acetaminophen Codrugs

In another approach, Omar and coworker utilized a well-known analgesic, acetaminophen, to mask the carboxylic acid group of NSAIDs (Figure 13.24) [64]. Although acetaminophen is relatively safe at therapeutic doses, large overdoses can produce the toxic metabolite, *N*-acetyl-*p*-benzoquinoneimine (NAPQI). Codrugs of acetaminophen with NSAIDs would reduce the g.i. adverse effects of NSAIDs and could also reduce the formation of the toxic metabolite NAPQI from acetaminophen. A series of ester-linked codrugs of acetaminophen with NSAIDs were synthesized and evaluated, and the stability of these codrugs was examined at pH 1.3 and 7.4 in nonenzymatic aqueous buffers and 80% human plasma. Results showed appreciable stability of the codrugs both in nonenzymatic simulated gastric fluid (pH 1.3) (half-life = 6.7–43 h) and in nonenzymatic simulated intestinal fluid (pH 7.4) (half-life

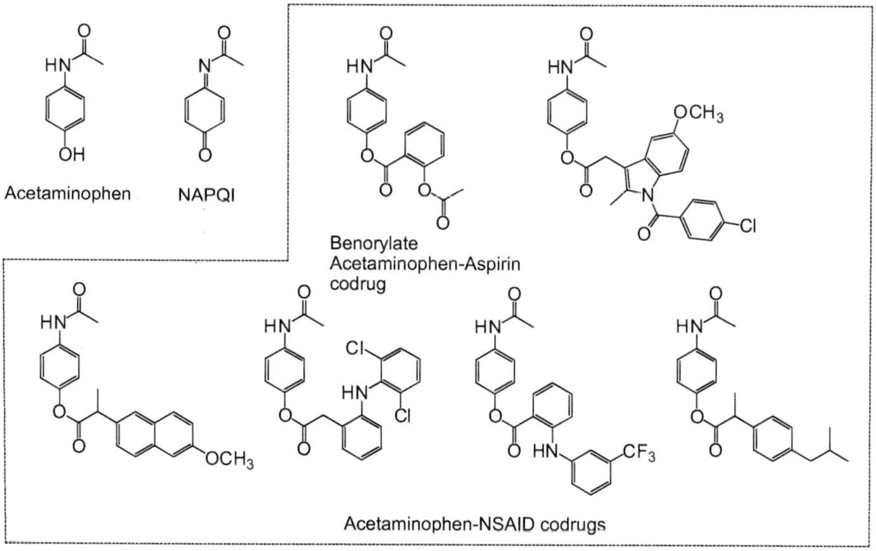


**Figure 13.24** A series of codrugs of acetaminophen and NSAIDs.

= 1.5–25 h). The codrugs exhibited much shorter half-lives in human plasma (half-life = 13.9–38.4 min) and in rat liver homogenate (half-life = 12.6–42.9 min). From the hydrolytic study, it was found that the susceptibility of the codrugs to enzymatic hydrolysis depends upon the type of NSAID covalently linked to the acetaminophen molecule. The aspirin-acetaminophen codrug having the smallest acyl moiety was found to be the most susceptible to enzymatic degradation. Codrugs with bulkier acyl moieties were found to be least susceptible to enzymatic hydrolysis. On the basis of *in vitro* data, the codrug of ibuprofen and acetaminophen was selected for bioavailability studies. No appreciable concentration of the codrug was detected in plasma after oral administration of the codrug, confirming very fast hydrolysis of the ester linkage *in vivo* compared to *in vitro* hydrolysis. Over a 24-h time course, the ibuprofen-acetaminophen codrug produced higher concentration of ibuprofen in the plasma compared to a physical mixture of the two parent drugs, indicating a higher bioavailability of the codrug due to improved lipophilicity.

A codrug of diclofenac and acetaminophen was chosen for an ulcerogenicity study and was compared with an equivalent physical mixture of the two parent drugs. Mice treated with a physical mixture of the two drugs showed significant damage of the mucous layer and ulceration of submucosal cells. However, mice chronically treated with the corresponding codrug did not show any significant gastric mucosal injury. The analgesic activities of the codrugs and the corresponding physical mixtures were analyzed using the mouse hot plate assay. The results showed a significant increase in the analgesic activity of the codrug over time, compared to the physical mixture of the parent drugs. All the synthesized codrugs showed significantly higher analgesic activity than the control groups (equivalent physical mixture of parent drugs).

### 13.7.3 Naproxen–Propyphenazone Codrugs

In another study aimed at suppressing the g.i. toxicity of NSAIDs without affecting their anti-inflammatory activity, codrugs of naproxen (NAP) and propyphenazone were synthesized and evaluated (Figure 13.25) [65]. NAP is a potent carboxylic acid-containing NSAID and has a moderate analgesic activity associated with g.i. irritation [66]. Previously reported alkyl ester and thioester prodrugs of NAP showed reduced g.i. erosive properties and similar anti-inflammatory activity, but significantly reduced analgesic potency [67]. On the other hand, propyphenazone is a nonacidic pyrazole drug with good analgesic and antipyretic activity and no anti-inflammatory activity [68]. The metabolism of propyphenazone is known to proceed via the formation of its active metabolite, 3-hydroxymethylpropyphenazone (HMP), which has similar activity to the parent drug [69, 70]. An NAP-propyphenazone codrug strategy was considered a rational approach to achieving an anti-inflammatory and synergistic analgesic effect with a reduction in g.i. irritation associated with the NSAID. Propyphenazone was first converted to HMP or 3-aminomethylpropyphenazone (AMP). In one of the codrug molecules, HMP was directly linked to NAP to afford the NAP-HMP codrug. In the second codrug design, HMP was linked to the endogenous amino acid glycine through an ester linkage, and the free amino group of glycine was then covalently linked to NAP via an amide bond. In the third codrug molecule, a different linker, glycolic acid, was used to link AMP and NAP. Since the carboxylic acid group of NAP is essential for its analgesic activity, the release of NAP from the various codrugs was studied initially in nonenzymatic aqueous buffer solutions at pH 1.2 and 7.4, and in liver homogenates having activated esterase enzymes. Stability studies of the codrugs in aqueous buffers showed significant stability (half-life = 60–91 h at pH 1.2 and 10–19 h at pH 7.4). The codrugs showed a high susceptibility toward hydrolysis in rat liver homogenate (half-life 54–85 min). The analgesic activity of the codrugs compared to equimolar doses of the

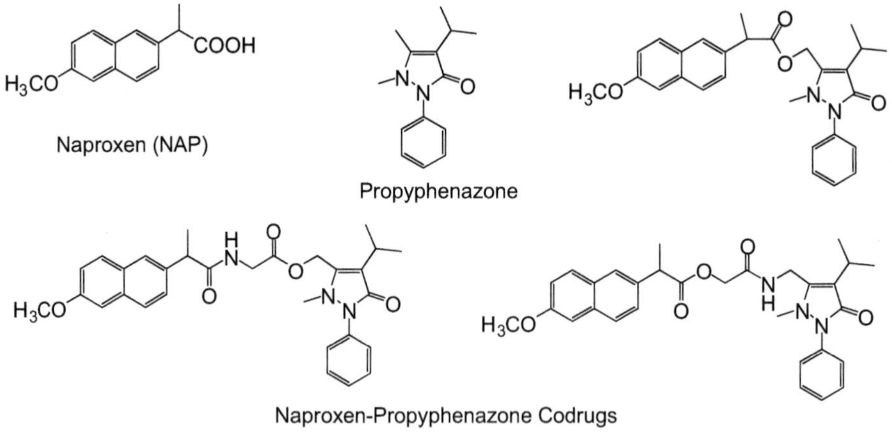


**Figure 13.25** A series of naproxen-propyphenazone codrugs.

two parent drugs was tested in the mouse hot plate assay. In a general trend, the codrugs showed improved analgesic activity over time compared to the parent drugs, reaching a maximum effective dose after about 4–6 h due to improved codrug bioavailability and efficient hydrolysis to the parent drugs. Comparative anti-inflammatory activity of the codrugs and NAP was determined by measuring the swelling of the paw after intraplantar injection of carrageenan in the rat. The codrug of NAP and HMP linked through glycolic acid also reduced inflammation in a pattern similar to an equimolar dose of NAP. This codrug was analyzed for its ulcerogenic activity and compared to those of the parent drugs, NAP and HMP. The NAP-treated mice, and to some extent the HMP-treated mice, showed complete damage of the mucous layer in addition to ulceration of the submucosal cells of the g.i. tract, while the codrug-treated group and the control group (treated with vehicle only) did not show any ulcerogenic activity.

### 13.7.4 Flurbiprofen–Amino Acid Codrugs

In another approach, the adverse g.i. effects of the NSAID, flurbiprofen, were reduced by masking the carboxylic acid group through the formation of an amide bond with a series of amino acids. The anti-inflammatory activity of amino acids against gelatin-induced hind paw edema in rats and their healing effect on gastric lesions produced by NSAIDs have been reported in literature [71]. Thus, conjugates of flurbiprofen with anti-inflammatory amino acids can be clearly considered as codrugs since they would produce amino acids as hydrolytic products having synergistic anti-inflammatory effects with NSAIDs, and would also afford g.i. protective effect against NSAIDs. By covalently linking appropriate amino acids to NSAIDs, codrugs with optimal polarity, solubility profile, and acid–base properties can be designed. Thus, a series of amide codrugs of flurbiprofen with methyl esters of L-tryptophan, L-histidine, L-phenylalanine, and DL-alanine (Figure 13.26) were synthesized and evaluated [72]. The stability of the codrugs was studied in hydrochloric acid buffer (pH = 1.2), phosphate buffer (pH = 7.4), and 80% human plasma.

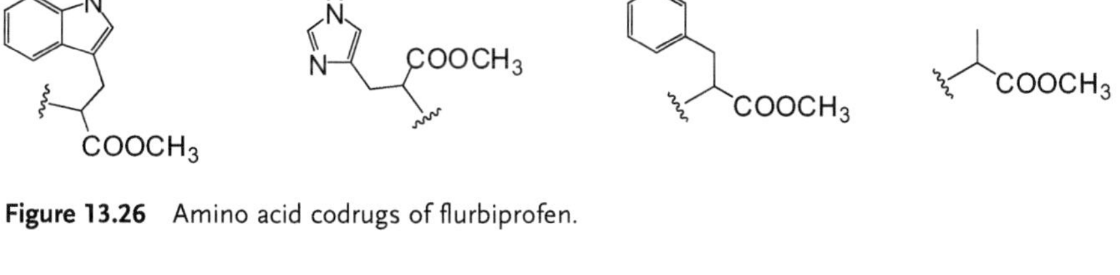


Figure 13.26 Amino acid codrugs of flurbiprofen.

The codrugs were found to be stable in hydrochloric acid buffer but underwent hydrolysis in phosphate buffer with half-life values ranging from 30.19 to 70.09 min. This result suggested that the codrugs were likely to be stable enough to be absorbed intact from the intestine. The comparatively shorter half-lives of the codrugs in plasma (ranging from 16.2 to 29.3 min) indicated that rapid production of the parent drugs in the systemic circulation was likely. Results from the evaluation of the anti-inflammatory properties of the codrugs revealed that flurbiprofen-phenylalanine and flurbiprofen-alanine codrugs were superior to flurbiprofen alone; the flurbiprofen–-tryptophan and flurbiprofen–histidine codrugs were comparable to flurbiprofen in terms of anti-inflammatory activity.

### 13.7.5
### NSAID–Chlorzoxazone Codrugs

In a recent study, an active muscle relaxant drug was used to mask the carboxylic acid group of NSAIDs via the formation of a codrug [73]. Chlorzoxazone is an active muscle relaxant and is marketed as a single component drug or in combination with NSAIDs. On the basis of these observations, codrugs of chlorzoxazone with three different NSAIDs were synthesized in an attempt both to minimize the adverse gastrointestinal effects of NSAIDs and to improve the pharmacokinetic properties of the parent drugs while retaining anti-inflammatory and skeletal muscle relaxant activities (Figure 13.27). Chlorzoxazone was first converted to the key intermediate, hydroxymethylchlorzoxazone, and then coupled with the carboxylic acid group of the appropriate NSAID to form ester-linked codrugs. Hydrolysis of these codrugs was studied in nonenzymatic aqueous buffers at pH 1.2 and 7.4 and in 80% human plasma. The hydrolysis data showed that the codrugs were sufficiently stable at pH 1.2 and 7.4 to be absorbed almost unchanged from the g.i. tract. The codrugs showed susceptibility to hydrolysis in 80% human plasma (half-life = 34–37 min). In the carrageenan-induced paw edema bioassay, ibuprofen and the ibuprofen-chlorzoxazone codrug showed the greatest inhibition of inflammation followed by the naproxen–chlorzoxazone and mefenamic acid–chlorzoxazone codrugs. The overall data showed that the codrugs exhibited comparable anti-inflammatory activity to their parent NSAIDs. The muscle relaxant activity of the codrugs in comparison with that of the muscle relaxant chlorzoxazone was examined using rat sciatic nerve tibialis

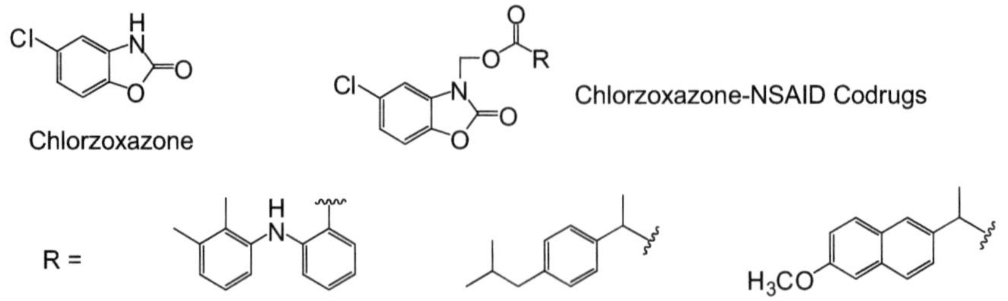


**Figure 13.27** A series of codrugs of chlorzoxazone with NSAIDs.

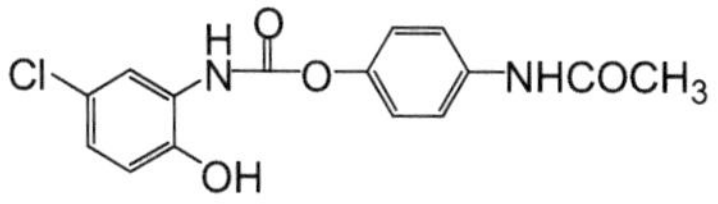

Figure 13.28 Codrug of chlorzoxazone and acetaminophen.

muscle preparation. Muscle relaxant activity was exhibited by all the codrugs, while that of the ibuprofen–chlorzoxazone codrug was comparable with chlorzoxazone. Importantly, the ibuprofen–chlorzoxazone codrug-treated animals showed far less damage to the mucous layer of the gastrointestinal tract compared to those treated by ibuprofen alone.

### 13.7.6 Acetaminophen–Chlorzoxazone Codrug

In a related study, a codrug molecule incorporating chlorzoxazone and acetaminophen has been reported (Figure 13.28) [74]. The main reason for the synthesis of this codrug was the observed synergistic effects of these two drugs when administered together. The rate of liberation of the parent drugs from this codrug was studied at pH 7.4 in phosphate buffer, and in human and rat plasma. The codrug regenerated chlorzoxazone and acetaminophen simultaneously and quantitatively under the experimental conditions. However, the codrug showed a higher susceptibility to the formation of parent drugs in phosphate buffer than in either human or rat plasma, indicating that the release of chlorzoxazone from the codrug did not need to be enzyme mediated.

## 13.8 Analgesic Codrugs of Opioids and Cannabinoids

There is a continuing need for analgesic medications that are able to provide high-efficacy pain relief while providing more favorable pharmacokinetics and reducing the possibility of undesirable side effects. Enhancement of the analgesic effect of opioids with cannabinoids has been previously described [75]. These two classes of drug work via opioid and cannabinoid receptors, which are found throughout the central and peripheral nervous system. Synergy between $\Delta^9$-THC and opioids is well documented in the literature [76, 77]. In addition, these two classes of drug produce similar effects on calcium levels and cyclic AMP accumulation through G-protein-mediated pathways. However, appropriate dosing of these active agents to their site of action, for example, the brain or spinal column, can be difficult because of their differential pharmacokinetics. A codrug approach can be useful in overcoming the differential physicochemical and pharmacokinetic properties of opioid and cannabinoid drugs. In addition, opioids exert their analgesic effect on nociceptive pain while cannabinoids are effective in modulating neuropathic pain. Thus, an opioid–

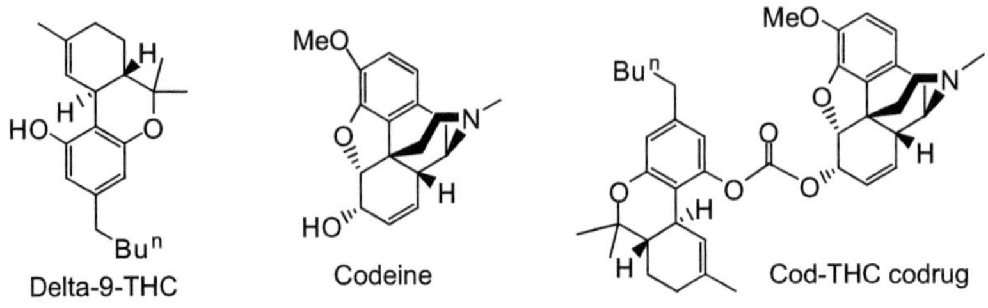


**Figure 13.29** Structures of delta-9-THC, codeine, and Cod-THC codrug.

cannabinoid codrug might be able to cover a broader range of pain. Keeping these points in mind, a series of opioid–cannabinoid codrugs were designed and synthesized, and a codrug of codeine and $\Delta^9$-THC (Cod-THC) was fully evaluated in pain models, stability indicating assays, and *in vivo* pharmacokinetic studies [78, 79] (Figure 13.29).

The effect of the Cod-THC codrug after oral administration in nociceptive and neuropathic pain models utilizing tail flick and chronic constriction injury pain models in the rat was evaluated. The oral efficacies of each of the parent drugs, codeine and $\Delta^9$-THC, were also compared with the Cod-THC codrug as pain modulators in the above pain models to determine their relative effectiveness. In both pain models, the codrug showed both improved effectiveness and more prolonged pain management properties, compared to the parent drugs (Figure 13.30).

The Cod-THC codrug was initially evaluated for its stability in buffers ranging from pH 1 to pH 9, in simulated gastric and intestinal fluids (SGF and SIF,

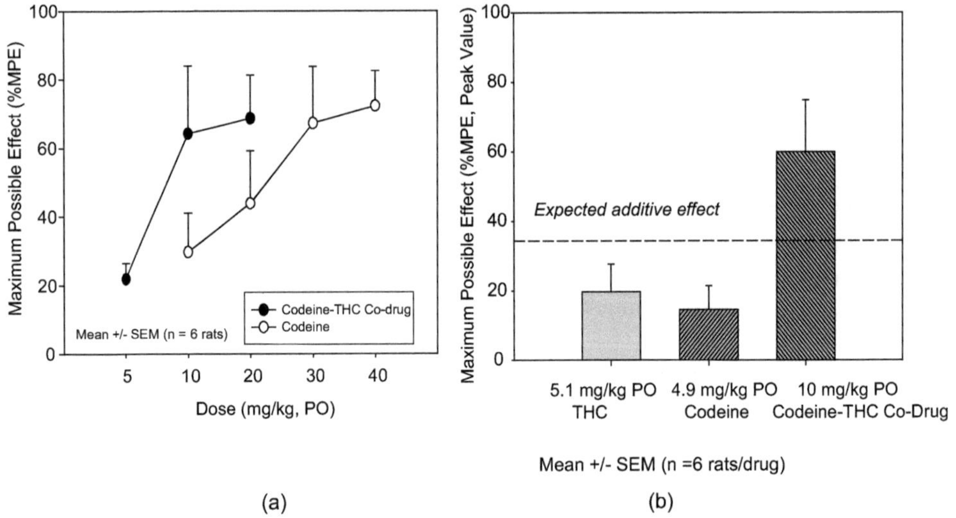


**Figure 13.30** (a) Dose–response curves for the antinociceptive effects of the codeine-THC codrug and codeine alone in the tail flick test. (b) Antihyperalgesic effect of codeine, THC, and the Cod-THC codrug in the chronic constriction nerve injury (CCI) model.

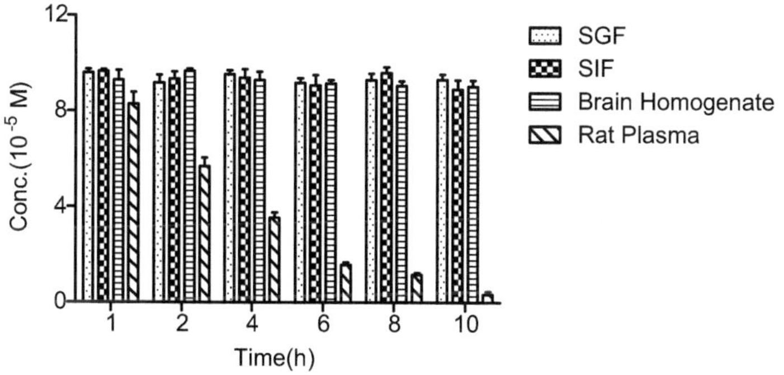


**Figure 13.31** Hydrolysis of the Cod-THC codrug under different enzymatic conditions.

respectively), and in rat plasma and brain homogenate. The codrug was found to have a favorable drug stability profile for oral administration, was stable in aqueous solutions over a wide range of physiologically relevant pH from 1 to 7.4, and was also stable in simulated gastric fluid, simulated intestinal fluid, and rat brain homogenate. In rat plasma, the codrug was hydrolyzed to the two parent drugs, codeine and $\Delta^9$-THC with a rate constant of 0.282/h (Figure 13.31).

The pharmacokinetic profile of the Cod-THC codrug was evaluated in the rat after oral administration and compared with the pharmacokinetic profile of an equimolar physical mixture of the parent drugs. Several groups have reported low bioavailability of THC (2–6%) and codeine (4–8%) after oral administration in rats due to poor absorption from the gastrointestinal tract [80, 81]. Rat plasma concentrations of the Cod-THC codrug were determined after oral and i.v. administration. The resulting data were compared with those obtained after oral administration of an equimolar physical mixture of the two parent drugs, codeine and $\Delta^9$-THC. The plasma concentrations of codeine and $\Delta^9$-THC were found to be much higher after oral administration of the codrug in the rat, compared to plasma concentrations of these drugs after oral administration of the equimolar physical mixture of the two parent drugs. The parent drugs were clearly released from the codrug molecule in 1:1 ratio in plasma, while administration of the physical mixture did not afford equimolar concentrations of codeine and $\Delta^9$-THC in the plasma (Figure 13.32). This is likely both due to the different pharmacokinetic profiles of the two parent drugs and due to the different pharmacokinetic profile of the Cod-THC codrug. Also, the parent drugs were present in plasma for a longer period of time after oral administration of codrug, likely due to the sustained release of the parent drugs from the codrug in the plasma.

## 13.9 Codrugs Containing Anti-HIV Drugs

The rapid spread of the human immunodeficiency virus (HIV), the etiological agent of acquired immunodeficiency syndrome (AIDS), has stimulated intensive efforts worldwide to develop chemotherapeutic agents effective against HIV.

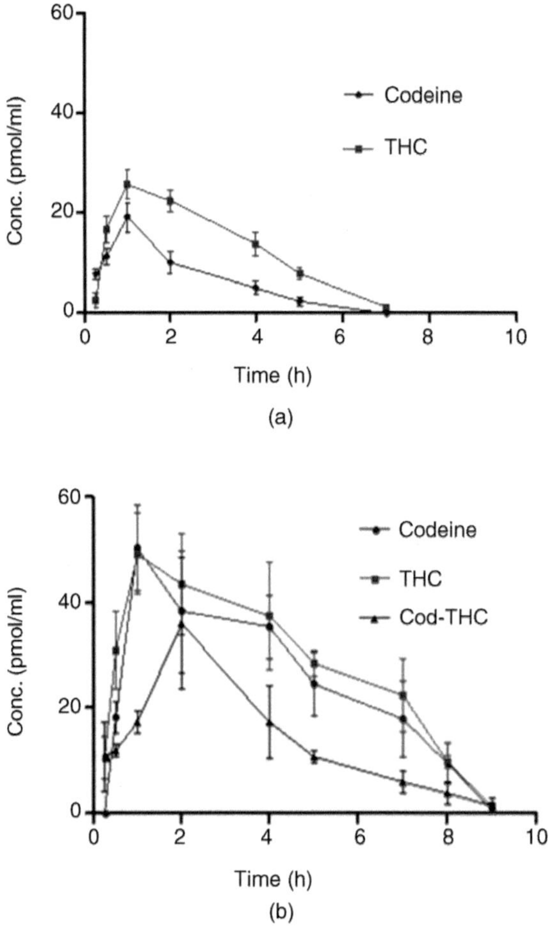


**Figure 13.32** Plasma concentrations of codeine, $\Delta^9$-THC, and Cod-THC codrug after administration of physical mixture of (a) codeine, 4.9 mg/kg, and $\Delta^9$-THC, 5.1 mg/kg (b) and Cod-THC codrug, 10 mg/kg.

2′,3′-Dideoxynucleosides (ddNs) are one of the most potent series of compounds active against HIV [82, 83]. The expression of activity of these drugs requires bioconversion into their corresponding 5′-*O*-triphosphate analogues [84–86]. The resulting triphosphate analogues may inhibit the replication of the virus by competitive inhibition of viral reverse transcriptase (RT) and/or by incorporation into and subsequent chain termination of the growing viral DNA strand [87]. Six drugs from the ddN family have been marketed: zidovudine (AZT, Retrovir), stavudine (d4T, Zerit), zalcitabine (ddC, Hivid), didanosine (ddI, Videx), lamivudine (3TC, Epivir), and abacavir (1592U89, Ziagen). AZT was the first drug to be approved by the FDA [88]. Some other families of compounds have also been approved by the FDA and are now commercially available as anti-HIV therapeutic agents; for example, nucleoside analogues (adefovir, dipivoxil), nonnucleoside reverse transcriptase inhibitors, also known as NNRTIs (nevirapine), and protease inhibitors (indinavir). AZT is still one of the most effective anti-HIV agents used, although it is the oldest compound approved by the FDA. Although AZT therapy has reduced the mortality rate and frequency of opportunistic infections in AIDS patients, it is associated with some adverse effects and unsuitable pharmacokinetic properties. These adverse effects are listed as follows:

- AZT administration is associated with significant dose-related toxicity leading to anemia and leucopenia [89, 90]
- Pharmacokinetic studies in phase I trials revealed that the plasma half-life of AZT was only 1 h [91], requiring frequent administration of AZT to maintain therapeutic plasma concentration of the drug.
- Bone marrow toxicity was caused by the high doses of AZT needed to achieve adequate concentrations in cerebrospinal fluid (CSF)
- AZT does not penetrate into brain tissue from the CSF [92] and thus causes no suppression of viral replication in the brain.

Designing lipophilic prodrugs of AZT is one approach both to increase its permeability through plasma membranes and to improve blood–brain barrier permeability. Combination therapy of AZT with other nucleoside derivatives, or certain NNRTIs, or different protease inhibitors, has been found to be more effective than AZT therapy alone [93]. On the basis of these observations and the need for improvements in chemotherapeutic agents to treat AIDS, a series of codrugs of AZT has been synthesized and evaluated.

### 13.9.1
### AZT–Retinoic Acid Codrug

Aggarwal *et al.* synthesized a series of mutual prodrugs of AZT with improved permeability properties to achieve higher concentrations of AZT both in the CNS and in the targeted HIV-infected cells. Among these was a codrug of retinoic acid and AZT linked through an ester moiety (Figure 13.33) [94]. Retinoic acid has previously been shown to inhibit HIV replication. The synthesized AZT-retinoic acid codrug and the parent drug AZT were partitioned between *n*-octanol and phosphate buffer (0.2 M, pH 7.4) to determine their partition coefficients (PCs), and the codrug (PC = 17.9) was found to be more lipophilic than AZT (PC = 1.2). The hydrolysis

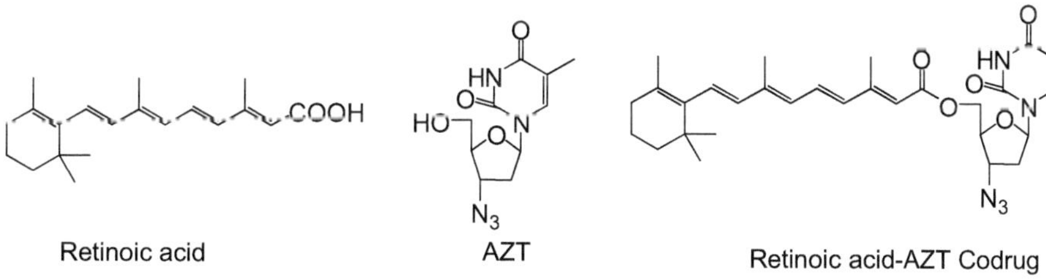


**Figure 13.33** Anti-HIV codrug of AZT.

of the codrug to the parent compounds was examined in phosphate buffer (pH = 7.4) and in human plasma. The codrug was found to be stable in phosphate buffer, and the half-life of the codrug was found to be 120 min in human plasma. The stability of the codrug was also studied upon incubation with hepatic microsomes isolated from rat. The half-life of the codrug was found to be 60 min, indicating relatively rapid and complete microsomal enzymatic hydrolysis to the two parent drugs. The extent of cell membrane permeability of AZT and the retinoic acid-AZT codrug was measured by comparing the uptake of the radiolabeled drugs into H9 cells. The data showed that the uptake of the retinoic acid–AZT codrug in H9 cells was highest among all the synthesized AZT derivatives and that the uptake of the retinoic acid–AZT codrug was four times the parent compound, AZT. The antiviral activity of the retinoic acid–AZT codrug and AZT against HIV-1 was determined *in vitro* in peripheral blood lymphocytes (PBL) obtained from HIV-seronegative donors. The codrug was found to have similar antiviral activity to AZT, although cellular uptake of the codrug was much higher than that of AZT, and this may indicate incomplete cellular hydrolysis of the codrug under *in vitro* conditions. Although retinoic acid is known to inhibit HIV replication, the codrug did not exhibit synergistic effects, most likely due to only partial release of retinoic acid.

## References


1 Hamad, M.O., Kiptoo, P.K., Stinchcomb, A.L., and Crooks, P.A. (2006) Synthesis and hydrolytic behavior of two novel tripartate codrugs of naltrexone and 6β-naltrexol with hydroxybupropion as potential alcohol abuse and smoking cessation agents. *Bioorganic & Medicinal Chemistry*, **14**, 7051–7061.

2 Silverman, R.B. (2004) *The Organic Chemistry of Drug Design and Drug Action*, 2nd edn, Elsevier, Oxford.

3 Howard, M., Al-Ghananeem, A., and Crooks, P.A. (2007) A novel chemical delivery system comprising an ocular sustained release formulation of a 3α, 17α, 21-trihydroxy-5β-pregnan-20-one-bis-5-flouroucil codrug. *Drug Development and Industrial Pharmacy*, **33**, 677–682.

4 Lipinski, C.A., Lombardo, F., Dominy, B.W., and Feeney, P.J. (2001) Experimental and computational approaches to estimate solubility and permeability in drug discovery and development settings. *Advanced Drug Delivery Reviews*, **46**, 3–26.

5 Baltzer, B., Binderup, E., von Daehne, W., Godtfredsen, W.O., Hansen, K., Nielsen, B., Sørensen, H., and Vangedal, S. (1980) Mutual pro-drugs of beta-lactam antibiotics and beta-lactamase inhibitors. *Journal of Antibiotics*, **10**, 1183–1192.

6 Hartley, S. and Wise, R. (1982) A three-way crossover study to compare the pharmacokinetics and acceptability of sultamicillin at two dose levels with that of ampicillin. *The Journal of Antimicrobial Chemotherapy*, **10**, 49–55.

7 Svartz, N. (1942) Salazopyrin, a new sulfanilimide preparation. *Acta Medica Scandinavica*, **110**, 577–598.

8 Das, K.M., Eastwood, M.A., McManus, J.P.A., and Sircus, W. (1973) Adverse reactions during salicylazosulfapyridine therapy and the relation with drug metabolism and acetylater phenotype. *New England Journal of Medicine*, **289**, 491–495.

9 Peppercorn, M.A. and Goldman, P. (1972) The role of intestinal bacteria in the metabolism of salicylazosulphapyridine. *Journal of Pharmacology and Experimental Therapeutics*, **181**, 555–562.

10 Azad Khan, A.K., Guthrie, G., Johnson, H.H., Truelove, S.C., and Williamson, D.

(1983) Tissue and bacterial splitting of sulphasalazine. *Clinical Science*, **64**, 349–354.

**11** Beales, D.L., Burry, H.C., and Graham, R. (1972) Comparison of aspirin and benorylate in the treatment of rheumatoid disease. *British Medical Journal*, **2**, 483–485.

**12** Robertson, A., Glynn, J.P., and Watson, A.K. (1972) The absorption and metabolism in man of 4-acetamidophenyl-2-acetoxybenzoate (benorylate). *Xenobiotica: The Fate of Foreign Compounds in Biological Systems*, **2**, 339–347.

**13** Howard-Sparks, M., Al-Ghananeem, A.M., Pearson, A.P., and Crooks, P.A. (2005) Evaluation of $O^{3\alpha}$-, $O^{21}$-di-($N^1$-methyloxycarbonyl-2,4-dioxo-5-fluoropyrimidinyl)17α-hydroxy-5β-pregnan-20-one as a novel potential antiangiogenic codrug. *Journal of Enzyme Inhibition and Medicinal Chemistry*, **20**, 417–428.

**14** Howard, M., Al-Ghananeem, A., and Crooks, P.A. (2007) A novel chemical delivery system comprising an ocular sustained release formulation of a 3α, 17α, 21-trihydroxy-5β-pregnan-20-one-bis-5-fluoroucil codrug. *Drug Development and Industrial Pharmacy*, **33**, 677–682.

**15** Ashton, P., Crooks, P.A., Cynkowski, T., Cynkowska, G., Riggs, R.M., and Guo, H. (2000) Means to achieve sustained release of synergistic drugs by conjugation. U.S. Patent No. 6,051,576 April 18, 2000.

**16** Machemer, R. (1988) Proliferative vitreoretinopathy (PVR): a personal account of its pathogenesis and treatment. *Investigative Ophthalmology & Visual Science*, **29**, 1771–1783.

**17** Cheng, C.K., Berger, A.S., Pearson, P.A., Ashton, P., and Jaffe, G.J. (1995) Intravitreal sustained-release dexamethasone device in the treatment of experimental uveitis. *Investigative Ophthalmology & Visual Science*, **36**, 442–453.

**18** Tano, Y., Sugita, G., Abrams, G., and Machemer, R. (1980) Inhibition of intraocular proliferations with intravitreal corticosteroids. *American Journal of Ophthalmology*, **89**, 131–136.

**19** Tano, Y., Chandler, D., and Machemer, R. (1980) Treatment of intraocular proliferation with intravitreal injection of triamcinolone acetonide. *American Journal of Ophthalmology*, **90**, 810–816.

**20** Blumenkranz, M., Ophir, A., and Claflin, A. (1981) A pharmacological approach to non-neoplastic intraocular proliferation. ARVO Abstracts. *Investigative Ophthalmology & Visual Science*, **20** (Suppl.), 200.

**21** Stern, W.H., Guerin, C.J., Erickson, P.A., Lewis, G.P., Anderson, D.H., and Fisher, S.K. (1983) Ocular toxicity of fluorouracil after vitrectomy. *American Journal of Ophthalmology*, **96**, 43–51.

**22** Berger, A.S., Cheng, C.K., Pearson, P.A., Ashton, P., Crooks, P.A., Cynkowski, T., Cynkowska, G., and Jaffe, G.J. (1996) Intravitreal sustained release corticosteroid-5-fluorouracil conjugate in the treatment of experimental proliferative vitreoretinopathy. *Investigative Ophthalmology & Visual Science*, **37**, 2318–2325.

**23** Algvere, P. and Bill, A. (1981) Effects of vitrectomy and phakectomy on the drainage of the vitreous compartment. Albrecht von Graefe's. *Archive for Clinical and Experimental Ophthalmology*, **216**, 253–260.

**24** Tingey, D.P., Schroeder, A., Epstein, M.P.M., and Epstein, D.L. (1992) Effects of topical ethacrynic acid adducts on intraocular pressure in rabbits and monkeys. *Archives of Ophthalmology*, **110**, 699–702.

**25** Epstein, D.I., Roberts, B.C., and Skinner, L.L. (1997) Nonsulfhydryl-reactive phenoxyacetic acids increase aqueous humor outflow facility. *Investigative Ophthalmology & Visual Science*, **38**, 1526–1534.

**26** Melamed, S., Kotas-Neumann, R., Barak, A., and Epstein, D.L. (1992) The affect of intracamerally injected ethacrynic acid on intraocular pressure in patients with glaucoma. *American Journal of Ophthalmology*, **113**, 508–512.

**27** Peczon, J.D. and Grant, W.M. (1968) Diuretic drugs in glaucoma. *American Journal of Ophthalmology*, **66**, 680–683.

**28** Shargel, L., Mutnick, A., Souney, P., Swanson, L., and Block, L. (1997) *Comprehensive Pharmacy Review*, Lippincott Williams & Wilkins, Baltimore, MD.

**29** Safran, A.B., Simona, F., Sansonetti, A., Pometta, D., and James, R. (1993) Topical timolol maleate might adversely affect serum lipoproteins. *International Ophthalmology*, **17**, 109–110.

**30** Volpicelli, J.R., Alterman, A.I., Hayashida, M., and O'Brien, C.P. (1992) Naltrexone in the treatment of alcohol dependence. *Archives of General Psychiatry*, **49**, 876–880.

**31** Rukstalis, M.R., Stromberg, M.F., O'Brien, C.P., and Volpicelli, J.R. (2000) 6-β-Naltrexol reduces alcohol consumption in rats. *Alcoholism, Clinical and Experimental Research*, **24**, 1593–1596.

**32** Wang, D., Raehal, K.M., Bilsky, E.J., and Sadee, W. (2001) Inverse agonists and neutral antagonists at mu opioid receptor (MOR): possible role of basal receptor signaling in narcotic dependence. *Journal of Neurochemistry*, **77**, 1590–6000.

**33** Volpicelli, J.R., Rhines, K.C., and Rhines, J.S. (1997) Naltrexone and alcohol dependence. Role of subject compliance. *Archives of General Psychiatry*, **54**, 737–743.

**34** Medical Economics (1996) *PDR Generics*, 2nd edn, Medical Economics, Montvale, NJ, pp. 2229–2233.

**35** Kiptoo, P.K., Hamad, M.O., Crooks, P.A., and Stinchcomb, A.L. (2006) Enhancement of transdermal delivery of 6-beta-naltrexol via a codrug linked to hydroxybupropion. *Journal of Controlled Release*, **113**, 137–145.

**36** Cooper, B.R., Wang, C.M., Cox, R.F., Norton, R., Shea, V., and Ferris, R.M. (1994) Evidence that the acute behavioral and electrophysiological effects of bupropion (Wellbutrin) are mediated by a noradrenergic mechanism. *Neuropsychopharmacology*, **11**, 133–141.

**37** Ascher, J.A., Cole, J.O., Colin, J.N., Feighner, J.P., Ferris, R.M., Fibiger, H.C., Golden, R.N., Martin, P., Potter, W.Z., and Richelson, E. (1995) Bupropion: a review of its mechanism of antidepressant activity. *Journal of Clinical Psychiatry*, **56**, 395–401.

**38** Sanchez, C. and Hyttel, J. (1999) Comparison of the effects of antidepressants and their metabolites on reuptake of biogenic amines and on receptor binding. *Cellular and Molecular Neurobiology*, **19**, 467–489.

**39** Slemmer, J.E., Martin, B.R., and Damaj, M.I. (2000) Bupropion is a nicotinic antagonist. *Journal of Pharmacological and Experimental Therapeutics*, **295**, 321–327.

**40** Kiptoo, P.K., Paudel, K.S., Hammell, D.C., Hamad, M.O., Crooks, P.A., and Stinchcomb, A.L. (2008) *In vivo* evaluation of a transdermal codrug of 6-β-naltrexol linked to hydroxybupropion in hairless guinea pigs. *Journal of Pharmaceutical Sciences*, **33**, 371–379.

**41** Hammell, D.C., Hamad, M., Vaddi, H.K., Crooks, P.A., and Stinchcomb, A.L. (2004) A duplex "Gemini" prodrug of naltrexone for transdermal delivery. *Journal of Controlled Release*, **97**, 283–290.

**42** Morganti, P. (1999) Skin hydration, in *Novel Cosmetic Delivery Systems* (eds E. Mandassi and E. Touitou), Marcel Dekker, New York, pp. 71–97.

**43** Thiele, J.J., Dreher, F., and Packer, L. (2000) Antioxidant defense system in skin, in *Cosmeceuticals* (eds P. Elsner and H. Maibach), Marcel Dekker, New York, pp. 145–177.

**44** Beijersbergen van Henegouwen, G.M.J., Junginger, H.E., and de Vries, H. (1995) Hydrolysis of RRR-α-tocopheryl acetate (vitamin E acetate) in the skin and its UV protecting activity (an *in vivo* study with the rat). *Journal of Photochemistry and Photobiology*, **29**, 45–51.

**45** Lampen, P., Pittermann, W., Heise, H.M., Schmitt, M., Jungmann, H., and Kietzmann, M. (2003) Penetration studies of vitamin E acetate applied from cosmetic formulations to the stratum corneum of an *in vitro* model using quantification by tape stripping, UV spectroscopy, and HPLC. *Journal of Cosmetic Science*, **54**, 119–131.

**46** Gensler, H.L., Aickin, M., Peng, Y.M., and Xu, M. (1996) Importance of the form of topical vitamin E for prevention of photocarcinogenesis. *Nutrition and Cancer*, **26**, 183–191.

47 Ostacolo, C., Marra, F., Laneri, S., Sacchi, A., Nicoli, S., Padula, C., and Santi, P. (2004) α-Tocopherol pro-vitamins: synthesis, hydrolysis and accumulation in rabbit ear skin. *Journal of Controlled Release*, **99**, 403–413.

48 Leppanen, J., Huuskonen, J., Nevalainen, T., Gynther, J., Taipale, H., and Jarvinen, T. (2002) Design and synthesis of a novel L-DOPA–entacapone codrug. *Journal of Medicinal Chemistry*, **45**, 1379–1382.

49 Stefano, D.A., Sozio, P., Iannitelli, A., Cocco, A., Orlando, G., and Ricciutelli, M. (2006) Synthesis and preliminary evaluation of L-DOPA/benserazide conjugates as dual acting codrugs. *Letters in Drug Design and Discovery*, **3**, 747–752.

50 Stefano, D.A., Sozio, P., Cocco, A., Iannitelli, A., Santucci, E., Costa, M., Pecci, L., Nasuti, C., Cantalamessa, F., and Pinnen, F. (2006) L-DOPA and dopamine-(*R*)-α-lipoic acid conjugates as multifunctional codrugs with antioxidant properties. *Journal of Medicinal Chemistry*, **49**, 1486–1493.

51 Stefano, D.A., Sozio, P., Cocco, A., Iannitelli, A., Santucci, E., Costa, M., Pecci, L., Nasuti, C., Cantalamessa, F., and Pinnen, F. (2007) Synthesis and study of L-DOPA-glutathione codrugs as new anti-Parkinson agents with free radical scavenging properties. *Journal of Medicinal Chemistry*, **50**, 2506–2515.

52 Piera, S., Iannitelli, A., Cerasa, S.L., Cacciatore, I., Cornacchia, C., Giorgioni, G., Ricciutelli, M., Nasuti, C., Cantalamessa, F., and Stefano, D.A. (2008) New L-DOPA codrugs as potential antiparkinson agents. *Archiv der Pharmazie: Chemistry in Life Sciences*, **341**, 412–417.

53 Stefano, D.A., Sozio, P., Iannitelli, A., Cocco, A., Orlando, G., and Ricciutelli, M. (2006) Synthesis and preliminary evaluation of L-DOPA/benserazide conjugates as dual acting codrugs. *Letters in Drug Design and Discovery*, **3**, 747–752.

54 Pinnen, F., Cacciatore, I., Cornacchia, C., Sozio, P., Cerasa, S.L., Iannitelli, A., Nasuti, C., Cantalamessa, F., Sekar, D., Gabbianelli, R., Falcioni, L.M., and Stefano, D.A. (2009) Codrugs linking L-DOPA and sulfur-containing antioxidants: new pharmacological tools against Parkinson's disease. *Journal of Medicinal Chemistry*, **52**, 559–563.

55 Biewenga, G.P., Haenen, G., and Bast, A. (1997) The pharmacology of the antioxidant lipoic acid. *General Pharmacology*, **29**, 315–331.

56 Packer, L., Witt, E.H., and Tritschler, H.J. (1995) Alpha-lipoic acid as a biological antioxidant. *Free Radical Biology & Medicine*, **19**, 227–250.

57 Haenen, G. and Bast, A. (1991) Scavenging of hypochlorous acid by lipoic acid. *Biochemical Pharmacology*, **42**, 2244–2246.

58 Grinberg, L., Fibach, E., Amer, J., and Atlas, D. (2005) *N*-Acetylcysteine amide, a novel cell-permeating thiol, restores cellular glutathione and protects human red blood cells from oxidative stress. *Free Radical Biology & Medicine*, **38**, 136–145.

59 Offen, D., Ziv, I., Sternin, H., Melamed, E., and Hochman, A. (1996) Prevention of dopamine-induced cell death by thiol antioxidants: possible implications for treatment of Parkinson's disease. *Experimental Neurology*, **141**, 32–39.

60 Martínez, M., Martínez, N., Hernández, A.I., and Ferrándiz, M.L. (1999) Hypothesis: can *N*-acetylcysteine be beneficial in Parkinson's disease? *Life Sciences*, **64**, 1253–1257.

61 Horwitz, L.D. (2003) Bucillamine: a potent thiol donor with multiple clinical applications. *Cardiovascular Drug Reviews*, **21**, 77–90.

62 Hammond, C.L., Lee, T.K., and Ballatori, N. (2001) Novel roles for glutathione in gene expression, cell death, and membrane transport of organic solutes. *Journal of Hepatology*, **34**, 946–954.

63 Otagiri, M. and Fukuhara, T.I. (1999) Improving the pharmacokinetic and pharmacodynamic properties of a drug by chemical conversion to a chimera drug. *Journal of Controlled Release*, **62**, 223–229.

64 Fadl, T.A. and Omar, F.A. (1998) Paracetamol (acetaminophen) esters of some non-steroidal anti-inflammatory carboxylic acids as mutual prodrugs with improved therapeutic index. *Inflammopharmacology*, **6**, 143–157.

65 Shehaa, M., Khedr, A., and Elsherief, H. (2002) Biological and metabolic study of naproxen–propyphenazone mutual prodrug. *European Journal of Pharmaceutical Sciences*, **17**, 121–130.

66 Shanbhag, V.R., Crider, A.M., Gokhale, R., Harpalani, A., and Dick, R.M. (1992) Esters and amide prodrugs of ibuprofen and naproxen: synthesis, antiinflammatory activity, and gastrointestinal toxicity. *Journal of Pharmaceutical Sciences*, **81**, 149–154.

67 Venuti, M.C., Young, J.M., Maloney, P.J., Johnson, D., and McGreevy, K. (1989) Synthesis and biological evaluation of omega-(*N*,*N*,*N*-tri-alkylammonium)alkyl esters and thioesters of carboxylic acid non-steroidal antiinflammatory agents. *Pharmaceutical Research*, **6**, 867–873.

68 Burne, K. (1986) Comparative pharmacology of non-opioid analgesics. *Medical Toxicology*, **1** (Suppl.), 1–9.

69 Goromaru, T., Matsura, H., Furuta, T., and Baba, S. (1984) Identification of isopropylantipyrine metabolites in rat and man by using stable isotope tracer techniques. *Chemical & Pharmaceutical Bulletin*, **32**, 3179–3186.

70 Neugebauer, M., Khedr, A., El-Rabbat, N., El-Kommes, M., and Saleh, G. (1997) Stereoselective metabolic study of famprofazone. *Biomedical Chromatography*, **11**, 356–361.

71 Meyers, B.E., Moonka, D.K., and Davis, R.H. (1979) The effect of selected amino acids on gelatin-induced inflammation in adult male mice. *Inflammation*, **3**, 225–233.

72 Gairola, N., Nagpal, D., Dhaneshwar, S.S., Dhaneshwar, S.R., and Chaturvedi, S.C. (2005) Synthesis, hydrolysis kinetics and pharmacodynamic profile of novel prodrugs of flurbiprofen. *Indian Journal of Pharmaceutical Sciences*, **67** (3), 369–373.

73 Abdel-Azeem, A.Z., Abdel-Hafez, A.A., El-Karamany, G.S., and Farag, H.H. (2009) Chlorzoxazone esters of some non-steroidal anti-inflammatory (NSAI) carboxylic acids as mutual prodrugs: design, synthesis, pharmacological investigations and docking studies. *Bioorganic & Medicinal Chemistry*, **17**, 3665–3670.

74 Vigroux, A. and Bergon, M. (1995) Synthesis of prodrugs and mutual prodrug of chlorzoxazone and acetaminophen based on masked benzoxazolone. *Bioorganic & Medicinal Chemistry Letters*, **5**, 427–430.

75 Cichewicz, D.L., Martin, Z.L., Smith, F.L., and Welch, S.P. (1999) Enhancement of μ opioid antinociception by oral $\Delta^9$-tetrahydrocannabinol: dose–response analysis and receptor identification. *The Journal of Pharmacology and Experimental Therapeutics*, **289**, 859–867.

76 Bloom, A.S. and Dewey, W.L. (1978) A comparison of some pharmacological actions of morphine and $\Delta^9$-tetrahydrocannabinol in the mouse. *Psychopharmacology*, **57**, 1432–2072.

77 Cichewicz, L.D. and McCarthy, E.A. (2002) Antinociceptive synergy between delta(9)-tetrahydrocannabinol and opioids after oral administration. *The Journal of Pharmacology and Experimental Therapeutics*, **304**, 1010–1015.

78 Holtman, J.R., Crooks, P.A., and Dhooper, H.K. (2006) Novel synergistic opioid-cannabinoid codrug for pain management. US Patent 2008/0176885A1.

79 Dhooper, H.K., Holtman, J., and Crooks, P.A. (2008) Preparation of a synergistic codrug of codeine and $\Delta^9$-THC as a potent antinociceptive agent. Twenty Second Annual Meeting and Exposition of the American Association of Pharmaceutical Scientists, November, 2008, Atlanta, GA.

80 Chiang, C.N. and Barnett, G. (1984) Marijuana effect and delta-9-tetrahydrocannabinol plasma level. *Clinical Pharmacology and Therapeutics*, **6**, 234–238.

81 Shah, J. and Mason, D.W. (1990) Pharmacokinetics of codeine after parenteral and oral dosing in the rat. *Drug Metabolism and Disposition: The Biological Fate of Chemicals*, **18**, 670–673.

82 Mitsuya, H. and Broder, S. (1986) Inhibition of the *in vitro* infectivity and cytopathic effect of human T-lymphotropic virus, type III/lymphadenopathy-associated virus (HTLV III/LAV) by 2′,3′-

dideoxynucleosides. *Proceedings of the National Academy of Sciences of the United States of America*, **83**, 1911–1915.
83 De Clercq, E. (1997) In search of a selective antiviral chemotherapy. *Clinical Microbiology Reviews*, **10**, 674–693.
84 Furman, P.A., Fyfe, J.A., St. Clair, M.H., Weinhold, K., Rideout, J.L., Freeman, G.A., Nusinoff-Lehrman, S., Bolognesi, D.P., Broder, S., Mitsuya, H., and Barry, D.W. (1986) Phosphorylation of 3′-azido-3′-deoxythymidine and selective interaction of the 5′-triphosphate with HIV reverse transcriptase. *Proceedings of the National Academy of Sciences of the United States of America*, **83**, 8333–8337.
85 Hao, Z., Cooney, D.A., Hartman, N.R., Perno, C.F., Fridland, A., De Vico, A.L., Sarngadharan, M.G., Broder, S., and Johns, D.G. (1988) Factors determining the activity of 2′,3′-dideoxynucleosides in suppressing human immunodeficiency virus *in vitro*. *Molecular Pharmacology*, **34**, 431–435.
86 Balzarini, J. and De Clercq, E. (1999) Nucleoside and nonnucleoside reverse transcriptase inhibitors active against HIV, in *Textbook of AIDS Medicine* (eds T.C. Merigan, J.G. Bartlett, and D. Bolognesi), Lippincott Williams & Wilkins, Baltimore, pp. 815–847.
87 Cheng, Y.C., Dutschman, G.E., Bastow, K.F., Sarngadharan, M.G., and Ting, R.Y.C. (1987) HIV reverse transcriptase: general properties and its interactions with nucleoside triphosphate analogues. *The Journal of Biological Chemistry*, **262**, 2187–2189.
88 Mitsuya, H., Weinhold, K.J., Furman, P.A., St. Clair, M.H., Nusinoff-Lehrman, S., Gallo, R.C., Bolognesi, D.P., Barry, D.W., and Broder, S. (1985) 3′-Azido-3′-deoxythymidine (BWA509U): an antiviral agent that inhibits the infectivity and cytopathic effect of human T-cell lymphotropic virus type III/ lymphadenopathy-associated virus *in vitro*. *Proceedings of the National Academy of Sciences of the United States of America*, **82**, 7096–7100.
89 Fischl, M.A., Richman, D.D., Grieco, M.H., Gottlieb, M.S., Volberding, P.A., Laskin, O.L., Leedom, J.M., Groopman, J.E., Mildvan, D., Schooley, R.T., Jackson, G.G., Durack, D.T., and King, D. (1987) The efficacy of azidothymidine (AZT) in the treatment of patients with AIDS and AIDS-related complex. A double blind, placebo-controlled trial. *The New England Journal of Medicine*, **317**, 185–191.
90 Richman, D.D., Fischl, M.A., Grieco, M.H., Gottlieb, M.S., Volberding, P.A., Laskin, O.L., Leedom, J.M., Groopman, J.E., Mildvan, D., Hirsch, M.S., Jackson, G.G., Durack, D.T., and Nusinoff-Lehrman, S. (1987) The toxicity of azidothymidine (AZT) in the treatment of patients with AIDS and AIDS-related complex. A double blind, placebo-controlled trial. *The New England Journal of Medicine*, **317**, 192–197.
91 Klecker, R.W., Collins, J.M., Yarchoan, R., Thomas, R., Jenkins, J.F., Broder, S., and Meyers, C.E. (1987) Plasma and cerebrospinal fluid pharmacokinetics of 3′-azido-3′-deoxythymidine: a novel pyrimidine analog with potential application for the treatment of patients with AIDS and related diseases. *Clinical Pharmacology and Therapeutics*, **41**, 407–412.
92 Terasaki, T. and Pardridge, W.M. (1988) Restricted transport of 3′-azido-3′-deoxythymidine and dideoxynucleosides through the blood-brain barrier. *The Journal of Infectious Diseases*, **158**, 630–632.
93 De Clercq, E. (1995) Toward improved anti-HIV chemotherapy: therapeutic strategies for intervention with HIV infections. *Journal of Medicinal Chemistry*, **38**, 2491–2517.
94 Aggarwal, S.K., Gogu, S.R., Rangan, S.R.S., and Agrawal, K.C. (1990) Synthesis and biological evaluation of prodrugs of Zidovudine. *Journal of Medicinal Chemistry*, **33**, 1505–1510.

# 14
# Soft Drugs

*Paul W. Erhardt and Michael D. Reese*

## 14.1
## Introduction

It is important to begin this chapter by emphasizing that although both prodrugs and soft drugs rely upon biotransformations to dictate their course of activities, soft drugs are not a class of prodrugs and prodrugs are not a class of soft drugs. Strategically, soft drugs are designed to be distinct types of agents, and their resulting constructs remain so upon implementation. So, why a chapter on soft drugs within a book about prodrugs: because both types of drugs rely upon biotransformations that draw from the same set of medicinal chemistry principles that are used during their structural design, synthetic assembly, and ultimately their clinical deployment. Each of these aspects will be made clear within the context of soft drugs during this discourse.

### 14.1.1
### Definition

The term "soft drug" (sometimes called "antedrug") was first introduced by Bodor [1] about 30 years ago to contrast Ariens' drug design concept of nonmetabolized "hard drugs," the latter intending to avoid problems caused by reactive species or active metabolites that are sometimes formed after *in vivo* administration of a standard drug [2]. While soft drugs are thus designed to prompt their own metabolism, these events are programmed to occur in a predictable manner that leads to inactive metabolites. In accord with this original theme while also borrowing from similar language that can be used to alternatively define prodrugs, an acceptable definition for today is as follows: *soft drugs are efficaciously active agents that have been constructed so as to contain a molecular feature that dictates a specified route and rate of bioconversion to efficaciously silent and nontoxic compounds* [3]. Just like for prodrugs, bioconversion generally has been accomplished by an enzymatically driven biotansformation, although with today's increasing levels of technical sophistication, a chemically driven event or any combination of both processes may also be programmed into

*Prodrugs and Targeted Delivery: Towards Better ADME Properties.* Edited by Jarkko Rautio

ISBN: 978-3-527-32603-7

either type of molecule. Opposite of prodrugs, which by definition are efficaciously inactive until they become activated by bioconversion, soft drugs are active molecules that become deactivated by this process. Thus, when the bioconversion is enzymatic, a soft drug can be thought of as undergoing a specified metabolic degradation to inactive metabolites at a programmed rate.

It also should be emphasized that inherent to this definition is the active role played in the design of these types of agents. Thus, compounds that happen to have a short half-life without intentionally being designed to display this profile, do not qualify as soft drugs. Instead, such compounds are simply short-acting compounds. By strict definition, exclusion of the latter still holds even when some attribute of their inherently fast metabolism is subsequently exploited clinically. Furthermore, there is no requirement for soft drugs to be necessarily short acting at all, a frequent misconception that is often embedded as representing the sole option toward deploying this drug design strategy. The relationships between a drug, prodrug, and soft drug are further contrasted schematically within Figure 14.1.

### 14.1.2 Prototypical Agent

Esmolol can be regarded as a classic example of a soft drug [4]. Its chemical structure and an account of its discovery are offered as a case study at the end of this chapter. To fully appreciate how the definition and unique pharmacokinetic properties of a soft drug are linked to the clinic from initial concept to final deployment, the pharmacological target and ultimate clinical profile for this prototypical example are described below. The description is done in a narrative style so that this section also can serve as an introduction to the case study that will then focus upon esmolol's translational research aspects.

#### 14.1.2.1 Backdrop

In the early-1960s, the clinical successes of propranolol (**1** in Figure 14.2) were serving to establish it as an effective antihypertensive agent and the "pioneer drug" within the category of beta-adrenergic receptor blocking agents [5]. The field of cardiovascular preventive medicine, just beginning to "bud" at about that time, would soon be joining these clinical successes rallied by this early "beta-blocker." As a result, numerous pharmaceutical companies were already deploying "analog-based drug discovery" [6, 7] to pursue additional compounds with enhanced pharmacological profiles. For most cardiac indications, the preferred profile typically being sought during this highly competitive era of active beta-blocker analogue campaigns was (i) selectivity for beta-1 receptors over alpha- and beta-2 receptors, (ii) low partial agonist or "intrinsic sympathomimetic activity," (iii) low membrane depressant or stabilizing activity, and (iv) a long duration of action conducive to once-a-day dosing.

#### 14.1.2.2 Clinical Challenge

Within the specific setting of acute myocardial infarction (MI), however, the seemingly beneficial use of beta-blockers to slow heart rate, and thus preserve

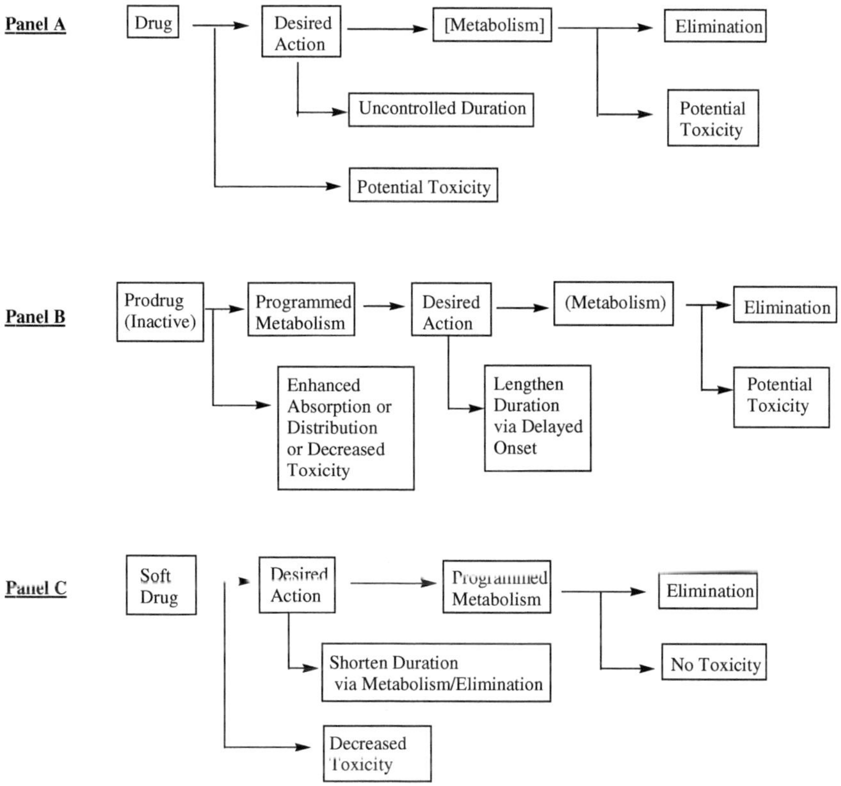


**Figure 14.1** Contrasting dispositions of a drug, prodrug, and soft drug [3]. Panel A depicts a generalized version of a standard drug's pattern of observed activities. Panel B depicts how a prodrug approach can be used to modify the entry side portion of a given drug's overall profile of actions. Panel C depicts how a soft drug approach can be used to modify the elimination side portion of a given drug's overall profile of action. Both prodrugs and soft drugs can be used to decrease toxicity. Note that while "programmed metabolism" events are typically devised for both prodrug and soft drug strategies, this key event can also utilize chemically driven (nonenzymatic) conversions that have been programmed into the molecule to take advantage of specific physiological or pathophysiological chemical environments that are encountered after administration.

ischemic cardiac tissue by lowering its energy and oxygen requirements, was accompanied by considerable reservation. This was because unhealthy cardiac muscle often relies upon beta-1 adrenergic drive to sustain contractility, and when the latter was inhibited at too high a level during the early use of beta-1 blockers, it occasionally resulted in heart block and death [8]. Therefore, in this particular indication, the clinical challenge became the need for an effective level of drug-induced beta-receptor antagonism to be finely balanced against the need to have a critical level of endogenous-driven beta-agonism. Further complicating this challenge was the fact that this combination was also in a dynamic state of flux associated with an acute emergency situation wherein the precise level of adrenergic tone across

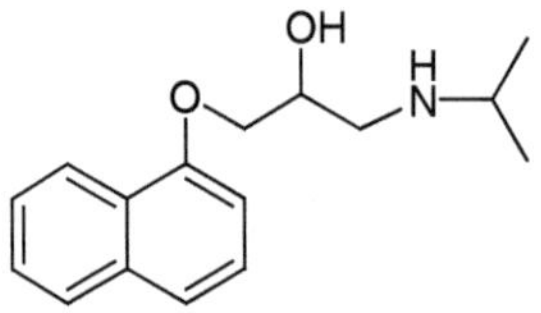


Propranolol, 1

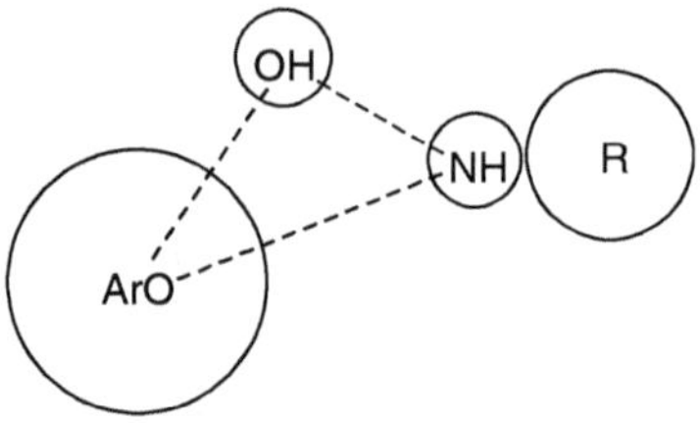


*beta*-Blocker
Pharmacophore

**Figure 14.2** Propranolol and the early beta-blocker pharmacophore [3]. As the "pioneer" (first successful) clinical agent for this important class of adrenergic drugs, propranolol (**1**) also served as the structural prototype for establishing early versions of the "aryloxypropanolamine" pharmacophore needed to antagonize beta-1 and beta-2 adrenergic receptors (itself being a nonselective beta-adrenergic blocking agent). This pharmacophore is grossly depicted as a single plane (dashed lines) established by three spatial regions consisting of (i) a lipophilic aryloxy moiety (ArO), (ii) a secondary hydroxyl group (OH), and (iii) a secondary amine bearing a lipophilic substituent (NH-R). While this topographical map has gradually evolved into a much higher level of sophistication, these three key regions in space as conveyed by this early cartoon have basically remained the same over the years.

the heart was very difficult to ascertain. This clinical paradigm is illustrated in Figure 14.3.

#### 14.1.2.3 **Pharmacological Target**

It was clear that the desired balance between adrenergic tone and its antagonism could be achieved and continually adjusted only if it were possible to titrate a beta-blocker's effects against some readily measurable parameter of cardiac function. This called for a short-acting version of propranolol that could be administered by the intravenous (iv) route, while the measurement of heart rate as a noninvasive "biomarker" was regarded as being a useful way to continually monitor the effects of such dosing. Not only could the level of blockade be readily adjusted for such a compound, if it were administered in too large an amount for a given patient, but also the short duration would allow the antagonistic effects to be quickly removed by simply stopping the drug infusion [8]. From clinical experience using dopamine, a naturally occurring short-acting renal vasodilator to effectively treat renal failure by iv infusion during late-stage shock, a half-life of about 10 min was envisioned to be ideal to precisely titrate the desired level of effect. Since the term "soft drug" had not yet been popularized, this new type of cardiovascular agent was dubbed an "ultra-short acting" beta-blocker.

Jumping across the translational research, which will be described later in the case study, the final embodiment that successfully addressed this clinical challenge by hitting the pharmacological target became the prototypical soft drug now known as esmolol. To complete the close connection between a given soft drug technology and its specific clinical indication, esmolol's pharmacology and clinical profile, as well as its deployment within the market, are summarized in the following section.

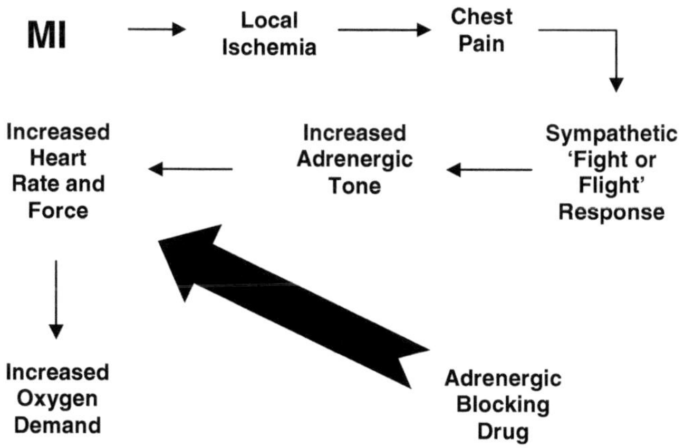


**Figure 14.3** Pathophysiology of acute myocardial infarction and its potential treatment with a beta-adrenergic receptor blocking agent [3]. Note that the body's natural "fight or flight" response can exacerbate the ischemic (low oxygen) damage during an MI because it increases the cardiac muscles' demand for oxygen. Alternatively, by attenuating heart rate and contractile force, a beta-blocker drug may be able to preserve cardiac tissue because oxygen demand will also be reduced. However, because the cardiac muscle is not healthy and its intrinsic beating properties may be compromised, it is important to maintain a certain level of beta-adrenergic tone (agonistic activity) in order to sustain heartbeats. Thus, in this critical setting, a delicate balance must be maintained between agonist drive and antagonist blockade of an adrenergic system that is in a very dynamic state of flux due to the ongoing pathophysiology and the body's misguided attempt to deal with it.

#### 14.1.2.4 **Pharmacology, Human Pharmacokinetic Profile, and Clinical Deployment**

Upon iv infusion to a dog animal model (Figure 14.4), esmolol quickly produces a pseudosteady state of beta-blockade and when the infusion is stopped, the effects of esmolol rapidly disappear with a half-life of about 10 min. Alternatively, propranol requires nearly 2 h to reach a pseudosteady state of blockade, and then dissipates only very slowly with a half-life of nearly 4 h.

In the clinic, esmolol has a distribution half-life of 2 min and an elimination half-life of 9 min. According to the most recent compilation of reports used for the package insert, esmolol hydrochloride is rapidly metabolized by enzymes chiefly residing in the cytosol of red blood cells.[1] Its volume of distribution is 3.4 l/Kg and its total clearance is 285 ml/Kg/min "which is greater than cardiac output; thus the metabolism of esmolol is not limited by the rate of blood flow to metabolizing tissues such as the liver, nor is it affected by hepatic or renal blood flow."[1] As expected from such a high rate of blood-based metabolism, less than 2% of the drug is excreted unchanged in the urine.[1] Within 24 h after infusion, approximately 73–88% of the total dose can be accounted for in the urine as the metabolite. Esmolol becomes about 55% bound to plasma proteins, while its metabolite is only 10% bound. The metabolite has been shown to have about 1/1500th the activity of esmolol in animal models, and in normal

1) Quote and details taken directly from package insert as provided by Bedford Laboratories™ for "Esmolol Hydrochloride Injection ready-to-use 10 mL vials."

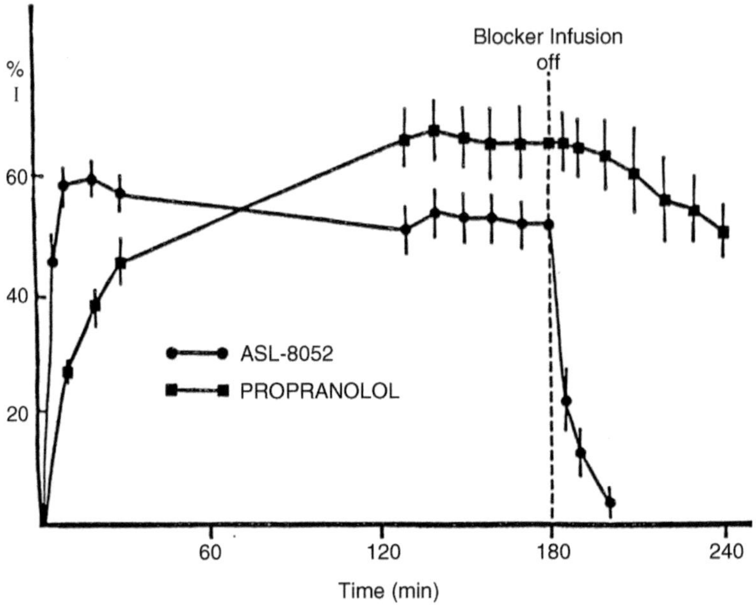


**Figure 14.4** Pharmacodynamic PK profile for esmolol versus propranolol [3]. A 3-h iv infusion of esmolol (designated above as "ASL-8052") versus propranolol in dogs (average of five animals for each drug) wherein percentage inhibition (% I) reflects beta-blockade of a standardized isoproterenol-induced tachycardia and the *x*-axis reflects time after the start of infusion. Note that the infusion for each agent was stopped at 180 min, such that the subsequent fall in activity of each curve reflects the half-life of each compound. The ultrashort-acting beta-blockade exhibited by esmolol compared to propranolol is striking. Its half-life achieves the pharmacological target value of 10 min. Error bars indicate ± one standard deviation.

volunteers its blood levels do not correspond to any significant level of beta-blockade. The metabolite has an elimination half-life of about 3.7 h and is excreted in the urine with a clearance approximately equivalent to the glomerular filtration rate.[1] Esmolol continues to be used clinically to control adrenergic tone across the heart in emergency room (ER) situations during critical care medicine of both very young and adult patients.[2] It also finds use for alleviating the adrenergic-burst-prompted trauma that can be experienced during intubation prior to surgery.

## 14.2 Indications

While the aforementioned example of an "ultra-short acting beta-blocker" effectively provides a glimpse of one prototypical agent, there are numerous other therapeutic

**2)** Esmolol enjoys a certain level of name recognition among the lay public in that its common use within emergency room settings has prompted the long-running television series entitled "ER" often to open its first scene with a physician shouting "Esmolol, STAT!" (STAT a medical acronym meaning immediately).

indications that could be well served by adopting a soft drug strategy. Many of these other uses are completely different from just making short-acting compounds. In all cases, however, the key feature remains that of programming a compound's metabolism so as to control its activity. Thus, a given parent drug (or new drug candidate) would be specifically modified so that its overall therapeutic profile is significantly enhanced (or becomes optimized for a new clinical indication), by incorporating a distinct soft drug construct into its chemical structure.

### 14.2.1
### A Huge Potential

More examples can be drawn by expanding the prototypical case cited above. Several other types of critical care drugs that are to be administered iv can be created via a soft drug strategy so as to provide for moment-to-moment control of their effects by readily adjusting their infusion drip rates. In addition to emergency room settings involving adult critical care patients, an entire line of such agents would be beneficial for the neonatal population in general [9–12].

Topical agents, including cosmetics and perfumes, as well as medications, could benefit by utilizing soft drug strategies wherein the so-modified products would be designed to quickly biodegrade and thus have no activity or side effects should they become absorbed into the systemic circulation. In addition to similar safety benefits, ocular agents could be designed to have specific durations of action; for example, an atropine-like dilator could be constructed so that its inconvenient light-sensitivity side effects would subside immediately after an eye has been examined [9–12].

More sophisticated constructs can be imagined by linking soft drug strategies with other technologies. For example, various drug delivery technologies could be partnered with soft drug approaches so as to localize a given drug's effects to the immediate vicinity of the injection, implant, or photoactivation site. Enhancing the selectivity of chemotherapeutic agents becomes possible by such a "dual technology" strategy. Similarly, these localization features could be incorporated into drugs used in surgical closure and wound-healing materials, such as antibiotics, growth inducers, or local pain killers. In all of these settings, the soft drugs would be designed to be quickly metabolized upon their departure from the immediate locale of the targeted biocompartment. These examples thus involve unique localization features that can be additionally instilled via soft drug approaches that go well beyond selectively administering the composite compound to the target area [9–12]. Finally, along these same lines and coming full circle with the overall theme of this book, one can imagine that a prodrug strategy could be used to target a certain biocompartment while simultaneously coupled with a soft drug strategy that could be used to further enhance its localization therein. A caveat for this type of combination construct, however, is that the prodrug would have to initially mask both the desired efficacious activity and the susceptibility to quick, programmed biodegradation until the "pro-soft prodrug's" arrival at the desired compartment wherein it would undergo a "dual bioactivation," that is, one for immediate activity and the other for subsequent programmed deactivation.

Alternatively, when a soft drug strategy is combined with delayed release formulation or delivery technologies, fine-tuning the rate of metabolism to match the rate of delivery into the general circulation would produce partnered technological systems capable of providing very consistent and prolonged, constant levels of medication in the blood. Again, a prodrug delivery approach could be used in place of a formulation technology with the same caveat as described above. In all of these cases, the general compartment would first be "primed" with active agent to initially establish the desired blood level that could then be precisely maintained by the so-described paired entry biodegradation technologies [9–12].

Many other smaller-market, therapeutic indications can be additionally imagined. The broad utility for potentially deploying soft drug technologies is further summarized in Table 14.1. Accompanying each setting listed in Table 14.1 is one or more parent drug that might be modified so as to achieve the desired soft drug properties.

### 14.2.2
### "To Market, To Market" [13]

From the wide array of potential soft drug applications, compounds for only a few indications have progressed all the way to the marketplace. Recall that we are not considering inherently short-acting agents such as epinephrine, dopamine, or

**Table 14.1** Clinical settings for which deployment of soft drug technologies could enhance existing therapeutic options [9–12].

| Settings | Exemplary parent drugs |
|---|---|
| 1. Weaning patients from a particular drug | Clonidine-like agents |
| 2. Eye examination drops | Atropine |
| 3. Neuromuscular blockade during surgery | Decamethonium, pancuronium |
| 4. Hypertensive crises (Raynaud's) | Prazosin, indoramin |
| 5. Consistent blood level when paired with sustained delivery technology | Phenytoin, carbamazapine |
| 6. ACE inhibitor for ER use | Enalaprilat |
| 7. Antihistamines for ER use | Diphenhydramine, famotidine |
| 8. Bronchopulmonary crises | Theophylline |
| 9. Anti-inflammatory for ER use | Indomethacin |
| 10. Antiarrhythmic for ER use | Lidocaine |
| 11. Vasodilator for ER use | Nifedipine, verapamil |
| 12. Localized action chemotherapeutics paired with localized administration or with photoactivation, sustained release, implants, sutures, or wound healing technologies or preparations | Various anticancer drugs, sulfamethoxazole, ampicillin, cephalexin, tetracycline |
| 13. Numerous topical agents, for example, psoriasis | Methotrexate |
| 14. Persistent pulmonary hypertension in newborns | Tolazoline |

procaine to be soft drugs even though their naturally quick metabolic degradation has been exploited very successfully in the clinic. Likewise, the numerous "drug wannabe" compounds [14] that may have made it to clinical testing but not yet to the stage of a market launch are also not being considered herein even though they may have been derived from a very significant amount of excellent work within the soft drug arena. Foremost in the area of both basic and applied soft drug research has been Bodor whose continuing efforts have gone on to eventually popularize the term that he initially introduced many years ago [1, 2, 15–17]. Representative medical uses that have received attention from Bodor and several other investigators include (i) additional beta-blockers for vascular [18–20], airway [21], and ocular [22, 23] indications; (ii) anticholinergic muscle relaxants [24] and ocular agents [25]; (iii) analgesics [26]; (iv) anti-inflammatory steroids [27, 28]; (v) antiarrhythmic agents [29, 30]; (vi) antimicrobials [1, 31]; (vii) ACE inhibitors [32]; (viii) calcium channel blockers [33]; and (ix) soft cannabinoids for ocular indications [34].

From this backdrop of potential use and ongoing basic research activities, a review of new chemical entities (NCEs) that actually entered the marketplace subsequent to the launch of esmolol (Brevibloc®) in 1987 suggests that only nine agents can be considered to be soft drugs. A few additional compounds take advantage of an inherently short duration of action, but they do not meet the intentionally programmed bioconversion drug design aspects of our strict definition. Alternatively, more than twice this number of NCEs appear to qualify as intentionally designed prodrugs. Table 14.2 lists the candidate soft drugs identified by our review. The accompanying Figure 14.5 provides each of their structures.

Leading this select group of NCEs with four entries are the anticholinergic muscle relaxant compounds **2–5** [35–38]. These compounds are designed to have a short duration of action similar to succinylcholine while serving as nondepolarizing neuromuscular junction blocking agents similar to *d*-tubocurarine. Characteristic structural features include (i) an acetylcholine-like pharmacophore consisting of a quaternary ammonium group connected to a simple ester arrangement via a two or three carbon linkage; (ii) a second quaternary ammonium group or an additional tertiary amine that becomes protonated at physiological pH, approximately 8 to 16 atoms away; and (iii) a bulky carbon skeleton either connecting or embedding the two positively charged moieties. With the ester portion of (i) serving to prompt a rapid biodegradation, (ii) providing binding to cholinergic receptors at the neuromuscular junction, and (iii) eliminating any intrinsic depolarizing activity, these compounds are administered as adjunct medications during intubation and as intravenous products for moment-to-moment control of muscle relaxation during surgery while exhibiting less side effects than their predecessor compounds.

The next largest group of entries contains three anti-inflammatory or antiallergy steroid compounds, namely, **6–8** [36, 39, 40]. These corticosteroids were derived from a considerable amount of preceding research that has, in turn, led to a large family of such agents. Characteristic structural features for these recent family members include esters placed at the 17 position of the D-ring within the prednisolone type of steroidal ring system. Compound **6** was introduced as a topical ointment for which the beneficial actions at the local inflammatory site are highly dissociated from any

**Table 14.2** Soft drugs identified from survey of all NCEs launched into the marketplace between 1987 and 2007 excluding esmolol (1987) that is discussed separately as a prototypical example and as a representative discovery case study. See Figure 14.5 for chemical structures..

| Cmpd. # | Name | Trade name | Company | Market launch | Indication | Lead Ref. |
|---|---|---|---|---|---|---|
| 2 | Mivacurium chloride | Mivacron | Wellcome | 1992 USA | Muscle Relaxant | [43] |
| 3 | Rocuronium bromide | Zemuron; esmeron | Organon | 1994 USA; UK | Muscle relaxant | [44] |
| 4 | Cisatracurium besylate | Nimbex | Glaxo Wellcome | 1995 USA | Muscle relaxant | [45] |
| 5 | Rapacuronium bromide | Raplon | Akzo Nobel | 1999 USA | Muscle relaxant | [46] |
| 6 | Betamethasone butyrate propionate | Antebate; antevate | Torii | 1994 Japan | Topical anti-inflam. | [47] |
| 7 | Loteprednol etabonate | Lotemax | Bausch & Lomb | 1998 USA | Opthalmic anti-inflam. | [48] |
| 8 | Fluticasone furoate | Veramyst | GSK | 2007 USA | Antiallergy | [49] |
| 9 | Remifentanil hydrochloride | Ultiva | Glaxo Wellcome | 1997 Germany | Analgesic | [50] |
| 10 | Landiolol | Onoact | Ono | 2002 Japan | Antiarrhythmic | [51] |

systemic side effects, presumably due to rapid biodegradation of compound **6** upon departure from its desired locale. Compound **7** is deployed as an ophthalmic suspension for inflammatory and allergic conditions of the eye. It has an improved safety profile compared to prior ophthalmic steroids due to its fast enzymatic transformation to an inactive metabolite upon its arrival in the systemic circulation. Finally, depending on the route of administration, it can be argued that compounds containing the unusual *S*-fluoromethyl carbothioate moiety like that within **8** should not be regarded as soft drugs because they rely upon the liver for their biodegradation and, as a result, they may be able to accumulate (**2**). Nevertheless, for **8**'s specific introduction to the marketplace as a nasal spray to treat allergic rhinitis, its discussion, if not classification, within the context of soft drugs seems quite justified. Following intranasal administration of **8**, most of the dose is actually swallowed. The carbothioate group rapidly undergoes extensive first-pass metabolism to its inactive carboxylate by the action of CYP3A4 located in the gut lining and liver such that there is negligible systemic exposure to active drug via the inadvertently obtained oral route. Likewise, systemic bioavailability from the airway passages has been estimated to be less than 0.5% with rapid metabolism again contributing favorably to this situation. Thus, the deliberate incorporation of a metabolic pharmacophore that leads to an efficaciously inactive and less toxic metabolite, even if not obtained perfectly in all of its potential clinical applications, certainly improves this agent's overall profile within the context of its usage described herein.

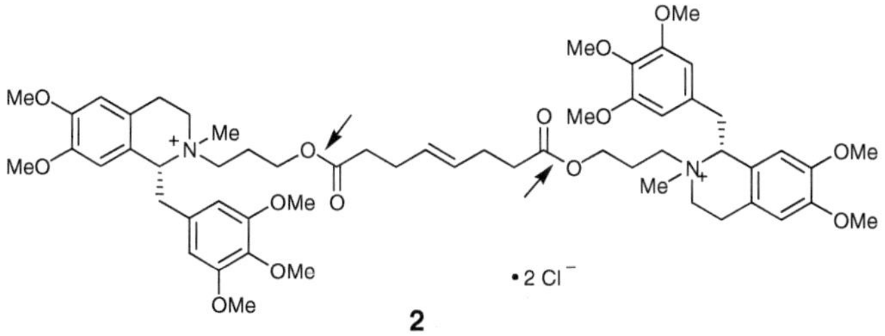

**2**

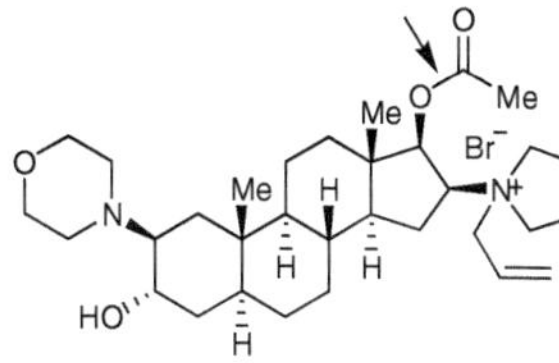

**3**

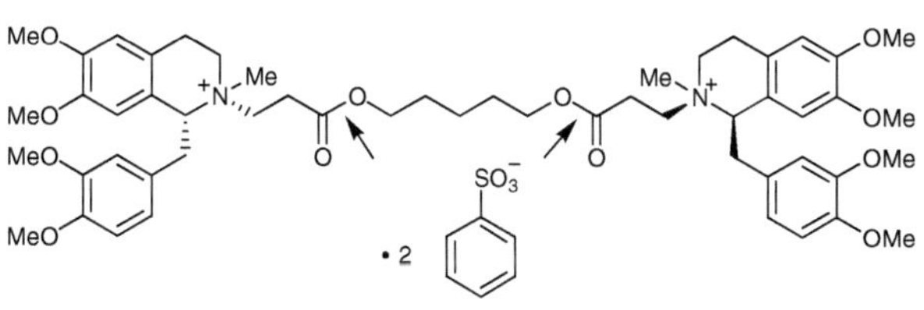

**4**

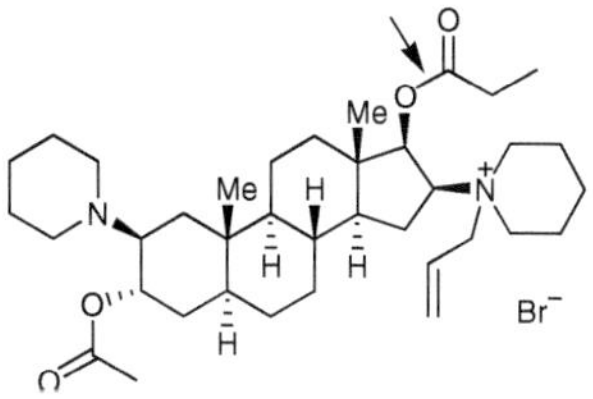

**5**

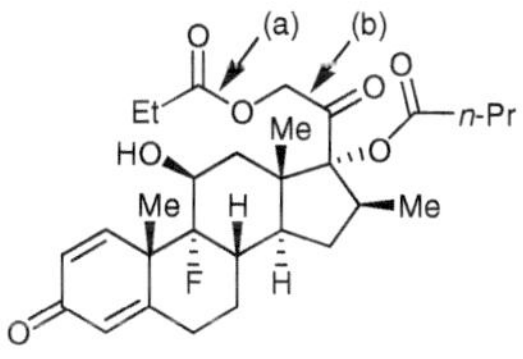

**6**

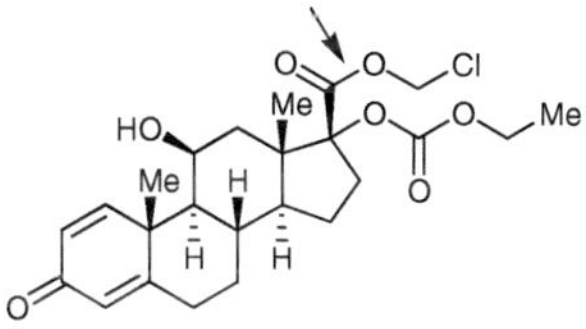

**7**

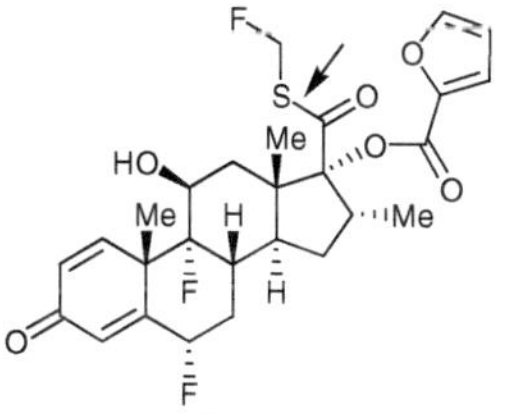

**8**

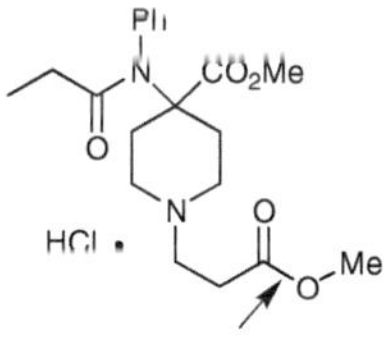

**9**

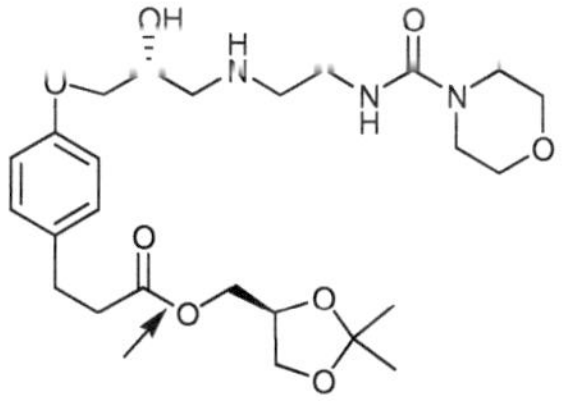

**10**

**Figure 14.5** Chemical structures of soft drugs identified from a survey of NCEs launched after the introduction of esmolol (1997) that ran until 2007. Arrows indicate "soft bonds" that are cleaved by intended metabolism. See Table 14.2 for additional details and main text for discussion. Note that compound **2** is a mixture of three stereoisomers and that in **6** metabolic hydrolysis (a) is followed by spontaneous collapse at (b).

The last two NCEs qualifying as candidates for soft drug status include an ultrashort-acting analgesic compound **9** [41], and perhaps fittingly as the final entry, an analogue of esmolol called landiolol, **10**, launched in 2002 [42]. Compound **9** is used by iv administration during general anesthesia and for the immediate management of postoperative pain. While its pharmacodynamic properties are similar to other μ agonists, **9**'s rapid onset and "offset" ($t_{1/2}$ of about 5 min) due to catabolism by general esterases afford a unique pharmacokinetic profile that is very useful for its indicated clinical settings. Compound **10** is indicated for uses similar to esmolol. Its β-blocking activity is more β1 selective than that of esmolol such that **10** is more cardioselective in its actions, although hypertension is proving to be its most frequent adverse event. The key structural feature for both of these final agents is the strategic incorporation of a simple ester moiety into the structural pharmacophore required for their desired efficacious activities.

## 14.3 Design Considerations

This section will highlight some of the most salient points associated with the design of soft drugs. For more in-depth treatment of this aspect, readers may refer to the chapter by Bodor and Buchwald and the accompanying chapter by our group within the latest edition of *Burger's Medicinal Chemistry* [2, 3].

### 14.3.1 General Requirements

A fundamental set of pharmacokinetic principles that must be adhered to during soft drug design is illustrated in Figure 14.6. First and foremost, if the rate of conversion of the soft drug via arrow (i) is not significantly faster than the sum of those associated with (ii), then the programmed control of the desired activity and a reduction in side-effect toxicity will not be obtained. Noting that this is a relative situation, such control can be approached both by slowing down the composite of pathways (ii) and by accelerating pathway (i). An equally important pharmacodynamic principle is that the chemical constructs added to the parent molecule so as to preferentially program the latter's conversion via pathway (i) must not significantly alter the parent compound's

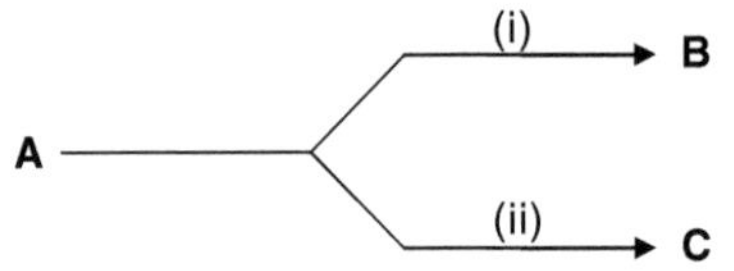


**Figure 14.6** Key pharmacokinetic relationships between metabolism and soft drugs. Soft drug **A** is active while metabolite **B** is inactive, nontoxic and, ideally, readily excreted. Metabolite **C** may be active, toxic, or lead to additional metabolites having such properties. Arrow (i) represents a metabolic pathway or chemically driven bioconversion that accomplishes the desired biodegradation. Arrow (ii) represents other metabolic and/or elimination pathways that can compete with (i). The goal in any soft drug design strategy is to have pathway (i) significantly predominate over the sum of all possible multiplicities of (ii) while also having the specific rate of (i) calibrated to a level of conversion that allows an optimal deployment of **A** within the clinic.

inherently efficacious activity, a requirement that is just the opposite of such considerations when designing prodrugs. Finally, the latter prompts the use of a fundamental medicinal chemistry principle that can be deployed when a new molecular construct is added to the parent compound, namely, that such adducts need to be placed within a neutral structure–activity region of the overall pharmacophore. Regions that can tolerate the soft drug adduct without a concomitant loss in potency will thus need to be defined by systematic structure–activity relationship (SAR) studies.

### 14.3.2 Enzymatic Aspects

Given these fundamental challenges associated with the design of soft drugs, it should be clear that the choice to be pursued for programming pathway (i) in an optimal manner becomes paramount. Furthermore, in addition to needing pathway (i) to dominate the metabolic competition from nondesirable pathways, it is also advantageous to design pathway (i) so that it is not subject to individual variation (genetic polymorphism) or to the potential for becoming involved in serious drug–drug interactions. In all of these regards, one of the most functionally prominent and diversity-tolerant broad category of human xenobiotic metabolizing enzymes are the hydrolases. Within this broad class, the subcategory of carboxylesterases contains the best candidates for manipulation during the design of both prodrug and soft drug strategies. In general, the carboxylesterases are metabolically aggressive toward a variety of ester arrangements while being subject to attenuation by "tailored" manipulation of their steric environments. They are ubiquitously distributed in plentiful amounts, which generally reduces their potential to become saturated and for their substrates to become involved in drug–drug interactions. Finally, they do not appear to be subject to high genetic polymorphisms in a manner that might compromise their eventual exploitation within the clinic. Thus, carboxylesterases represent an excellent starting point for pathway (i) during the early stages of considering a soft drug design strategy. History reveals that the carboxylic ester pathways have, indeed, been repeatedly pursued and often successfully exploited for both prodrug and soft drug purposes [52]. Similarly so for more recent surveys [53], including the one conveyed herein with respect to NCEs entering the marketplace over the last 20 years. For a further discourse of the esterases relative to the design of both prodrugs and soft drugs, readers may consult Refs [2, 3], as well as an entire text that has recently been dedicated to this topic [54].

### 14.3.3 Chemical Structural Aspects

As appreciated long ago by Hansch, one of the key paths traversed during a given drug's "random walk" throughout the body is that of xenobiotic metabolism that, in turn, is governed by the drug's overall physicochemical properties coupled to its distinct chemical structure [55, 56]. By analogy to Lipinski's "rule of five" that specifically pertains to a drug's ability to permeate membranes by passive processes [57], an elementary and generally useful "rule of thumb" related to physicochemical properties can likewise be applied to drug metabolism. Because this particular "rule" operates with such a high degree of certainty compared to all other rules that might be devised for predicting metabolism of a given xenobiotic, it has previously been referred to as "drug metabolism's rule of one" [3, 58, 59]. The rule pertains to the impact of steric features upon drug metabolism rates. From the start, it has been cast in conjunction with the hydrolysis of esters because of the dominant role that the latter typically play during biotransformation when compared to other chemical functional groups that may be found on a given xenobiotic [60, 61]. Within the context of esters, the portions of this "rule" that are the most relevant for the present discourse are as follows:

1) If there is a simple ester present in the molecule, it will typically get hydrolyzed as the predominant metabolic pathway unless it is sterically hindered.
2) All metabolic processes are exquisitely sensitive to steric features wherein the rate for any given event tends to be inversely proportional to the immediate steric environment at its biotransformation site.

The simplicity of this rule should be readily apparent in that it derives from the fundamental physical law that "no two bodies can occupy the same space at the same time." However, it is the rule's subtleties that become important for a medicinal chemist embarking upon a soft drug campaign. For example, after constructing an ester moiety within a parent "drug wannabe" based upon the previous delineation of an amenable structural space from a directed library that was assessed during hit follow-up chemistry, "metabolism's rule of one" suggests that it generally becomes quite feasible to fine-tune the hydrolysis rate according to systematic structural manipulation of the ester's immediate steric environment. While it should be apparent that one can often slow down reactions, including a given metabolic process, by steric inhibition, perhaps not so obvious is that it remains possible to deploy the logic of this rule to increase the hydrolysis rate of an added ester moiety. This interesting situation is further exemplified in Section 14.4. Continuing more specifically at this point, not only can the metabolic rate at a given enzyme be altered by a substrate's overall steric features but also can the selectivity for one esterase versus another be influenced by where such steric factors are explicitly constructed within the substrate. For example, CES1 versus CES2 selectivity can be so manipulated in a preferential manner by focusing upon the steric features placed either on the "alcohol side" or on the "carbonyl side" of the ester's acyloxy moiety [3].

Because other practical considerations during the design of soft drugs can be simultaneously influenced by the steric environment constructed around the moiety destined to drive path (i) in Figure 14.6, it is worthwhile to additionally track these variables while systematically defining the SAR between metabolic bioactivation rate and steric features. These factors include sufficient chemical stability to enable process and eventual manufacturing scale synthesis, "user-friendly" purification, and formulation of drug substance, as well as convenient storage and shelf life of the finished product [62]. Likewise, since steric impediments can be assembled with varying degrees of hydrophilicity that are very much under the control of the medicinal chemist, it becomes advantageous to simultaneously consider this physicochemical parameter during soft drug design so as to enhance, rather than detract from, the range of net polarity desired for optimum aqueous solubility and/or membrane penetration properties.

In terms of polarity, as long as lipophilic or hydrophilic extremes are not positioned within the immediate vicinity of the target enzyme's active site, the resulting impact upon metabolic rate should still track well to correlations directed primarily toward the systematic exploration of steric features. Alternatively, soft drug constructs containing highly polar groups will need to be investigated as their own distinct series relative to the specific enzyme associated with their pathway (i) process of biodegradation. For example, incorporation of a carboxylic acid group (which can ionize at physiological pH) too close to a carboxylester prodrug moiety represents a hydrophilic extreme that can dramatically attenuate the metabolic rates for substrates that depend upon carboxylesterases. Alternatively, incorporation of a phosphatyl moiety, even so close as to be part of the target ester linkage itself, is still subject to rapid hydrolysis when designing toward serum phosphatases to serve as pathway (i). Finally, close incorporation of amides and simple amines capable of protonating at physiological pH can sometimes lead to dramatic increases in metabolic rates relative to certain carboxylesterases. Examples for the latter include the simple aminoalkyl arrangement $RCO_2(CH_2)_2N(CH_2CH_3)_2$ that is normally present in procaine, an ultrashort-acting local anesthetic agent. Analogues of this arrangement have been used as soft drug moieties for some of the NCEs previously shown on Table 14.2. Thus, to be on the "safest ground" in terms of establishing steric-related SAR for a targeted carboxylesterase within the structural context of a given parent scaffold responsible for the desired efficacy, it remains prudent to construct the "soft drug wannabe" ester appendages in a manner that does not place ionizable groups too close to the prodrug moiety. Each type of "soft drug wannabe" ester and each substituted version of a given ester type having an additional ionizable group can then be examined as their own series by adopting the same constraints and using the preceding results as a growing baseline for rigorously assessing the importance of steric factors in a systematic manner. For a further discourse about ester groups and other types of less common moieties that can be deployed for bioconversion of both prodrugs and soft drugs, readers may consult Ref. [3].

A final, key chemical design aspect involves deciding where to place the potential bioconversion moieties within the parent structure. It has already been emphasized that for the specific case of soft drugs, this relationship must be constructed in such a manner that the inherent efficacy-related pharmacophore remains functionally undisturbed until the conversion event has taken place. With that as a fundamental principle, two very different strategies can be entertained. For cases where a parent drug's metabolism is already known, a metabolic "soft spot" can be converted into an ester linkage such that the latter then gains complete domination over all other metabolic possibilities. Because of its reliance upon a prior point of nonprogrammed metabolism, this useful strategy is called "retrometabolism-based drug design." This phrase again having been popularized by Bodor, readers may consult Ref. [2] for more detailed discussions about this particular strategy as delivered by its "founder." Alternatively and independent of the state of prior knowledge about the parent system's metabolism, soft drug design can be undertaken in a completely *ab initio* manner by either systematic exploration across the parent molecule or by a rational structural investigation driven by a specific hypothesis. The latter is exemplified in detail by the esmolol case study conveyed immediately below.

## 14.4 Case Study: The Discovery of Esmolol

As described in Section 1.2, the clinical need for an agent to attenuate adrenergic tone and address arrhythmias during critical cardiac conditions led to the pharmacological target called an "ultra-short acting beta-blocker." The latter's pharmacodynamic properties were supposed to reflect the efficacy afforded by the pioneer beta-adrenergic receptor blocking agent known as propranolol (shown as structure **1** in Figure 14.2). However, instead of having a long duration of action like **1**, the PK profile of the new agent was supposed to be dictated by a programmed ultrashort half-life of about 10 min. Because of the latter, the new agent's level of activity could thus be under moment-to-moment control via ready adjustment of its iv infusion drip rate. The remainder of this section describes how this clinical concept was translated into a novel composition of matter that hit the pharmacological target so precisely that it eventually became both a successfully marketed NCE and a classic example of a prototypical soft drug design construct, with all events transpiring well before such terminology had ever become popularized [3].

### 14.4.1 Internal Esters

Initially, another pioneer drug served as an additional starting point for drug design, this time to pursue the ultrashort-acting PK profile. As shown in Figure 14.7, procaine is a naturally short-acting anesthetic agent that is rapidly deactivated by esterase-mediated hydrolysis because its aryl and amino pharmacophoric elements get completely severed from their requisite contiguous arrangement. Combining the relevant "structural space" from **1** so as to retain its efficacy, with that of procaine so as to prompt a short duration of action, resulted in a "double analog-based design construct" that took the form of target compound **11** shown below in Figure 14.8.

By analogy to procaine, it was anticipated that metabolic hydrolysis of **11**'s ester would fragment the requisite beta-blocker pharmacophore. Portrayed in Figure 14.2, the key components of this pharmacophore are an aryloxy moiety, a secondary alcohol, and a secondary amino group, all displayed in a distinct 3D spatial arrangement usually specified by connection to a flexible three-carbon scaffold [5].

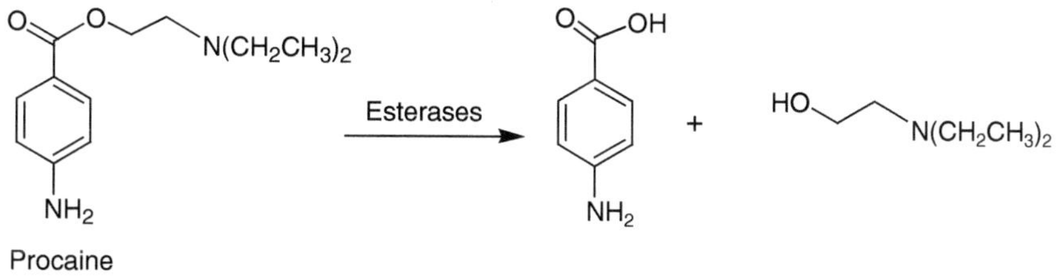


**Figure 14.7** Metabolic hydrolysis of procaine [3]. Esterases sever the requisite pharmacophore needed for its anesthetic action by converting procaine into two inactive fragments. Since this process is accomplished very rapidly in the body by these ubiquitous enzymes, procaine naturally exhibits an ultrashort duration of action after parenteral administration.

Disruption of this pharmacophore would deactivate such compounds. Because an ester linkage was to be incorporated within the requisite "aryloxypropanolamine" pharmacophore, these types of target molecules were called "internal esters" [3, 4, 63]. Previous SAR indicated that an increase in the oxypropyl chain's length by one carbon did not dramatically alter the interaction with beta-receptors. Thus, this useful bit of "neutral SAR" data gained from the literature suggested that the addition of a carbonyl moiety to create the desired ester linkage should also be an acceptable modification.

Unfortunately, these seemingly simple types of structures proved stubborn to synthesize. This was due, in part, to their propensity to undergo rapid side-product reactions that become problematic whenever the amine is not protonated. Although these side-product problems would eventually be solved [4, 64], an immediate solution to these difficulties was needed, including the possibility of pursuing different design constructs.

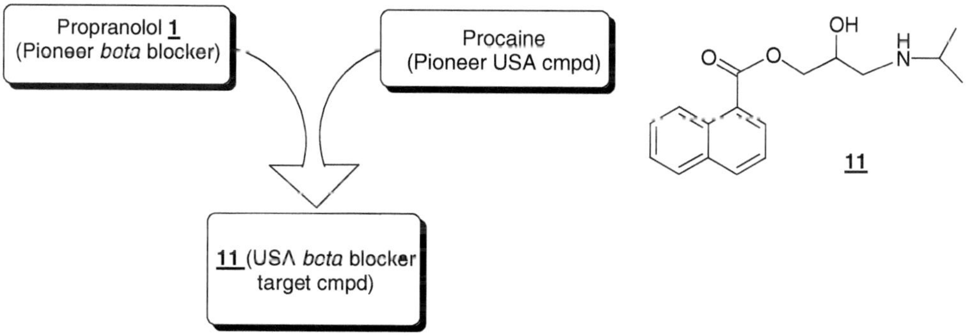


**Figure 14.8** Initial design of beta-blockers having an internal ester [3, 4]. The unique starting point for the rational design of these compounds (denoted as cmpd) was able to draw from two different prototypical structures: propranolol (**1** in Figure 14.2) for its beta-blocking activity and procaine (shown in Figure 14.7) for its ultrashort acting ("USA") duration of action.

### 14.4.2
### External Esters

The following medicinal chemistry logic and hypothesis led to an alternative design strategy. By virtue of their lipophilic nature, it was assumed that the aryloxy and typical *N*-aliphatic substituent portions of the beta-blocker pharmacophore interacted with the beta-receptor in a hydrophobic manner, for example, within distinct pockets that preferred lipophilic groups. Thus, while the presence of a "neutral" ester moiety placed in either of these areas of the parent drug molecule might be tolerated, it was hypothesized that the acid resulting from ester hydrolysis, upon further ionization at physiological pH and then likely accompanied by solvation with a cluster of water molecules, would represent an "extreme" that would not be well tolerated. These new target molecules are shown in Figure 14.9 as compounds **12** and **13**. Since their ester moieties had now been placed outside of the requisite beta-blocking pharmacophore, such compounds were called "aryl-" and "N-external esters," respectively. Because later reviews have not always conveyed this key conceptual design step in a clear manner, it becomes worthwhile to re-emphasize here that this critical aspect of the overall strategy pertaining to the discovery of esmolol was based upon what can be called a "lipophilic versus hydrophilic hypothesis." It had nothing to do with the metabolism observed for metoprolol (an ether-containing beta-blocker that has a long duration of action) or with any resemblance to "external" amide appendages as was present in practolol (which has a several-hour-long half-life) [65, 66]. Eventually proving to be a successful "umpolung" of a physicochemical property, when correctly appreciated this fundamental design concept has useful ramifications for prodrug/soft drug design constructs of today and for the future.

### 14.4.3
### "Square Pegs and Round Holes"

Although compound **13** provided certain synthesis challenges in terms of controlling the degree of N-alkylation [67], several compound representatives for both of these new series were able to be prepared quickly [68–70]. The resulting increase in the overall lipophilicity for these types of esters when placed on a naphthyl system analogous to **1**, however, proved to lower aqueous solubility to the point that biological

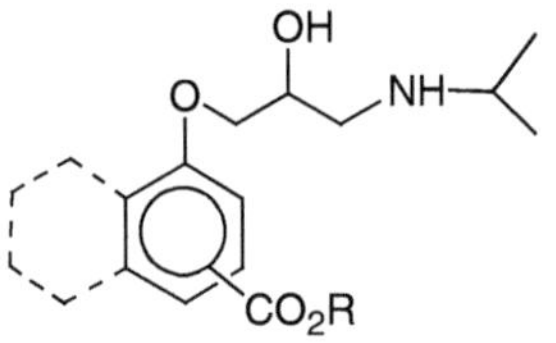


**12**

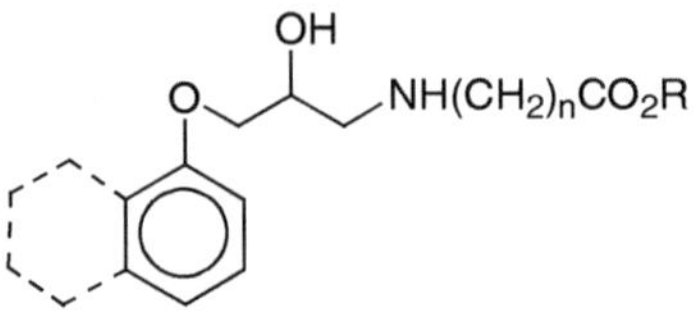


**13**

**Figure 14.9** General external ester target molecules [3, 4, 63]. For both the aryl- (**12**) and N-external esters (**13**), the dashed-line ring is intended to also represent a naphthalene system that would then be most analogous in design to the prototypical beta-blocker propranolol (**1** in Figure 14.2).

assessment became problematic. The single phenyl ring system was therefore deployed as an alternative scaffold because it provided a perfectly adequate aryl pharmacophoric element while having higher aqueous solubility. However, when a single-ring system was left unsubstituted, significant intrinsic sympathomimetic activity (ISA) became problematic. Given the earlier synthetic difficulties encountered with the internal esters ("strike one"), at this point the poor behavior toward testing the external esters encountered first with the low aqueous solubility naphthyl series and immediately followed by the second ISA-problematic series of N-external esters ("strikes two and three") almost caused the entire ultrashort-acting beta-blocker program to be dropped. After nearly a year into this program with nothing to show, management had begun to consider the effort to obtain ultrashort-acting drugs to be equivalent to trying to "put a square peg into a round hole." Rightly so, they wanted literature precedent indicating that the rational design and successful obtainment of a compound could be accomplished for any case of an ultrashort-acting agent. Still "ahead of its time" in this regard, however, the only examples to be found for this type of PK profile related to naturally short acting compounds ("accidental soft drugs" so to speak) rather than to any intentionally devised agents.

### 14.4.4
### Surrogate Scaffolds for Testing Purposes and a "Glimmer of Hope"

To address the ISA issues, a series of nonester-substituted phenyl aryloxypropanolamine systems was quickly prepared and examined to find a more suitable scaffold to allow true exploration of the uncharted structural space associated with the N-external ester constructs. This series is depicted in Figure 14.10. After measuring beta-blocker potency, overall lipophilicity via partition coefficient, and level of ISA, an *ortho*-methyl-phenyl ring was chosen for series **13**. Note that the ring in **12** is inherently substituted via its external ester placement, and so it did not show significant problems with ISA. Importantly, in both **12** and **13**, these types of esters were found to retain their potency as beta-blockers.

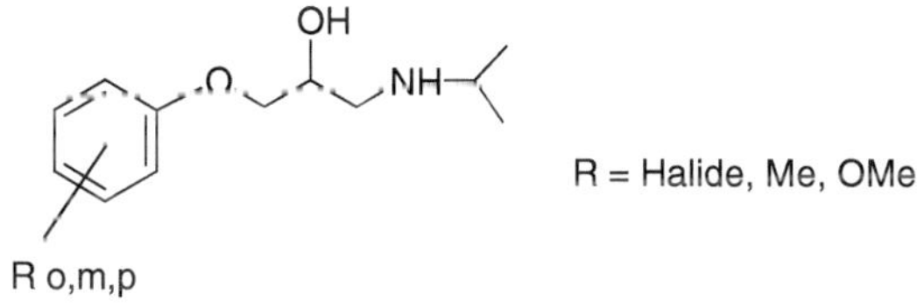


**Figure 14.10** Identification of a surrogate scaffold for exploring the N-external ester concept [3, 4]. Approximately, a dozen compounds were prepared and tested for beta-blocking potency, relative lipophilicity via partition coefficient, and ISA effects. An "*ortho*-methyl-phenyl" system was selected because of its high beta-blocker activity, acceptably low relative lipophilicity, and absence of ISA. This scaffold was then deployed with the N-external ester types of target series previously shown as **13** (Figure 10.9) and ultimately demonstrated for the first time that external ester constructs could indeed be utilized to create ultrashort-acting beta-blockers.

Even more important for the fundamental hypothesis and novel design strategy, however, the carboxylic acid (anticipated metabolite) versions of these constructs were found to be essentially inactive. As mentioned for **13**, a substituted phenyl ring was required to eliminate ISA for the N-external esters. In both **12** and **13**, the effects of aromatic substitution followed the pattern where *ortho*-substituents enhanced potency greater than *meta*-substituents that were more active than those placed in a *para*-position. Furthermore, the fall in potency was much greater for beta-2 receptors than for beta-1 receptors. Thus, while the *para*-substituted series had an overall lower potency, they were more selective for beta-1 in their actions. This efficacy-related SAR trend was in accord with that suggested by the existing literature for nonester-containing β-blockers [5]. In addition, another structure–metabolism relationship (SMR) was beginning to be conceptualized and it would soon lead to a second important medicinal chemistry-derived hypothesis that also can still be very useful for today's prodrug/soft drug design constructs. This concept stems from early observations associated with a comparison of the half-life data for some of the initial aryl external ester compounds, namely, **14** and **15** as shown in Figure 14.11. Compound **14**, in particular, began to demonstrate a significantly shortened half-life. However, in terms of the overall program, while management now acknowledged that the 30-min half-life was "close," they were also quick to reiterate that the target value was actually 10 min and that there was still "no cigar" from all of this "basic research stuff." Thus, the programmatic "chop-block" continued to loom ominously over the entire "USAβB" project.

### 14.4.5
### A "Goldilocks" Compound Called Esmolol

For **14** and **15**, the half-lives for beta-blocking activity in an *in vivo* dog model were found to be 30 and 60 min, respectively. Speculating that this difference reflected steric effects, it was hypothesized that hydrolysis might be even quicker for esters having less steric hindrance. But how can one construct a simple ester system smaller than the methanol partner that is already present as part of this arrangement in compound **14**?

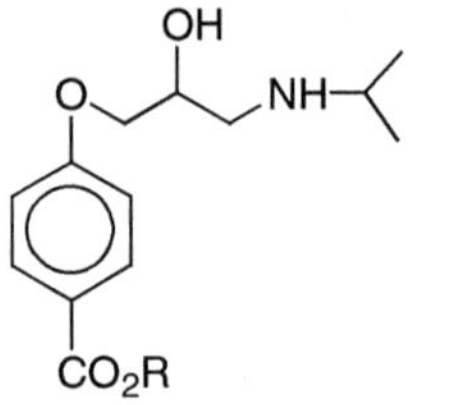


| | R | $t_{1/2}$ (min) |
|---|---|---|
| 14 | $CH_3$ | 30 |
| 15 | $CH_2CH_3$ | 60 |

**Figure 14.11** Early-stage aryl-external esters [3, 4]. In addition to suggesting that this type of construct could be used to create ultrashort-acting beta-blockers, these particular compounds prompted a key hypothesis about the potential importance of steric effects in relation to metabolic hydrolysis rates. Eventually manipulated in a manner that proved to be successful, this hypothesis was later formalized as the key feature within what we have come to call "metabolism's rule of one."

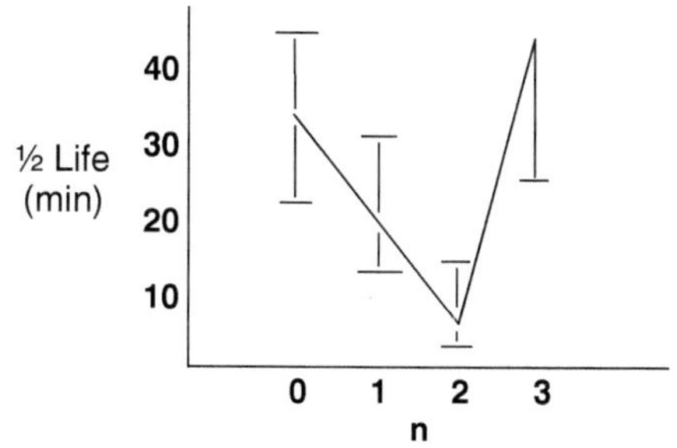


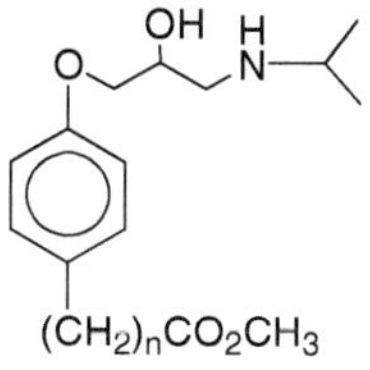


**16**

**Figure 14.12** Proposed relief of steric impediment caused by the phenyl ring system [3, 4, 69]. The correlation between biological half-life in minutes and added methylene unit spacers (*n*) was assessed by measuring 80% recovery from 50% beta-blockade of isoproterenol-induced tachycardia (agonist effect) after iv administration to anesthetized dogs (five animals per reading). Error bars indicate ± standard deviation. Note that when $n = 0$, then **16** is the same as **14** and when $n = 2$, then **16** is what later came to be called esmolol. The seeming paradox observed for $n = 3$ is discussed in the chapter.

Since that is not possible from the alcohol side of the ester, one might instead focus attention upon the carbonyl side of the ester. And so came the notion that it might be advantageous to further distance the entire ester linkage from its proximity to the neighboring (bulky) phenyl ring. To address this hypothesis, compound series **16** was prepared wherein methylene "spacers" were sequentially added between the ester's carboxyl group and its attached phenyl ring. These compounds and their corresponding half-life data are shown in Figure 14.12 [69]. The *Goldilocks* nature[3] of **16**, where only $n = 2$ is "just right" for the desired duration, likely reflects the removal of the steric impediment caused by the aryl ring and thus supports the hypothesis behind the design of this series. Likewise, the paradox observed for **16** when $n = 3$ could reflect conformational folding of the *para*-substituent such that its ester group tends to reside closer to the overall bulk displayed by the entire aryloxypropanolamine system. Alternatively, drawing from today's increased knowledge of the various carboxylesterases, compound **16** might be so long as to become sterically hindered by the "rear" wall of these enzymes' active sites [3]. Either way, at this point in the esmolol story, the "Goldilocks compound" clearly demonstrated much more than just a "glimmer of hope" for the overall program, and the image of the "chop-block" was beginning to fade away.

The pharmacokinetic profile exhibited by **16**$n = 2$ (initially designated as "ASL-8052" and destined to become "esmolol") was depicted in Figure 14.4. This figure also shows the marked superiority of this analogue over propranolol for this type of clinical indication. Ultimately, the desired 10-min half-life was reproduced in humans. Further illustrating the importance of this exquisite inverse relationship uncovered between enzymatic hydrolysis rates and steric bulk is the fact that all the attempts to increase metabolic hydrolysis rates by constructing "good (electronic) leaving group"

**3)** Given the unique half-life for esmolol (16 with $n = 2$; 10 min) compared to either the higher or lower homologues ($n = 3$ or $n = 1$ being too long), this result has been referred to as the "Goldilocks effect." The term "Goldilocks" is derived from an Anglo-Saxon fairytale and in this context means "just right."

esters had only a negligible influence upon this process [68, 69]. Presumably, once Mother Nature is freed from steric constraints and gains proper access to a potential substrate, "she" needs no further assistance to lower the transition state energy for effecting an enzymatic conversion with high precision and efficiency. More details about esmolol's clinical profile have been provided in Section 14.1.

### 14.4.6
### "Esmolol Stat"[2)]

As stated previously, esmolol is used to control adrenergic tone across the heart in emergency room situations during critical care medicine of both very young and adult patients.[1)] It also finds use for alleviating the adrenergic-burst-prompted trauma that can be experienced during intubation prior to surgery. During the later stages of esmolol clinical development, this type of drugs, that is, drugs having a deliberately appended functional group that is constructed to program a specified metabolic deactivation pathway and rate, came to be known as "soft drugs" [60]. Thus, in the end, esmolol itself has become a "pioneer soft drug" for which the template portrayed in bold-faced atoms in Figure 14.13 can now serve as an effective starting point for "soft analog-based drug design" [3, 63].

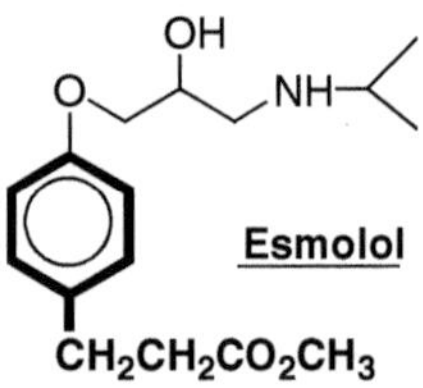


**Figure 14.13** "Short-acting" pharmacophore derived from esmolol [3, 4, 63]. The substructure in bold represents a generally useful soft drug design construct. It can be deployed as a potential design element for ultrashort activity as long as the arrangement can be placed within a parent compound in an efficaciously innocuous manner (retention of activity), coupled with the likelihood that upon hydrolysis the parent molecule's pharmacophore is either severed or the conversion leads to an "external" carboxylic acid moiety that is not tolerated by the biological surface associated with efficacy. Similarly, this short-acting pharmacophore can also be generally useful for the design of prodrug constructs whenever its arrangement can be introduced in a manner that inactivates the parent drug coupled with the knowledge that subsequent hydrolysis will occur to effect bioactivation back to the parent molecule. A simple example of the latter would be to mask a nonsterically hindered primary alcohol (required as part of a parent drug's efficacious pharmacophore) as its ester wherein the carboxylic acid to be deployed is a phenylpropionic acid, perhaps further substituted on the phenyl ring to achieve some other beneficial physicochemical property for the overall system. In this prodrug example, the methyl alcohol portion of the esmolol ester would thus be replaced by the aliphatic primary alcohol of the parent compound. Once a baseline is established for this metabolic pharmacophore deployment within a new structural context as either a soft drug or a prodrug construct, then the additional use of steric features to fine-tune the observed hydrolysis rate can be further manipulated to allow final hybridization of the new system to a specifically desired PK profile.

### 14.4.7 Case Study Summary and Some Take-Home Lessons for Today

The discovery of esmolol initially took advantage of a combination of analogue-based drug design from two different types of pioneer drugs, namely, propranolol for efficacy and procaine for an ultrashort duration of action. During soft drug design and experimental investigations, a novel medicinal chemistry hypothesis pertaining to a "lipophilic umpolung" led to a significant departure from procaine's internal ester structure and prompted investigation on the external ester constructs. The latter, in turn, eventually led to esmolol as the "Goldilocks" arrangement upon subsequent exploration of another key hypothesis pertaining to the inverse relationship between enzymatic ester hydrolysis rates and steric factors (now part of "metabolism's rule of one"). In addition to demonstrating several of the chemical and metabolic principles that are useful for the design of soft drugs and prodrugs, some of the hurdles traversed during the discovery of esmolol provide useful lessons for today's medicinal chemists who often are confronted by problems associated with a lead compound's overall PK profile [16, 60]. These final comments are listed below in a summary fashion under headings common to the jargon of today's drug discovery process [16, 60]. Taken together, these comments convey the important role that creative medicinal chemistry can play both toward establishing useful fundamental principles and toward the practical improvement or specific tailoring of selected therapeutic entities.

#### 14.4.7.1 Compound Libraries

While the attributes of a "drug-like" profile are in no way to be minimized, the first and foremost properties for a proposed test series during early drug discovery is certainly their "assay-likable" profile, that is, if a compound cannot be tested you would not get a result, or even worse, it may be perceived that one has an inactive compound and erroneously derive a negative SAR data point. Indeed, for the case of esmolol, the entire research program was almost halted when its first two series of target compounds were either too insoluble or too plagued by ISA to be able to be effectively screened.

Likewise, while "preferred scaffolds" and "privileged structures" generally refer to the attributes of such molecules relative to their potential clinical performance as drug candidates, this concept need not be so restrictive. For example, it may be useful to think in terms of the various preclinical testing steps to exploit attributes to examine a specific hypothesis that will be ultimately reapplied to the actual lead series. This was done for esmolol when the N-external esters served as important testing surrogates to help confirm the merits of the overall "external esters hypothesis" and to firmly establish that it is not necessarily required to fragment a pharmacophore in order to eliminate activity.

Although the redundancy of close homologues within a compound library may detract from "molecular diversity," their inclusion should not be precluded altogether, and certainly their pursuit should not be regarded as a mundane operation once a lead has been selected. Additional comments in this regard are provided Section 14.4.7.3.

#### 14.4.7.2 **Biological Testing**

While high-throughput screening (HTS) can work its way through huge libraries of test compounds in short order, it also pays to periodically check template representatives in an *in vivo* setting as early as possible during the screening process. In this case study, the discovery of esmolol actually relied upon a dog model to immediately ascertain overall metabolic stability. Although time consuming, this allowed the entire *in vivo* hydrolytic complement to be discerned, rather than quickly conducting a biochemical battery of discrete enzymatic assays. Had the latter been undertaken, SAR would have been very likely to have crossed back and forth from one test system to another for various molecular series, perhaps even to the extent of being noninterpretable as a composite of data relative to the key hypotheses being explored.

#### 14.4.7.3 **SAR**

The sole production of efficacy-associated "positive hit" data as typically derived from HTS methods can seriously detract from creative problem-solving medicinal chemistry. Note that verification of the key hypothesis leading to the pursuit of the external esters was actually gleaned from the novel "negative SAR" data found for the proposed carboxylic acid metabolites, with the anticipated "neutral SAR" data associated with the esters also falling nicely into place.

While hydrophilic/hydrophobic and/or substituent electronic properties may be important for various selected interactions with a given biological surface, steric effects are by far the most reliable and universally applicable parameter when trying to monitor and exploit SMR. Recall that the esmolol ester family was essentially nonresponsive to the electronics of the "leaving group." Alternatively, it was exquisitely sensitive to localized steric parameters in terms of enzymatic hydrolysis rates. Indeed, the inverse relationship between the degree of steric bulk and the rate of drug metabolism within such localized vicinities is generally so much reliable compared to any other attempted physicochemical correlation that it does indeed deserve to be considered as "metabolism's rule of one," just as was advocated during several of the earlier discourses in this chapter.

Finally, the importance of pursuing methyl, ethyl, propyl, and so on as a medicinal chemist fine-tunes a lead is worth mentioning again in this category, that is, the "Goldilocks" nature of esmolol with its distinct 10-min half-life was found to reside only at $n = 2$ within series **16**. With esmolol still saving lives daily within ERs across the globe, what more can be said about the potential merits of carefully conducting such systematic molecular scrutiny in a deliberately methodical manner?

## 14.5 Summary

Soft drugs represent a unique class of compounds that are distinct from prodrugs. Although both rely upon drug alterations that are programmed to occur *in vivo* to dictate their course of efficacious actions, soft drugs are active agents that get converted into inactive compounds while prodrugs are inactive compounds that get converted into active agents. The design strategies that can be deployed to control the desired drug alteration step for both soft drugs and prodrugs draw from the same set of fundamental medicinal chemistry principles. Generally, these molecular constructs involve prompting esterases to affect a selected hydrolysis at a specified rate after strategically placing ester functionalities into the parent drug molecules. Several subtle but key features associated with these types of molecular incorporations have been elaborated within the body of this chapter.

Discovered in the late-1970s and eventually marketed in 1987, esmolol represents a prototypical soft drug for which the story of its translational research provides several "take home" lessons that remain useful today both for the pursuit of such agents and for medicinal chemistry drug design and development activities in general. Even though numerous clinical indications can be entertained for the beneficial use of soft drug strategies, a survey of the NCEs entering the marketplace since the launch of esmolol suggests that only about nine of such compounds qualify as soft drugs. More than twice that number qualify as prodrugs. Thus, while the potential offered by the composite of these strategies would seem to be receiving reasonable attention during the course of today's drug discovery process, the potential of soft drugs, in particular, still appears to be underutilized.

## References


1 Bodor, N. (1977) Soft drugs, in *Design of Biopharmaceutical Properties Through Prodrugs and Analogs* (ed. E.B. Roche) Academy of Pharmaceutical Sciences, Washington D.C., pp. 98–135.

2 Bodor, N. and Buchwald, P. (2003) Retrometabolism-based drug design and targeting, in *Burger's Medicinal Chemistry, Drug Discovery and Development*, 6th edn (ed. D.J. Abraham), John Wiley & Sons, Inc., New York, pp. 533–608.

3 Erhardt, P.W., Khupse, R., Sarver, J.G., and Trendel, J.A. (2010) Prodrugs: strategic deployment, metabolic considerations and chemical design principles, in *Burger's Medicinal Chemistry, Drug Discovery and Development*, 7th edn (ed. D.J. Abraham and D.P. Rotella). John Wiley & Sons, Inc., New York, pp. 1–71.

4 Erhardt, P.W. (1993) Esmolol, in *Chronicles of Drug Discovery*, vol. **3** (ed. D. Lednicer) ACS Books, Washington, D.C, pp. 191–206.

5 Erhardt, P.W. and Matos, L. (2006) Selective beta-adrenergic receptor blocking agents, in *Analogue-Based Drug Discovery* (eds J. Fischer and C.R. Ganellin), Wiley-VCH Verlag GmbH, Weinheim, pp. 193–232.

6 Fischer, J. and Ganellin, C.R. (eds) (2006) *Analogue-Based Drug Discovery*, Wiley-VCH Verlag GmbH, Weinheim.

7 Fischer, J. and Ganellin, C.R. (eds) (2010) *Analogue-Based Drug Discovery II*, Wiley-VCH Verlag GmbH, Weinheim.

8 Zaroslinski, J., Borgman, R.J., O'Donnell, J.P., Anderson, W.G., Erhardt, P.W., Kam, S.T., Reynolds, R.D., Lee, R.j., and Gorczynski, R.J. (1982) Ultra short acting beta-blockers: a proposal for the treatment of the critically ill patient. *Life Sciences*, **31**, 899–907.

9 Erhardt, P.W. (2000) Aralkyl ester soft drugs. U.S. Patent filed 2000 with Divisional and CIPs still issuing.

10 Erhardt, P.W. (2004) Aralkyl ester soft drugs divisional I: clonidine indication. US Patent 6750238 B1.

11 Erhardt, P.W. and Aouthmany, M.M. (2004) Aralkyl ester soft drugs CIP I: methods and compositions for treating persistent pulmonary hypertension. US Patent 6756047 B2.

12 Erhardt, P.W. (2007) Aralkyl ester soft drugs divisional II: phenytoin indication. US Patent 7164017 B2.

13 The phrase "to market, to market" has been borrowed from the chapters dedicated to this topic within the running series *Annual Reports in Medicinal Chemistry*, ACS Publishing, Washington D.C.

14 Erhardt, P. (2009) Drug discovery, in *Pharmacology: Principles and Practice* (eds M. Hacker, W.S. Messer Jr. and K.A. Bachmann), Elsevier, Oxford, pp. 473–559.

15 Bodor, N., Kaminski, J.J., and Selk, S. (1980) Soft drugs. 1. Labile quaternary ammonium salts as soft antimicrobials. *Journal of Medicinal Chemistry*, **23** (5), 469–474.

16 Bodor, N. and Kaminski, J.J. (1980) Soft drugs. 2. Soft alkylating compounds as potential antitumor agents. *Journal of Medicinal Chemistry*, **23** (5), 566–569.

17 Bodor, N., Woods, R., Raper, C., Kearney, P., and Kaminski, J.J. (1980) Soft drugs. 3. A new class of anticholinergic agents. *Journal of Medicinal Chemistry*, **23** (5), 474–480.

18 Lin, Y.-T., Wu, B.-N., Wu, J.-R., Lo, Y.-C., Chen, L.-C., and Chen, I.-J. (1996) Vasomolol: an ultra short-acting and vasorelaxant vanilloid type β1-adrenoceptor antagonist. *Journal of Cardiovascular Pharmacology*, **28** (1), 149–157.

19 Atarashi, H., Kuruma, A., Yashima, M., Saitoh, H., Ino, T., Endoh, Y., and Hayakawa, H. (2000) Pharmacokinetics of landiolol hydrochloride, a new ultra-short acting β-blocker, in patients with cardiac arrhythmias. *Clinical Pharmacology and Therapeutics*, **68** (2), 143–150.

20 Hwang, S.-K., Juhasz, A., Yoon, S.-H., and Bodor, N. (2000) Soft Drugs. 12. Design, synthesis, and evaluation of soft bufuralol analogs. *Journal of Medicinal Chemistry*, **43** (8), 1525–1532.

21 Waldeck, B. (1995) β-Adrenoceptor agonists after terbutaline. *Pharmacology & Toxicology*, **77** (Suppl. 3), 25–29.

22 Stampfli, H.F. and Quon, C.Y. (1995) Polymorphic metabolism of flestolol and other ester containing compounds by a carboxylesterase in New Zealand white rabbit blood and cornea. *Research Communications in Molecular Pathology and Pharmacology*, **88** (1), 87–97.

23 Bodor, N., Elkoussi, A., Zuobi, K., and Kovacs, P. (1996) Synthesis and pharmacological activity of adaprolol enantiomers: a new soft drug for treating glaucoma. *Journal of Ocular Pharmacology and Therapeutics*, **12** (3), 387.

24 Savarese, J.J., Ali, H.H., Basta, S.J., Embree, P.B., Scott, R.P.F., Sunder, N., Weakly, J.N., Wastila, W.B., and El-Sayad, H.A. (1988) The clinical neuromuscular pharmacology of mivacurium chloride (BW B1090U): a short-acting nondepolarizing ester neuromuscular blocking drug. *Anesthesiology*, **68** (5), 723–732.

25 Juhasz, A., Huang, F., Ji, F., Buchwald, P., Wu, W.M., and Bodor, N. (1998) Design and evaluation of new soft anticholinergic agents. *Drug Development Research*, **43** (2), 117–127.

26 Haidar, S.H., Moreton, J.E., Liang, Z., Hoke, J.F., Muir, K.T., and Eddington, N.D. (1997) Evaluating a possible pharmacokinetic interaction between remifentanil and esmolol in the rat. *Journal of Pharmaceutical Sciences*, **86** (11), 1278–1282.

27 Orgel, H.A., Meltzer, E.O., Bierman, C.W., Bronsky, E., Connell, J.T., Lieberman, P.L., Nathan, R., Pearlman, D.S., Pence, H.L., Slavin, R.G. *et al.* (1991) Intranasal fluocortin butyl in patients with perennial rhinitis: a 12-month efficacy and safety study including nasal biopsy. *The Journal of Allergy and Clinical Immunology*, **88** (2), 257–264.

28 Howes, J. and Novack, G.D. (1998) Failure to detect systemic levels, and effects of loteprednol etabonate and its metabolite, PJ-91, following chronic ocular administration. *Journal of Ocular Pharmacology and Therapeutics*, **14** (2), 153–158.

29 Chorvat, R.J., Black, L.A., Ranade, V.V., Barcelon-Yang, C., Stout, D.M., Brown, B.S., Stampfli, H.F., and Quon, C.Y. (1993) Mono- and bis (aminomethyl)phenylacetic acid esters

as short-acting antiarrhythmic agents. *Journal of Medicinal Chemistry*, **36** (17), 2494–2498.

**30** Morey, T.E., Seubert, C.N., Raatikainen, M.J.P., Martynyuk, A.E., Druzgala, P., Milner, P., Gonzalez, M.D., and Dennis, D.M. (2001) Structure–activity relationships and electrophysiological effects of short-acting amiodarone homologs in guinea pig isolated heart. *The Journal of Pharmacology and Experimental Therapeutics*, **297** (1), 260–266.

**31** Graffner-Nordberg, M., Kolmodin, K., Aqvist, J., Queener, S.F., and Hallberg, A. (2001) Design, synthesis, computational prediction, and biological evaluation of ester soft drugs as inhibitors of dihydrofolate reductase from Pneumocystis carinii. *Journal of Medicinal Chemistry*, **44** (15), 2391–2402.

**32** Baxter, A.J.G., Carr, R.D., Eyley, S.C., Fraser-Rae, L., Hallam, C., Harper, S.T., Hurved, P.A., King, S.J., and Meghani, P. (1992) (*R*)-2-(3-Mercapto-2(*S*)-methyl-1-oxopropoxy)-3-(methylthio)propanoic acid (FPL 66564), the first ultra-short-acting angiotensin converting enzyme inhibitor. *Journal of Medicinal Chemistry*, **35** (20), 3718–3720.

**33** Kieler-Jensen, N., Jolin-Mellgard, A., Nordlander, M., and Ricksten, S.-E. (2000) Coronary and systemic hemodynamic effects of clevidipine, an ultra-short-acting calcium antagonist, for treatment of hypertension after coronary artery surgery. *Acta Anaesthesiologica Scandinavica*, **44** (2), 186–193.

**34** Buchwald, A., Derendorf, H., Ji, F., Nagaraja, N.Y., Wu, W.-M., and Bodor, N. (2002) Soft cannabinoid analogues as potential anti-glaucoma agents. *Die Pharmazie*, **57** (2), 108–114.

**35** Strupczewski, J.D. and Ellis, D.B. (1993) To market, to market – 1992. *Annual Reports in Medicinal Chemistry*, **28**, 325–341.

**36** Cheng, X.-M. (1995) To market, to market – 1994. *Annual Reports in Medicinal Chemistry*, **30**, 295–317.

**37** Cheng, X.-M. (1996) To market, to market – 1995. *Annual Reports in Medicinal Chemistry*, **31**, 337–355.

**38** Gaudilliere, B. and Berna, P. (2000) To market, to market – 1999. *Annual Reports in Medicinal Chemistry*, **35**, 331–356.

**39** Gaudilliere, B. (1999) To market, to market – 1998. *Annual Reports in Medicinal Chemistry*, **34**, 317–338.

**40** Hegde, S. and Schmidt, M. (2008) To market, to market – 2007. *Annual Reports in Medicinal Chemistry*, **43**, 455–497.

**41** Galatsis, P. (1997) To market, to market – 1996. *Annual Reports in Medicinal Chemistry*, **32**, 305–326.

**42** Boyer-Joubert, C., Lorthiois, E., and Moreau, F. (2003) To market, to market – 2002. *Annual Reports in Medicinal Chemistry*, **38**, 347–374.

**43** Wrigley, S.R., Jones, R.M., Harrop-Griffiths, A.W., and Platt, M.W. (1992) Mivacurium chloride: a study to evaluate its use during propofol-nitrous oxide anaesthesia. *Anaesthesia*, **47** (8), 653–657.

**44** Wicks, T.C. (1994) The pharmacology of rocuronium bromide (ORG 9426). *AANA Journal*, **62** (1), 33–38.

**45** Hunter, J.M. (1995) New neuromuscular blocking drugs. *The New England Journal of Medicine*, **332** (25), 1691–1699.

**46** Onrust, S.V. and Foster, R.H. (1999) Rapacuronium bromide: a review of its use in anesthetic practice. *Drugs*, **58** (5), 887–918.

**47** Koshiyama, Y., Maekawa, Y., Kojima, T., Kariya, K., Muto, T., Ohtani, H., Ueda, N., Kanno, S., Uchiyama, H., Tamegaya, M., and Oda, M. (1994) Topical anti-inflammatory activity with weak systemic side effects of betamethasone butyrate propionate (BBP) on paper disk granuloma in rats. *Oyo Yakuri (Pharmacometrics)*, **47** (5), 489–493.

**48** Dell, S.J., Shulman, D.G., Lowry, G.M., and Howes, J. (1997) A controlled evaluation of the efficacy and safety of loteprednol etabonate in the prophylactic treatment of seasonal allergic conjunctivitis. *American Journal of Ophthalmology*, **123** (6), 791–797.

**49** Sorbera, L.A., Serradell, N., and Bolos, J. (2007) Fluticasone furoate. *Drugs Future*, **32** (1), 12–16.

50 Feldman, P.L., James, M.K., Brackeen, M.F., Bilotta, J.M., Schuster, S.V., Lahey, A.P., Lutz, M.W., Johnson, M.R., and Leighton, H.J. (1991) Design, synthesis, and pharmacological evaluation of ultrashort- to long-acting opioid analgesics. *Journal of Medicinal Chemistry*, **34** (7), 2202–2206.

51 Sugiyama, A., Takahara, A., and Hashimoto, K. (1999) Electrophysiologic, cardiohemodynamic and β-blocking actions of a new ultra-short-acting β-blocker, ONO-1101, assessed by the *in vivo* canine model in comparison with esmolol. *Journal of Cardiovascular Pharmacology*, **34** (1), 70–77.

52 Lin, J.H. and Lu, A.Y. (1997) Role of pharmacokinetics and metabolism in drug discovery and development. *Pharmacological Reviews*, **49**, 403–449.

53 Ettmayer, P., Amidon, G.L., Clement, B., and Testa, B. (2004) Lessons learned from marketed and investigational prodrugs. *Journal of Medicinal Chemistry*, **47** (10), 2393–2404.

54 Testa, B. and Mayer, J.M. (eds) (2003) *Hydrolysis in Drug and Prodrug Metabolism*, Verlag Helvetica Chimica Acta, Zurich, Switzerland.

55 Hansch, C. and Fujita, T.J. (1964) P-σ-π analysis. A method for the correlation of biological activity and chemical structure. *Journal of the American Chemical Society*, **86**, 1616–1626.

56 Hansch, C. and Leo, A. (1979) *Substituent Constants for Correlation Analysis in Chemistry and Biology*, John Wiley & Sons, Inc., New York, NY.

57 Lipinski, C.A., Lombardo, F., Dominy, B.W., and Feeney, P.J. (1997) Experimental and computational approaches to estimate solubility and permeability in drug discovery and development settings. *Advanced Drug Delivery Reviews*, **23**, 3–25.

58 Erhardt, P.W. (2009) Drug discovery, in *Pharmacology: Principles and Practice* (eds M. Hacker, K. Bachmann, and W. Messer), Elsevier, Oxford, UK, pp. 475–560.

59 Erhardt, P.W. and Proudfoot, J.R. (2007) Drug discovery: historical perspective, current status and outlook, in *Comprehensive Medicinal Chemistry II* (eds J.B. Taylor and D.J. Triggle), Elsevier, Oxford, UK, pp. 29–96.

60 Erhardt, P. (2002) Medicinal chemistry in the new millennium: a glance into the future. *Pure and Applied Chemistry*, **74**, 703–785.

61 Erhardt, P. (1998) Drug metabolism data: past and present status. *Medicinal Chemistry Research*, **8** (78), 400–421.

62 Beaumont, K., Webster, R., Gardner, I., and Dack, K. (2003) Design of ester prodrugs to enhance oral absorption of poorly permeable compounds: challenges to the discovery scientist. *Current Drug Metabolism*, **4**, 461–485.

63 Erhardt, P. (2006) Case study: 'esmolol stat', in *Analog-Based Drug Discovery* (eds J. Fischer and R. Ganellin), Wiley-VCH Verlag GmbH, Weinheim, Germany, pp. 233–246.

64 Kam S.T., Martier, W.L., Mai, K.X., Barcelon-Yang, C., Borgman, R.J., O'Donnell, J.P., Stampfli, H.S., Sum, C.Y., Anderson, W.G., Gorczynski, R.J., and Lee, R.J. (1984) [(Arylcarbonyl)oxy] propanolamines. 1. Novel beta-blockers with ultrashort duration of action. *Journal of Medicinal Chemistry*, **27**, 1007–1016.

65 Bodor, N. and Buchwald, P. (2000) Soft drug design: general principles and recent applications. *Medicinal Research Reviews*, **20**, 58–101.

66 Gringauz, A. (1997) *Introduction to Medicinal Chemistry. How Drug Act and Why*, John Wiley & Sons, Inc., New York.

67 Erhardt, P.W. (1983) Benzylamine and dibenzylamine revisited. Syntheses of N-substituted aryloxypropanolamines exemplifying a general route to secondary aliphatic amines. *Synthetic Communications*, **13**, 103.

68 Erhardt, P.W., Woo, C.M., Gorczynski, R.J., and Anderson, W.G. (1982) Ultra-short-acting beta-adrenergic receptor blocking agents. 1. (Aryloxy) propanolamines containing esters in the nitrogen substituent. *Journal of Medicinal Chemistry*, **25**, 1402–1407.

69 Erhardt, P.W., Woo, C.M., Anderson, W.G., and Gorczynski, R.J. (1982) Ultra-short-acting β-adrenergic receptor

blocking agents. 2. (Aryloxy) propanolamines containing esters on the aryl function. *Journal of Medicinal Chemistry*, **25**, 1408–1412.

70 Erhardt, P.W., Woo, C.M., Matier, W.L., Gorczynski, R.J., and Anderson, W.G. (1983) Ultra-short-acting beta-adrenergic receptor blocking agents. 3. Ethylenediamine derivatives of (aryloxy) propanolamines having esters on the aryl function. *Journal of Medicinal Chemistry*, **26**, 1109–1112.

# Part Four
# Preclinical and Clinical Consideration for Prodrugs

*Prodrugs and Targeted Delivery: Towards Better ADME Properties.* Edited by Jarkko Rautio

ISBN: 978-3-527-32603-7

# 15
# Pharmacokinetic and Biopharmaceutical Considerations in Prodrug Discovery and Development

*John P. O'Donnell*

## 15.1
## Introduction

Optimization of drug efficacy is based on successful delivery to its site of action. Drug concentrations act directly at key receptors through inhibition (as an antagonist) or through stimulation (as an agonist). The magnitude and duration of response is influenced by the amount of time that drug remains at the site of action, the affinity for the drug at the targeted receptor, and level of drug concentration achieved. The study of drug concentration over time in living systems is called pharmacokinetics. In this aspect, the process for which concentrations rise and fall in the body are influenced by absorption, distribution, metabolism, and excretion (ADME) of the drug of interest. While the consideration of drug concentration and duration at the site of action is key to understanding its activity of therapeutic interest, the potential for off-target pharmacology must also be considered in terms of safety of the dosing regimen. Thus, the goal of delivering effective drug concentrations to yield a desired therapeutic effect must be tempered by safety considerations. Prodrugs enable the effective delivery of active compound to its site of action at the appropriate concentrations required for efficacy. The types of prodrug strategies utilized are becoming as varied as the classes of active drugs themselves. A recent comprehensive review of successful prodrug strategies discusses the developing expertise in this science and the expansion of chemical space that can be pursued for drug discovery and development [1]. This chapter will introduce the basic concepts of phamacokinetics and ADME properties that influence the success of a prodrug strategy.

## 15.2
## Understanding Pharmacokinetic/Pharmacodynamic Relationships

A simple consideration of optimizing the pharmacokinetic profile/regimen for efficacy can be observed with compounds used in the treatment of bacterial infections. Depending on their mechanism of action, some drug classes such as

*Prodrugs and Targeted Delivery: Towards Better ADME Properties.* Edited by Jarkko Rautio

ISBN: 978-3-527-32603-7

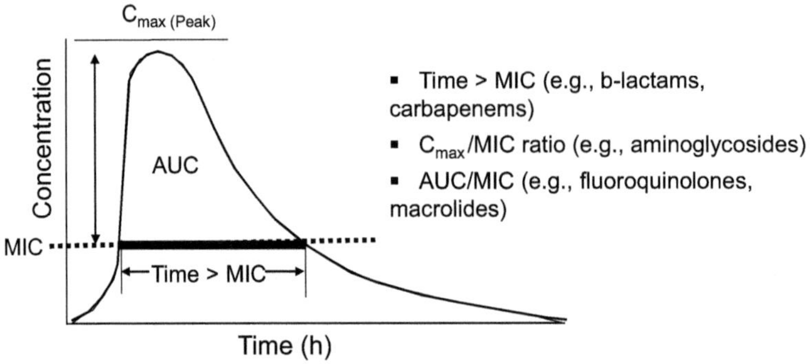


**Figure 15.1** PK/PD driver relationships for drug efficacy.

fluoroquinolones and aminoglycosides exhibit concentration-dependent killing (activity increases with increased concentration) while other classes such as β-lactams demonstrate time-dependent activity where optimum pathogen killing is achieved by maintaining drug concentration above a minimum inhibition concentration (MIC). Three major PK/PD driver relationships emerge in this analysis – $C_{max}$/MIC, AUC/MIC, and $T>$ MIC (Figure 15.1) [2]. In this aspect, the plasma concentration or the tissue concentration versus time profile should be considered based on maximizing therapeutic value without compromising safety. In the case of β-lactams, further increases in drug concentration beyond a minimum inhibitory concentration are of diminished value. Dosing paradigms for β-lactams that infuse and hold drug concentrations for a set duration (30–40% $T>$ MIC, typical) will demonstrate the optimum activity and unnecessarily high concentrations will be avoided to ensure a safe therapeutic regimen. Other classes of antibacterial agents such as aminoglycosides can be optimized by achieving higher $C_{max}$ concentrations. These differences will translate to very different plasma concentration versus time profiles. Thus, an effective pharmacokinetic profile for a particular therapy needs to be understood as part of a successful prodrug strategy.

## 15.3 Pharmacokinetics

While a review of fundamental pharmacokinetics is not the intent of this chapter, a basic understanding of concepts such as clearance (CL), volume of distribution ($V$), half-life ($t_{1/2}$), and bioavailability ($F$) is important because they relate to the pharmacokinetic profile target for a compound of interest. Conceptually, clearance is the volume of fluid from which drug is eliminated per unit time. The volume of distribution is the mathematical representation of the apparent volume that the drug is dissolved within the body. The actual volume of water within a human is 0.6 l/kg [3]. For a set amount of drug, the initial concentration will be lower for a compound that exhibits a high volume of distribution compared to one with a low volume of distribution. Half-life of drug elimination is related to volume of distribution and clearance by the following expression:

$$T_{1/2} = \ln 2 \times \left(\frac{V}{CL}\right)$$

Thus, it follows that half-life will increase with an increase in volume of distribution and/or reduction of clearance. While the individual parameters of clearance and volume of distribution dictate drug concentration, half-life is an important consideration in dosing regimen. Short half-life drugs will often need to be dosed more frequently to achieve adequate concentrations at the site of activity, particularly for compounds whose pharmacodynamics is characterized as time dependent. While these concepts are important for the disposition of the parent or the active drug itself, they are equally important in the consideration of prodrugs since the clearance and volume of distribution of the prodrugs may be quite different than their active moieties. In particular, a prodrug would need to be sufficiently bioconverted to their active products prior to direct elimination of the prodrug themselves.

For oral prodrugs, the concept of bioavailability is an important consideration in the development of a prodrug strategy. For an active compound, oral bioavailability can be established from determining the area under curve (AUC) following intravenous and oral administrations of the compound (ideally in a crossover fashion):

$$\mathrm{F} = \frac{\mathrm{AUC_{PO}} \times \mathrm{Dose_{IV}}}{\mathrm{AUC_{IV}} \times \mathrm{Dose_{PO}}}$$

While the doses do not necessarily need to be the same, a key assumption is that the clearance is the same after oral and IV dosing. Related to the concept of oral bioavailability is the "first-pass effect," which is the sequential impact of absorption, intestinal metabolism, and processing in the liver on oral bioavailability. It can be estimated as:

$$F_{\mathrm{PO}} = (1 - f_{\mathrm{abs}}) \times (1 - f_{\mathrm{gut}}) \times (1 - f_{\mathrm{hepat}})$$

where $F_{\mathrm{PO}}$ represents oral bioavailability, $f_{\mathrm{abs}}$ represents the fraction of dose not absorbed, $f_{\mathrm{gut}}$ represents the fraction of drug cleared from the gut wall via metabolism and $f_{\mathrm{hepat}}$ represents the fraction of drug cleared from the liver via metabolism and/or secretion into bile. Alternately, oral bioavailability is often expressed in terms of the fraction of dose remaining following absorption and metabolism/excretion in the gut and liver:

$$F_{\mathrm{PO}} = F_{\mathrm{abs}} \times F_{\mathrm{gut}} \times F_{\mathrm{hepat}}$$

where $F_{\mathrm{abs}} = (1 - f_{\mathrm{abs}})$, $F_{\mathrm{gut}} = (1 - f_{\mathrm{gut}})$, and $F_{\mathrm{hepat}} = (1 - f_{\mathrm{hepat}})$. If gut metabolism and urinary excretion is minimal, $f_{\mathrm{hepat}}$ can be estimated as a ratio of total drug CL and blood flow to the liver ($Q_{\mathrm{H}}$) where $f_{\mathrm{hepat}} = \mathrm{CL}/Q_{\mathrm{H}}$. Oral bioavailability can then be simplified to:

$$F_{\mathrm{PO}} = F_{\mathrm{abs}} \times \left(1 - \frac{\mathrm{CL}}{Q_{\mathrm{H}}}\right)$$

where $Q_H$ is hepatic blood flow (~20 ml/min/kg for a human). In this aspect, it is important to consider the impact of hepatic and/or intestinal metabolism on overall bioavailability of a compound or the active (parent) moiety of a prodrug. Early in the discovery process, promising compounds are often pursued as oral agents due to convenience of administration. Upon finding poor oral bioavailability, it was often mistakenly thought that poor absorption is the main reason for low exposure and a strategy to make a lipophilic, hydrolyzable prodrug is pursued aggressively. While this may indeed be the case, compounds that demonstrate poor intestinal and/or hepatic stability due to metabolic processing are not desirable candidates for a prodrug strategy, unless the prodrug is capable of surviving metabolism through the intestine and liver. Compounds whose metabolic clearance approaches hepatic blood should be avoided as candidates for an oral prodrug strategy. While the dose extraction due to $f_{gut}$ may be difficult to estimate *in vivo*, $f_{hepat}$ can be determined for active parent from *in vivo* studies in preclinical species equipped with jugular and portal vein catheters [4]. In this case, $f_{hepat}$ can be determined as:

$$f_{hepat} = 1 - \left(\frac{AUC_{hpv}}{AUC_{IV}}\right)$$

where $AUC_{hpv}$ represents the area under curve following administration of dose directly into the portal vein and $AUC_{IV}$ is the area under curves established following intravenous delivery of the same dose. The advantage of evaluating $f_{hepat}$ *in vivo* is that it includes both metabolic clearance and biliary excretion contributions to $f_{hepat}$. Extrapolation and scalability of these findings from preclinical species to humans, however, is subject to further elucidation of the clearance mechanism(s) involved for the compound being investigated. Species differences in clearance can often lead to an inaccurate prediction of human pharmacokinetics. Alternately, an estimate of metabolic clearance in the liver can be carried out *in vitro* using liver subfractions such as microsomes and hepatocytes. An initial evaluation of the metabolic stability of the active parent using these *in vitro* reagents would be prudent to ensure that the compound is sufficiently stable to survive first pass. The fraction of dose remaining after first-pass metabolism in the liver can be estimated as:

$$F_{hepat} = 1 - \left(\frac{fu \times CL_{int}}{Q_H + fu \times CL_{int}}\right)$$

where $fu$ is the free fraction of the drug, $CL_{int}$ is the free intrinsic clearance established in the *in vitro* system, and $Q_H$ is hepatic blood flow [5, 6]. It follows that a compound with high intrinsic clearance ($fu^*CL_{int} \gg Q_H$) that hepatic clearance becomes blood flow dependent and $F_{hepat}$ approaches zero. Thus, an oral prodrug strategy for a compound with high intrinsic clearance could be problematic, particularly if a significant portion of the dose is converted to active parent in the gut or in the portal bloodstream. The importance of characterization of the ADME properties of the active parent early in the discovery cycle cannot be underestimated since these data are integral in the development of a successful prodrug approach. Improvement in physicochemical properties to improve oral absorption offers little for a compound that undergoes extensive metabolism in the liver.

## 15.4
## Tools for the Prodrug Scientist

The complexities associated with prodrug delivery require a balance of *in vivo* and *in vitro* approaches in a drug discovery and development setting [7]. Screening efforts conducted using *in vitro* stability, permeability, and transporter experiments provide the opportunity to streamline evaluation of multiple analogues in a cost-effective manner. In addition, these experiments are increasingly being evaluated with human tissues and/or cell lines such as Caco-2 expressing relevant enzymes and transporters of clinical interest. Stably transfected cell lines expressing specific human transporters such as PEPT1, MCT-1, and P-glycoprotein (MDR1) are commonly used for targeted oral delivery, and for understanding the potential for nonabsorptive efflux liabilities [8, 9]. Alternately, the complex, dynamic environment associated with the *in vivo* system is impossible to reproduce in its entirety. Intestinal enzymes important for the conversion of prodrugs such as carboxylesterases, amidases, aminopeptidases, and phosphatases are expressed ubiquitously in mammalians [10–15] allowing for evaluation of prodrug performance in a suitable preclinical species. While substrate affinity and expression of hydrolytic enzymes and transporters often varies among species, some such as PEPT1 are highly conserved in sequence, distribution, and activity. For instance, regional expression of PEPT1 in rats closely resembles that of humans with higher expression in the proximal portion of the small intestine and minimal expression in the colon [16, 17]. Several studies have demonstrated similar substrate affinity and activity between the two species particularly with regard to the absorption of oral β-lactams. Human absorption across several drug classes in general has been shown to correlate with rats, however, this analysis has not been fully evaluated for prodrugs [18]. In addition to supporting formulation development, *in vivo* models such as the intestinal-vascular access ported (IVAP) dog model can be used to further understand regional absorption and first-pass metabolism. This approach, for instance, has been used to elucidate the contributions of first-pass losses in the gut ($f_{gut}$) and liver ($f_{hepat}$) for verapamil [19] and the absorption window of the nucleoside 2′,3′-dideoxyinosine [20]. Care must be taken, however, in the interpretation of absorption data obtained in dogs due to the potential for higher paracellular absorption compared to those obtained in other species [21].

### 15.4.1
### Bioanalytical Assay Development

Bioanalytical and metabolite identification support is critical for the development of an effective prodrug program. The analysis of active parent concentrations alone provides limited information, unless of course the prodrug works extremely well, converting rapidly and quantitatively to the targeted compartment. At a minimum, assays to determine intact prodrug and active parent concentrations are necessary to evaluate prodrug distribution and conversion efficiency. In addition, a better understanding of oral bioavailability and its dependence on $f_{gut}$ and $f_{hepat}$ following oral, intravenous, and intraportal delivery can be achieved with prodrug and active parent

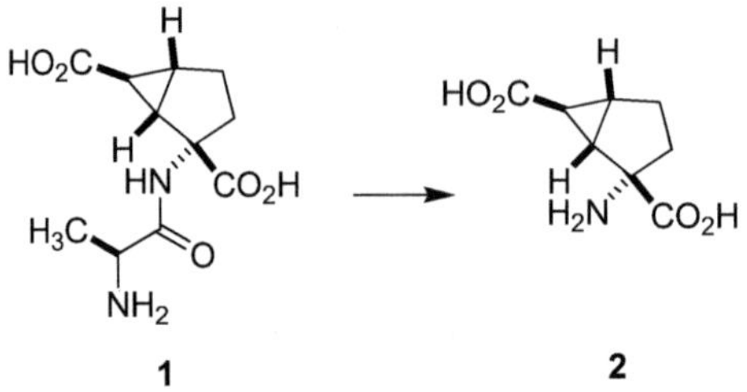

**Figure 15.2** Conversion of LY544344 to LY354740.

concentrations. *In vivo* pharmacokinetic studies with LY544344 (**1**), a prodrug of the Group II metabotopic glutamate receptor agonist LY354740 (**2**), demonstrated only 3% of the $C_{max}$ of LY354740 in the portal vein suggesting rapid and near complete conversion during absorption of the compound (Figure 15.2) [22]. These data were consistent with *in vitro* evaluation of the prodrug in jejunal homogenate where extensive hydrolysis of the prodrug was observed [23]. It is important to note that monitoring of intact prodrug as well as active parent is typically required for regulatory submissions that include toxicokinetic evaluation in GLP toxicology studies even when prodrug levels may be minimal due to rapid metabolic conversion. Diligence with respect to stabilizing blood samples and developing a robust analytical assay for a prodrug prone to hydrolyze in the blood may be problematic. In our experience, whole-blood assays with immediate quenching and cooling of the sample in an appropriate stabilizing buffer are required to quantify levels of circulating prodrug. The use of EDTA as an anticoagulant and preservative helps due to its ability to inhibit metallopeptidase activity, but this typically is insufficient for long-term stability of the sample. Dilution of the sample with a low pH buffer (~4–5) typically will provide the necessary storage stability required should reassay of the sample be required.

### 15.4.2
### Use of Radiolabel

A greater level of understanding prodrug disposition is achieved with the use of radiolabeled compound. Insufficient physicochemical properties, nonproductive metabolism and excretion of intact prodrug can be major reasons for prodrug failure. The use of radioalabeled compound provides quantitative assessments of mass balance, absorption, and metabolite formation. Availability of radiolabel may also provide better resolution with Caco-2 permeability and uptake assays where a better mechanistic understanding of carrier-mediated processes is warranted. Ideally, the active parent is labeled in a metabolically stable position so its fate can be determined following conversion from the prodrug. At times, it may be appropriate to use a dual label or conduct a separate *in vivo* study with the radiolabel incorporated on the prodrug side chain to further understand its metabolic and excretory fate. This work would be encouraged for novel or potentially reactive prodrug side chains where the safety of the agent is unknown. For oral prodrug approaches, the fraction of radiolabeled dose excreted in urine serves as a measure of $F_{abs}$ since absorption is required for radiolabel to be excreted into the urine. Alternately $F_{abs}$ can be estimated by drug administration in separate oral and intravenous studies and quantifying the amount of unchanged drug excreted in the urine from each study. The ratio of unchanged drug excreted in the urine from oral and intravenous administration is equivalent to $F_{abs}$. This estimate, however, is based on the assumption that clearance is route independent, which may not entirely accurate given the complexities associated with prodrug disposition.

## 15.5 Enzymes Involved with Prodrug Conversion

### 15.5.1 Carboxylesterases

Hydrolase activity plays an important function in the conversion of prodrugs to their pharmacologically active parent compounds. The abundance of ester containing prodrugs on the market is attributed to the catalytic efficiency of these enzymes in the conversion of esters of hydroxyl, phenolic, and carboxyl compounds [10]. Carboxylesterases play a predominant role in the hydrolysis of prodrug esters such as angiotensin-converting enzyme inhibitors, for example, temocapril (**3**) [24] and antitumor agents, for example, irinotecan (CPT-11, **4**) [25] and capecitabine (**5**) (Figure 15.3) [26]. The majority of carboxylesterases fall within two isozyme families, CES1 and CES2, which are characterized by their substrate specificity, tissue distribution, immunological properties and gene regulation [14]. In humans, hCE-1, a CES1 isozyme, is distributed throughout many tissues with the notable exception of the intestine. However, the human CES2 isozymes hCE-2 and hiCE are expressed throughout the intestine, liver, and kidney [27]. In general, hCE-1 catalyzes the hydrolysis of esters with large acyl and small alcohol moieties, whereas hCE-2 can hydrolyze esters of smaller acyl and larger alcohol groups [14, 28]. Thus, a compound such as temocapril with its small alcohol group and large acyl group is hydrolyzed predominantly by hCE-1, while CPT-11 with its bulky alcohol group is hydrolyzed almost exclusively by hCE-2. Both families of carboxylesterases are extensively expressed in mammalian species; however, notable differences do exist. For instance, there is minimal hydrolase activity in the small intestine of dog, which can have important implications for the use of this species in the evaluation of ester prodrugs [13]. Hydrolase activity in the small intestine of humans and rats, however, is similar with exclusive expression of CES2 isozymes and similar distribution along the length of the intestine [15]. Human carboxylesterases are expressed differently between colon carcinoma and adjacent normal tissue with hCE-1 and hCE-2 more abundant in normal tissues. The expression pattern of CES isozymes in Caco-2 monolayers is very different from the human intestine and much more consistent with human liver containing much higher levels of hCE-1 than hCE-2 [29]. Thus,

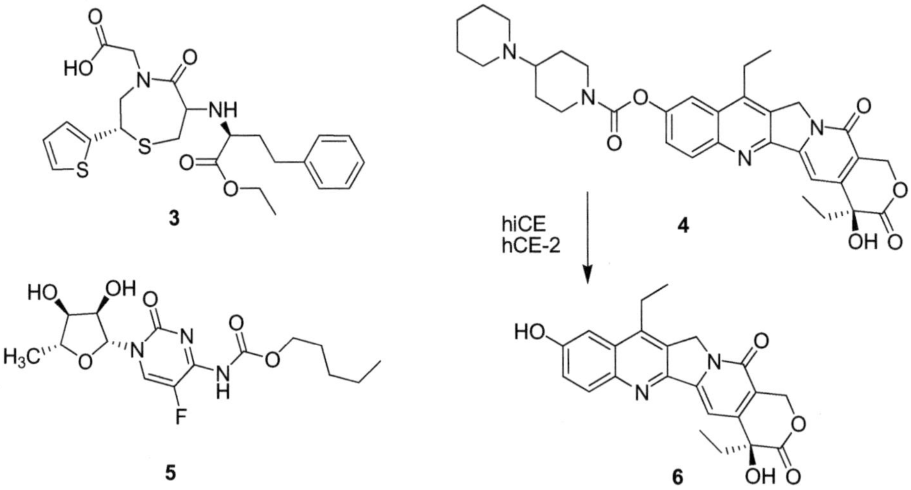


**Figure 15.3** Common prodrug substrates (**3**, **4**, and **5**) for carboxylesterases.

screening efforts of ester prodrugs in Caco-2 monolayers may be somewhat misleading due to this difference in carboxylesterase expression.

Irinotecan (CPT-11) is a prodrug of the topoisomerase I inhibitor SN-38 (ethyl-10-hydroxy-camptothecin, **6**). SN-38 demonstrates potent antitumor activity and is being developed for the treatment of lymphoma, colorectal, lung, gastric, ovarian, and cervical cancer. CPT-11 undergoes hydrolytic activation by carboxylesterases ubiquitously expressed throughout the body. While CPT-11 is a substrate for human carboxylesterase hCE-1, hCE-2, hiCE, and human butylcholinesterase, the highest catalytic efficiency is achieved with hCE-2 and hiCE that share an identical coding sequence with the exception of nine amino acids [30]. Expression of hiCE is highest in the small intestine where its expression in the brush border membrane is responsible for localized conversion of CPT-11 to SN-38. A major side effect of the therapy includes delayed diarrhea that presumably is caused in part from the efficient conversion of CPT-11 by hiCE. Cloning of hiCE from human intestinal tissue biopsies into COS-7 cells confirmed conversion of CPT-11 to SN-38 and increased sensitivity to cytotoxicity, providing a plausible explanation for this observed side effect [30]. Alternately, the major metabolite of SN-38 is a glucuronidated conjugate that is eliminated in bile and ultimately deposited back into the small intestine. Gut flora is capable of cleaving the glucuronide moiety to reform SN-38 leading to localized toxicity in the small intestine. Excretion of CPT-11 directly into bile has been observed following intravenous dosing and therefore the toxicity can be manifested irrespective of route of administration. In order to improve the tolerability and reduce dose-limiting toxicity, several strategies are being pursued including selective inhibition of hiCE with small-molecule approaches as well as potential ADEPT approaches with hCE-2 to effectively modulate and localize the hydrolysis of CPT-11 to SN-38 [31].

The differences in substrate specificity can be used advantageously in the design of a prodrug program if the SAR is fully understood. One such example was the development of the tumor selective prodrug of 5-fluorouracil (5-FU), which was designed to pass intact through the intestinal epithelium and undergo sequential conversion to 5-FU via catalysis by enzymes localized in the liver and tumor tissue [32]. In this aspect, *in vitro* assessments in crude carboxylesterase preparations from human intestine and liver were effectively used to assess prodrug stability of a number of $N^4$-substituted 5′-deoxy-5-fluorocytidine derivatives (**7**). Upon hydrolysis of these prodrugs (Figure 15.4), the product 5′-deoxy-5-fluorocytidine (5′-DFCR, **8**) is readily converted to 5′-deoxy-fluorouridine (5′-DFUR, **9**) via cytidine deaminase found within the liver and tumor tissues. Further metabolism by thymidine phosphorylase ultimately releases 5-FU (**10**) within the tumor itself.

From analysis of several $N^4$-substituted analogues, the $N^4$-alkoxycarbonyl group of compounds emerged as a prodrug series that maintained good stability against human intestinal carboxylesterases, yet were readily hydrolyzable by the isoform(s) in the liver. The reaction was sensitive to chain length with the C4–C6 alkyl chain length rendering the greatest susceptibility to the human liver enzyme. In monkey tissue, the optimum chain length was C8. Slightly higher susceptibility was noted for chain lengths of C3 through C5 in mouse liver tissue, reiterating the species differences in substrate affinity for carboxylesterase activity. To further characterize and identify a lead candidate for development, several of the carbamate prodrugs were evaluated in oral pharmacokinetic studies in monkeys. From these studies, the C5 alkyl chain length analogue (capecitabine) emerged as the prodrug with the highest AUC and Cmax of 5′-DFUR circulating in plasma. In studies using crude tissue homogenates from mice, monkeys, and humans, the compound demonstrated excellent specificity for liver carboxylesterase compared to esterase activity observed in the intestine (Figure 15.5). Intact prodrug concentrations were also very low suggesting that once the prodrug was absorbed, efficient conversion to 5′-DFUR occurred readily in the

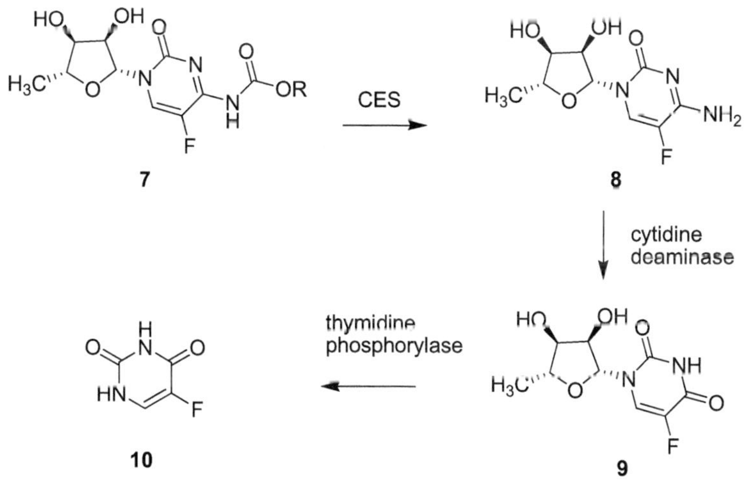


**Figure 15.4** Tissue selective conversion of $N^4$-substituted 5′-deoxy-5-fluorocytidine derivatives to 5-fluorouracil.

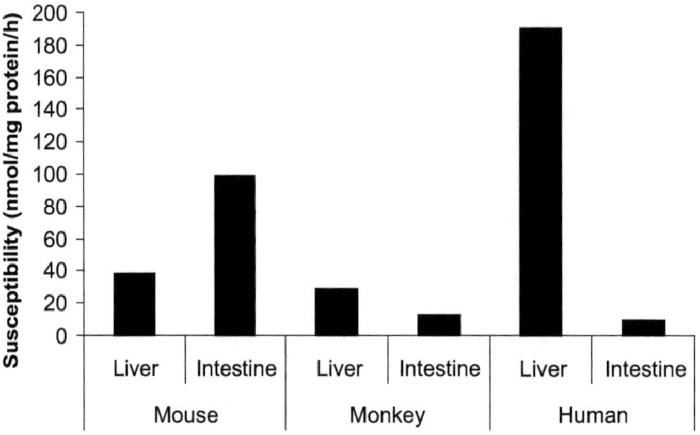


**Figure 15.5** Susceptibility of capecitabine to carboxylesterase activity in the liver and intestine of mice, monkeys, and humans.

liver. Higher tumor selectivity of capecitabine administered orally compared to 5-FU administered IP was also demonstrated using an HCT116 human colon cancer xenograft model in mice as suggested by 5-FU levels in tumors. Taken collectively, the identification of a novel fluoropyrimidine carbamate with selective stability in the presence of intestinal and liver carboxylesterases was achieved through the use of *in vitro* stability assessments in relevant human tissue and through preclinical oral pharmacokinetic evaluation to confirm the optimized absorption and ultimate conversion of capecitabine to the antitumor agent 5-FU [33].

### 15.5.2
### Alkaline Phosphatase

In addition to prodrug strategies to increase permeability for optimized oral bioavailability, several strategies have been pursued to improve compound solubility, thus enabling greater dose loading in parenteral formulations, as well as the potential to improve dissolution properties of orally administered agents. In this aspect, it is important to consider the biopharmaceutical properties of the active parent compound. It is estimated that nearly 40% of drug candidates identified in combinatorial screening efforts have solubility less than 10 μM [33].

While several solubilizing prodrugs exist for parenteral delivery, far fewer have been developed for oral administration. In terms of the Biopharmaceutical Classification System (BCS) [34], a drug is considered highly soluble when it can be fully dissolved at its highest dose in 250 ml of buffer over the pH encountered within the GI tract – thus ensuring that the dose is in solution for absorption. While the use of cosolvents, solubilizing excipients, and/or reduction of particle size can improve dissolution, the solubility of a compound may be too low for delivery at the dose required for the therapeutic indication. The use of phosphate esters is a common approach to improving the solubility of a compound as these esters are readily hydrolyzed by alkaline phosphatases that are expressed throughout

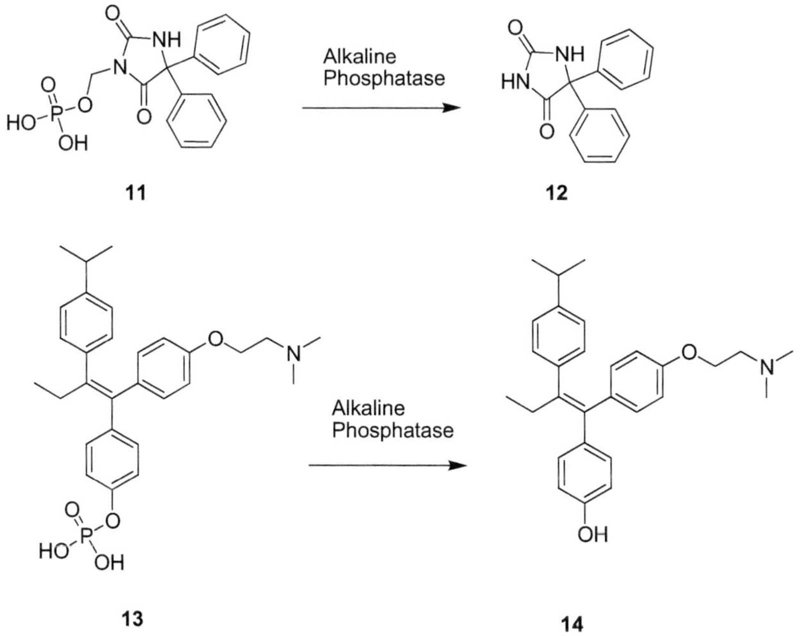

**Figure 15.6** Conversion of phosphate prodrugs by alkaline phosphatase.

the body [35]. The improvement in solubility afforded with this approach can be profound. Fosphenytoin (**11**), the phosphate ester of phenytoin (**12**, Figure 15.6), improves its solubility from ~25 μg/ml to more than 140 mg/ml [36] enabling an effective parenteral delivery of phenytoin for the treatment of acute seizures. The conversion of phosphate esters is catalytically efficient as nearly quantitative formation of phenytoin is achieved in humans with this prodrug strategy [37].

The use of phosphate esters as oral prodrugs is made possible by the expression of alkaline phosphatase on the brush border membrane of the intestinal epithelium. Solubilized prodrug reaches the brush border membrane where the phosphate group is hydrolyzed to yield the more lipophilic active parent, which then is able to permeate across the cell membrane. The higher concentrations achieved at the brush border membrane should theoretically improve absorptive flux. The water-soluble phosphate prodrug ester miproxifene phosphate (TAT-59, **13**; sol. = 52 μg/ml at pH 7.4) is an example of an oral prodrug approach using a solubilizing strategy (Figure 15.6). The active parent compound DP-TAT-59 (**14**) is nearly insoluble with a solubility of <1 μg/ml [38]. Although DP-TAT-59 exhibits a clearance of around 40% of hepatic blood flow in rats, the prodrug achieved nearly 30% bioavailability in that species. In addition, dose–linear pharmacokinetics has been achieved in clinical trials with TAT-59 [39]. The oral phosphate prodrug approach, however, has not been nearly as successful as phosphate prodrug strategies pursued for parenteral administration. It has been suggested that enzyme-mediated precipitation may attenuate improvements with increased solubilization [40]. The propensity for prodrug precipitation will depend on the rates of conversion, the extent of supersaturation, and the required dose of the prodrug.

### 15.5.3
### Cytochrome P450

Cytochrome P450s are a superfamily of heme containing enzymes involved in the oxidation of compounds. These enzymes are expressed in several tissues of the body including the liver, intestine, kidney, and the lung. Those expressed in the liver are of particular importance due to their role in the oxidation of xenobiotics, particularly following oral administration. The major isoforms responsible for the metabolism of drugs include 3A4, 3A5, 2C9, 2C19, 2D6, 1A2, and 2E1. The predominant isoform 3A4 is expressed in high levels in the liver and to lesser extent in the intestine and therefore can contribute substantially to $f_{hepat}$ and $f_{gut}$ of absorbed substrates. The use of P450s as prodrug-converting enzymes is often sought out for liver-targeting approaches. One example is pradefovir (**15**), a prodrug of the antiviral agent, adefovir (**16**). In spite of the improved bioavailability afforded by the use of a dipivoxil prodrug of adefovoir, the prodrug exhibits dose-limiting nephrotoxicity. Since adefovir was developed to treat hepatitis B, ideally a prodrug specifically targeting the liver with limited distribution to other organs would help increase the efficacy and safety of adefovir. A series of prodrugs, designed to be activated by enzymatic oxidation by P450 in hepatocytes, were synthesized for targeted delivery of adefovir [41]. Pradefovir emerged as lead candidate consisting of a cyclic ester prodrug of the phosphonate moiety of adefovir. Stable to esterase activity, the ring system is oxidized by P450 3A4 to yield a ring opened product that undergoes further β-elimination to yield free adefovir and an aryl vinyl ketone (Figure 15.7). In clinical trials, pradefovir demonstrated superior efficacy compared to adefovir dipivoxil with lower systemic concentrations [42].

The utility of this approach has been extended for compounds exhibiting alcohol functionalities [43]. Similar liver-target approaches have been applied in the development of MB07811 a prodrug of the phosphonate-containing thyroid hormone receptor agonist MB07344 [44]. The prodrug was designed to release the active parent in the liver in order to avoid extrahepatic side affects associated with this class of compounds. In preclinical species, the absorbed prodrug had undergone extensive first-pass metabolism in the liver as designed with oral bioavailability ranging from 3 to 10%. Extensive intrinsic clearance was also characterized *in vitro* with liver microsomes, suggesting MB07811 is an ideal prodrug candidate for the targeted delivery of MD07344 to the liver (Figure 15.8).

## 15.6
## Use of the Caco-2 System for Permeability and Active Transport Evaluation

While historically the use of animal PK studies has been the standard for which prodrug selection and development has been conducted, the use of *in situ* and *in vitro* model systems is becoming increasingly popular to gain insight into the

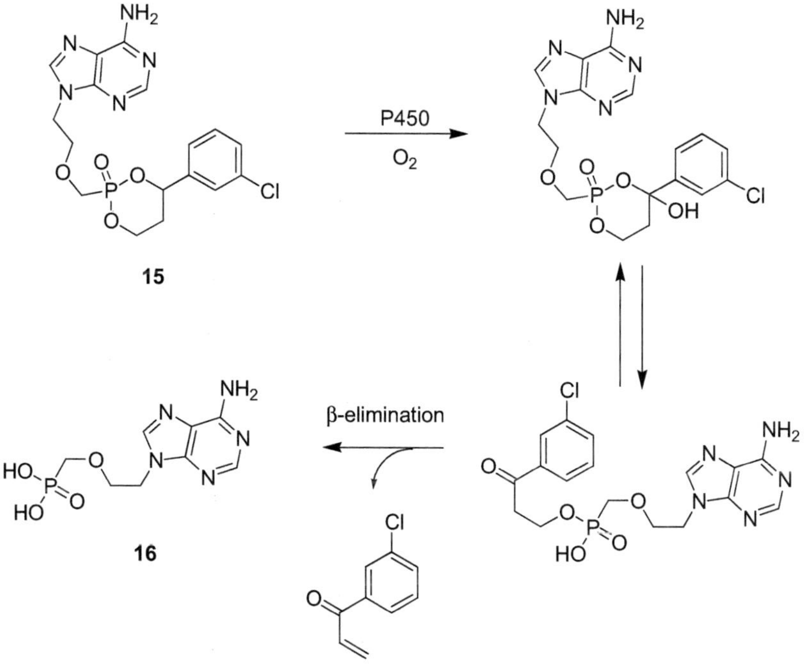


Figure 15.7 Cleavage mechanism of pradefovir.

mechanism(s) of prodrug performance. The Caco-2 transwell assay in particular has been used retrospectively to understand clinical success and failure of oral prodrugs advanced to human trials. In addition to being a relevant cell-based tool for understanding passive permeability of compounds, the expression of key

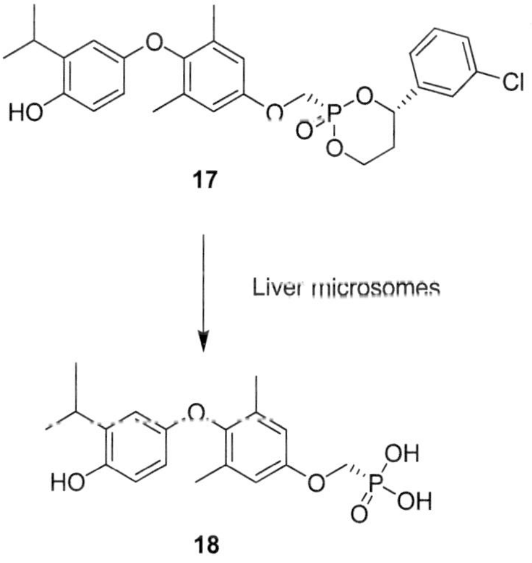


Figure 15.8 Liver-mediated conversion of MB07811 to MB07344.

transporters, allows the investigator to understand whether active transport processes may play a role in the absorption of a particular compound or prodrug. Caco-2 is a human intestinal carcinoma cell line that is cultured to form a monolayer that expresses a variety of apical (luminal side) and basolateral (portal circulation side) transporters such as the peptide transporter PEPT1 (apical), MDR1, also known as P-glycoprotein (apical), and several MRP transporters expressed on both apical and basolateral membranes. Depending on the location and the function of these transporters, they can serve to carry substrates in and out of the cell, and more importantly, dictate the overall flux of a compound – either in the absorptive or in the exsorptive direction. Because these transporters are expressed in the small intestine of humans and more is known about their substrate affinity, they have become prime targets for oral prodrug delivery. The ability to assess this effectively *in vitro* using the Caco-2 cell line provides the investigator the ability to streamline prodrug screening and selection.

The localization and substrate specificity of these transporters becomes an important aspect in the optimization of an effective prodrug strategy. The interplay of transporters and prodrug-converting enzymes should not be underestimated. Although it has often been suggested that oral prodrugs are converted in the bloodstream or in the liver following absorption, an increasing amount of evidence has suggested that extensive conversion occurs within the gut enterocyte, well prior to distribution into the portal circulation. Additionally, while the study of apical transporters such as PEPT1 and P-glycoprotein (Pgp) has been investigated extensively, we are just beginning to learn about the role of basolateral transporters in drug absorption and efflux.

Recent literature is rich with successful examples of prodrug strategies used in the delivery of nucleoside analogues for the treatment of antiviral infections and anticancer chemotheraphy [45]. These compounds are quite polar with anionic groups, which make them difficult for absorption via the oral route. In particular, acyclic nucleoside phosphonates such as adefovir have very poor oral availability due to their anionic phosphonate moieties. Strategies to mask the negatively charged phosphonate group of adefovir resulted in the discovery of a bis(pivaloyloxymethyl) prodrug (**19**), which improved the log $P$ value of adefovir from $-4.11$ to 2.48. This prodrug demonstrated bioavailability from 36 to 45% compared to less than 12% for free adefovir administered orally [46, 47]. Additional characterization of the absorption/conversion of the dipivoxil prodrug in Caco-2 studies demonstrated the formation of the monoester in addition to adefovir itself [48]. Adefovir dipivoxil (Figure 15.9) appeared to be a substrate for a Pgp in Caco-2 studies with preferential efflux to the apical pole that was attenuated in the presence of the Pgp inhibitor verapamil [49]. In addition, the monoester and adefovir itself were also substrates for apical efflux via a non-Pgp transporter.

The role of Pgp-mediated efflux as a potential barrier to absorption of prodrugs and other compounds is a subject of considerable debate. In general, drug concentrations in the intestine are typically well in excess of $K_M$ values established in the transport kinetics of this apical transporter and saturation would be anticipated. Compounds exhibiting poor permeability due to less than optimum physicochemical properties,

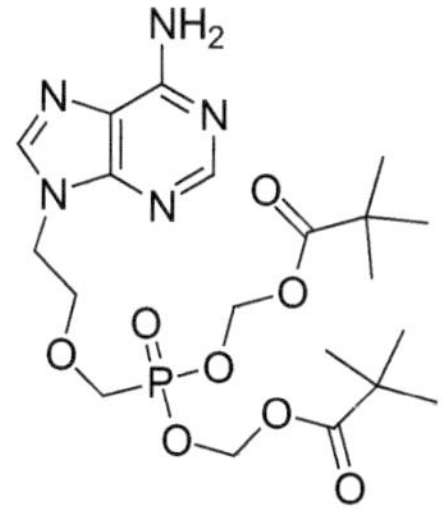

**19**

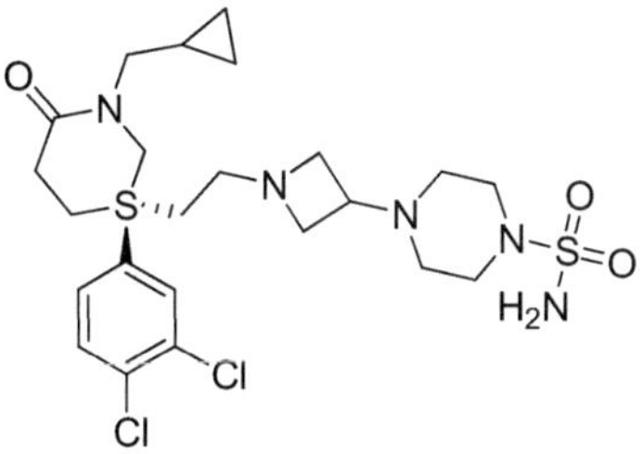

**20**

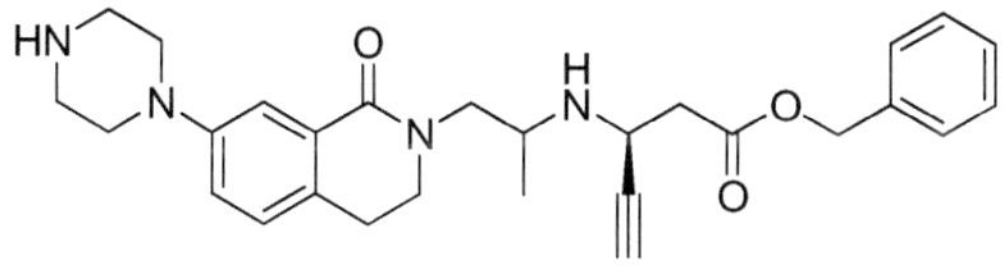

**21**

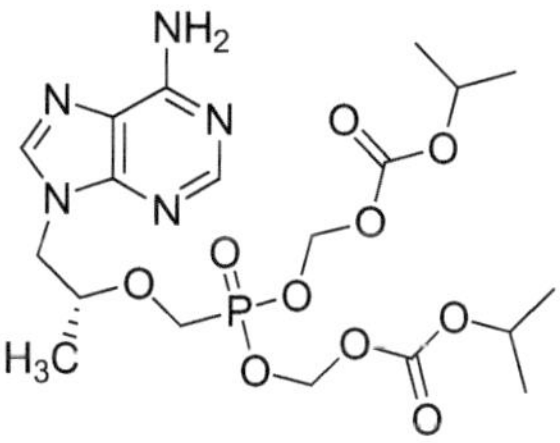

**22**

**Figure 15.9** Substrates for the apical efflux transporter Pgp.

however, could account for subsaturating concentrations within the enterocyte that are readily effluxed by Pgp back into the intestinal lumen. Expression of Pgp is lowest in the duodenum compared to the jejunum and the ileum, thus creating the potential for a limited absorption window confined to the proximal portion of the small intestine [50]. Additionally, given the common overlap in substrate specificity between Pgp and P450 3A4 expressed in the intestinal epithelium, it has been suggested that this transport/metabolism interplay works in concert to increase the overall clearance of compounds at the gut wall [51–53]. While asymmetric transport (basolateral to apical flux/apical to basolateral flux ratio > 2) of compounds evaluated in Caco-2 can serve to implicate apical efflux due potentially to Pgp as a barrier to absorption, more convincing data can be obtained *in vivo* using MDR1 knockout mice. The $NK_2$ receptor antagonist UK-224,671 (**20**, Figure 15.9) demonstrated evidence for apical efflux as suggested by asymmetric transport in Caco-2 with a B to A/A to B ratio of 13 [54]. This compound was further evaluated in mdr1a(−/−) and mdr1a/b (−/−) mice that are deficient in the expression of Pgp. In wild-type mice a bioavailability of <2% was observed, while Pgp knockout mice demonstrated a bioavailability of 22%. Although fewer examples exist for prodrugs, the benzyl ester of the zwitterionic fibrinogen receptor antagonist L-767,679 was determined to be a substrate for Pgp in Caco-2 experiments (Figure 15.9) [55]. The prodrug L-775,318 (**21**) demonstrated asymmetric transport favoring the apical pole. Apical transport demonstrated saturable kinetics and was markedly reduced by Pgp inhibitors verapamil and quinidine, providing further evidence that Pgp was the specific transporter involved. Interestingly, the addition of verapamil not only attenuated apical efflux of L-775,318 in Caco-2 but also inhibited its hydrolysis by rat esterase in intestinal S9 fractions. While reduction of hydrolysis of L-775,318 would theoretically increase the amount of prodrug available for Pgp efflux, a rapid increase in intracellular concentrations could saturate its transport kinetics ($K_M \sim 400\,\mu M$). This combined with Pgp inhibition directly with verapamil likely contributed to the enhanced absorption of L-775,318 observed in rat *in situ* intestinal loop studies.

The interplay of esterase activity and Pgp efflux was also studied in the development of tenofovir disoproxil fumarate (**22**, Figure 15.9). Similar to the dipivoxil ester prodrug of adefovir, tenofovir disoproxil fumarate is a substrate for Pgp as suggested by asymmetric flux and transport polarity affects observed in the presence of cyclosporine A using the Caco-2 system [56]. The addition of ester mixtures and strawberry extract was shown to improve the absorption of tenofovir equivalents in Caco-2, primarily with the appearance of intact prodrug appearing in the basolateral chamber. These data suggest that the improved transcellular absorption is due to inhibition of prodrug hydrolysis afforded with the ester mixtures and strawberry extract. Similar to L-775,318, rapid increase in the level of tenofovir disoproxil fumarate in the enterocyte could also potentially saturate its apical efflux by Pgp.

## 15.7
## XP13512: Improving PK Performance by Targeting Active Transport

The discovery of additional absorptive nutrient transporters in the digestive tract has provided several opportunities for targeted prodrug delivery. A recent example of targeting specific transporters is the oral prodrug of gabapentin, XP13512 (**23**). Gabapentin (Neurontin®, **24**) is a structural analogue of GABA and has been used in the treatment of epilepsy [57] and a variety of other neurological disorders [58]. The compound demonstrates dose-dependent bioavailability that decreases from 60% to less than 35% at therapeutic dose levels that are used for the treatment of neuropathic pain [59]. Saturable absorption is thought to be the mechanism underlying the dose-dependent exposure observed for the drug, thus providing subtherapeutic concentrations in some patients [60]. In addition to the comparatively poor absorption in some patients, the short half-life (5–7 h) leads to required dosing of three to four times a day, which increases patient noncompliance [61]. A more prolonged exposure would be beneficial for the drug's activity and improve the dose regimen. Attempts to invent a sustained formulation, however, have been unsuccessful due to incomplete absorption of the drug in the lower portion of the intestinal tract. XP13512 was designed to have consistently high absorption at all portions of the intestinal tract via targeting a high-capacity transporter that is expressed throughout the entire intestine and colon. Substrate affinity and transport of X13512 was verified *in vitro* by uptake studies with cells expressing the sodium-dependent multivitamin transporter (SMVT) or the monocarboxylate transporter type 1 (MCT-1) transporters that are expressed throughout the intestinal tracts of rats and humans (Figure 15.10) [62]. The boost in bioavailability afforded through oral administration of X13512 was demonstrated in oral preclinical pharmacokinetic studies in rats and monkeys [63]. Bioavailability of gabapentin increased 3.2-fold following oral administration of

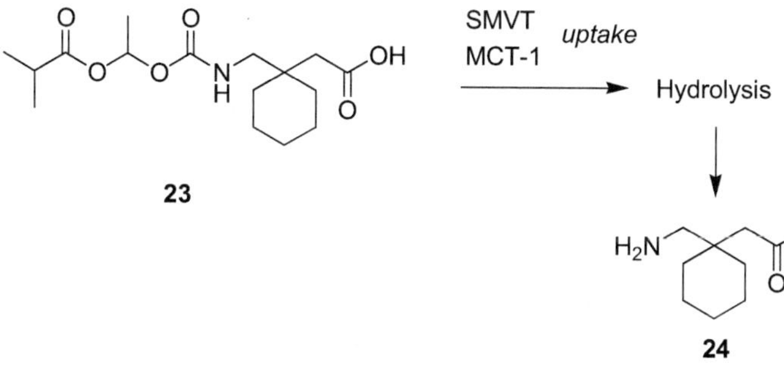


**Figure 15.10** Uptake and conversion of XP13512.

XP13512 compared to commercial capsules of Neurontin. No evidence of saturation was observed for either species at doses as high as 5000 mg/kg in rats. In addition, no stereoselectivity was observed in the transport and conversion of XP13512 thus allowing for development of the racemic compound. Intracolonic delivery of XP13512 in both rats and monkeys confirmed a 17- and 32-fold relative increase in gabapentin exposure via the prodrug, respectively. Expansion of the absorption window into the colon would enable sustained release formulation development and potentially reduce dosing frequency in the clinic. Prodrug stability studies *ex vivo* in rat, in monkey, and in human tissue suggested similar rates of conversion, suggesting metabolic conversion in humans would behave similarly to that observed preclinically.

Based on compelling *in vitro* and *in vivo* preclinical studies, XP13512 was advanced to clinical trials for pharmacokinetic evaluation. In human trials, XP13512 yielded dose-proportional increases in gabapentin exposure (Figure 15.11) with consistently high bioavailability (>68%) over the dose range evaluated (350–2800 mg) [64]. By contrast, standard doses of gabapentin bioavailability decreased from 65% at 200 mg

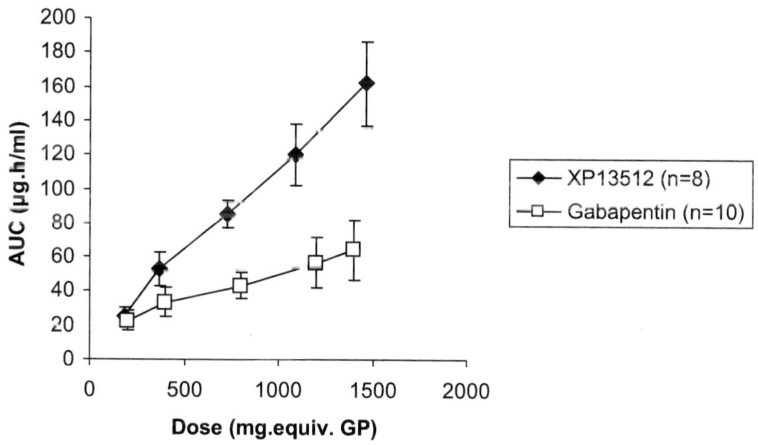


**Figure 15.11** Dose linearity of gabapentin versus XP13512 in humans.

to 27% at 1400 mg. A sustained release (XR) formulation was also evaluated. Similar to what was found with the immediate release formulation, dose-proportional increases in exposure were observed throughout the dose range. Bioavailability generally increased from 60 to 80% when the prodrug was administered with food. Based on these clinical findings, it is anticipated that a successful sustained release formulation can be made using XP13512, which will enable lower dosing frequency, decreased variability in compound exposure, and greater patient compliance for the various neuropathic treatment options being pursued for gabapentin.

## 15.8 Prodrug Absorption: Transport/Metabolic Conversion Interplay

When dealing with prodrugs, the added complexity of compound stability and conversion to the active moiety is something that needs to be considered in the analysis of Caco-2 data. The preconceived notion that prodrugs pass through the intestinal epithelium and are hydrolyzed preferentially in the blood or in the plasma is quite often not the case at all. For instance, it has been shown that Caco-2 cells themselves express an abundance of esterases and amidases with varied substrate affinity and capacity. A common strategy for a prodrug approach is to increase the permeability of the molecule through the addition of a hydrolyzable lipophilic moiety. While the more lipophilic prodrug affords passive permeation through the apical or the luminal side of the intestinal epithelial cell wall, rapid hydrolysis within the cell via an esterase or an amidase yields the much more polar active moiety with insufficient physicochemical properties to permeate out of the basolateral membrane into circulation and instead accumulates within the cell where it could potentially be further metabolized to an inactive molecule.

### 15.8.1 Pivampicillin

Pivampicillin (PIVA, **25**) is a successful lipophilic prodrug of the antibiotic ampicillin (**26**). While ampicillin itself is orally available, its bioavailability is limited to ~30–50%. While previous studies have suggested ampicillin may be a substrate for the apical transporter PEPT1 [65], recent data have suggested that this compound is likely absorbed paracellularly [66]. Esterification of the carboxylic acid moiety with the pivaloyloxymethylester partially masks the overall zwitterionic charge of the compound at neutral pH and increases lipophilicity to improve passive permeation of the compound. In this manner, bioavailability of nearly 90% is achievable in humans. Retrospective analysis of the compound using the Caco-2 system revealed the more complex nature of the absorption mechanism and eventual conversion of the prodrug to ampicillin [67]. Upon addition of PIVA to the apical (luminal) side of the Caco-2 monolayer, high concentrations of amipicillin were observed within the cell and in the basolateral chamber after a 3 h incubation. Only limited amounts of intact PIVA were detected in the basolateral side. Incubation of ampicillin itself on the apical side resulted in significantly less apical-to-basolateral transport of ampicillin compared to PIVA. The transport and release of ampicillin from PIVA added to the apical pole was not affected by inhibitors of PEPT1 and OCTN2 transporters, however, depletion of ATP or addition of bis-(4-nitrophenyl)-phosphate (BNPP; an esterase inhibitor) resulted in substantially less amount of ampicillin transported to the basolateral pole. Taken collectively, the data suggested that rapid hydrolysis and accumulation of ampicillin occurred within Caco-2 cells following passive permeation of PIVA. The fact that flux of ampicillin was limited through the depletion of ATP or inhibition of esterase activity further suggested that an active transporter on the basolateral membrane was responsible for transporting ampicillin preferentially to the basolateral pole. In addition, a phthalimidomethylester of ampicillin (PIMA, **27**), which is less susceptible to enzymatic hydrolysis, was evaluated in parallel with PIVA (Figure 15.12). The transport efficiency of ampicillin via the PIMA prodrug was very poor and similar to the observed transport of ampicillin when added to the apical pole itself, further suggesting that efficient hydrolysis of the ester prodrug is a prerequisite for the efficient formation and transport of ampicillin through the basolateral membrane. Cell-loading experiments were conducted with PIVA (1 h incubation of PIVA in the apical chamber, followed by transferring the loaded cells to fresh apical and basolateral buffer) to evaluate the disappearance of PIVA and ampicillin due hydrolytic activity and transport processes. These experiments were conducted at 37 and 4 °C to further distinguish enzyme-mediated processes (transport/metabolism) versus passive permeability. While clearance of PIVA was rapid at both 37 and 4 °C, ampicillin clearance was much slower at 37 °C and no clearance of ampicillin could be discerned at 4 °C. Using the same cell-loading protocol, the efflux of ampicillin was nearly twofold higher through the basolateral pole than the apical pole, which is consistent with vectoral transport in the absorptive direction. Efflux of ampicillin could effectively be inhibited by probenecid (nonselective transport inhibitor) as well as MK-571 (a selective MRP transporter inhibitor) suggesting an MRP-type transporter was likely responsible for the basolateral efflux of ampicillin.

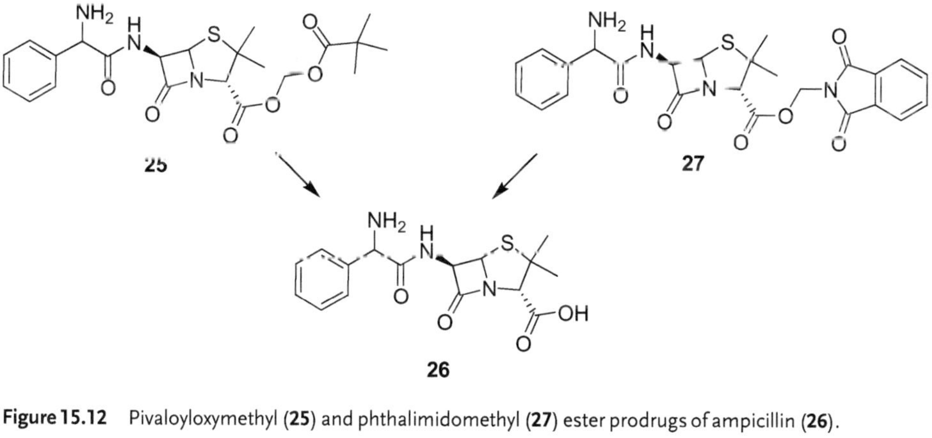

**Figure 15.12** Pivaloyloxymethyl (**25**) and phthalimidomethyl (**27**) ester prodrugs of ampicillin (**26**).

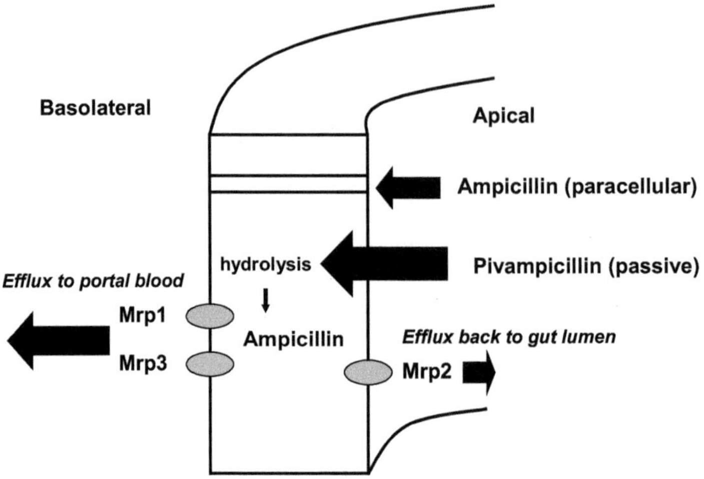


**Figure 15.13** Proposed absorption of pivampicillin.

Taken collectively, these data suggest that the enhanced absorption of ampicillin via its pivaloyloxymethylester prodrug is mediated by passive diffusion through the apical membrane, rapid hydrolysis, and accumulation of ampicillin within the enterocyte and active transport preferentially to the basolateral pole via an MRP-type transporter (Figure 15.13).

### 15.8.2
### Valacyclovir

The apical peptide transporter PEPT1 has been commonly targeted for prodrug approaches [8, 22, 45, 68, 69]. This transporter recognizes di- and tripeptides as well as pharmacologically active peptidomimetics such as β-lactam antibiotics and ACE inhibitors [70, 71]. Retrospective examination of the PEPT1 transport-mediated absorption of ACE inhibitors and β-lactam antibiotics led to the development of prodrug strategies including the use of stabilized dipeptides. Dipeptides D-Asp-Ala, D-Glu-Ala, Asp-Sar, and Glu-Sar have been utilized as prodrug moieties for model benzyl alcohols, purines, and pyrimidine analogues [72–74]. These model prodrugs were shown to be transported across Caco-2 monolayers via PEPT1 with higher affinity for the transporter correlating with increased drug lipophilicity [74]. In addition, di- and monoamino acid-linked L-dopa prodrugs have demonstrated enhanced permeability in both rat perfusion and Caco-2 studies with the improvement attenuated in the presence of Gly-Gly and Gly-Sar [75, 76].

One of the most successful and comprehensively studied prodrug approaches specifically targeted for carrier-mediated delivery is the antiviral prodrug valacyclovir (VACV, **28**) used in the treatment of varicella zoster virus disease. This L-valyl ester of acyclovir (**29**) is an oral prodrug capable of achieving plasma levels that are comparable to levels achieved intravenously (Figure 15.14). The mean absolute bioavailability achieved in humans with VACV is 54%, providing three- to fivefold

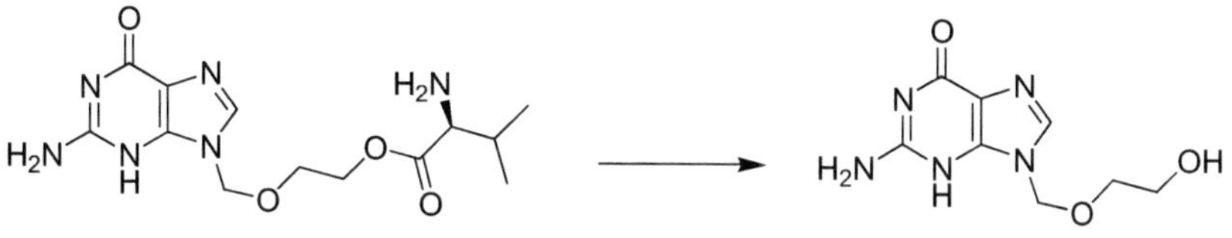

**Figure 15.14** Valacyclovir, the L-valyl ester of acyclovir.

greater exposure than orally administered acyclovir [77]. The prodrug emerged from an initial screening of 18 amino acid esters with the L-isomer demonstrating greater performance compared to its D-isomer [78].

Enhanced stereoselective performance suggested a role for transport-mediated absorption of the prodrug. Several laboratories have implicated PEPT1 and/or organic anion (OAT) and organic cation (OCTs) as the key active transporters responsible for VACV absorption in humans and animals [79]. More recent work, however, has suggested a role for the human oligopeptide transporter HPT1 based on a positive correlation of gene expression for this transporter compared to individual absorption (as suggested by higher $C_{max}$ and AUC values) [80]. Interestingly, in this same study, no significant correlation of VACV $C_{max}$ and AUC values could be made with PEPT1 or (OCT/OAT) transporter expression levels. In addition, high negative correlations were observed with the efflux pumps MDR1 (P-glycoprotein) and MRP2, and cytochrome P450 3A4 suggesting a potential role of these transporters/enzymes in maintaining intracellular levels of acyclovir. Recognition and transport of VACV by HPT1 was confirmed *in vitro* with uptake experiments using transiently HPT1-expressing HeLa cells. Uptake of [$^3$H]-VACV by HPT1 expressing HeLa cells was 1.8-fold greater than normal HeLa cells. In addition, HeLa cells overexpressing PEPT1 demonstrated 1.6-fold greater uptake compared to normal cells confirming affinity of VACV for PEPT1 as well. Interestingly, physiologically based pharmacokinetic modeling and advanced compartment absorption and transit (ACAT) simulations were consistent with VACV absorption mediated by a transporter uniformly expressed throughout the GI tract [81]. Since PEPT1 has been shown to have greater expression more proximally in the duodenum with less expression further down into the jejunum and ileum [82], the involvement of HPT-1 and other potential transporters such as peptide transporters PTR3 and PHT1 seems plausible. Additionally, while valacyclovir appears to be a substrate for both PEPT1 and HCT-1, the higher expression of HCT-1 compared to PEPT1 may explain its dominant role in the transport of valacyclovir in humans [80]. Single-pass perfusion procedure (SPIP) models in the rat suggested a role for OAT and OCT in the absorption of VACV based on inhibition of uptake by *p*-amino hippuric acid (PAH) and quinine [79]. In humans, however, no positive correlations of the expression of these transporters were observed with the absorption of VACV, suggesting that active transport of this prodrug may be mediated by different transporters in other species. These data suggest that extrapolation of absorption mediated by active transport processes in preclinical species to humans must done with caution.

## 15.9 Preabsorptive Degradation

While *in vitro* investigations with Caco-2 and other cell lines help to further clarify the mechanism for which prodrugs are recognized, metabolized and delivered to systemic circulation, stability within the stomach and luminal environment may play a significant role in determining the amount of prodrug available for absorption. The pH environment varies significantly along the GI tract with very low acidic pH in the fasted stomach to comparatively basic pH in the lower GI tract. In the duodenum where the vast majority of absorption takes place for passively permeable compounds, the pH ranges from 5 to 7 and is typically around 6.5. The pH in the jejunum and ileum rises to 7.5 and is close to 8 near the colon. Lipophilic prodrugs with "activated" esters (spaced with oxo-methylene spacers to facilitate hydrolysis) are often base labile and therefore will often present with a limited absorption window because of prodrug degradation in the higher pH environment of the lower GI tract.

### 15.9.1 Cephalosporin Prodrugs

In addition to chemical stability, enzymatic stability in the stomach and intestine become important considerations for prodrug design. Peptidases, lipases, trypsin, and chymotrypsin found within the pancreatic secretions transferred to the small intestine to aid in digestion have the capability of hydrolyzing susceptible prodrugs. Prodrugs of cephalosporin antibiotics have been shown to be hydrolytically unstable in human intestinal juice (Figure 15.15) [83]. Incubations of cefuroxime axetil (**30**) and cefpodoxime proxetil (**31**) in duodenal secretions obtained from human volunteers demonstrated accelerated degradation compared to pH 7.4 phosphate buffer. Bioavailability of diastereomeric mixtures of cephalosporin esters is generally around 40 to 50% and it has been suggested that preabsorptive degradation of the prodrug is responsible for the less than complete oral bioavailability of these agents. Initial investigations suggested base catalyzed isomerization of the Δ3-cephalosporin ester

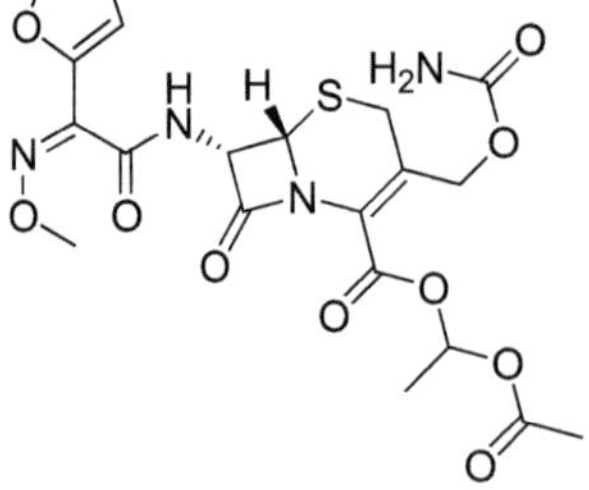

**30**

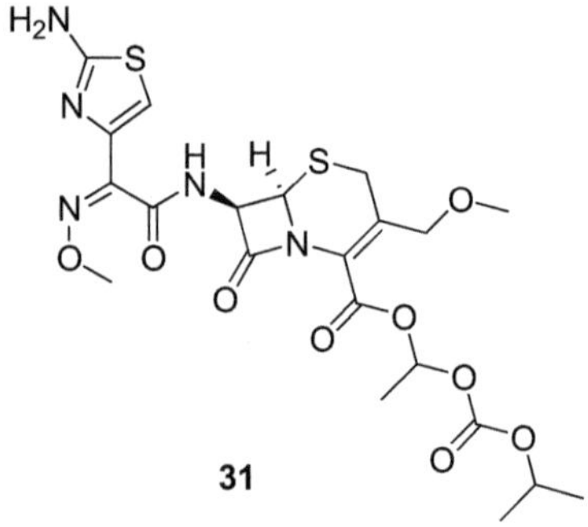

**31**

**Figure 15.15** Cephalosporin prodrugs that undergo intestinal degradation.

to the hydrolytically labile Δ2-cephalosporin ester to yield the inactive Δ2-cephalosporin carboxylate as a plausible explanation [84]. At pH 6.0, the Δ2-cephalosporin ester is significantly more unstable compared to the Δ3 ester. Therefore, the extent of bioavailability would simply be a function of the kinetics of isomerization of the Δ3- cephalosporin ester to the Δ2 ester. Incubations with cefuroxime axetil and cefpodoxime proxetil in human intestinal juice, however, showed that spontaneous isomerization to the Δ2 isomer was significantly slower than hydrolysis to the Δ3-cephalosporin carboxylate. Thus, enzymatic hydrolysis was the main determinant in the significantly higher levels of the pharmacologically active Δ3-cephalosporin carboxylate compared to the minor amounts of the Δ2 isomer formed through isomerization. Stereoselectivity observed in the hydrolysis of the diastereomeric ester mixtures further suggested a role for intestinal enzymes in prodrug degradation.

### 15.9.2 Sulopenem Prodrugs PF-00398899, PF-03709270, and PF-04064900

Sulopenem (**32**) is a broad-spectrum penem antibiotic currently in Phase II evaluation for the treatment of respiratory tract infections. The lack of oral absorption as demonstrated in preclinical studies necessitated the development of an oral prodrug program. The first lead candidate, PF-00398899 (**33**) was a lipophilic prodrug ester that was progressed through a discovery screening strategy based primarily on physicochemical properties and improved absorption in oral rodent pharmacokinetic and efficacy studies (Figure 15.16). The prodrug demonstrated bioavailability in excess of 50% in rats, 24% in monkeys, and demonstrated nearly equivalent efficacy as sulopenem dosed parenterally in mice. PF-00398899, however, produced less than 15% bioavailability through the dose range evaluated in the clinic (400–1000 mg). Accelerated degradation in porcine pancrelipase preparations *in vitro* suggested preabsorptive degradation of the prodrug could contribute to the low bioavailability observed in human clinical trials. Porcine pancrelipase was used as a surrogate for human intestinal juice and as an upfront screen to prioritize backup prodrug candidates. Those compounds exhibiting half-lives in excess of 15 min in porcine pancrelipase were then evaluated in human intestinal juice at multiple prodrug concentrations in order to derive Michaelis–Menten parameters that could be used in biopharmaceutical-based pharmacokinetic (BBPK) model [85]. Two prodrugs emerged from this *in vitro* approach: PF-03709270 (sulopenem etzadroxil, **34**) and PF-04064900 (**35**). These two prodrugs demonstrated half lives in excess of 20 min in porcine pancrelipase and had intrinsic clearances of 0.07 and 0.13 ml/min in human intestinal juice (Table 15.1), which compare favorably to the higher clearance of 0.38 ml/min determined for PF-00398899. In addition, the $K_M$ values determined for PF 03709270 and PF-04064900 were readily saturable at 105 and 91 μM, respectively. No apparent $K_M$ could be determined for PF-00398899 due to solubility limitations; however, at concentrations as high as 300 μM its degradation half-life was 3.01 min compared to 38.5 and 21.1 min for PF-03709270 and PF-04064900, respectively. Both diastereoisomers of cefpodoxime proxetil were evaluated as controls based on the findings of stereoselective hydrolysis of this prodrug in human intestinal juice [83].

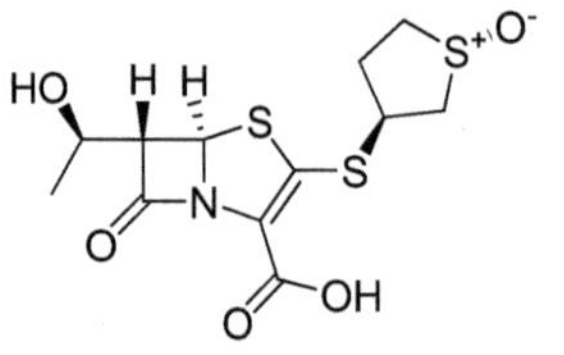

32

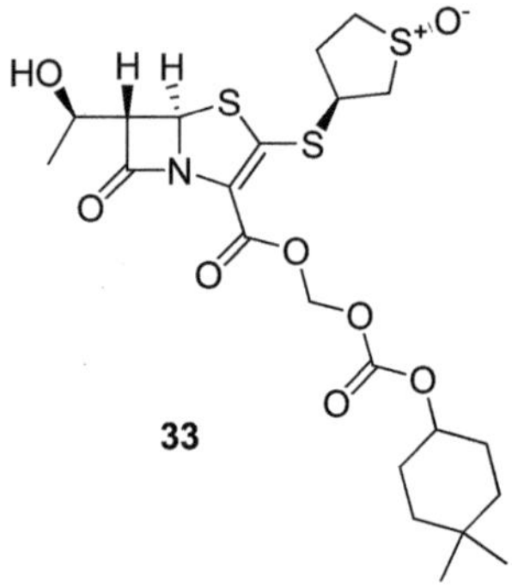

33

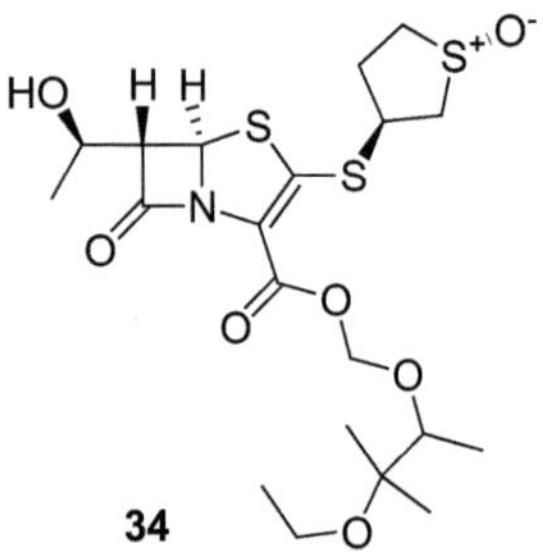

34

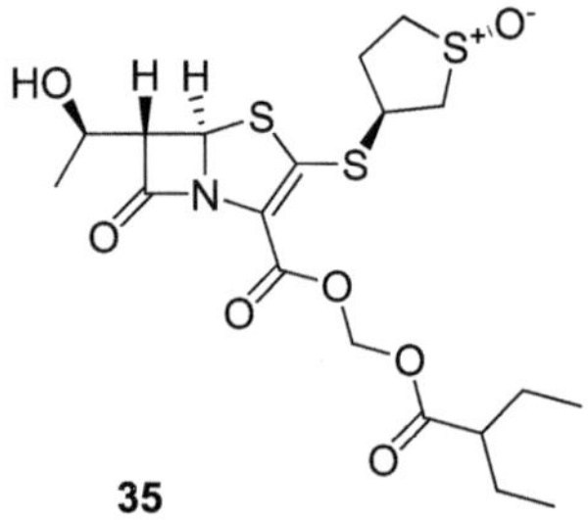

35

**Figure 15.16** Sulopenem and its oral prodrugs.

## 15.10
## Biopharmaceutical-Based PK Modeling for Prodrug Design

Studies assessing the stability of sulopenem prodrugs in human intestinal juice suggested that the concentration of prodrug in solution could make a significant impact on the fraction of dose degraded prior to absorption. Key biopharmaceutical properties such as particle size, solubility, dissolution rate, gut transit time, and absorption rate work in combination to determine concentrations in the gut and liver

**Table 15.1** Kinetic parameters for stability of sulopenem prodrugs and cefpodoxime proxetil diastereomers in human intestinal juice.

| Compound | Half-life ($T_{1/2}$) at 300 μM (min) | $K_M$ (μM) | $V_{max}$ (nmoles/min) | $CL_{int}$ (mL/min) |
|---|---|---|---|---|
| PF-00398899 | 3.01 | >300 | 114 | 0.38 |
| PF-04064900 | 21.1 | 105 | 13.6 | 0.13 |
| PF-03709270 | 38.5 | 91 | 6.40 | 0.07 |
| Cefpodoxime proxetil (isomer 1) | 4.62 | >300 | 84.0 | 0.28 |
| Cefpodoxime proxetil (isomer 2) | 27.7 | >300 | 6.40 | 0.06 |

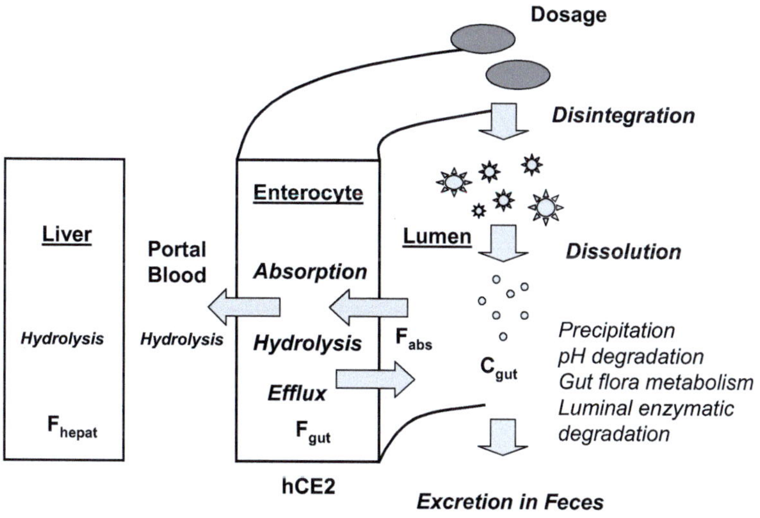


**Figure 15.17** The combined role of prodrug physicochemical properties and physiological processes dictating overall compound exposure and transfer during absorption.

and ultimately dictate the levels of active parent in systemic circulation (Figure 15.17). For instance, compounds with low solubility or slow dissolution may produce concentrations below the $K_M$ for luminal enzymes that degrade them. Compounds with higher solubility on the other hand may dissolve readily with saturating concentrations and thus reduce the amount of dose degraded in the lumen as well as potentially achieve greater flux due to the higher concentration gradient established at the site of absorption.

To help characterize this, a pharmacokinetic-based compartment model similar to the compartmental absorption and transit (CAT) model developed by Yu and Amidon [86] was developed to predict the absorption potential of prodrugs within the sulopenem program. Michaelis–Menten parameters associated with luminal stability were combined with biopharmaceutical properties and physiological parameters to predict fraction absorbed. A summary of the model is shown in Figure 15.18. More ACAT models such as GastroPLUS are now used routinely for *in silico* predictions of fraction of dose absorbed and bioavailability, however, the approach taken here within our laboratory was sufficient for advancing prodrugs with enhanced luminal stability to clinical trials. In addition, while the current ACAT model used in GastroPLUS considers chemical degradation within the gut lumen, the metabolic degradation is confined within the enterocyte. Our model incorporates both chemical degradation and enzymatic degradation described by a capacity-limited Michaelis–Menten function prior to absorption into the enterocyte. Simple passive absorption with no impact from carrier-mediated transport is considered.

Using the BBPK model, the predicted fractions of dose absorbed for PF-03709270 and PF-04064900 were 63 and 82%, respectively, at the clinical dose of 1200 mg. In

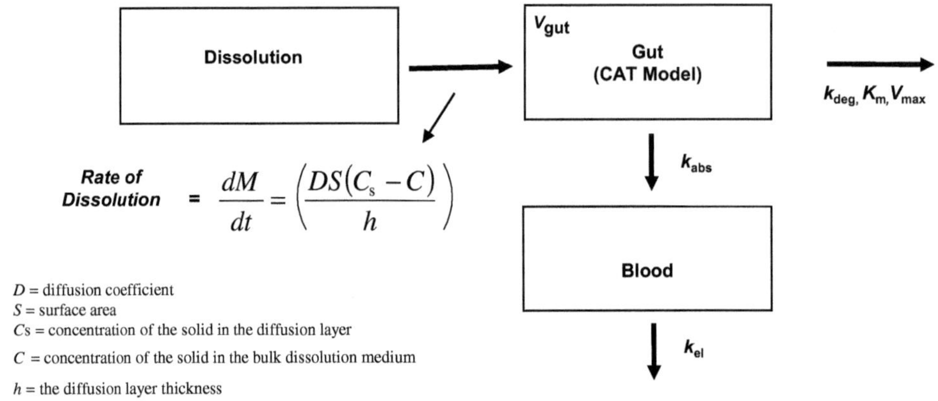


$$\frac{dC_{gut}}{dt} = \frac{1}{V_{gut}} \bullet \frac{dM}{dt} - (k_{abs} + k_{deg}) \bullet C_{gut} - \frac{V_{max} \bullet C_{gut}}{K_m + C_{gut}}$$

$$\frac{dC_{blood}}{dt} = k_{abs} \bullet C_{gut} - k_{el} \bullet C_{blood}$$

**Figure 15.18** Biopharmaceutical-based pharmacokinetic model to estimate fraction absorbed of sulopenem prodrugs.

clinical FIH studies, mean observed bioavailabilities of 25 and 39% were determined for sulopenem following oral administration PF-03709270 and PF-04064900, respectively. In addition, based on the *in vitro* stability data of PF-00398899 and its physiochemical properties, a predicted fraction of dose absorbed of 20% was estimated using the BBPK model for the clinical dose of 1000 mg. A mean bioavailability of 11% was observed in clinical trials.

These data collectively are consistent with approximately 50% of the absorbed dose being metabolized or degraded in the enterocyte ($f_{gut}$) and/or liver ($f_{hepat}$). As previously highlighted, "first-pass" metabolism could drastically reduce the effectiveness of an oral prodrug strategy if the metabolism is extensive. Clearance of sulopenem is 5 ml/min/kg, half of which is renal excretion of unchanged drug. The remaining 2.5 ml/min/kg, however, is only 12.5% of hepatic blood flow suggesting either the model estimates for $F_{abs}$ were inaccurate or the prodrug alters the clearance of sulopenem. An estimate of first-pass extraction of PF-03709270 was established from two clinical studies evaluating the pharmacokinetics of sulopenem following oral administration of PF-03709270 at 2000 mg and urinary excretion of total radioactivity following oral administration of [$^{14}$C]PF-03709270 at the same 2000 mg dose. Bioavailability of sulopenem following oral administration of a 2000 mg dose of PF-03709270 was comparatively low at 20.1%. Urinary excretion, however, of total radioactivity following administration of the same dose with a radiolabel incorporated on the sulopenem core structure was 44.3% of the total dose administered.

Since only absorbed material can be excreted in urine, the 44.3% of the dose quantified in the urine serves as a measure of the total amount of dose absorbed ($F_{abs} = 44.3\%$). This value compares favorably to ~50% $F_{abs}$ estimated using the BBPK model for a 2000 mg dose suggesting the model provides a reasonable estimate of absorbed prodrug. Caco-2 studies with PF-03709270 and PF-040640900 suggested these prodrugs are substrates for Pgp and may be potentially effluxed, however, the involvement of Pgp in limiting $F_{abs}$ at the gut concentrations achieved *in vivo* seems unlikely based on *in vitro* study results (data not shown).

Alternately, nonproductive metabolism could account for the difference in oral bioavailability and fraction of dose absorbed. An estimate of the fraction of dose surviving first pass can be determined as:

$$F_{gut} \times F_{hepat} = \frac{F_{po}}{F_{abs}} \text{ or } F_{gut} \times F_{hepat} = \frac{20.1\%}{44.3\%} = 45.4\%$$

This suggests that nearly 50% of the absorbed PF-03709270 does not generate circulating concentrations of sulopenem. Interestingly, experiments with both sulopenem and PF-03709270 were carried out in human liver and intestinal microsomes as well as hepatocytes where sulopenem was shown to be stable and consistent with the low hepatic clearance of <2.5 ml/min/kg estimated *in vivo*. Incubations with PF-03709270 demonstrated rapid and quantitative conversion to sulopenem in liver S9 fractions; however, very low hydrolytic activity was observed in intestinal microsomes. These *in vitro* data suggested an ideal situation where a lipohilic prodrug ester of a metabolically stable active parent could permeate the intestinal epithelium intact and hydrolyze to active in the portal blood and/or liver prior to distribution into systemic circulation. The disparate results, however, with clinical data suggesting higher first-pass extraction than would be anticipated suggests an important gap in understanding the metabolic fate of PF-03709270 *in vivo*.

Structural elucidation of metabolites identified in the plasma of human subjects receiving PF-03709270 and from preclinical ADME studies performed with sulopenem and PF-03709270 provided valuable insight into the metabolic discrepancies between the *in vitro* and the *in vivo* settings. In addition to the major β-lactam hydrolyzed metabolite generated via dipeptidase, several other metabolites were detected that were consistent with reduction of the sulfoxide moiety of sulopenem. These reduced metabolites were more abundant in the urine of rats following oral administration of [$^{14}$C]PF-03709270 compared to IV administration of [$^{14}$C]sulopenem (Figure 15.19). The fecal metabolite profile in rats demonstrated the vast majority of metabolites to be reduced to the sulfide suggesting this reduction occurs readily in the GI tract presumably mediated by the gut flora [87]. Interestingly, both rat and human plasma PK profiles of total radioactivity revealed a bimodal distribution with $C_{max}$ ~ 1 h postdose and a secondary peak at 4 h postdose. Separate metabolite identification studies of the plasma radioactivity that made up each of these peaks were completed to determine whether there was a difference in the type and/or abundance of specific metabolites. Indeed, the secondary peak at 4 h postdose demonstrated an abundance of reduced metabolites suggesting reduction of the dose further down in the distal portion of the GI tract where gut flora activity

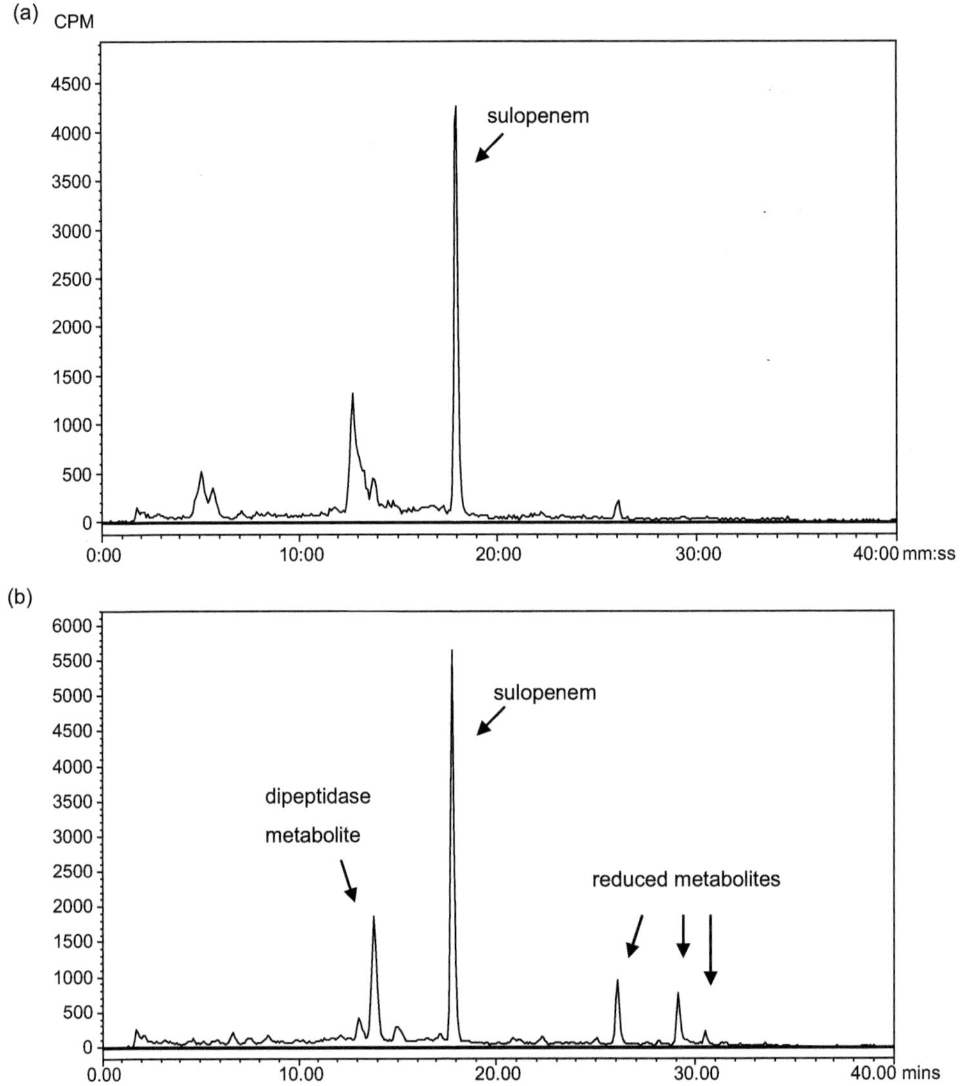


**Figure 15.19** Urinary metabolite profiles in rats following (a) intravenous administration of [$^{14}C$]-sulopenem or (b) oral administration of [$^{14}C$]-PF-03709270.

would be higher. While the BBPK modeling would suggest the reduced sulfide is absorbed as intact prodrug, the absorption of the free sulfide cannot be ruled out.

In addition to reduction of the sulfide moiety, metabolites consistent with hydrolysis of the β-lactam ring were also prevalent. Initial data suggested this metabolic clearance is localized in the kidneys and mediated via renal dipeptidase and would not impact first-pass loss of the active parent. Follow-up studies with freshly prepared monkey and rat intestinal tissue homogenates, however, suggested extensive hydrolysis of the β-lactam ring of sulopenem. This reaction was not observed in human intestinal and liver microsomes due to peptidase inhibitors that are often added in the preparation of microsomes to maintain the integrity of the reagent. Based on these retrospective analyses, there is compelling evidence that extensive first-pass metabolism via gut flora and human intestinal dipeptidase precluded major improvements in sulopenem oral bioavailability provided by increased absorption of its prodrug ester. A proposed representation of PF-03709270 absorption and metabolism in the intestine is shown in Figure 15.20 based on the data generated to date. While improved stability against pancreatic enzymes is realized, dissolved dose is subject to further metabolism by gut flora to yield hydrolyzed prodrug as well as reduction of the sulfoxide to yield the sulfide.

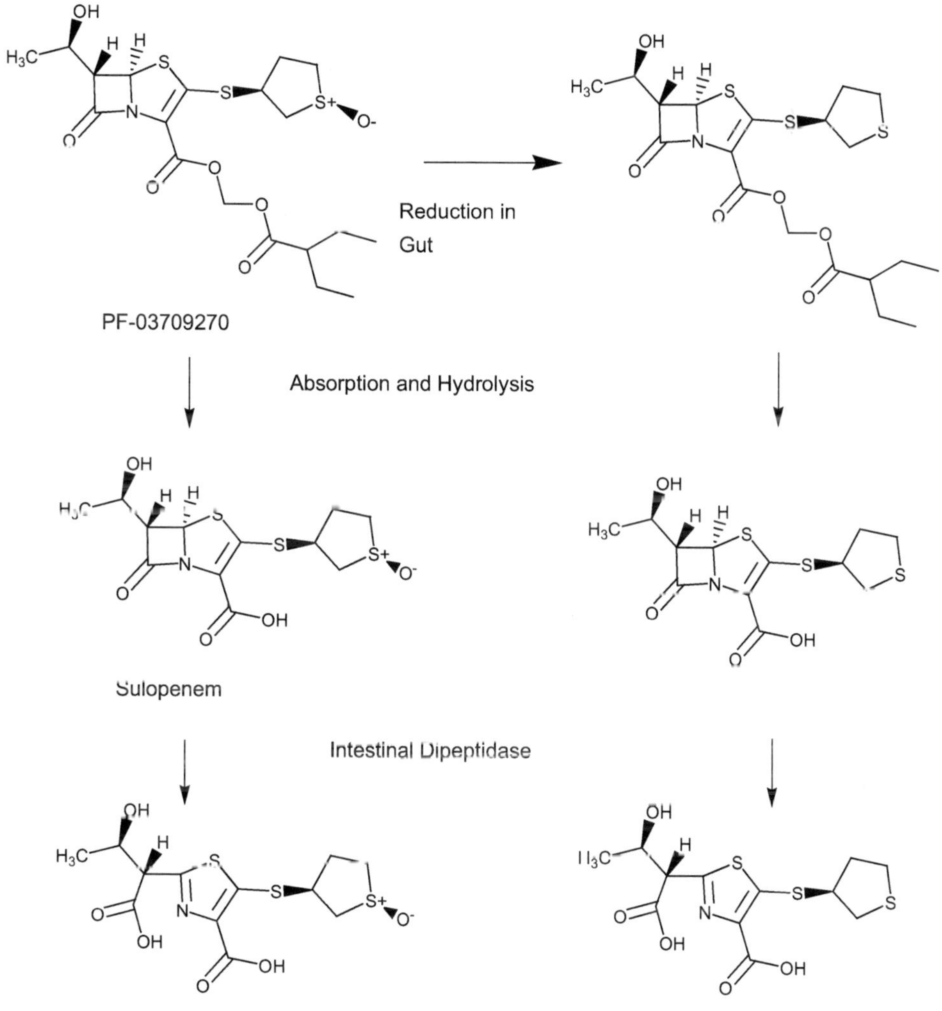


**Figure 15.20** Proposed metabolites following oral administration of [$^{14}$C]-PF-03709270.

Passive absorption of intact PF-03709270 and its sulfide metabolite yields high levels of sulopenem and the sulfide following hydrolysis of the prodrug ester – a reaction that appears to be catalytically efficient based on the observation of no intact prodrug in the basolateral pole of Caco-2 studies. Intact sulopenem and its sulfide metabolite are subject to hydrolysis of the β-lactam ring via dipeptidase activity within the enterocyte-limiting bioavailability improvement afforded with the lipophilic prodrug ester. Reduction of the sulfoxide by gut flora and hydrolysis of the prodrug due to the increasing pH environment of the lower GI tract creates a narrow absorption window for delivering optimum exposure of sulopenem.

Despite the comparatively low bioavailability achieved with PF-03709270 and PF-04064900, the exposure achieved with 1000 mg of PF-03709270 has been shown to be sufficient for establishing efficacy in human Phase II clinical trials [88]. Additionally, the comparatively moderate fraction absorbed achieved with these prodrugs improves the tolerability of sulopenem by reducing the amount of active antibiotic reaching the distal portion of the GI tract where it could act to disrupt the balance of gut flora.

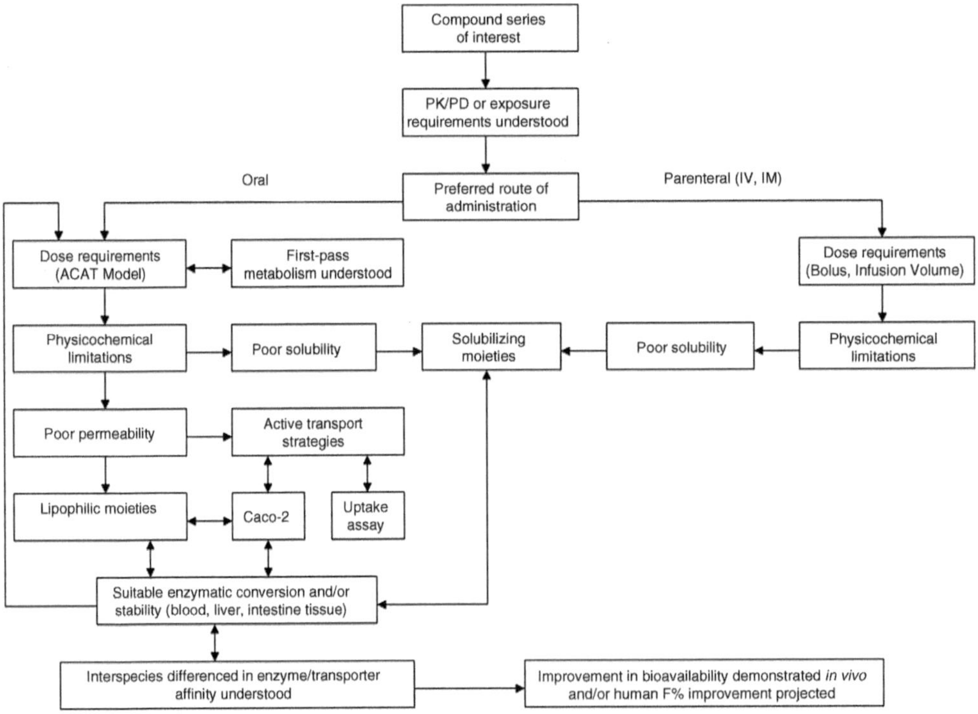


**Figure 15.21** Proposed considerations for an effective prodrug screening strategy.

## 15.11 Conclusions

Incorporation of prodrug strategies in the development of NCEs that present with suboptimal properties for required exposure is becoming an integral part of the discovery process today. Retrospective evaluation of successful prodrugs as well as a contemporary understanding of passive and carrier-mediated transport processes, enzymatic conversion, and biopharmaceutical considerations have provided the medicinal chemist the knowledge needed to increase the odds of success. A fundamental understanding of the pharmacokinetic/pharmacodynamic relationship to drug efficacy is critical to determining the type of strategy to pursue. The effective use and prioritization of *in vitro* and *in vivo* studies detailed in this chapter and summarized in Figure 15.21 is encouraged to enable a viable prodrug screening effort.

## References


1 Rautio, J., Kumpulainen, H., Heimbach, T., Oliyai, R., Oh, D, J arvinen, T., and Savolainen, J. (2008) Prodrugs: design and clinical applications. *Nature Reviews*, **7**, 255–270.

2 Craig, W. (1998) Pharmacokinetic/pharmacodynamic parameters: rationale for antimicrobial dosing of mice and men. *Clinical Infectious Diseases*, **26**, 1–12.

3 Davies, B. and Morris, T. (1993) Physiological parameters in laboratory animals and humans. *Pharmaceutical Research*, **10** (7), 1093–1096.

4 Griffiths, R., Lewis, A., and Jeffrey, P. (1996) Models for drug absorption *in situ* and in conscious animals, in *Models for Assessing Drug Absorption and Metabolism* (eds R. Borchard and T. Smith), Plenum Press, New York, pp. 67–81.

5 Rane, A., Wilkinson, G.R., and Shand, D.G. (1977) Prediction of hepatic extraction ratio from *in vitro* measurement of intrinsic clearance. *Journal of Pharmacology and Experimental Therapeutics*, **200**, 420–424.

6 Obach, R.S., Baxter, J.G., Liston, T.E., Silber, B.M., Jones, B.C., MacIntyre, F., Rance, D.J., and Wastall, P. (1997) The prediction of human pharmacokinetic parameters from preclinical and *in vitro* metabolism data. *Journal of Pharmacology and Experimental Therapeutics*, **283**, 46–58.

7 Beaumont, K., Webster, R., Gardner, I., and Dack, K. (2003) Design of ester prodrugs to enhance oral absorption of poorly permeable compounds: challenges to the discovery scientist. *Current Drug Metabolism*, **4**, 461–485.

8 Han, H-k., Rhie, J.K., Oh, D-M., Saito, G., Hsu, C-P., Stewart, B.H., and Amidon, G.L. (1999) CHO/hPEPT1 Cells overexpressing the human peptide transporter (hPEPT1) as an alternate *in vitro* model for peptidomimetic drugs. *Journal of Pharmaceutical Sciences*, **88** (3), 347–350.

9 Landowski, C.P., Vig, B.S., Song, X., and Amidon, G.L. (2005) Targeted delivery to PEPT1-overexpressing cells: acidic, basic, and secondary floxuridine amino acid ester prodrugs. *Molecular Cancer Therapy*, **4** (4), 659–667.

10 Liederer, B.M. and Borchardt, R.T. (2005) Enzymes involved in the bioconversion of ester based prodrugs. *Journal of Pharmaceutical Sciences*, **95** (6), 1177–1195.

11 Sato, T. and Hosokawa, M. (1998) The mammalian carboxylesterases: from molecules to function. *Annual Reviews of Pharmacological Toxicology*, **38**, 257–288.

12 Brodin, B., Nielsen, C.U., Steffansen, B., and Frockjaer, S. (2002) Transport

of peptidomimetic drugs by intestinal di/tri peptide transporter, PepT1. *Pharmacological Toxicology*, **90**, 285–296.

13 Imai, T. (2006) Human carboxylesterase isozymes: catalytic properties and rational drug design. *Drug Metabolism and Pharmacokinetics*, **21**, 173–185.

14 Imai, T., Taketani, M., Shii, M., Hosokawa, M., and Chiba, K. (2006) Substrate specificity of carboxylesterase isozymes and their contribution to hydrolase activity in human liver and small intestine. *Drug Metabolism and Disposition*, **34** (10), 1734–1741.

15 Taketani, M., Shii, M., Ohura, K., Ninomiya, S., and Imai, T. (2007) Carboxylesterase in the liver and small intestine of experimental animals and human. *Life Sciences*, **81**, 924–932.

16 Englund, G., Rorsman, F., Ronnblom, A., Karlbom, U., Lazorova, L., Grasjo, J., Kindmark, A., and Artursson, P. (2006) Regional levels of drug transporters along the human intestinal tract: co-expression of ABC and SLC transporters and comparison with Caco-2 cells. *European Journal of Pharmaceutical Sciences*, **29**, 269–277.

17 Lu, H. and Klaassen, C. (2006) Tissue distribution and thyroid hormone regulation of Pept1 and Pept2 MRNA in rodents. *Peptides*, **27**, 850–857.

18 Chiou, W.L. and Barve, A. (1998) Linear correlation of the fraction of oral dose absorbed of 64 drugs between humans and rats. *Pharmaceutical Research*, **15** (11), 1792–1795.

19 Lee, Y.H., Perry, B.A., Lee, H.S., Kunta, J.R., Sutyak, J.P., and Sinko, P.J. (2001) Differential of gut and hepatic first-pass effect of drugs. 1. Studies of verapamil in ported dogs. *Pharmaceutical Research*, **18**, 1721–1728.

20 Sinko, P.J., Sutyak, J.P., Leesman, G.D., Hu, P., Makhey, V.D., Yu, H., and Smith, C.L. (1997) Oral absorption of anti-AIDs nucleoside analogues. 3. Regional absorption and the *in vivo* permeability of 2′,3′-dideoxyinosine in an intestinal-vascular access port (IVAP) dog model. *Biopharmaceutics and Drug Disposition*, **18** (8), 697–710.

21 He, Y-L., Murby, S., Warhurst, G., Gifford, L., Walker, D., Ayrton, J., Eastmond, R., and Rowland, M. (1998) Species differences in size discrimination in the paracellular pathway reflected by the oral bioavailability of poly(ethylene glycol) and D-peptides. *Journal of Pharmaceutical Sciences*, **87**, 626–633.

22 Perkins, E.J. and Abraham, T. (2007) Pharmacokinetics, metabolism, and excretion of the intestinal peptide transporter 1 (SLC15A1)-targeted prodrug (1*S*,2*S*,5*R*,6*S*)-2-[(2′*S*]-(2-amino) propionyl]aminobicyclo[3.1.0]hexen-2,6-dicarboxylic acid (LY544344) in rats and dogs: assessment of first-pass bioactivation and dose linearity. *Drug Metabolism and Disposition*, **35**, 1903–1909.

23 Bueno, A.B., Collado, I., Dios, A.d., Dominguez, C., Martin, J.A., Martin, L.M., Martinez-Grau, M.A., Montero, C., Pedregal, C., and Catlow, J. (2005) Dipeptides as effective prodrugs of the unnatural amino acid (+)-2-aminobicyclo[3.1.0]hexane-2,6-dicarboxylic acid (LY354740, a selective Group II metabotropic glutamate receptor agonist. *Journal of Medicinal Chemistry*, **48**, 5305–5320.

24 Takai, S., Mutsuda, A., Usami, Y., Adachi, T., Sugiyama, T., Katagiri, Y., Tatematsu, M., and Hirano, K. (1997) Hydrolytic profile for ester- or amide linkage by carboxylesterases pI 5.3 and 4.5 from human liver. *Biological Pharmaceutical Bulletin*, **20**, 869–873.

25 Humerickhouse, R., Lohrbach, K., Ki, L., Bosron, W.F., and Dolan, M.E. (2000) Characterization of CPT-11 hydrolysis by human carboxylesterase isoforms hCE-1 and hCE-2. *Cancer Research*, **60**, 1189–1192.

26 Tabata, T., Katoh, M., Tokudome, S., Nakajima, M., and Yokoi, T. (2004) Identification of the cytosolic carboxylesterase catalyzing 5′-deoxy-5-fluorocytidine formation from capecitabine in human liver. *Drug Metabolism and Disposition*, **32**, 1103–1110.

27 Xu, G., Zhang, W., Ma, M.K., and McLeod, H.L. (2002) Human

carboxylesterase 2 is commonly expressed in tumor tissue and is correlated with activation of irinotecan. *Clinical Cancer Research*, **8**, 2605–2611.
28 Sato, T., Taylor, P., Bosron, W.F., Sanghani, P., Hosokawa, M., and Du, B.N. (2002) Current progress on esterases: from molecular structure to function. *Drug Metabolism and Disposition*, **30**, 488–493.
29 Imai, T., Imoto, M., Sakamoto, H., and Hashimoto, M. (2005) Identification of esterases expressed in Caco-2 cells and effects of their hydrolyzing activity in predicting human intestinal absorption. *Drug Metabolism and Disposition*, **33**, 1185–1190.
30 Khanna, R., Morton, C.L., Danks, M.K., and Potter, P. (2000) Proficient metabolism of irinotecan by human intestinal carboxylesterase. *Cancer Research*, **60**, 4725–4728.
31 Danks, M.K., Morton, C.L., Krull, E.J., Cheshire, P.J., Richmond, L.B., Naeve, C.W., Pawlik, C.A., Houghton, P.J., and Potter, P. (1999) Comparison of activation of CPT-11 by rabbit and human carboxylesterase for use in enzyme/prodrug therapy. *Clinical Cancer Research*, **5**, 917–924.
32 Shimma, N., Umeda, I., Arasaki, M., Murasaki, C., Masubuchi, K., Kohchi, Y., Miwa, M., Ura, M., Sawada, N., Tahara, H., Kuruma, I., Horii, I., and Ishitsuka, H. (2000) The design and synthesis of a new tumor-selective fluoropyrimidine carbamate, capecitabine. *Bioorganic and Medicinal Chemistry*, **8**, 1697–1706.
33 Lipinski, C. (2002) Poor solubility: an industry wide problem in drug discovery. *American Pharmaceutical Reviews*, **5**, 82–85.
34 Amidon, G.L., Lennernas, H., Shah, V.P., and Crison, J.R. (1995) A theorctical basis for a biopharmaceutic drug classification: the correlation of *in vitro* drug product dissolution and *in vivo* bioavailability. *Pharmaceutical Research*, **12** (3), 413–420.
35 Heimbach, T., Fleisher, D., and Kaddoumi, A. (2007) in *Prodrugs: Challenges and Rewards. Part 1* (eds V.J. Stella *et al.*) AAPS Press/Springer, New York, pp. 115–212.
36 Varia S.A., Schuller, S., Sloan, K.B., and Stella, V.J. (1984) Phenytoin prodrugs III: water soluble prodrugs for oral and/or parenteral use. *Journal of Pharmaceutical Sciences*, **73**, 1068–1073.
37 Boucher, B.A. (1996) Fosphenytoin: a novel phenytoin prodrug. *Pharmacotherapy*, **16**, 777–791.
38 Heimbach, T., Oh, D-M., Li, L.Y., Forsberg, M., Savolainen, J., Leppanen, J., Matsunaga, Y., Flynn, G., and Fleisher, D. (2003) Absorption rate limit considerations for oral phosphate prodrugs. *Pharmaceutical Research*, **20** (6), 848–856.
39 Masuda, H., Ikeda, K., Nagamachi, N., Nagayama, S., and Kawaguchi, Y. (1998) Metabolic Fate of TAT-59 (4th report) species difference, dose response and protein binding. *Yakuri to Chiryo*, **26**, 809–828.
40 Heimbach, T., Oh, D-M., Li, L.Y., Rodriguez-Hornedo, N., Garcia, G., and Fleisher, D. (2003) Enzyme-mediated precipitation of parent drugs from their phosphate prodrugs. *International Journal of Pharmaceutics*, **261**, 81–92.
41 Erion, M.D. *et al.* (2004) Design, synthesis, and characterization of a series of cytochrome P(450)3A-activated prodrugs (HepDirect prodrugs) useful for targeting phosphonate-based drugs to the liver. *Journal of the American Chemical Society*, **126**, 5154–5163.
42 Erion, M.D., Bullough, D.A., Lin, C.C., and Hong, Z. (2006) HepDirect prodrugs for targeting nucleotide-based antiviral drugs to the liver. *Current Opinion of Investigational Drugs*, **7**, 109–117.
43 Huttunen, K.M., Mahonen, N., Leppanen, J., Vepsalainen, J., Juvonen, R.O., Raunio, H., Kumpulainen, H., Jarvinen, T., and Rautio, J. (2007) Novel cyclic phosphate prodrug approach for cytochrome P450-activated drugs containing an alcohol functionality. *Pharmaceutical Research*, **24** (4), 679–687.
44 Fujitaki, J.M., Cable, E.E., Ito, B.R., Zhang, B-H., Hou, J., Yang, C., Bullough, D.A., Ferro, J.L., van Poelje, P.D., Linemeyer, D.L., and Erion, M.D. (2008) Preclinical pharmacokinetics of a HepDirect

prodrug of a novel phosphonate-containing thyroid hormone receptor agonist. *Drug Metabolism and Disposition,* **36**, 2393–2403.

45 Li, F., Maag, H., and Alfredson, T. (2008) Prodrugs of nucleoside analogues for improved oral absorption and tissue targeting. *Journal of Pharmaceutical Sciences,* **97** (3), 1109–1134.

46 Braditch-Crovo, P., Toole, J., Hendrix, C.W., Cundy, K.C., Ebeling, D., Jaffe, H.S., and Lietman, P.S. (1997) Anti-human immunodeficiency virus (HIV) activity, safety, and pharmacokinetics of adefovir dipivoxil (9-[2-(bis-(pivaloyloxymethyl)-phosphonylmethoxyethyl]adenine) in HIV infected patients. *Journal of Infectious Diseases,* **176**, 406–413.

47 Cundy, K.C., Barditch-Crovo, P., Walker, R.E., Collier, A.C., Ebling, D., Toole, J., and Jaffe, H.S. (1995) Clinical pharmacokinetics of adefovir in human immunodeficiency virus type 1-infected patients. *Antimicrobial Agents and Chemotherapy,* **39**, 2401–2405.

48 Annaert, P., Kinget, R., Naesens, L., Clercq, E.d., and Augustijns, P. (1997) Transport, uptake, and metabolism of the bis(pivaloyloxymethyl)-ester prodrug of 9-(2-phosphonylmethoxyethyl)adenine in an *in vitro* cell culture system of the intestinal mucosa (Caco-2). *Pharmaceutical Research,* **14** (4), 492–496.

49 Annaert, P., Gelder, J.V., Naesens, L., Clercq, E.D., den Mooter, G.V., Kinget, R., and Augustijns, P. (1998) Carrier mechanisms involved in the transepithelial transport of bis(POM)-PMEA and its metabolites across Caco-2 monolayers. *Pharmaceutical Research,* **15** (8), 1168–1173.

50 Mouly, S. and Paine, M.F. (2003) *Pharmaceutical Research,* **20** (10), 1595–1598.

51 Wacher, V.J., Salphati, L., and Benet, L. (1996) Active secretion and enterocytic drug metabolism barriers to drug absorption. *Advanced Drug Delivery Reviews,* **20**, 99–112.

52 Lampen, A., Zhang, Y., Hackbarth, I., Benet, L.Z., Sewing, K.F., and Christians, U. (1998) Metabolism and transport of the macrolide immunosuppressant sirolimus in the small intestine. *Journal of Pharmacology and Experimental Therapeutics,* **285**, 1104–1112.

53 Hebert, M.F. (1997) Contributions of hepatic and intestinal metabolism and P-glyciprotein to cyclosporin and tacrolimus oral drug delivery. *Advanced Drug Delivery Reviews,* **27**, 201–214.

54 Beaumont, K., Harper, A., Smith, D.A., and Bennett, J. (2000) The role of P-glycoprotein in determining the oral absorption and clearance of the NK2 antagonist, UK-224,671. *European Journal of Pharmaceutical Sciences,* **12**, 41–50.

55 Prueksaritanont, T., Deluna, P., Gorham, L.M., Ma, B., Cohn, D., Pang, J., Xu, X., Leuing, K., and Lin, J.H. (1998) *In vitro* and *in vivo* evaluations of intestinal barriers for the zwitterion L-767,679 and its carboxyl ester prodrug L-775,318. *Drug Metabolism and Disposition,* **26** (6), 520–527.

56 Gelder, J.V., Deferme, S., Naesens, L., Clercq, E.D., den Mooter, G.V., Kinget, R., and Augustijns, P. (2002) Intestinal absorption enhancement of the ester prodrug tenofovir disoproxil fumarate through modulation of the biochemical barrier by defined ester mixtures. *Drug Metabolism and Disposition,* **30**, 924–930.

57 McLean, M.J. (1999) Gabapentin in the management of convulsive disorders. *Epilepsia,* **40** (Suppl. 6), S39–S40.

58 Pollack, M.H., Matthews, J., and Scott, E.L. (1998) Gabapentin as a potential treatment for anxiety disorders. *American Journal of Psychiatry,* **155**, 992–993.

59 Gidal, B.E., Radulovic, L.L., Kruger, S., Rutecki, P., Pitterle, M., and Brockbrader, H.N. (2000) Inter- and intra-subject variability in gabapentin absorption and absolute bioavailability. *Epilepsy Research,* **40**, 123–127.

60 Stewart, B.H., Kugler, A.R., Thompson, P.R., and Brockbrader, H.N. (1993) A saturable transport mechanism in the intestinal absorption of gabapentin is the underlying cause of the lack of proportionality between increasing dose and the drug levels in plasma. *Pharmaceutical Research,* **10**, 276–281.

61 McLean, M.J. (1995) Gabapentin. *Epilepsia*, **36** (Suppl. 2), S73–S76.

62 Cundy, K.C., Branch, R., Chernov-Rogan, T., Dias, T., Estrada, T., Hold, K., Koller, K., Li, X., Mann, A., Panuwat, M., Raillard, S.P., Upadhyay, S., Wu, Q.Q., Xiang, J-N., Yan, H., Zerangue, N., Zhou, C.X., Barrett, R.W., and Gallop, M.A. (2004) XP13512 [(+/−)-1-([(α-isobutanoyloxyethoxy) carbonyl]aminomethyl)-1-cyclohexane acetic acid, a novel gabepentin prodrug. I. design, synthesis, enzymatic conversion to gabapentin, and transport by intestinal solute transporters. *Journal of Pharmacology and Experimental Therapeutics*, **311** (1), 315–323.

63 Cundy, K.C., Annamalai, T., Bu, L., Vera, J.D., Estrela, J., Luo, W., Shirsat, P., Torneros, A., Yao, F., Zou, J., Barrett, R.W., and Gallop, M.A. (2004) XP13512 [(+/−)-1-([(α-isobutanoyloxyethoxy) carbonyl]aminomethyl)-1-cyclohexane acetic acid], a novel gabapentin prodrug. II. Improved oral bioavailability, dose proportionality, and colonic absorption compared with gabapentin in rats and monkeys. *Journal of Pharmacology and Experimental Therapeutics*, **311** (1), 324–333.

64 Cundy, K.C., Sastry, S., Luo, W., Zou, J., Moors, T.L., and Canafax, D.M. (2008) Clinical pharmacokinetics of XP13512, a novel transported prodrug of gabapentin. *Journal of Clinical Pharmacology*, **48**, 1378–1388.

65 Nakashima, E., Tsuji, A., Kagatani, S., and Yamana, T. (1984) Intestinal absorption mechanism of amino-β-lactam antibiotics. III. Kinetics of carrier mediated transport across the rat small intestine *in situ*. *Journal of Pharmacobiological Dynamics*, **7**, 452–464.

66 Lafforgue, G., Arellano, C., Vachoux, C., Woodley, J., Philibert, C., Dupouy, V., Bousquet-Melou, A., Gandia, P., and Houin, G. (2008) Oral absorption of ampicillin: role of paracellular route vs. PepT1 transporter. *Fundamental Clinical Pharmacology*, **22** (2), 189–201.

67 Chanteux, H., Bambeke, F.V., Mingeot-Leclercq, M-P., and Tulkens, P.M. (2005) Accumulation and oriented transport of ampicillin in Caco-2 cells from its pivaloyloxymethylester prodrug, pivampicillin. *Antimicrobial Agents and Chemotherapy*, **49** (4), 1279–1288.

68 Oh, D.M., Han, H.K., and Amidon, G.L. (1999) Drug transport and targeting. Intestinal transport. *Pharmaceutical Biotechnology*, **12**, 59–88.

69 Varma, M.V.S., Eriksson, A.H., Sawada, G., Pak, Y.A., Perkins, E.J., and Zimmerman, C.L. (2009) Transepithelial transport of the Group II metabotropic glutamate 2/3 receptor agonist (1*S*,2*S*,5*R*,6*S*)-2-aminobicyclo[3.1.0] hexane-2,6-dicarboxylate (LY354740) and its prodrug (1*S*,2*S*,5*R*,6*S*)-2-[(2′-amino) propionyl]aminobicyclo[3.1.0]hexane-2,6-dicarboxylate (LY544344). *Drug Metabolism and Disposition*, **37**, 211–220.

70 Eddy, E.P., Wood, C., Miller, J., Wilson, G., and Hidalgo, I.J. (1995) A comparison of the affinities of dipeptides and antibiotics for the di/tripeptide transporter in Caco-2 cells. *International Journal of Pharmaceutics*, **115**, 79–86.

71 Brodin, B., Nielsen, C.U., Steffansen, B., and Frokjaer, F. (2002) Transport of peptidomimetic drugs by the intestinal di/tri-peptide transporter PepT1. *Pharmacological Toxicology*, **90**, 285–296.

72 Friedrichsen, G.M., Jacobsen, P., Taub, M.E., and Begtrup, M. (2001) Application of enzymatically stable dipeptides for enhancement of intestinal permeability. Synthesis and *in vitro* evaluation of dipeptide-coupled compounds. *Bioorganic Medicinal Chemistry*, **9**, 2625–2632.

73 Thomsen, A.E., Friedrichsen, G., Sorensen, A.H., Andersen, R., Neilsen, C.U., Brodin, B., Begtrup, M., Frokjaer, S., and Steffansen, B. (2003) Prodrugs of purine and pyrimidine analogues for the intestinal di/tripeptide transporter PepT1: affinity for hPepT1 in Caco-2 cells, drug release in aqueous media and *in vitro* metabolism. *Controlled Release*, **86**, 279–292.

74 Nielsen, C.U., Andersen, R., Brodin, B., Frokjaer, S., and Taub, M.E. (2001) Dipeptide model prodrugs for the intestinal oligopeptide transporter. Affinity for and transport via hPepT1 in

the human intestinal Caco-2 cell line. *Journal of Controlled Release*, **76**, 129–138.

75 Bai, J.P.F. (1995) pGlu-L-Dopa-Pro: a tripeptide prodrug targeting the intestinal peptide transporter for absorption and tissue enzymes for conversation. *Pharmaceutical Research*, **12**, 1101–1104.

76 Tamai, I., Nakanishi, T., Nakahara, H., Sai, Y., Ganapathy, V., Leibach, F.H., and Tsuji, A. (1998) Improvement of L-dopa absorption by dipeptidyl derivatization utilizing peptide transporter PepT1. *Journal of Pharmaceutical Sciences*, **87**, 1542–1546.

77 Soul-Lawton, J., Seaber, E., On, N., Wootton, R., Rolan, P., and Posner, J. (1995) Absolute bioavailability and metabolic disposition of valacyclovir, the L-valyl ester of acyclovir, following oral administration to humans. *Antimicrobial Agents and Chemotherapy*, **39**, 2759–2764.

78 Beauchamp, L.M., Orr, G.F., Miranda, P.d., Doucette, M., Burnette, T., and Krenitsky, T.A. (1992) Amino acid ester prodrugs of acyclovir. *Antiviral Chemistry and Chemotherapy*, **3**, 157–164.

79 Sinko, P.J. and Balimane, P.V. (1998) Carrier-mediated intestinal absorption of valacyclovir, the L-valyl ester prodrug of acyclovir. 1. Interactions with peptides, organic anions and organic cations in rats. *Biopharmaceutics and Drug Disposition*, **19**, 209–217.

80 Landowski, C.P., Sun, D., Foster, D.R., Menon, S.S., Barnett, J.L., Welage, L.S., Ramachandran, C., and Amidon, G.L. (2003) Gene expression in the human intestine and correlation with oral valacyclovir pharmacokinetic parameters. *Journal of Pharmacology and Experimental Therapeutics*, **306**, 778–786.

81 Bolger, M.B., Lukacova, V., and Woltosz, W.S. (2009) Simulations of Nonlinear Dose Dependence for Substrates of Influx and Efflux Transporters in the Human Intestine. *The AAPS journal*, **11**(2), 353–363.

82 Herrera-Ruiz, D., Wang, Q., Gudmundsson, O.S., Cook, T.J., Smith, R.L., Faria, T.N., and Knipp, G.T. (2001) Spatial expression patterns of peptide transporters in the human and rat gastrointestinal tracts, Caco-2 *in vitro* cell culture model and multiple human tissues. *AAPS Pharmaceutical Sciences*, **3**, E9.

83 Stoeckel, K., Hofheinz, W., Laneury, J.P., Duchene, P., Shedlofsky, S., and Blouin, R. (1998) Stability of cephalosporin prodrug esters in human intestinal juice: implications for oral bioavailability. *Antimicrobial Agents and Chemotherapy*, **42** (10), 2602–2606.

84 Richter, W.F., Chong, Y.H., and Stella, V.J. (1990) On the mechanism of isomerization of cephalosporin esters. *Journal of Pharmaceutical Sciences*, **79**, 185–186.

85 O'Donnell, J.P., Brighty, K., Engtrakul, J., Fichtner, M., Gootz, T., Hardink, J., Hazra, A., Lamb, L., Lo, J., Marfat, A., Marra, A., McLeod, D., Monahan, R., Price, L., Smith, W., Soma, K., Sutton, S., and Winton, J. (2008) Biopharmaceutical-based pharmacokinetic modeling of sulopenem prodrugs: impact of luminal stability on fraction of dose absorbed. 48th Annual Interscience Conference on Antimicrobial Agents and Chemotherapy (ICAAC) and the Infectious Diseases Society of America (IDSA) 46th Annual Meeting, Washington, DC, Abstract F1-352.

86 Yu, L.X. and Amidon, G.L. (1999) A compartmental absorption and transit model for estimating oral drug absorption. *International Journal of Pharmaceutics*, **186**, 119–125.

87 Strong, H.A., Oates, J., Sembi, J., Renwick, A.G., and George, C.F. (1984) Role of the gut flora in the reduction of sulfinpyrazone in humans. *Journal of Pharmacology and Experimental Therapeutics*, **230** (3), 726–732.

88 Forrest, A., Hazra, A., Girard, D., Finegan, S., O'Donnell, J., and Soma, K. (2008) PK/PD analysis to select PF-03709270 (PF) doses, with & without probenecid (P) for Phase 2b trials. 48th Annual Interscience Conference on Antimicrobial Agents and Chemotherapy (ICAAC) and the Infectious Diseases Society of America (IDSA) 46th Annual Meeting, Washington DC, Abstract A-034.

# 16
# The Impact of Pharmacogenetics on the Clinical Outcomes of Prodrugs[1)]

*Jane P.F. Bai, Mike Pacanowski, Atiqur Rahman, and Lawrence L. Lesko*

## 16.1
## Introduction

Pharmacogenetics is the study of how genetic variation impacts the pharmacokinetics, pharmacodynamics, or clinical outcomes of drug therapy and seeks to predict how an individual or individual subgroup is likely to respond to a particular medication. Genetic variations related to drug response often reside with drug metabolizing enzymes, transporters, and receptors. For drugs where responses are closely related to drug exposure, pharmacokinetic variability may ultimately affect the drug's clinical efficacy and safety. For instance, warfarin is an anticoagulant drug that targets vitamin K epoxide reductase (VKORC1) and is metabolized by cytochrome P-450 2C9 (CYP2C9). Single-nucleotide polymorphisms (SNPs) in the *VKORC1* gene confer sensitivity, while *CYP2C9* SNPs modulate exposure. SNPs in these genes account for the majority of pharmacodynamic variability (i.e., INR) in warfarin response and have been associated with higher rate of bleeding [1]. Applying pharmacogenetics in the clinical use of the drug has the potential to minimize response heterogeneity and improve the risk–benefit ratio.

A prodrug is an inactive precursor to an active drug. Prodrugs are usually developed to improve the bioavailability and delivery of the active drug by (1) increasing its aqueous solubility or membrane permeability, (2) reducing its hepatic or intestinal first-pass metabolism, or (3) targeting delivery of active drug to a specific organ via an organ-specific transporter for uptake or via an organ-specific enzyme for release of active drug. The pharmacologically active molecule is released upon being metabolized *in vivo*, and the enzymes involved in releasing active drugs from their inactive precursors could reside in the intestine, liver, plasma, or a specific organ, such as brain or kidney. On the other hand, many prodrugs that are commonly used in clinical practice were not designed so strategically, but were successfully developed into a medication because the metabolites are therapeutically active.

1) *Disclaimer*: The article represents the views of the authors and not the offical position of the US Food and Drug Administration.

*Prodrugs and Targeted Delivery: Towards Better ADME Properties*. Edited by Jarkko Rautio

ISBN: 978-3-527-32603-7

Tamoxifen and clopidogrel are such examples where the major active metabolite was characterized after the drug came into routine use.

The enzymes involved in prodrug activation can be polymorphic and subject to interindividual variability in activity. For example, genetic variation in CYP450 enzymes is known to affect the disposition and response of many drugs. Variability in prodrug-activating enzyme activity, either due to varying protein expression or due to intrinsic activity, could ultimately result in high variations in the systemic exposure of active drugs. Accumulating evidence suggests that polymorphisms of prodrug-activating enzymes contribute substantially to variability in prodrug exposure, and by extension, the clinical efficacy and safety of these compounds.

This chapter will highlight several examples in which drug-metabolizing enzyme polymorphisms have demonstrated effects on the systemic exposure and responses to prodrugs, including clopidogrel, codeine, tamoxifen, capecitabine, tegafur, irinotecan, and cyclosphosphamide, in hope of providing scientists with understanding how pharmacogenetics impacts clinical response by a prodrug. For each prodrug, the impact of genetic polymorphisms of prodrug-activating enzymes on its systemic exposure, efficacy, and safety is summarized. Furthermore, implications of such lessons learned on drug development will be highlighted.

## 16.2 Clopidogrel and CYP2C19

Clopidogrel is a thienopyridine antiplatelet drug that has become the standard of care to prevent cardiovascular events in patients with acute or recent myocardial infarction (MI), recent stroke, or peripheral artery disease. At the time clopidogrel was first approved, it was known to be a prodrug of an active metabolite that irreversibly inhibits the platelet ADP receptor, P2Y12 [2]. However, the active metabolite has a highly unstable thiol group, which has made it difficult to quantify, and the metabolic pathway and structure of the active metabolite were not elucidated until several years after its approval [3, 4]. In recent years, assay methods have been developed to quantify the active metabolite, which has led to a greater understanding of clopidogrel disposition and response [5].

The active metabolite of clopidogrel is formed in two sequential steps. Following oral administration, the parent compound is rapidly absorbed. The majority (85%) of the inactive prodrug is converted *in vivo* to the inactive carboxylic acid metabolite [6]. Multiple CYP450 enzymes including CYP1A2, CYP2B6, CYP2C9, CYP2C19, and CYP3A4/5 convert the remaining parent compound first to an intermediate, 2-oxo-clopidogrel and then to the active thiol metabolite, as shown in Figure 16.1 [4, 7–9]. This metabolite is then free to bind to the platelet ADP receptor. Based on the redundancy of this activation pathway, complete loss of function in any one enzyme, ostensibly, will not necessarily result in complete loss of active metabolite generation.

Variability in the response to clopidogrel is well documented. It has been reported that approximately one-third of patients have less than a 10% change in platelet aggregation following routine loading doses of clopidogrel [10]. Many factors may

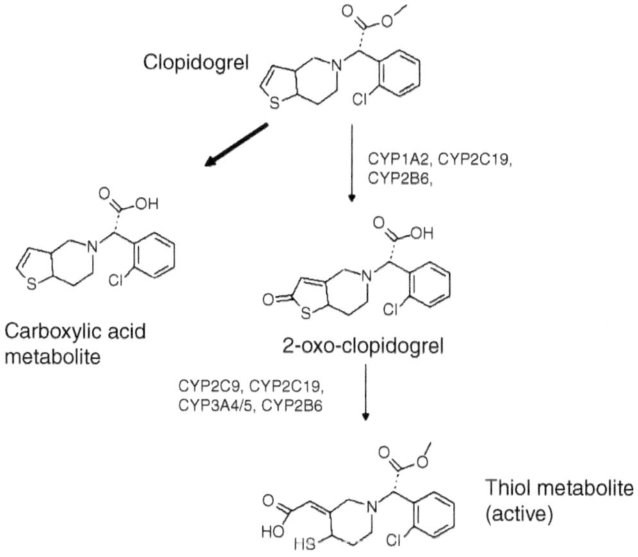


**Figure 16.1** Activation pathways of clopidogrel.

contribute to this response variability, including patient adherence to therapy, comorbid disease states such as diabetes, or genetic factors. It is becoming increasingly recognized that pharmacokinetic differences in active metabolite formation, as determined by CYP2C19 metabolic activity, account for a portion of the variability [11].

CYP3A4 and CYP3A5 have been shown to be the major CYP450 enzymes involved in clopidogrel metabolism in *in vitro* experiments [7]. Drug interaction studies with CYP3A4 inhibitors such as ketoconazole and verapamil demonstrated reduced antiplatelet responses [12, 13]. However, extending these findings to genetic polymorphism has not been as consistent. Angiolillo *et al.* evaluated several polymorphisms in *CYP3A4*, demonstrating that the IVS10 + 12G > A polymorphism was associated with greater response in terms of ADP-mediated glycoprotein IIb/IIIa activation [14]. This was not replicated in other pharmacodynamic studies [12, 15–17]. Although it is known that *CYP3A5* also has common loss-of-function polymorphisms, pharmacokinetic and pharmacodynamic studies have not demonstrated a consistent effect on clopidogrel disposition or response [16–21].

CYP2C19 has surfaced as a major determinant of clopidogrel pharmacokinetics and pharmacodynamics. More than a dozen studies have been published that describe a significant impact of *CYP2C19* polymorphisms, particularly the *2 allele, on the antiplatelet responses to clopidogrel. These findings have since been extended to drug interactions with CYP2C19 inhibitors, namely, the proton pump inhibitors [22, 23].

Due to the instability of the active metabolite, initial studies characterized genotypic differences in the parent compound disposition. In Korean subjects, Kim *et al.* [24] reported that parent compound exposure (area under the concentration–time curve, AUC) was approximately two- and threefold higher in intermediate and poor metabolizers, respectively, relative to extensive metabolizers after a 300 mg loading dose and 75 mg maintenance dose. Consistent with higher parent compound exposures and the inferred reduction in active metabolite generation, antiplatelet responses were 31% lower in intermediate metabolizers and 41% lower in poor metabolizers following the loading dose. Similar findings were observed after 6 days at the maintenance dose.

Upon developing assay methods for the active metabolite, Umemura *et al.* undertook a single-dose study of 300 mg on 47 Japanese subjects [25]. In this study, the ratio of active metabolite exposure relative to extensive metabolizers was 0.67 (95% confidence interval (CI), 0.51–0.83) for intermediate metabolizers and 0.61 (95% CI, 0.45–0.82) for poor metabolizers. Active metabolite exposure was moderately but significantly correlated with two measures of antiplatelet response, and patients with one or two *2 or *3 alleles demonstrated significantly diminished antiplatelet responses.

The most comprehensive study conducted to date evaluated active metabolite disposition and response with a pooled analysis across several clinical pharmacology studies. The investigators evaluated variation not only in *CYP2C19* but also in *CYP1A2*, *CYP2B6*, *CYP2C9*, and *CYP3A4/5*. The first report captured the results of two studies evaluating 300 mg loading doses in a total of 89 subjects [19]. The AUC and $C_{max}$ of the active metabolite of clopidogrel was almost 50% lower in patients carrying a *2 allele of *CYP2C19*. Poor response (defined as <20% inhibition of platelet aggregation) was significantly more prevalent among *CYP2C19*2* carriers (13 of 18 subjects). In a subsequent report [9], the same pharmacogenetic analysis strategy was applied to six other clinical pharmacology studies at 300 and 600 mg loading doses and 75 mg maintenance doses. Pooled analysis revealed a 32% lower AUC for the active metabolite and 9% absolute difference in the change in platelet aggregation. Interestingly, in the first report, *CYP2C9* also demonstrated a significant relationship with clopidogrel exposure and response, while in the second report, *CYP2B6* and *CYP3A5* also appeared to contribute but less than *CYP2C19*. These data highlight that *CYP2C19* is a major source of variability, although variant alleles of other genes may contribute.

While relatively few studies have evaluated the pharmacogenetics of the active metabolite exposure, numerous studies have replicated the heterogeneity of pharmacodynamic responses by *CYP2C19* genotype in diverse patient populations [9, 16, 17, 21, 22, 24–28]. Most studies used ADP-mediated platelet aggregation as the response measure, although pharmacogenetic effects have also been replicated using a variety of other methods, such as point-of-care testing with *VerifyNow* (Accumetrics). Considering the totality of evidence, antiplatelet responses following loading and maintenance doses of clopidogrel tended to be 30–50% lower in individuals carrying one or two reduced function alleles (intermediate or poor metabolizers). Poor metabolizers generally demonstrated the lowest responses.

Based on the redundancy of the activation pathway, it is possible that reduced CYP2C19-mediated metabolism might be overcome by increasing the dose [27].

Gladding *et al.* [27] conducted a pharmacogenetic study of both the standard 75 mg maintenance dose and a higher, 150 mg maintenance dose. Patients with reduced function alleles of *CYP2C19*, specifically the *2 or *4 alleles, had lower responses, but reduced metabolizers treated with the higher dose had greater antiplatelet responses compared to those who were treated with the standard dose. While the study was small, it supports the hypothesis that dose adjustment may be an effective strategy to manage the pharmacogenetic interaction. Future studies should determine the impact of a pharmacogenetic strategy on clinical outcomes and how effective dose adjustment strategy is in individuals with two reduced function alleles.

As an extension of the clinical pharmacology findings for CYP2C19, reduced CYP2C19 function was also associated with reduced clinical efficacy of clopidogrel in acute coronary syndrome patients. A retrospective analysis of 1477 patients in the clopidogrel cohort of the TRITON-TIMI 38 trial demonstrated that those with reduced function alleles of *CYP2C19*, approximately 30% of the population, were at higher risk for the combined end point of death, myocardial infarction and stroke (8% versus 12.1%; hazard ratio (HR) 1.53, 95% CI 1.07–2.19) [9]. These patients were also at higher risk for stent thrombosis (0.8% versus 2.6%; HR = 3.09, 95% CI, 1.19–8.00). Other cohort studies in percutaneous coronary intervention populations from France [29, 30], Germany [28], and Italy [26] have produced similar results for incident cardiovascular events and stent thrombosis. Taken together, loss of CYP2C19 activity may lead to diminished efficacy in approximately one-third population.

### 16.2.1 Summary

Clopidogrel is a prodrug with a complex activation pathway that is mediated by multiple polymorphic enzymes. The characteristics of the active metabolite were described extensively after clopidogrel had been on the market for nearly a decade. Data are now available to support a significant pharmacogenetic interaction between CYP2C19 and clopidogrel. As CYP2C19 is not the only CYP450 enzyme involved in the interaction, it is plausible that knowledge of CYP450 genotypes, and perhaps transporters, could further identify individuals who are likely to have diminished clopidogrel active metabolite exposure and antiplatelet responses. Future strategies to compensate for reduced CYP450-mediated activation may focus on dosing given the redundancy of the activation pathway of clopidogrel, or alternative therapies without polymorphic metabolic pathways.

## 16.3 Codeine and CYP2D6

Codeine is a prodrug that is converted to morphine, an active analgesic, *in vivo* by CYP2D6. Morphine itself is also a prodrug, with the main active moiety being the M6-glucuronide conjugate that is generated by a UDP-glucuronosyltransferase isomer in subfamily 2B (UGT2B7), as illustrated in Figure 16.2 [31, 32]. The gene encoding

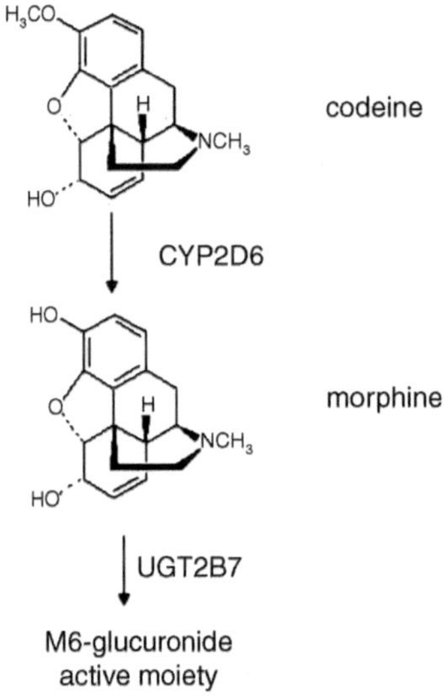


**Figure 16.2** Activation pathway of codeine.

CYP2D6 is highly polymorphic, with over 50 alleles documented [33]. Duplication of the *CYP2D6* gene can occur, resulting in ultrarapid metabolism of CYP2D6 substrates [34]. UGT2B7 is also polymorphic, and the C>T substitution at nucleotide 802 (*2) in its encoding gene, *UGT2B7*, has been associated with higher M6-glucuronide concentrations [35]. Thus, as it relates to codeine, it is possible that patients either may lack an effect in the setting of CYP2D6 dysfunction due to diminished conversion to morphine or may have hyperresponsiveness and toxicity in the setting of *UGT2B7*2* or *CYP2D6* gene duplication events due to greater generation of morphine.

Codeine is frequently prescribed following childbirth and generally regarded as compatible with breastfeeding [36]. However, of mothers taking codeine while breastfeeding, 24% reported drowsiness in the infant [37]. Several cases of severe opiate toxicity in neonates being breastfed by codeine-treated mothers have been reported in recent years [37–39]. Genotype analysis of the mothers revealed that they were ultrarapid metabolizers for CYP2D6. In two of these cases, the mothers were evaluated also for *UGT2B7*2* and were found to be carriers of this higher function allele. Thus, the increased generation of morphine and its active metabolite may have precipitated acute and potentially life-threatening toxicity in these infants. The FDA revised the codeine label to include information on this potential risk to breastfeeding infants.

Similar to the observations for breastfeeding infants, opiate toxicity has been reported in children and adults receiving codeine as an antitussive or analgesic. In one report, twins treated with codeine both experienced severe toxicity: one died and the other developed severe apnea requiring mechanical ventilation [40]. Both cases had duplication of extensive metabolizer genes. Another report followed for a child receiving codeine after tonsillectomy, which resulted in apnea and brain injury [41].

In adult ultrarapid metabolizers, urinary recovery of O-demethylated products of codeine is approximately twice that of extensive metabolizers [42]. Subsequent pharmacokinetic studies demonstrated that the concentrations of morphine and the M6-glucuronide conjugate are increased 45% in ultrarapid metabolizers [43]. This translates to higher adverse event rates, such as sedation [43]. Dalen *et al.* reported the occurrence of severe epigastric pain and euphoria in a CYP2D6 extensive metabolizer (genotyped and phenotyped) woman [44], although more severe cases have been reported. Gasche *et al.* [39] described a patient who became unresponsive 12 h following a dose of codeine, which was accompanied by respiratory depression. Further assessment found that he had very high M6-glucuronide concentrations and at least three copies of a functional CYP2D6 gene. The patient recovered following administration of naloxone [39].

Duplication of normal function alleles has the potential to lead to ultrarapid metabolism, but it should be noted that many *CYP2D6* gene duplication events are for nonfunctional alleles [33, 34]. Depending on the ethnic population studied, gene duplication events, not considering the underlying functionality, have been reported at frequencies of up to 10%. In individuals of European descent, the duplicated gene is generally functional, whereas in African-American individuals, the duplication is more commonly not functional [33, 34].

At the other end of the spectrum, reduced CYP2D6 function may result in lack of codeine efficacy. The database pertaining to studies on differences in analgesic efficacy is relatively small. The initial studies demonstrated that morphine was not detectable in poor metabolizers, whereas the active moiety could be quantified in the majority of extensive metabolizers [45–51]. O-Demethylation of codeine was clearly followed a bimodal distribution, and it was actually being developed as a probe drug for the activity of CYP2D6 [50]. A study in women following hysterectomy had only one poor metabolizer, but that patient did not experience any response to patient-controlled analgesia with codeine. While low concentrations of morphine metabolites (i.e., M6-glucuronide) associated with decreased efficacy in another study, a significant relationship between CYP2D6 phenotype and analgesic responses could not be delineated [45]. The largest study of analgesic efficacy was carried out in 96 children randomized to morphine or codeine following adenotonsillectomy. Morphine and its metabolites were undetectable in 36% of the children given codeine, and intermediate/poor CYP2D6 metabolizers generated significantly less morphine [52]. Poor metabolizers required significantly more rescue analgesia in the early postoperative period, but again, pain scores did not differ.

Since clinical pain is a highly subjective phenotype, one might also look at alternative phenotypes for evidence of a pharmacogenetic interaction. Pharmacodynamic studies using laser stimulation [49], electrical stimulation [53], and the cold presser test [47, 54] have all shown that pain thresholds are relatively unchanged with codeine in poor metabolizers, but analgesia is not affected in extensive metabolizers [55]. The findings of these studies are also supported by low or no detectable morphine in the blood of poor metabolizers [49]. Beyond pain phenotypes, others have shown that the typical opiate-induced gastrointestinal [54, 56], pruritic [54], neurologic [54], respiratory, and miotic effects [46] are also less apparent in poor metabolizers compared to extensive metabolizers. On the basis of these findings, it is evident that CYP2D6 genotype/phenotype affects the responsiveness to codeine.

### 16.3.1
### Summary

Taken together, differences in CYP2D6 metabolic capacity clearly have implications for the use of prodrugs such as codeine. Severe and sometimes life-threatening toxicities have been reported in individuals with gene duplication, which illustrates the importance of CYP2D6 genotype/phenotype on the safety of prodrug substrates. Conversely, lack of efficacy for CYP2D6 prodrugs may be common given the high prevalence of intermediate and poor metabolism. Similar to what has been described in other sections of this chapter, targeted use of drugs in individuals who have the ability to form the active metabolite may reduce heterogeneity in drug response and improve the overall safety/efficacy profile of the prodrug.

## 16.4
## Tamoxifen and CYP2D6

Tamoxifen is a hormonal agent prescribed for the prevention and treatment of breast cancer. In 1977 when this drug was introduced on the market, tamoxifen, 4-hydroxytamoxifen (4-OH TAM), and *N*-desmethyltamoxifen (*N*-Des TAM) were considered to be the active moieties responsible for the pharmacologic effect of the agent [57]. However, recent publications have established 4-hydroxy-*N*-desmethyltamoxifen (endoxifen), a secondary metabolite, as the key pharmacologic entity responsible for the antitumor activity of tamoxifen [58–60].

Tamoxifen is a substrate for a number of cytochrome P-450 enzymes including CYP3A, CYP2C9, CYP2B6, and CYP2D6 enzymes. The primary pathway for metabolism of tamoxifen is CYP3A-mediated formation of *N*-desmethyltamoxifen (Figure 16.3) [61]. Endoxifen is formed via metabolism of two primary metabolites, *N*-Des TAM and 4-OH TAM. The primary pathway for the formation of endoxifen is CYP2D6-mediated metabolism of *N*-Des TAM, and a minor pathway includes CYP3A-mediated metabolism of 4-OH TAM. The primary metabolite, 4-OH TAM, and secondary metabolite, endoxifen, have approximately 100-fold greater affinity for estrogen receptors than tamoxifen and is approximately 30–100-fold more potent in suppressing estrogen-dependent cell proliferation than tamoxifen. Since plasma concentrations of endoxifen are 5–10 times higher than those of 4-OH TAM, endoxifen is considered the metabolite that is predominantly responsible for the antitumor effect of tamoxifen [59, 60].

A number of enzymes involved in the activation and disposition of tamoxifen are polymorphic in nature and are expressed at different levels in individuals. However, CYP2D6 is the predominant polymorphic enzyme that determines the level of endoxifen systemic exposure. As noted in Section 16.3, the gene coding CYP2D6 is polymorphic with over 50 alleles resulting in a wide range of enzyme activity

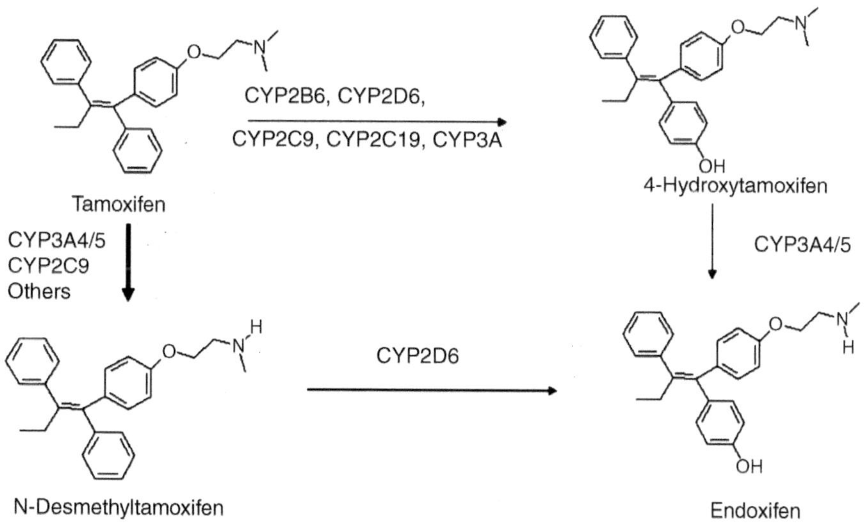


**Figure 16.3** Selected transformation pathways of tamoxifen and the main CYP enzymes involved. The relative contribution of each pathway to the overall oxidation of tamoxifen is shown by the thickness of the arrow, and the principal P450 isoforms responsible are highlighted in larger fonts. Adapted from Ref. [61].

[33, 62]. Approximately, 5–10% of the Caucasian population, 2–8% of African-Americans, and 1% of Asians are poor metabolizers of drugs metabolized by CYP2D6. The null (no activity) alleles are *CYP2D6*3, *4, *5, *6, *7, *8, *11, *12, *13, *14, *15, *16, *19, *20, *38, *40, *42,* and **44,* whereas *CYP2D6*9, *10, *17, *36, *37,* and **41* are alleles with reduced enzyme activity [27, 63, 64]. Laboratory tests are available to identify *CYP2D6* genotype. The most common nonfunctional alleles associated with no CYP2D6 activity are *CYP2D6 *4* and **5*; the most frequent dysfunctional alleles associated with reduced CYP2D6 activity are **10* in Asians, **17* in African-Americans, and **41* in Caucasians. Patients with two nonfunctional alleles (homozygous) have low or no CYP2D6 activity and those with one nonfunctional allele (heterozygous) have intermediate activity. Duplication of *CYP2D6* gene results in ultrarapid metabolism of tamoxifen and increased level of endoxifen.

Clinical studies have demonstrated lower levels of endoxifen in patients who carry variant alleles of *CYP2D6* or use moderate and strong CYP2D6 inhibitors while on tamoxifen treatment [65–68]. Median steady state plasma concentrations of endoxifen in patients treated with tamoxifen 20 mg daily for more than 8 weeks were significantly lower (36.7 ng/ml versus 52.3 ng/ml, $p = 0.003$) in 11 patients with *CYP2D6* null alleles (absence of any activity) compared to 86 patients with functional alleles [65]. A clinical study conducted by Lim *et al.* in Korean patients taking tamoxifen for more than 8 weeks showed that steady-state concentration of endoxifen was less than half (7.9 ng/ml versus 19.9 ng/ml) in patients with *CYP2D6 *10/*10* genotype compared to patients with wild-type alleles [67]. A pharmacokinetic study by Borges *et al.* demonstrated that patients carrying at least one variant allele of *CYP2D6* had mean endoxifen concentrations that were 55% of those patients who were homozygous for wild-type *CYP2D6* genotype, while patients homozygous for *CYP2D6* *4/*4 genotype had mean endoxifen concentrations that were 26% of the wild type [68].

The effects of CYP2D6 inhibitors on tamoxifen exposure and response are consistent with the genetic effects of low or nonfunctional alleles of *CYP2D6*. Patients using CYP2D6 inhibitors had 58% lower endoxifen concentration compared to patients not using CYP2D6 inhibitors [68]. In another study, mean paroxetine (strong CYP2D6 inhibitor)-mediated reduction of endoxifen concentrations was 64% (95% CI, 39–89%) in women who were wild type for *CYP2D6* and 24% (95% CI, 23–71%) in women with a variant allele ($p = 0.03$) [66]. Plasma endoxifen concentration significantly decreased from 12.4 ng/ml before paroxetine coadministration to 5.5 ng/ml afterward ($p = 0.004$) [66].

Clinical studies have explored the relationship between *CYP2D6* genotype and clinical response to tamoxifen treatment. Schroth *et al.* conducted a clinical study including 1580 consecutively collected retrospective German cohort and prospectively collected patients from the US North Central Cancer Treatment Group (NCCTG) [69]. The patients had stage I, II, or III primary estrogen positive (ER+) primary breast cancer, who received tamoxifen monotherapy in the adjuvant setting. The tumor recurrence rates at the 9-year follow-up were 14.9% for extensive metabolizers, 20.9% for heterozygous metabolizers, and 29% for poor metabolizers [69]. Another study that included 280 ER+ breast cancer patients who did not receive tamoxifen, but received adjuvant chemotherapy or no drug therapy, had no differential clinical outcome in tumor recurrence and relapse free time, indicating that CYP2D6 is a predictive, but not a prognostic, biomarker in tamoxifen treatment outcome. Goetz *et al.* conducted a retrospective review of a prospective adjuvant tamoxifen trial in which 190 postmenopausal breast cancer patients received 20 mg tamoxifen once daily for 5 years following surgery [61]. Patients with *CYP2D6*4/*4* genotype had worse disease-free survival compared to patients with one variant alleles or both wild-type alleles (adjusted HR = 1.86; $p = 0.089$). Newman *et al.* studied breast cancer patients carrying *BRCA1* and *BRCA2* mutations and treated with tamoxifen after surgery [70]. Patients who are poor metabolizers of CYP2D6 and carried *BRCA2* mutations had worse overall survival (median survival, 7 versus 28 years; adjusted HR = 9.7; 95% CI, 2.3–41.0; $p = 0.008$). Effect of *CYP2D6*10* allele (lower enzyme activity) on survival outcome after tamoxifen treatment in pre- and postmenopausal women was studied by Xu *et al.* [71]. Patients with *CYP2D6*10/10* genotype had a significantly shorter disease-free survival (HR = 4.7; 95% CI, 1.1–20.0) compared to patients carrying wild-type alleles or one variant **10* allele. *CYP2D6*10/*10* genotype was not associated with disease-free survival in patients who were not treated with tamoxifen establishing that *CYP2D6*10* genotype is not a prognostic factor for clinical response.

A Swedish study including 677 postmenopausal, estrogen receptor-positive breast cancer patients demonstrated that patients with *CYP2D6*4/*4* genotype had a borderline significant ($p = 0.055$) improvement in recurrence-free survival; however, in a subset of patients who were treated with tamoxifen for 2 or 5 years, there were no differences in recurrence risk between patients carrying *CYP2D6**4* allele and patients carrying wild-type alleles [72]. The result of this study is a deviation from other studies that investigated the relationship between *CYP2D6* polymorphism and tamoxifen clinical outcome. Another study by Nowell *et al.* in 167 pre- and post-menopausal breast cancer women demonstrated no association between *CYP2D6**4/*4* genotype and overall survival [73].

A retrospective analysis of 1659 patients treated with tamoxifen showed that the risk for breast cancer recurrence was significantly higher (7.5% versus 14.0%; HR = 1.92; 95% CI, 1.36–2.73; $p = 0.0002$) for patients who used moderate to potent CYP2D6 inhibitors compared to patients who did not use any CYP2D6 inhibitor [74]. The use of weak CYP2D6 inhibitors, such as citalopram, escitalopram, and fluvoxamine, was not associated with increased risk for breast cancer recurrence. An analysis of 225 patients of the NCCTG trial conduced by Goetz *et al.* determined the association of CYP2D6 phenotype and breast cancer outcomes [75]. CYP2D6 poor metabolizers were defined as women (i) homozygous for the **4* allele (**4/*4*), (ii) **4*/wild-type and coadministration of a moderate or potent inhibitor, or (iii) homozygous for the wild-type genotype and coadministration of a potent inhibitor. Compared to extensive metabolizers, poor metabolizers had significantly shorter time to breast cancer recurrence (HR = 3.2; 95% CI, 1.37–7.55; $p = 0.007$), to relapse-free survival (HR = 2.69; 95% CI, 1.34–5.37; $p = 0.005$), and to disease-free survival. The 2-year relapse-free survival rates were 98% for extensive metabolizers and 68% for poor metabolizers.

## 16.4.1
## Summary

Endoxifen is the predominant pharmacological active moiety contributing to the treatment effect of tamoxifen. Endoxifen is a secondary metabolite of tamoxifen formed mostly by CYP2D6 from *N*-desmethyltamoxifen. *CYP2D6* polymorphism results in varying levels of endoxifen in breast cancer patients with CYP2D6 poor metabolizers having significantly low levels of endoxifen compared to CYP2D6 extensive metabolizers. Also, patients taking strong CYP2D6 inhibitors while treated with tamoxifen achieve low levels of endoxifen. A number of clinical studies from various regions of the world provide evidence, although not entirely consistent, that tamoxifen treated breast cancer patients with deficient CYP2D6 enzyme activity because of variant allele in *CYP2D6* gene or the use of moderate and strong CYP2D6 inhibitors are at increased risk for breast cancer recurrence. Patients taking CYP2D6 strong inhibitors such as paroxetine and fluoxetine while on treatment with tamoxifen are at increased risk for breast cancer recurrence. Although there is no study that evaluates the association between endoxifen levels in patients and tamoxifen treatment outcome, scientific and clinical evidence indicates that response to tamoxifen is related to endoxifen exposure as demonstrated by increased breast cancer recurrence risk in patients who are likely to achieve low levels of endoxifen because of CYP2D6 polymorphism or the use of strong CYP2D6 inhibitors while on treatment with tamoxifen.

## 16.5 Fluorouracil Prodrugs and Carboxylesterase

Developed more than 50 years ago, fluorouracil (5-FU) remains the drug of choice for the treatment of colorectal and other cancers. 5-FU drug undergoes extensive first-pass metabolism when taken orally, and even when administered intravenously, its shortcomings include a short half-life and rapid elimination from the systemic circulation. Over the years, several 5-FU prodrugs were developed to overcome these shortcomings, such as capecitabine, tegafur, floxuridine, and doxifluridine. These prodrugs are activated and converted to 5-FU via different activation pathways involving different enzymes. Capecitabine and tegafur are reviewed herein to illustrate the impact of polymorphisms of prodrug-activating enzymes on the variability of the ultimate clinical efficacy of 5-FU. Adapted from Ref. [76], the conversion pathway of capecitabine and tegafur each to 5-FU and subsequent metabolism of 5-FU are illustrated in Figure 16.4. Clearly, variability in the clinical efficacy and safety of these prodrugs is unavoidable in light of the polymorphisms of enzymes involved in their activation.

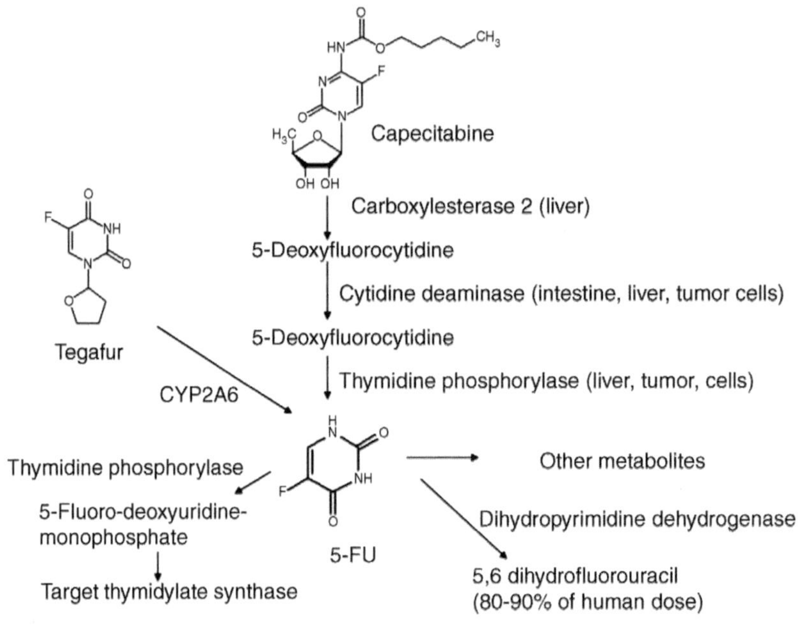


**Figure 16.4** Activation pathways of 5-FU prodrugs and 5-FU metabolism.

## 16.5.1
## Capecitabine and Carboxylesterase

Capecitabine, a triple prodrug of 5-FU, is approved as the first-line monotherapy for the treatment of metastatic colorectal cancer and breast cancers, and by design it should be converted to 5-FU mainly in tumor cells [77]. Once administered, capecitabine is first converted by hepatic carboxylesterase 2 (CES2) to 5′-deoxyfluorocytidine, which is then converted to 5′-deoxyfluorouridine by cytidine deaminase in liver, intestine, and tumor cells. Capecitabine, 5′-deoxyfluorocytidine, and 5′-deoxyfluorouridine are pharmacologically inactive. The active drug, 5-FU, is finally released from 5′-deoxyfluorouridine by thymidine phosphorylase in the liver and tumor cells. In tumor cells, its target is thymidylate synthase. Inactivation of 5-FU by dihydropyrimidine dehydrogenase occurs mainly in the liver (approximately 85%).

Human pharmacokinetic studies of oral capecitabine showed a high degree of variability in the release of 5-FU from capecitabine. After two repeated oral doses of capecitabine at 666 or 1225 mg/m$^2$, the coefficients of variation (CV%) for the $C_{max}$ and AUC values of capecitabine, 5′-deoxyfluorocytidine, 5′-deoxyfluorouridine, and 5-FU were all more than 30% [78]. Genetic association studies with clinical efficacy or toxicity of capecitabine have largely focused on the target enzyme of 5-FU, thymidylate synthase, and on dihydropyrimidine dehydrogenase that metabolizes 5-FU [76, 77, 79–81]. The role of thymidine phosphorylase in the clinical efficacy of capecitabine seems to be rather complex since this enzyme is not only involved in the release of 5-FU from capecitabine but is also known as the platelet-derived endothelial cell growth factor (the angiogenesis factor), which reportedly promoted tumor growth and was linked to poor prognosis of colorectal cancer [82].

Variability in the systemic exposure of capecitabine, intermediate metabolites and 5-FU following oral capecitabine could be caused by polymorphisms of CES2, cytidine deaminase, and thymidine phosphorylase, which are involved in the sequential steps of 5-FU release from capecitabine. Disappointingly, much less attention was paid to these three enzymes. So far, only one report investigated the association between *CES2* gene and clinical efficacy of capecitabine [77]. In this study, 136 advanced breast or colorectal cancer patients were treated with oral capecitabine. Patients were genotyped for 14 different polymorphisms in the genes encoding CES2 and dihydroprimidine dehydrogenase to determine their relationship with capecitabine efficacy. Polymorphisms in two regions of the *CES2* gene, 5′ untranslated region (5′UTR) and exon 3, were genotyped, and only the 5′UTR region showed a statistical association with tumor response rate. Patients with the 5′UTR 823 C/G polymorphism of *CES2* had a higher rate of response (time to progression of disease) to capecitabine than the wild-type carriers (8.7 month, 59, 95% CI: 40–75% versus 5.3 month, 32, 95%: 22–44%, $p = 0.015$). The variant alleles in exon 3 were of very low frequency (2% or less) in the study population, resulting in no statistical association. Likewise, no statistical association with clinical response rate in patients receiving capecitabine was found for *DPYD* (encoding dihydropyrimidine dehydrogenase). In regard to *TYMS* (encoding thymidylate synthase), 42% of patients carrying the TSER 2R allele and 32% of patients homozygous for the TSER3R allele responded to capecitabine treatment ($p = 0.7$), TSER is the enhancer region of *TYMS* with 2R representing two repeats of 28-bp tandem and 3R three repeats. No significant association was observed between *TYMS* genotype and capecitabine clinical outcome.

Garcia *et al.* reported a study of 26 cervical cancer patients, in which *TYMS* was genotyped. Gene expressions of *DPYD* and *TYMP* (encoding thymidine phosphorylase) in tumors were also determined [80]. Low treatment response (partial response in four patients, stable disease state in nine patients, and the rest worse) led to an early clinical trial termination, so no correlations with clinical outcomes were established for these enzymes. Garcia *et al.* reported another study of 27 patients with platinum-sensitive ovarian cancer or platinum-sensitive primary peritoneal cancer [79]. A low response rate led to an early trial termination as well. According to the investigators, "*TYMS* genotype or expression of *DPYD* or *TYMP* was not associated with any of the severe toxicities." Thymidylate synthase expression was found, however, associated with severe nausea/vomiting. Unfortunately, these small studies with no significant clinical efficacy do not provide meaningful information. In a study involving 67 patients with metastatic colorectal cancer, the association between the efficacy of the capecitabine plus irinotecan regimen and expression of *TYMP*, *TYMS*, and *DPYD* genes each was studied [83]. Only thymidine phosphorylase expression was associated with tumor response with an odds ratio of 4.77. The association between *TYMP* polymorphisms and its expression was not studied, nor was the relationship between *TYMP* genotype and clinical tumor response. The mRNA levels of *TYMP* and *DPYD* were, however, found to correlate with each other in primary tumor and metastatic tumor in another study of 91 patients [84]. In this study, the lack of association of *TYMS* or *TYMP* gene expression with the parameter of "time to treatment failure" was attributed to lower capecitabine doses in some subjects. The authors further hypothesized that increased release of 5-FU by increased *TYMP* expression could be offset by increased metabolism of 5-FU caused by higher *DPYD* expression. Interesting, patients with *TYMS* mRNA below the median level had a significantly longer survival; this observation was consistent with what was reported by others [76].

Since 5-FU is metabolized by dihydropyrimidine dehydrogenase (encoded by the *DPYD* gene), its systemic exposure is inversely related to dihydropyrimidine dehydrogenase activity. Dihydropyrimidine dehydrogenase activity in tumor cells is expected to be a determinant of patients' response to 5-FU treatment while that in the liver affects the 5-FU treatment-related severe toxicity. Accumulated evidence indicates an association between the clinical efficacy and toxicity of 5-FU and the dihydropyrimidine dehydrogenase activity [85]. Several reports have investigated the relation between *DPYD* polymorphism and 5-FU toxicity. In a study of 487 French Caucasian cancer patients receiving 5-FU, the splice site variant IVS14 + 1G>A or 2846A>T SNP was associated with lower systemic clearance and higher exposure to 5-FU and with early experience of grade 3–4 toxicity compared to the SNPs of

1590T>C, 85T>C, or wild type [86]. The association of the splice variant IVS14 + 1 G>A of *DPYD* with the toxicity (grade 3 or grade 4) of 5-FU was also reported in another study of 573 German cancer patients receiving 5-FU [87]. Prompted by accumulated evidences, the labels of capecitabine and 5-FU have been updated and warn that these drugs are contraindicated for patients with dihydropyrimidine dehydrogenase deficiency.

#### 16.5.1.1 **Summary**

Only a limited number of studies ever investigated any association between the clinical efficacy of capecitabine and the *CES2* polymorphism. These studies involved only a small number of patients; therefore, it is difficult to establish a meaningful statistical association between *CES2* gene variants or *TYMP* expression and capecitabine clinical outcomes. Capecitabine and 5-FU are contraindicated for patients with dihydropyrimidine dehydrogenase deficiency.

### 16.5.2
### Tegafur and CYP2A6

Several *in vitro* studies have been conducted to mechanistically delineate the release of 5-FU from tegafur. An *in vitro* study using human liver microsomes and cytosol revealed that tegafur was converted to 5-FU by microsomal CYP450 at low concentrations and by cytosolic thymidine phosphorylase (TP) at high concentrations [88]. On the basis of these *in vitro* studies, CYP2A6, CYP1A2, and CYP2C8 were reported to be involved in converting tegafur to 5-FU [89]. A recent study concluded that conversion of tegafur to 5-FU mainly involved CYP2A6 in the human liver [90]. As a result, association of *CYP2A6* gene polymorphisms with the clinical outcome of tegafur treatment regimens has been the focus of pharmacogenetic interaction studies.

Tegafur and 5-chloro-2,4-dihydroxypyridine, an inhibitor of dihydropyrimidine dehydrogenase, were administered orally in a study of five patients with gastric cancer, and one patient who carried *CYP2A6** *4A* (deletion of *CYP2A6*) and *CYP2A6* * *11* (670T>C) alleles had approximately four times higher tegafur AUC than other patients [91]. This result is consistent with the fact that *CYP2A6** *11* is known to have lower enzyme activity than the wild type. Fujita *et al.* studied the association of *CYP2A6* genotype and tegafur pharmacokinetics in 54 patients with solid tumors [92]. The null or much less active *CYP2A6* alleles tested in this study included *4, *4A, *7, and *9. The frequencies of wild type (*1/*1), one-variant genotype (*1/variant), and two-variant genotype (variant/variant) in the target population were 22.2, 38.9, and 38.9%, respectively. Oral clearance of tegafur was significantly lower in those patients who carried two variant *CYP2A6* alleles. Interestingly, the $AUC_{0-8}$ of 5-FU, however, did not correlate with *CYP2A6* genotype. In another report of 46 nonsmall-cell lung cancer patients, *CYP2A6** *4C* heterozygotes or homozygotes had a significantly higher AUC of tegafur (1.5-fold higher; $p < 0.05$) and lower $C_{max}$ of 5-FU than wild-type carriers [93]. In this study, the *CYP2A6* genotype frequencies in the study population were 17.4% for

*1/*1, 60.8% for *1/variant, and 21.6*% for variant/variant where variant alleles included *4C, *7, and *9.

#### 16.5.2.1 Summary

CYP2A6 is involved in converting tegafur to 5-FU. *CYP2A6* variants seem to be related to lower clearance, or higher AUC, of tegafur and consequently contribute to lower systemic exposure to 5-FU.

## 16.6 Irinotecan and Carboxylesterase 2

Irinotecan is clinically used in combination with 5-FU and oxaliplatin to treat colorectal, ovarian, stomach, and lung cancers. Irinotecan is a prodrug activated to its active metabolite, SN-38, by carboxylesterases; and SN-38 is mainly eliminated via glucuronidation by UDP-glucuronosyl-transferase 1A1 (UGT1A1) (Figure 16.5). In the human liver, carboxylesterase 2 (CES2) reportedly had higher activity activating irinotecan than carboxylesterase 1 (CES1) [94]. In a study of 60 human liver samples, 11 single nucleotide polymorphisms of *CES2* (the gene encoding CES2) were identified, but none of them affected the amino acid sequence of CES2 or its activity in irinotecan activation [95]. A study in 176 Japanese cancer patients, the nonsynonymous SNP of 100C>T (Arg34Trp, *2) was detected and the patients heterozygous for Arg34Trp had substantially reduced AUC ratios between irinotecan and its active metabolite (SN-38) plus SN-28-glucuronide [96]. This result is

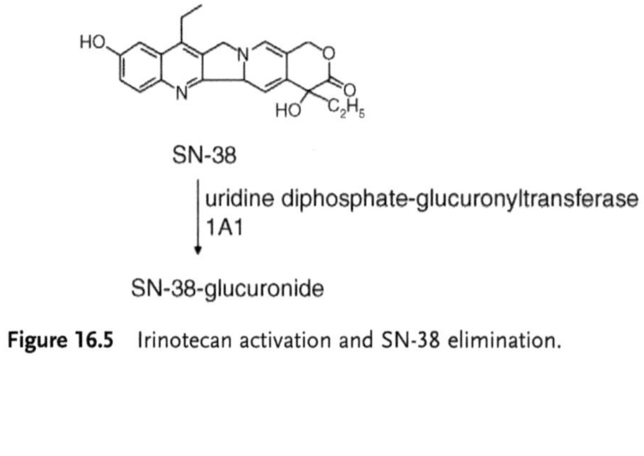


Figure 16.5 Irinotecan activation and SN-38 elimination.

consistent with a report that the 100C>T (R34W) SNP was functionally deficient in Japanese population [97].

In a study concerning the 830C>G polymorphism located in the 5′ untranslated [97] region of *CES2* gene, the G allele had a frequency of 8.2% in 104 Caucasian colorectal patients [98]. It was concluded that the *CES2* 830C>G genotype was not related to the therapeutic efficacy (tumor response, event-free survival) or toxicity of irinotecan. One likely contributing factor is that there were only five heterozygotes and one homozygote among those who received irinotecan. However, this possible explanation was ruled out by the observation, using 12 human liver samples of 830GG and 830CG genotypes, that allele G did not significantly affect the function or activity of CES2. *CES2* and *CES1* genes were determined in another study involving 65 patients with solid tumors treated with irinotecan, among whom the *CES1* 1440 A>T wild type had a frequency of 100% and the *CES1* 1525 A>C and *CES2* 1647 C>T wild types each had a frequency of 99% [99]. Due to the low frequencies of variant alleles of *CES1* and *CES2*, the impact of *CES1* or *CES2* polymorphism on the pharmacokinetics of irinotecan or SN-38 could not be meaningfully determined.

SN-38 is metabolized to SN-38-glucuronide by uridine diphosphate glucuronyl transferase 1A1 (UGT-1A1). SN-38 is associated with irinotecan treatment-related severe toxicity of delayed diarrhea (grade 3/4) and hematotoxicity (neutropenia). According to a recent review by *Schulz et al.* [100], the *UGT1A1 *28* polymorphism has been the focus of studies to understand the genetic basis of the clinical efficacy and safety of irinotecan. *UGT1A1 *28 allele* is related to the number of TA (thymine–adenine) insertions in the TATAA element of the 5′-promoter region of *UGT-1A1*; the normal allele has 6 TA insertions while the variant allele 7 TA insertions. The 7 TA variant allele (*UGT1A1 *28*) reportedly caused a 70% reduction in the transcription of *UGT1A1*. Patients carrying the *UGT1A1 *28* genotype have a higher exposure of SN-38 as a result of lower UGT1A1 activities and less inactivation of SN-38 to SN-38-glucuronide. The accumulated evidences of UGT1A1 activity impacting the clinical safety of irinotecan have prompted the Food and Drug Administration to update the label of irinotecan with a statement of "Individuals who are homozygous for the *UGT1A1* 28* allele are at increased risk for neutropenia following initiation of CAMPTOSAR treatment" and recommends a reduced initial dose for patients homozygous for the *UGT1A1* 28* allele.

### 16.6.1
### Summary

In the Japanese population, the nonsynonymous SNP, 100C>T (Arg34Trp, *2) in *CES2*, is related to absence of CES2 activity and reduced conversion of irinotecan to its active metabolite. More studies are needed to determine whether the *CES2* 830C>G genotype is related to irinotecan clinical outcomes. The initial dose of irinotecan should be reduced for those who are *UGT1A1 *28* homozygotes or heterozygotes.

## 16.7 Others

### 16.7.1 ACE Inhibitors and CES

Imidapril is an ester prodrug of imidaprilat, an angiotensin-converting enzyme (ACE) inhibitor, for treating essential hypertension. Imidapril was reportedly activated to imidaprilat by hepatic CES1, not CES2. A study of 62 patients with mild to moderate essential hypertension showed that the rate of blood pressure normalization in these patients was 55% [101]. While the reasons why some patients did not respond to imidapril are still unknown, attempts have been made to understand the impact of the functional polymorphisms of the enzymes involved in converting imidapril to imidaprilat. The systemic exposures of imidapril and imidaprilat following oral imidapril are highly variable. A study on 10 hypertensive patients showed that mean (SD) steady-state AUC values of imidapril and imidaprilat were 123 (34) ng ml/h and 240 (55) ng ml/h, respectively [102]. Naturally, *CES1* polymorphisms could be another source that could cause variability in the clinical response of oral imidapril. In a study of 105 Japanese hypertensive patients, clinical response rates to oral imidapril were found to differ as a function of polymorphism in the promoter region, -816 A>C [103]. The A/C and C/C genotypes had a significantly higher response rate than the A/A genotype ($p = 0.03$). The -816C allele increased nonresponse rates approximately twofold. There are many ACE inhibitors that share a common feature with imidapril, that is, structurally being carboxyl esters and needing activation to the acid form by hepatic enzymes. These compounds include trandolapril, benazepril, cilazapril, delapril, enalarpil, fosinopril, lisinopril, pentopril, perindopril, quinapril, spirapril, and ramipril [104]. More studies are needed to understand whether polymorphisms of CES genes impact the clinical variability of ACE inhibitors.

### 16.7.2 Cyclophosphamide and CYP2B6/CYP2C19

Cyclosphosphamide is a prodrug for treating cancers and systemic lupus erythematosus (SLE). Several CYP450 enzymes, such as CYP2B6, CYP3A4, and CYP2C19, have been implicated in its activation to active metabolites, 4- hydroxylcyclophosphamide and aldophosphamide [105, 106]. *CYP2B6* and *CYP2C19* are highly polymorphic, and their variant alleles have reduced or no activity compared to the wild type (Figure 16.6).

Pulsed intravenous cyclophosphamide is a standard protocol for treating SLE. In a study of 62 patients with lupus nephritis treated with cyclosphosphamide, common variants of *CYP2B6*, *2C19*, *2C9*, and *3A5* were genotyped [107]. *CYP2C19**2 carriers were found to have a lower risk of premature ovarian failure, a potentially devastating adverse effect of cyclophosphamide therapy, while *CYP2B6**5 or *CYP2C19**2 homozygotes had a higher probability of developing end-stage renal disease [107]. In

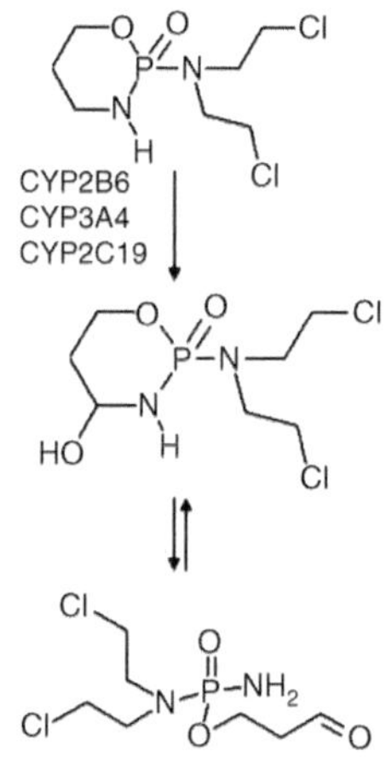


**Figure 16.6** Activation pathway of cyclophosphamide.

another study of 35 SLE patients treated with cyclosphosphamide, *CYP2C19**2 homozygotes or heterozygotes had a significantly lower risk of developing ovarian toxicity compared to the wild type. The lack of association between *CYP2B6**5 and the risk of developing ovarian toxicity was likely due to a small sample size [108].

#### 16.7.2.1 **Summary**

ACE inhibitors have variable systemic exposure, so understanding whether *CES1* variants would cause clinical variability should be helpful to manage high blood pressure. Cyclophosphamide is an important drug for treating SLE, understanding how variants of *CYP2B6* and *CYP2C19* affect its efficacy and toxicity is essential for better targeted treatment.

## 16.8 Drug Development Implication

The clinical outcomes of clopidogrel, codeine, morphine, tegafur, and tamoxifen have been instructive in that proactive characterization of the enzymes involved in prodrug activation accounted for some of the variability in drug exposure and response. Targeting the right population or optimizing doses accordingly could help avoid unwanted adverse effects or lack of efficacy in patients with specific genetic traits. Prodrug discovery has been and will continue to be an important aspect of drug development. As the attrition rate in drug discovery and development increases, prodrug strategies to extend the patent period through new uses of old drugs are becoming more popular than ever. Pharmaceutical scientists should be prepared to undertake the new challenges of not only discovering new chemical entities with adequate bioavailability and therapeutic efficacy but also actively targeting drugs and prodrugs to specific populations for the best efficacy and least adverse events.

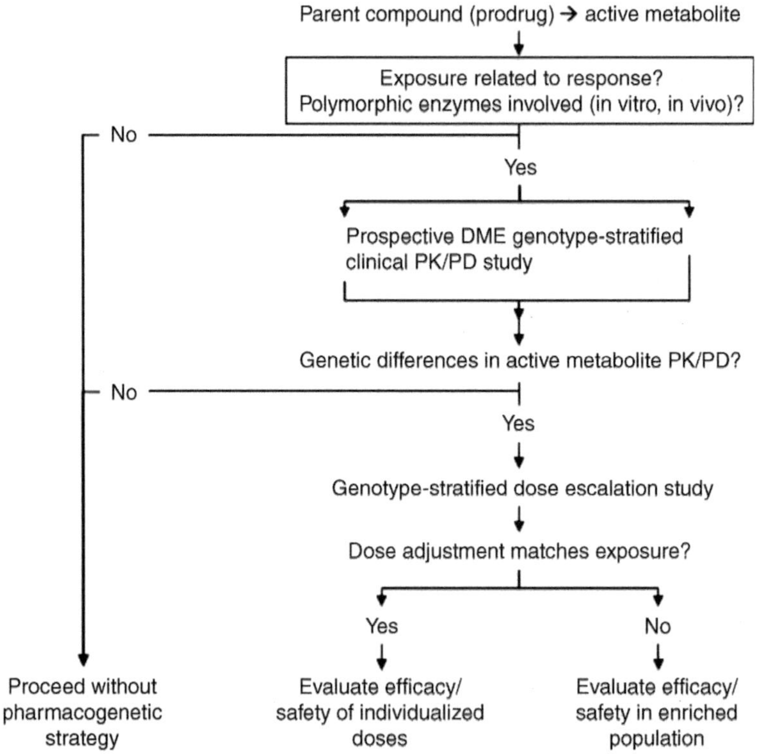


**Figure 16.7** Precision medicine.

As illustrated in Figure 16.7, pharmacogenetics could be included in early drug discovery and development phase. That is, detailed *in vitro* characterization of the enzymes involved in prodrug activation should be performed in order to predict the variability of systemic exposure of a prodrug and its active metabolite(s) in humans. Along with our knowledge of the gene polymorphisms and functional activities of variant alleles of specific prodrug-activating enzyme(s), such *in vitro* information should be used in the planning of phase I pharmacokinetic studies so that the impact of pharmacogenetics on the variability of the systemic exposure of a prodrug and its active metabolite(s) could be adequately determined. Thereafter, the phase II dose ranging studies in the target population with adequate enzymatic activities to activate prodrugs could then be meaningfully conducted in preparation for the phase III clinical trials in a larger target population.

Development of drugs with a high benefit/risk ratio is challenging, but strategies could be adopted to implement precision medicine so that the right patient population is targeted for the best benefit while the rest are avoided to prevent lack of efficacy or occurrence of severe adverse events. Strategic drug development might include (1) mechanistically characterizing conversion of a prodrug to its active drug or metabolism of a drug to its active metabolite(s), (2) genotyping the patients in early clinical trials to determine the association between the genotypes of prodrug-activating enzymes and clinical responses (systemic exposure, efficacy, and adverse effects), and (3) conducting clinical trials and determining the right dosing regimens in the target population with the desired genotypes for adequately activating prodrugs. Such strategies will help implement precision medicine with the benefit of reducing the attrition rate of drug development.

## 16.9 Conclusions

Prodrugs require activation by metabolizing enzymes in order to be therapeutically effective. Due to the fact that prodrug-activating enzymes are frequently polymorphic, individual therapeutic responses could be highly variable. Patients who are not able to produce active metabolites due to the presence of nonfunctional prodrug-activating enzymes may not have any therapeutic benefits of the prodrug prescribed. In contrast, patients who have duplicated copies, or carry a superfunctional genotype, of a prodrug-activating enzyme may produce a much higher amount of active metabolite(s), resulting in better efficacy, or adverse effects, at standard doses. Therefore, it is important to recognize the potential for interindividual variability in prodrug exposure or responses early in development to identify strategies to minimize pharmacokinetic or pharmacodynamic heterogeneity. A purposeful, targeted development toward drugs with less polymorphic activating enzymes or appropriate selection or dosing of genetically defined patient subsets of the population may enhance the efficacy and safety of prodrugs.

## References


1 Kamali, F. and Wynne, H. (2009) Pharmacogenetics of Warfarin. *Annual Review of Medicine*, **61** (1), 63–75.
2 Hollopeter, G., Jantzen, H.M., Vincent, D., Li, G., England, L., Ramakrishnan, V., Yang, R.B., Nurden, P., Nurden, A., Julius, D. *et al.* (2001) Identification of the platelet ADP receptor targeted by antithrombotic drugs. *Nature*, **409**, 202–207.
3 Pereillo, J.M., Maftouh, M., Andrieu, A., Uzabiaga, M.F., Fedeli, O., Savi, P., Pascal, M., Herbert, J.M., Maffrand, J.P., and Picard, C. (2002) Structure and stereochemistry of the active metabolite of clopidogrel. *Drug Metabolism and Disposition: The Biological Fate of Chemicals*, **30**, 1288–1295.
4 (a) Savi, P., Pereillo, J.M., Uzabiaga, M.F., Combalbert, J., Picard, C., Maffrand, J.P., Pascal, M., and Herbert, J.M. (2000) Identification and biological activity of the active metabolite of clopidogrel. *Thrombosis and Haemostasis*, **84**, 891–896. (b) Dansette, P.M., Libraire, J., Bertho, G., and Mansui, D. (2009) Metabolic oxidative cleavage of thiol esters: evidence for the formation of sulfenic acid intermediates in the bioactivation of the antithrombotic prodrugs ticlopidine and clopidogrel, *Chem. Res. Toxicol.*, **22**, 369–373.
5 Jinnai, T., Horiuchi, H., Makiyama, T., Tazaki, J., Tada, T., Akao, M., Ono, K., Hoshino, K., Naruse, Y., Takahashi, K. *et al.* (2009) Impact of CYP2C19 polymorphisms on the antiplatelet effect of clopidogrel in an actual clinical setting in Japan. *Circulation Journal*, **73**, 1498–1503.

6 Caplain, H., Donat, F., Gaud, C., and Necciari, J. (1999) Pharmacokinetics of clopidogrel. *Seminars in Thrombosis and Hemostasis*, **25** (Suppl. 2), 25–28.

7 Clarke, T.A. and Waskell, L.A. (2003) The metabolism of clopidogrel is catalyzed by human cytochrome P450 3A and is inhibited by atorvastatin. *Drug Metabolism and Disposition: The Biological Fate of Chemicals*, **31**, 53–59.

8 Savi, P., Combalbert, J., Gaich, C., Rouchon, M.C., Maffrand, J.P., Berger, Y., and Herbert, J.M. (1994) The antiaggregating activity of clopidogrel is due to a metabolic activation by the hepatic cytochrome P450-1A. *Thrombosis and Haemostasis*, **72**, 313–317.

9 Mega, J.L., Close, S.L., Wiviott, S.D., Shen, L., Hockett, R.D., Brandt, J.T., Walker, J.R., Antman, E.M., Macias, W., Braunwald, E. *et al.* (2009) Cytochrome P-450 polymorphisms and response to clopidogrel. *The New England Journal of Medicine*, **360**, 354–362.

10 De Miguel, A., Ibanez, B., and Badimon, J.J. (2008) Clinical implications of clopidogrel resistance. *Thrombosis and Haemostasis*, **100**, 196–203.

11 Roden, D.M. and Stein, C.M. (2009) Clopidogrel and the concept of high-risk pharmacokinetics. *Circulation*, **119**, 2127–2130.

12 Farid, N.A., Payne, C.D., Small, D.S., Winters, K.J., Ernest, C.S., 2nd, Brandt, J.T., Darstein, C., Jakubowski, J.A., and Salazar, D.E. (2007) Cytochrome P450 3A inhibition by ketoconazole affects prasugrel and clopidogrel pharmacokinetics and pharmacodynamics differently. *Clinical Pharmacology and Therapeutics*, **81**, 735–741.

13 Siller-Matula, J.M., Lang, I., Christ, G., and Jilma, B. (2008) Calcium-channel blockers reduce the antiplatelet effect of clopidogrel. *Journal of the American College of Cardiology*, **52**, 1557–1563.

14 Angiolillo, D.J., Fernandez-Ortiz, A., Bernardo, E., Ramirez, C., Cavallari, U., Trabetti, E., Sabate, M., Hernandez, R., Moreno, R., Escaned, J. *et al.* (2006) Contribution of gene sequence variations of the hepatic cytochrome P450 3A4 enzyme to variability in individual responsiveness to clopidogrel. *Arteriosclerosis, Thrombosis, and Vascular Biology*, **26**, 1895–1900.

15 Fontana, P., Hulot, J.S., De Moerloose, P., and Gaussem, P. (2007) Influence of CYP2C19 and CYP3A4 gene polymorphisms on clopidogrel responsiveness in healthy subjects. *Journal of Thrombosis and Haemostasis*, **5**, 2153–2155.

16 Geisler, T., Schaeffeler, E., Dippon, J., Winter, S., Buse, V., Bischofs, C., Zuern, C., Moerike, K., Gawaz, M., and Schwab, M. (2008) CYP2C19 and nongenetic factors predict poor responsiveness to clopidogrel loading dose after coronary stent implantation. *Pharmacogenomics*, **9**, 1251–1259.

17 Frere, C., Cuisset, T., Morange, P.E., Quilici, J., Camoin-Jau, L., Saut, N., Faille, D., Lambert, M., Juhan-Vague, I., Bonnet, J.L. *et al.* (2008) Effect of cytochrome P450 polymorphisms on platelet reactivity after treatment with clopidogrel in acute coronary syndrome. *The American Journal of Cardiology*, **101**, 1088–1093.

18 Suh, J.W., Koo, B.K., Zhang, S.Y., Park, K.W., Cho, J.Y., Jang, I.J., Lee, D.S., Sohn, D.W., Lee, M.M., and Kim, H.S. (2006) Increased risk of atherothrombotic events associated with cytochrome P450 3A5 polymorphism in patients taking clopidogrel. *Canadian Medical Association Journal*, **174**, 1715–1722.

19 Brandt, J.T., Close, S.L., Iturria, S.J., Payne, C.D., Farid, N.A., Ernest, C.S., 2nd, Lachno, D.R., Salazar, D., and Winters, K.J. (2007) Common polymorphisms of CYP2C19 and CYP2C9 affect the pharmacokinetic and pharmacodynamic response to clopidogrel but not prasugrel. *Journal of Thrombosis and Haemostasis*, **5**, 2429–2436.

20 Giusti, B., Gori, A.M., Marcucci, R., Saracini, C., Sestini, I., Paniccia, R., Valente, S., Antoniucci, D., Abbate, R., and Gensini, G.F. (2007) Cytochrome P450 2C19 loss-of-function polymorphism, but not CYP3A4

IVS10 + 12G/A and P2Y12 T744C polymorphisms, is associated with response variability to dual antiplatelet treatment in high-risk vascular patients. *Pharmacogenetics and Genomics*, **17**, 1057–1064.

**21** Hulot, J.S., Bura, A., Villard, E., Azizi, M., Remones, V., Goyenvalle, C., Aiach, M., Lechat, P., and Gaussem, P. (2006) Cytochrome P450 2C19 loss-of-function polymorphism is a major determinant of clopidogrel responsiveness in healthy subjects. *Blood*, **108**, 2244–2247.

**22** Shuldiner, A.R., O'Connell, J.R., Bliden, K.P., Gandhi, A., Ryan, K., Horenstein, R.B., Damcott, C.M., Pakyz, R., Tantry, U.S., Gibson, Q. *et al.* (2009) Association of cytochrome P450 2C19 genotype with the antiplatelet effect and clinical efficacy of clopidogrel therapy. *The Journal of the American Medical Association*, **302**, 849–857.

**23** Gilard, M., Arnaud, B., Cornily, J.C., Le Gal, G., Lacut, K., Le Calvez, G., Mansourati, J., Mottier, D., Abgrall, J.F., and Boschat, J. (2008) Influence of omeprazole on the antiplatelet action of clopidogrel associated with aspirin: the randomized, double-blind OCLA (Omeprazole Clopidogrel Aspirin) study. *Journal of the American College of Cardiology*, **51**, 256–260.

**24** Kim, K.A., Park, P.W., Hong, S.J., and Park, J.Y. (2008) The effect of CYP2C19 polymorphism on the pharmacokinetics and pharmacodynamics of clopidogrel: a possible mechanism for clopidogrel resistance. *Clinical Pharmacology and Therapeutics*, **84**, 236–242.

**25** Umemura, K., Furuta, T., and Kondo, K. (2008) The common gene variants of CYP2C19 affect pharmacokinetics and pharmacodynamics in an active metabolite of clopidogrel in healthy subjects. *Journal of Thrombosis and Haemostasis*, **6**, 1439–1441.

**26** Giusti, B., Gori, A.M., Marcucci, R., Saracini, C., Sestini, I., Paniccia, R., Buonamici, P., Antoniucci, D., Abbate, R., and Gensini, G.F. (2009) Relation of cytochrome P450 2C19 loss-of-function polymorphism to occurrence of drug-eluting coronary stent thrombosis. *The American Journal of Cardiology*, **103**, 806–811.

**27** Gladding, P., Webster, M., Zeng, I., Farrell, H., Stewart, J., Ruygrok, P., Ormiston, J., El-Jack, S., Armstrong, G., Kay, P. *et al.* (2008) The pharmacogenetics and pharmacodynamics of clopidogrel response: an analysis from the PRINC (Plavix Response in Coronary Intervention) trial. *JACC: Cardiovascular Interventions*, **1**, 620–627.

**28** Sibbing, D., Stegherr, J., Latz, W., Koch, W., Mehilli, J., Dorrler, K., Morath, T., Schomig, A., Kastrati, A., and von Beckerath, N. (2009) Cytochrome P450 2C19 loss-of-function polymorphism and stent thrombosis following percutaneous coronary intervention. *European Heart Journal*, **30**, 916–922.

**29** Collet, J.P., Hulot, J.S., Pena, A., Villard, E., Esteve, J.B., Silvain, J., Payot, L., Brugier, D., Cayla, G., Beygui, F. *et al.* (2009) Cytochrome P450 2C19 polymorphism in young patients treated with clopidogrel after myocardial infarction: a cohort study. *Lancet*, **373**, 309–317.

**30** Simon, T., Verstuyft, C., Mary-Krause, M., Quteineh, L., Drouet, E., Meneveau, N., Steg, P.G., Ferrieres, J., Danchin, N., and Becquemont, L. (2009) Genetic determinants of response to clopidogrel and cardiovascular events. *The New England Journal of Medicine*, **360**, 363–375.

**31** Coffman, B.L., Rios, G.R., King, C.D., and Tephly, T.R. (1997) Human UGT2B7 catalyzes morphine glucuronidation. *Drug Metabolism and Disposition: The Biological Fate of Chemicals*, **25**, 1–4.

**32** Madadi, P. and Koren, G. (2008) Pharmacogenetic insights into codeine analgesia: implications to pediatric codeine use. *Pharmacogenomics*, **9**, 1267–1284.

**33** Ingelman-Sundberg, M. (2005) Genetic polymorphisms of cytochrome P450 2D6 (CYP2D6): clinical consequences, evolutionary aspects and functional diversity. *The Pharmacogenomics Journal*, **5**, 6–13.

**34** Gaedigk, A., Ndjountche, L., Divakaran, K., Dianne Bradford, L., Zineh, I.,

Oberlander, T.F., Brousseau, D.C., McCarver, D.G., Johnson, J.A., Alander, S.W. *et al.* (2007) Cytochrome P4502D6 (CYP2D6) gene locus heterogeneity: characterization of gene duplication events. *Clinical Pharmacology and Therapeutics*, **81**, 242–251.

**35** Sawyer, M.B., Innocenti, F., Das, S., Cheng, C., Ramirez, J., Pantle-Fisher, F.H., Wright, C., Badner, J., Pei, D., Boyett, J.M. *et al.* (2003) A pharmacogenetic study of uridine diphosphate-glucuronosyltransferase 2B7 in patients receiving morphine. *Clinical Pharmacology and Therapeutics*, **73**, 566–574.

**36** American Academy of Pediatrics Committee on Drugs (2001) Transfer of drugs and other chemicals into human milk. *Pediatrics*, **108**, 776–789.

**37** Madadi, P., Ross, C.J., Hayden, M.R., Carleton, B.C., Gaedigk, A., Leeder, J.S., and Koren, G. (2009) Pharmacogenetics of neonatal opioid toxicity following maternal use of codeine during breastfeeding: a case–control study. *Clinical Pharmacology and Therapeutics*, **85**, 31–35.

**38** Koren, G., Cairns, J., Chitayat, D., Gaedigk, A., and Leeder, S.J. (2006) Pharmacogenetics of morphine poisoning in a breastfed neonate of a codeine-prescribed mother. *Lancet*, **368**, 704.

**39** Gasche, Y., Daali, Y., Fathi, M., Chiappe, A., Cottini, S., Dayer, P., and Desmeules, J. (2004) Codeine intoxication associated with ultrarapid CYP2D6 metabolism. *The New England Journal of Medicine*, **351**, 2827–2831.

**40** Hermanns-Clausen, M., Weinmann, W., Auwarter, V., Ferreiros, N., Trittler, R., Muller, C., Pahl, A., Superti-Furga, A., and Hentschel, R. (2009) Drug dosing error with drops: severe clinical course of codeine intoxication in twins. *European Journal of Pediatrics*, **168**, 819–824.

**41** Voronov, P., Przybylo, H.J., and Jagannathan, N. (2007) Apnea in a child after oral codeine: a genetic variant – an ultra-rapid metabolizer. *Paediatric Anaesthesia*, **17**, 684–687.

**42** Yue, Q.Y., Alm, C., Svensson, J.O., and Sawe, J. (1997) Quantification of the O- and N-demethylated and the glucuronidated metabolites of codeine relative to the debrisoquine metabolic ratio in urine in ultrarapid, rapid, and poor debrisoquine hydroxylators. *Therapeutic Drug Monitoring*, **19**, 539–542.

**43** Kirchheiner, J., Schmidt, H., Tzvetkov, M., Keulen, J.T., Lotsch, J., Roots, I., and Brockmoller, J. (2007) Pharmacokinetics of codeine and its metabolite morphine in ultra-rapid metabolizers due to CYP2D6 duplication. *The Pharmacogenomics Journal*, **7**, 257–265.

**44** Dalen, P., Frengell, C., Dahl, M.L., and Sjoqvist, F. (1997) Quick onset of severe abdominal pain after codeine in an ultrarapid metabolizer of debrisoquine. *Therapeutic Drug Monitoring*, **19**, 543–544.

**45** Poulsen, L., Riishede, L., Brosen, K., Clemensen, S., and Sindrup, S.H. (1998) Codeine in post-operative pain. Study of the influence of sparteine phenotype and serum concentrations of morphine and morphine-6-glucuronide. *European Journal of Clinical Pharmacology*, **54**, 451–454.

**46** Caraco, Y., Sheller, J., and Wood, A.J. (1996) Pharmacogenetic determination of the effects of codeine and prediction of drug interactions. *The Journal of Pharmacology and Experimental Therapeutics*, **278**, 1165–1174.

**47** Poulsen, L., Brosen, K., Arendt-Nielsen, L., Gram, L.F., Elbaek, K., and Sindrup, S.H. (1996) Codeine and morphine in extensive and poor metabolizers of sparteine: pharmacokinetics, analgesic effect and side effects. *European Journal of Clinical Pharmacology*, **51**, 289–295.

**48** Chen, Z.R., Somogyi, A.A., Reynolds, G., and Bochner, F. (1991) Disposition and metabolism of codeine after single and chronic doses in one poor and seven extensive metabolisers. *British Journal of Clinical Pharmacology*, **31**, 381–390.

**49** Sindrup, S.H., Brosen, K., Bjerring, P., Arendt-Nielsen, L., Larsen, U., Angelo, H.R., and Gram, L.F. (1990) Codeine increases pain thresholds to copper vapor laser stimuli in extensive but not poor metabolizers of sparteine. *Clinical Pharmacology and Therapeutics*, **48**, 686–693.

50 Yue, Q.Y., Svensson, J.O., Alm, C., Sjoqvist, F., and Sawe, J. (1989) Codeine O-demethylation co-segregates with polymorphic debrisoquine hydroxylation. *British Journal of Clinical Pharmacology*, **28**, 639–645.

51 Chen, Z.R., Somogyi, A.A., and Bochner, F. (1988) Polymorphic O-demethylation of codeine. *Lancet*, **2**, 914–915.

52 Williams, D.G., Patel, A., and Howard, R.F. (2002) Pharmacogenetics of codeine metabolism in an urban population of children and its implications for analgesic reliability. *British Journal of Anaesthesia*, **89**, 839–845.

53 Desmeules, J., Gascon, M.P., Dayer, P., and Magistris, M. (1991) Impact of environmental and genetic factors on codeine analgesia. *European Journal of Clinical Pharmacology*, **41**, 23–26.

54 Eckhardt, K., Li, S., Ammon, S., Schanzle, G., Mikus, G., and Eichelbaum, M. (1998) Same incidence of adverse drug events after codeine administration irrespective of the genetically determined differences in morphine formation. *Pain*, **76**, 27–33.

55 Somogyi, A.A., Barratt, D.T., and Coller, J.K. (2007) Pharmacogenetics of opioids. *Clinical Pharmacology and Therapeutics*, **81**, 429–444.

56 Mikus, G., Trausch, B., Rodewald, C., Hofmann, U., Richter, K., Gramatte, T., and Eichelbaum, M. (1997) Effect of codeine on gastrointestinal motility in relation to CYP2D6 phenotype. *Clinical Pharmacology and Therapeutics*, **61**, 459–466.

57 NOLVADEX (tamoxifen citrate) AstraZeneca Pharmaceuticals LP, W. Delaware. Available at http://www.fda.gov/cder/foi/label/2006/017970s054lbl.pdf.

58 Desta, Z., Ward, B.A., Soukhova, N.V., and Flockhart, D.A. (2004) Comprehensive evaluation of tamoxifen sequential biotransformation by the human cytochrome P450 system *in vitro*: prominent roles for CYP3A and CYP2D6. *The Journal of Pharmacology and Experimental Therapeutics*, **310**, 1062–1075.

59 Johnson, M.D., Zuo, H., Lee, K.H., Trebley, J.P., Rae, J.M., Weatherman, R.V., Desta, Z., Flockhart, D.A., and Skaar, T.C. (2004) Pharmacological characterization of 4-hydroxy-*N*-desmethyl tamoxifen, a novel active metabolite of tamoxifen. *Breast Cancer Research and Treatment*, **85**, 151–159.

60 Lim, Y.C., Desta, Z., Flockhart, D.A., and Skaar, T.C. (2005) Endoxifen (4-hydroxy-*N*-desmethyl-tamoxifen) has anti-estrogenic effects in breast cancer cells with potency similar to 4-hydroxy-tamoxifen. *Cancer Chemotherapy and Pharmacology*, **55**, 471–478.

61 Goetz, M.P., Rae, J.M., Suman, V.J., Safgren, S.L., Ames, M.M., Visscher, D.W., Reynolds, C., Couch, F.J., Lingle, W.L., Flockhart, D.A. *et al.* (2005) Pharmacogenetics of tamoxifen biotransformation is associated with clinical outcomes of efficacy and hot flashes. *Journal of Clinical Oncology*, **23**, 9312–9318.

62 Human Cytochrome P450 (CYP) Allele Nomenclature Committee web site http://www.cypalleles.ki.se/cyp2d6.htm.

63 Ozawa, S., Soyama, A., Saeki, M., Fukushima-Uesaka, H., Itoda, M., Koyano, S., Sai, K., Ohno, Y., Saito, Y., and Sawada, J. (2004) Ethnic differences in genetic polymorphisms of CYP2D6, CYP2C19, CYP3As and MDR1/ABCB1. *Drug Metabolism and Pharmacokinetics*, **19**, 83–95.

64 Sachse, C., Brockmoller, J., Bauer, S., and Roots, I. (1997) Cytochrome P450 2D6 variants in a Caucasian population: allele frequencies and phenotypic consequences. *American Journal of Human Genetics*, **60**, 284–295.

65 Gjerde, J., Hauglid, M., Breilid, H., Lundgren, S., Varhaug, J.E., Kisanga, E.R., Mellgren, G., Steen, V.M., and Lien, E.A. (2008) Effects of CYP2D6 and SULT1A1 genotypes including SULT1A1 gene copy number on

tamoxifen metabolism. *Annals of Oncology*, **19**, 56–61.

**66** Stearns, V., Johnson, M.D., Rae, J.M., Morocho, A., Novielli, A., Bhargava, P., Hayes, D.F., Desta, Z., and Flockhart, D.A. (2003) Active tamoxifen metabolite plasma concentrations after coadministration of tamoxifen and the selective serotonin reuptake inhibitor paroxetine. *Journal of the National Cancer Institute*, **95**, 1758–1764.

**67** Lim, H.S., Ju Lee, H., Seok Lee, K., Sook Lee, E., Jang, I.J., and Ro, J. (2007) Clinical implications of CYP2D6 genotypes predictive of tamoxifen pharmacokinetics in metastatic breast cancer. *Journal of Clinical Oncology*, **25**, 3837–3845.

**68** Borges, S., Desta, Z., Li, L., Skaar, T.C., Ward, B.A., Nguyen, A., Jin, Y., Storniolo, A.M., Nikoloff, D.M., Wu, L. *et al.* (2006) Quantitative effect of CYP2D6 genotype and inhibitors on tamoxifen metabolism: implication for optimization of breast cancer treatment. *Clinical Pharmacology and Therapeutics*, **80**, 61–74.

**69** Schroth, W., Goetz, M.P., Hamann, U., Fasching, P.A., Schmidt, M., Winter, S., Fritz, P., Simon, W., Suman, V.J., Ames, M.M. *et al.* (2009) Association between CYP2D6 polymorphisms and outcomes among women with early stage breast cancer treated with tamoxifen. *The Journal of the American Medical Association*, **302**, 1429–1436.

**70** Newman, W.G., Hadfield, K.D., Latif, A., Roberts, S.A., Shenton, A., McHague, C., Lalloo, F., Howell, S., and Evans, D.G. (2008) Impaired tamoxifen metabolism reduces survival in familial breast cancer patients. *Clinical Cancer Research*, **14**, 5913–5918.

**71** Xu, Y., Sun, Y., Yao, L., Shi, L., Wu, Y., Ouyang, T., Li, J., Wang, T., Fan, Z., Fan, T. *et al.* (2008) Association between CYP2D6 *10 genotype and survival of breast cancer patients receiving tamoxifen treatment. *Annals of Oncology*, **19**, 1423–1429.

**72** Wegman, P., Elingarami, S., Carstensen, J., Stal, O., Nordenskjold, B., and Wingren, S. (2007) Genetic variants of CYP3A5, CYP2D6, SULT1A1, UGT2B15 and tamoxifen response in postmenopausal patients with breast cancer. *Breast Cancer Research*, **9**, R7.

**73** Nowell, S.A., Ahn, J., Rae, J.M., Scheys, J.O., Trovato, A., Sweeney, C., MacLeod, S.L., Kadlubar, F.F., and Ambrosone, C.B. (2005) Association of genetic variation in tamoxifen-metabolizing enzymes with overall survival and recurrence of disease in breast cancer patients. *Breast Cancer Research and Treatment*, **91**, 249–258.

**74** Aubert, RE., Stanek, EJ., Yao, J. *et al.* (2009) Risk of breast cancer recurrence in women initiating tamoxifen with CYP2D6 inhibitors. Abstract #CRA508. ASCO Annual Meeting Proceedings, p. 9s.

**75** Goetz, M.P., Knox, S.K., Suman, V.J., Rae, J.M., Safgren, S.L., Ames, M.M., Visscher, D.W., Reynolds, C., Couch, F.J., Lingle, W.L. *et al.* (2007) The impact of cytochrome P450 2D6 metabolism in women receiving adjuvant tamoxifen. *Breast Cancer Research and Treatment*, **101**, 113–121.

**76** Maring, J.G., Groen, H.J., Wachters, F.M., Uges, D.R., and de Vries, E.G. (2005) Genetic factors influencing pyrimidine-antagonist chemotherapy. *The Pharmacogenomics Journal*, **5**, 226–243.

**77** Ribelles, N., Lopez-Siles, J., Sanchez, A., Gonzalez, E., Sanchez, M.J., Carabantes, F., Sanchez-Rovira, P., Marquez, A., Duenas, R., Sevilla, I. *et al.* (2008) A carboxylesterase 2 gene polymorphism as predictor of capecitabine on response and time to progression. *Current Drug Metabolism*, **9**, 336–343.

**78** Reigner, B., Verweij, J., Dirix, L., Cassidy, J., Twelves, C., Allman, D., Weidekamm, E., Roos, B., Banken, L., Utoh, M. *et al.* (1998) Effect of food on the pharmacokinetics of capecitabine and its metabolites following oral administration in cancer patients. *Clinical Cancer Research*, **4**, 941–948.

**79** Garcia, A.A., Blessing, J.A., Lenz, H.J., Darcy, K.M., Mannel, R.S., Miller, D.S., and Husseinzadeh, N. (2005) Phase II clinical trial of capecitabine in ovarian carcinoma recurrent 6–12 months after completion of primary chemotherapy, with exploratory TS, DPD, and TP correlates: a Gynecologic Oncology Group study. *Gynecologic Oncology*, **96**, 810–817.

80 Garcia, A.A., Blessing, J.A., Darcy, K.M., Lenz, H.J., Zhang, W., Hannigan, E., and Moore, D.H. (2007) Phase II clinical trial of capecitabine in the treatment of advanced, persistent or recurrent squamous cell carcinoma of the cervix with translational research: a Gynecologic Oncology Group study. *Gynecologic Oncology*, **104**, 572–579.

81 Grau, J.J., Caballero, M., Monzo, M., Munoz-Garcia, C., Domingo-Domenech, J., Navarro, A., Conill, C., Campayo, M., and Bombi, J.A. (2008) Dihydropyrimidine dehydrogenases and cytidine-deaminase gene polymorphisms as outcome predictors in resected gastric cancer patients treated with fluoropyrimidine adjuvant chemotherapy. *Journal of Surgical Oncology*, **98**, 130–134.

82 Moghaddam, A., Zhang, H.T., Fan, T.P., Hu, D.E., Lees, V.C., Turley, H., Fox, S.B., Gatter, K.C., Harris, A.L., and Bicknell, R. (1995) Thymidine phosphorylase is angiogenic and promotes tumor growth. *Proceedings of the National Academy of Sciences of the United States of America*, **92**, 998–1002.

83 Meropol, N.J., Gold, P.J., Diasio, R.B., Andria, M., Dhami, M., Godfrey, T., Kovatich, A.J., Lund, K.A., Mitchell, E., and Schwarting, R. (2006) Thymidine phosphorylase expression is associated with response to capecitabine plus irinotecan in patients with metastatic colorectal cancer. *Journal of Clinical Oncology*, **24**, 4069–4077.

84 Uchida, K., Danenberg, P.V., Danenberg, K.D., and Grem, J.L. (2008) Thymidylate synthase, dihydropyrimidine dehydrogenase, ERCC1, and thymidine phosphorylase gene expression in primary and metastatic gastrointestinal adenocarcinoma tissue in patients treated on a phase I trial of oxaliplatin and capecitabine. *BMC Cancer*, **8**, 386.

85 van Kuilenburg, A.B. (2004) Dihydropyrimidine dehydrogenase and the efficacy and toxicity of 5-fluorouracil. *European Journal of Cancer*, **40**, 939–950.

86 Morel, A., Boisdron-Celle, M., Fey, L., Soulie, P., Craipeau, M.C., Traore, S., and Gamelin, E. (2006) Clinical relevance of different dihydropyrimidine dehydrogenase gene single nucleotide polymorphisms on 5-fluorouracil tolerance. *Molecular Cancer Therapeutics*, **5**, 2895–2904.

87 Schwab, M., Zanger, U.M., Marx, C., Schaeffeler, E., Klein, K., Dippon, J., Kerb, R., Blievernicht, J., Fischer, J., Hofmann, U. *et al.* (2008) Role of genetic and nongenetic factors for fluorouracil treatment-related severe toxicity: a prospective clinical trial by the German 5-FU Toxicity Study Group. *Journal of Clinical Oncology*, **26**, 2131–2138.

88 Komatsu, T., Yamazaki, H., Shimada, N., Nagayama, S., Kawaguchi, Y., Nakajima, M., and Yokoi, T. (2001) Involvement of microsomal cytochrome P450 and cytosolic thymidine phosphorylase in 5-fluorouracil formation from tegafur in human liver. *Clinical Cancer Research*, **7**, 675–681.

89 Komatsu, T., Yamazaki, H., Shimada, N., Nakajima, M., and Yokoi, T. (2000) Roles of cytochromes P450 1A2, 2A6, and 2C8 in 5-fluorouracil formation from tegafur, an anticancer prodrug, in human liver microsomes. *Drug Metabolism and Disposition: The Biological Fate of Chemicals*, **28**, 1457–1463.

90 Kajita, J., Fuse, E., Kuwabara, T., and Kobayashi, H. (2003) The contribution of cytochrome P450 to the metabolism of tegafur in human liver. *Drug Metabolism and Pharmacokinetics*, **18**, 303–309.

91 Daigo, S., Takahashi, Y., Fujieda, M., Ariyoshi, N., Yamazaki, H., Koizumi, W., Tanabe, S., Saigenji, K., Nagayama, S., Ikeda, K. *et al.* (2002) A novel mutant allele of the CYP2A6 gene (CYP2A6*11) found in a cancer patient who showed poor metabolic phenotype towards tegafur. *Pharmacogenetics*, **12**, 299–306.

92 Fujita, K., Yamamoto, W., Endo, S., Endo, H., Nagashima, F., Ichikawa, W., Tanaka, R., Miya, T., Araki, K., Kodama, K. *et al.*

(2008) CYP2A6 and the plasma level of 5-chloro-2, 4-dihydroxypyridine are determinants of the pharmacokinetic variability of tegafur and 5-fluorouracil, respectively, in Japanese patients with cancer given S-1. *Cancer Science*, **99**, 1049–1054.

**93** Kaida, Y., Inui, N., Suda, T., Nakamura, H., Watanabe, H., and Chida, K. (2008) The CYP2A6*4 allele is determinant of S-1 pharmacokinetics in Japanese patients with non-small-cell lung cancer. *Clinical Pharmacology and Therapeutics*, **83**, 589–594.

**94** Humerickhouse, R., Lohrbach, K., Li, L., Bosron, W.F., and Dolan, M.E. (2000) Characterization of CPT-11 hydrolysis by human liver carboxylesterase isoforms hCE-1 and hCE-2. *Cancer Research*, **60**, 1189–1192.

**95** Charasson, V., Bellott, R., Meynard, D., Longy, M., Gorry, P., and Robert, J. (2004) Pharmacogenetics of human carboxylesterase 2, an enzyme involved in the activation of irinotecan into SN-38. *Clinical Pharmacology and Therapeutics*, **76**, 528–535.

**96** Kim, S.R., Sai, K., Tanaka-Kagawa, T., Jinno, H., Ozawa, S., Kaniwa, N., Saito, Y., Akasawa, A., Matsumoto, K., Saito, H. *et al.* (2007) Haplotypes and a novel defective allele of CES2 found in a Japanese population. *Drug Metabolism and Disposition: The Biological Fate of Chemicals*, **35**, 1865–1872.

**97** Kubo, T., Kim, S.R., Sai, K., Saito, Y., Nakajima, T., Matsumoto, K., Saito, H., Shirao, K., Yamamoto, N., Minami, H. *et al.* (2005) Functional characterization of three naturally occurring single nucleotide polymorphisms in the CES2 gene encoding carboxylesterase 2 (HCE-2). *Drug Metabolism and Disposition: The Biological Fate of Chemicals*, **33**, 1482–1487.

**98** Bellott, R., Le Morvan, V., Charasson, V., Laurand, A., Colotte, M., Zanger, U.M., Klein, K., Smith, D., Bonnet, J., and Robert, J. (2008) Functional study of the 830C>G polymorphism of the human carboxylesterase 2 gene. *Cancer Chemotherapy and Pharmacology*, **61**, 481–488.

**99** Mathijssen, R.H., Marsh, S., Karlsson, M.O., Xie, R., Baker, S.D., Verweij, J., Sparreboom, A., and McLeod, H.L. (2003) Irinotecan pathway genotype analysis to predict pharmacokinetics. *Clinical Cancer Research*, **9**, 3246–3253.

**100** Schulz, C., Boeck, S., Heinemann, V., and Stemmler, H.J. (2009) UGT1A1 genotyping: a predictor of irinotecan-associated side effects and drug efficacy? *Anti-Cancer Drugs*, **20**, 867–879.

**101** Palma Gamiz, J.L., Pego, M., Contreras, E.M., Anglada, M.P., Martinez, J.O., Esquerra, E.A., and Sagastagoitia Gorostiza, J.D. (2006) A twelve-week, multicenter, randomized, double-blind, parallel-group, noninferiority trial of the antihypertensive efficacy and tolerability of imidapril and candesartan in adult patients with mild to moderate essential hypertension: the Iberian Multicenter Imidapril Study on Hypertension (IMISH). *Clinical Therapeutics*, **28**, 2040–2051.

**102** Takai, S., Matsuda, A., Usami, Y., Adachi, T., Sugiyama, T., Katagiri, Y., Tatematsu, M., and Hirano, K. (1997) Hydrolytic profile for ester- or amide-linkage by carboxylesterases pI 5.3 and 4.5 from human liver. *Biological & Pharmaceutical Bulletin*, **20**, 869–873.

**103** Geshi, E., Kimura, T., Yoshimura, M., Suzuki, H., Koba, S., Sakai, T., Saito, T., Koga, A., Muramatsu, M., and Katagiri, T. (2005) A single nucleotide polymorphism in the carboxylesterase gene is associated with the responsiveness to imidapril medication and the promoter activity. *Hypertension Research*, **28**, 719–725.

**104** Song, J.C. and White, C.M. (2002) Clinical pharmacokinetics and selective pharmacodynamics of new angiotensin converting enzyme inhibitors: an update. *Clinical Pharmacokinetics*, **41**, 207–224.

**105** Huang, Z., Roy, P., and Waxman, D.J. (2000) Role of human liver microsomal CYP3A4 and CYP2B6 in catalyzing N-dechloroethylation of cyclophosphamide and ifosfamide. *Biochemical Pharmacology*, **59**, 961–972.

**106** Lee, J.M., Park, S., Shin, D.J., Choi, D., Shim, C.Y., Ko, Y.G., Kim, J.S., Shin, E.S., Chang, C.W., Lee, J.E. *et al.* (2009) Relation of genetic polymorphisms in the cytochrome P450 gene with clopidogrel resistance after drug-eluting stent implantation in Koreans. *The American Journal of Cardiology*, **104**, 46–51.

**107** Takada, K., Arefayene, M., Desta, Z., Yarboro, C.H., Boumpas, D.T., Balow, J.E., Flockhart, D.A., and Illei, G.G. (2004) Cytochrome P450 pharmacogenetics as a predictor of toxicity and clinical response to pulse cyclophosphamide in lupus nephritis. *Arthritis and Rheumatism*, **50**, 2202–2210.

**108** Singh, G., Saxena, N., Aggarwal, A., and Misra, R. (2007) Cytochrome P450 polymorphism as a predictor of ovarian toxicity to pulse cyclophosphamide in systemic lupus erythematosus. *The Journal of Rheumatology*, **34**, 731–733.

# Index



*Prodrugs and Targeted Delivery: Towards Better ADME Properties.* Edited by Jarkko Rautio

ISBN: 978-3-527-32603-7

***b***